Maternal Newborn
NURSING CARE PLANS

SECOND EDITION

Edited by

Carol J. Green, PhD, MN, RN, CNE
Professor
Graceland University School of Nursing
Independence, Missouri

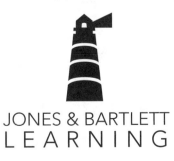

JONES & BARTLETT
LEARNING

World Headquarters

Jones & Bartlett Learning
40 Tall Pine Drive
Sudbury, MA 01776
978-443-5000
info@jblearning.com
www.jblearning.com

Jones & Bartlett Learning Canada
6339 Ormindale Way
Mississauga, Ontario L5V 1J2
Canada

Jones & Bartlett Learning International
Barb House, Barb Mews
London W6 7PA
United Kingdom

Jones & Bartlett Learning books and products are available through most bookstores and online booksellers.
To contact Jones & Bartlett Learning directly, call 800-832-0034, fax 978-443-8000, or visit our website,
www.jblearning.com.

Substantial discounts on bulk quantities of Jones & Bartlett Learning publications are available to corporations, professional associations, and other qualified organizations. For details and specific discount information, contact the special sales department at Jones & Bartlett Learning via the above contact information or send an email to specialsales@jblearning.com.

The authors, editor, and publisher have made every effort to provide accurate information. However, they are not responsible for errors, omissions, or for any outcomes related to the use of the contents of this book and take no responsibility for the use of the products and procedures described. Treatments and side effects described in this book may not be applicable to all people; likewise, some people may require a dose or experience a side effect that is not described herein. Drugs and medical devices are discussed that may have limited availability controlled by the Food and Drug Administration (FDA) for use only in a research study or clinical trial. Research, clinical practice, and government regulations often change the accepted standard in this field. When consideration is being given to use of any drug in the clinical setting, the health care provider or reader is responsible for determining FDA status of the drug, reading the package insert, and reviewing prescribing information for the most up-to-date recommendations on dose, precautions, and contraindications, and determining the appropriate usage for the product. This is especially important in the case of drugs that are new or seldom used.

Production Credits
Publisher: Kevin Sullivan
Acquisitions Editor: Amanda Harvey
Editorial Assistant: Rachel Shuster
Production Editor: Amanda Clerkin
Associate Marketing Manager: Katie Hennessy
V.P., Manufacturing and Inventory Control: Therese Connell
Composition: Shawn Girsberger
Cover Design: Scott Moden
Cover Image: © Artbox/age fotostock
Printing and Binding: Malloy, Inc.
Cover Printing: Malloy, Inc.

Library of Congress Cataloging-in-Publication Data
Green, Carol J.
    Maternal newborn nursing care plans / [edited by] Carol J. Green.—2nd ed.
        p. ; cm.
    Includes bibliographical references and index.
    ISBN 978-0-7637-7742-5
    1. Maternity nursing. 2. Nursing care plans.   I. Title.
    [DNLM: 1. Maternal-Child Nursing—methods. 2. Patient Care Planning. 3. Infant, Newborn. 4. Nursing Assessment—methods.
5. Pregnancy Complications—nursing. 6. Pregnancy. WY 157.3]
    RT49.G746 2012
    610.73—dc22
                                                                            2010040547
6048

Printed in the United States of America
15 14 13 12 11   10 9 8 7 6 5 4 3 2

CONTENTS

PREFACE

Change is the common denominator in today's healthcare environment and will continue to be in the near future. As such, I've attempted to integrate important components from clinical practice and education into the care plans in this book. For example, this edition addresses:

1. *Shorter hospital stays and home care:* Care plans and interventions are included for home care.
2. *Standardized nursing languages (NANDA and NIC):* Nursing interventions with rationales are included in *every* care plan.
3. *Emphasis on health promotion:* Normal pregnancy, labor and birth, postpartum, and newborn care are emphasized.
4. *Standardized care plans:* Students/nurses are taught how to modify standardized care plans to individualize care. This will facilitate their ability to better function in today's healthcare environment while still remaining true to the goal of nursing, which is to meet the unique needs of each patient.
5. *Emphasis on collaborative practice:* Descriptions of medical tests, treatments, and collaborative care plans are included for *every* topic. Nursing care plans for *both* collaborative problems (potential complications of medical diagnoses) and nursing diagnoses are also included.
6. *Emphasis on independent nursing actions:* New to this edition are independent nursing actions. These are actions that nurses can take without specific physician orders that may protect patient safety or prevent common complications from diseases or conditions.

This book can be used in a variety of academic levels and practice settings, including undergraduate nursing courses in maternity or maternal–child nursing, or in the clinical component of an integrated curriculum. Students will use it in preparation for clinical patient-care experiences, but it could also be used as an ancillary text in maternity courses. It is versatile enough for use by nurses in practice—for planning care for individual patients or for developing institutional standards of care and collaborative pathways for clinics, hospitals, physicians' offices, and birthing centers.

Students in all program types must learn to assess, plan, deliver, and evaluate care for normal pregnancy, delivery, and recovery—both for mother and baby. Most schools (and the NCLEX exam) also include the abnormal conditions included in the outline section of this book. Nearly all nursing students must learn to use the nursing process. This book facilitates that learning as well. This book is *not* intended as a vehicle for learning any of the associated psychomotor skills.

Overview of Chapters

Chapter 1—Explains how to use this book to combine standardized and individualized care plans; provides a case study exercise illustrating care planning.

Chapter 2—Provides generic nursing diagnosis care plans for nursing diagnoses that are used frequently in other chapters/topics.

Chapter 3—Provides generic care plans for collaborative problems found to occur frequently in other conditions and topics in the book. For example, the generic care plan for Potential Complication: Hemorrhage in this chapter is referred to in Gestational Trophoblastic Disease.

Chapter 4—Provides plans of care to be used in all three trimesters of normal pregnancy.

Chapter 5—Addresses pregnancy complicated by medical (e.g., prenatal anemia) and other (e.g., adolescence) conditions.

Chapter 6—Provides collaborative and nursing diagnosis care plans for 13 gestational complications (e.g., ectopic pregnancy, hyperemesis gravidarum).

Chapter 7—Provides care plans for use during normal labor and birth; it includes care plans for women undergoing amniotomy, induction/augmentation of labor, and epidural anesthesia/analgesia.

Chapter 8—Provides collaborative and nursing diagnosis care plans for intrapartal complications and commonly used procedures, such as external version and forceps- or vacuum-assisted birth.

Chapter 9—Focuses on the healthy woman during the postpartum period. It provides care plans for use from the first 4 hours after delivery through 6 weeks postpartum. It also includes care after cesarean birth, and a care plan for the first home visit.

Chapter 10—Provides collaborative and nursing diagnosis care plans for complications that occur during the postpartum period (e.g., postpartum hemorrhage).

Chapter 11—Provides plans of care for the newborn from birth through 2 days. Long-term needs of the normal newborn are addressed in the normal postpartum care plans.

Chapter 12—Provides collaborative and nursing diagnosis care plans for 11 common neonatal complications.

I hope that you will enjoy using this book, and I will be pleased to receive feedback that will allow me to continue improving it to meet your needs.

Carol J. Green, PhD, MN, RN, CNE

MATERNAL NEWBORN NURSING CARE PLANS CONTRIBUTORS

Judith J. Hilton, PhD, RNC, CNE
Professor of Nursing
Lenoir-Rhyne University
Hickory, North Carolina

Jeanne Linhart, MN, RN, FNP-BC
Professor of Nursing
Rockland Community College
Suffern, New York

Harriet (Hatsie) Pearson Mallicoat, MN, BSN, BA
Microbiology
Family Nurse Practitoner-Certified
Certified Nurse Midwife
Private Practice
Olathe, Kansas

Allison L. Scott, MSN, RN, PNP-BC, IBCLC
Instructor of Nursing
University of Arkansas, Eleanor Mann School of Nursing
Fayetteville, Arkansas

Cindy Waits, MSN, RN, CLC
Assistant Professor in Nusing (Obstetrics)
Graceland University
Independence, Missouri

Dawn L. Viets, MSN, RN, NNP-BC
Neonatal Nurse Practitioner
NICU Clinical Manager
Centerpoint Medical Center
Independence, Missouri

INTRODUCTION

HOW TO USE THIS BOOK

According to the American Nurses Association (ANA), *nursing* is "the protection, promotion, and optimization of health and abilities, prevention of illness and injury, alleviation of suffering… through the diagnosis and treatment of human responses to actual or potential health problems" (ANA, 2004, p. 7). A care plan is a guide for delivering care.

Standardized and Individualized Care Plans

Most nurses work under some system of managed care, in which collaborative (interdisciplinary) practice has become the norm. Furthermore, most patient care is given according to preplanned, computerized, or preprinted standards of care or a collaborative pathway—documents that outline the common, shared needs of all patients with a particular condition. For example, all women with gestational hypertension must have their blood pressure monitored; all women receiving magnesium sulfate for eclampsia require monitoring of their reflexes and $MgSO_4$ levels. For this reason, the care plans in this book are organized according to clinical conditions (e.g., medical diagnoses or treatments such as normal labor, cesarean birth, and amniocentesis). Refer to the table of contents in the front of the book for a list of the care plans included in this text.

Many of the needs of childbearing women can be met with a common set of interventions, so standardized plans are an efficient approach. However, nurses must not overlook individual needs—those that are not easily predicted on the basis of the medical diagnosis and that may be unique to a particular woman. Nurses should use nursing diagnoses and interventions to individualize preprinted plans and address individual needs for care.

Creating a Care Plan

The following are steps to take when using this book to plan care for a patient:

1. Identify the appropriate clinical condition or medical diagnosis (e.g., antepartum bleeding, normal labor, mastitis) for the woman.
2. Locate the medical diagnosis/condition in the table of contents and turn to that page.
3. Read the introductory material as needed to become familiar with the medical diagnosis/condition. This information is brief and is not intended to replace your primary textbook.
4. Within that main section, refer to the subsection titled "Collaborative (Standardized) Care for All Women With" (the medical diagnosis or condition you identified) for a description of the care that is needed for all women with that condition. The standardized collaborative care plans in this subsection may refer to one or more generic care plans included in Chapters 2 and 3.
5. To individualize care for a particular woman, refer to the subsection titled "Individualized (Nursing Diagnosis) Care Plans" (NDCPs). This subsection includes nursing diagnoses that are often, but not always, seen with the condition. Your nursing assessment will provide the information you need to choose the appropriate nursing diagnoses from this subsection. These NDCPs may also refer you to one or more of the generic care plans in Chapters 2 and 3.
6. The generic care plans in Chapters 2 and 3 represent common nursing diagnoses and collaborative problems that tend to occur frequently in the care of childbearing women, regardless of their medical diagnosis. For example, the nursing diagnosis, *Activity Intolerance*,[1] is often seen in women with anemia, cardiac disease, and antepartum hemorrhage. Therefore, information that is appropriate for all women with Activity Intolerance,[1] *regardless* of their medical diagnosis or of the cause of their Activity Intolerance,[1] was placed in this generic care plan in Chapter 2. As another example, "Potential Complication: Preterm Labor," in Chapter 3, is a potential complication of gestational hypertension, antepartum infections, and premature rupture of membranes; it includes certain interventions necessary for assessing and preventing hypertension in *all* pregnant women, regardless of the medical diagnosis that put them at risk for hypertension. It therefore can be used with the topics "Pregnant Adolescent," "Gestational Diabetes," and so forth. The collaborative care plans (see step 4) and the individualized NDCPs (see step 5) will refer you to the generic care plans when it is appropriate to use them. This eliminates the need to repeat generic information countless times in various topics.

Components of Care Plans in This Book

Clinical Condition or Topic

Each care plan (or topic) begins with a discussion of the topic, problem, medical diagnosis, or clinical condition (e.g., gestational diabetes, postpartum infection). This section includes a brief overview of the pathophysiology of the condition and enough other information to provide an understanding of the associated nursing and collaborative care needs.

Key Nursing Activities

This section provides an overview, a sort of road map for the care of a woman with the topic condition. These specific activities are, in very general terms, the most important focuses of nursing activity related to the topic of the care plan.

Etiologies and Risk (or Related) Factors

This section provides an overview of the etiology (cause) of the condition, if known. Risk factors refer to those conditions that place the woman at increased risk for the condition or diagnosis (e.g., previous placenta previa, age greater than 35 years, and multiparity are risk factors for antepartum hemorrhage).

Signs and Symptoms

The subjective and objective signs and symptoms (clinical manifestations) commonly associated with the clinical condition (topic) are listed in this section. The only chapter that does not contain a signs and symptoms section is Chapter 2, the generic NDCP chapter.

Diagnostic Studies

Studies commonly used to diagnose the condition are provided in this section, along with rationales and/or specific laboratory values.

Medical Management

Medical management (or treatment) of the condition pertains to those actions that must be performed or prescribed by a physician, midwife, or nurse practitioner, such as treatments, diagnostic tests, and medications.

Collaborative Problems

Collaborative problems include the potential physiologic complications that are always associated with the topic/condition (e.g., women receiving epidural anesthesia must be monitored for hypotension because it is a common complication of this type of anesthesia).

Collaborative (Standardized) Care for All Women With [the Problem or Clinical Condition]

Collaborative problems are *potential* problems, so the nursing care in this section consists of focus assessments and preventive nursing activities that are appropriate for all women with the clinical condition (e.g., focus assessments for all women having hemorrhage will include monitoring heart rate, blood pressure and pulse pressure, and assessing for visible bleeding). A rationale is provided for each nursing activity.

Individualized (Nursing Diagnosis) Care Plans

These nursing diagnoses and interventions are frequently, but not always, associated with the clinical condition and are not addressed by the collaborative plan of care (e.g., many, but not all, women with preterm labor have a nursing diagnosis of Anxiety[1]). Each of the nursing diagnosis care plans includes the following:

- *Nursing Diagnosis (e.g., Risk for Postpartum Infection, Anxiety[1]).* This includes the North American Nursing Diagnosis Association (NANDA) title.
- *Related Factors.* These are factors that may be contributing to the condition (e.g., fear of fetal compromise contributes to a woman's anxiety).
- *Goals, Outcomes, and Evaluation Criteria.* These are outcome statements that can be used as evaluation criteria. They are not in standardized language. The nurse should choose any of these that apply to the woman and individualize them based on assessment data. For example, the text may list a goal of 1–2 cm per day for uterine involution; however, for a multigravid woman or a woman with postpartum infection, this may not be achievable.
- *NIC Interventions.* These are standardized language intervention labels and definitions from the *Nursing Interventions Classification* (NIC) (Bulechek, Butcher, & Dochterman, 2008) and are linked to the identified nursing diagnoses. No specific nursing actions are noted for NIC titles. The nurse should choose those that are appropriate for the given woman. In this text, the NIC labels provide general direction for nursing care; more detailed guidance is found in the section called "Nursing Activities." The number after each NIC label indicates its place in the NIC taxonomy and may be used for computer coding.[2]
- *Nursing Activities.* These are nursing activities that are most likely to result in desired patient outcomes. They are not written in standardized language and are quite specific. Nonetheless, the nurse should individualize them further for each woman. For example, the text may say to "encourage oral fluids," but for a particular woman, the nurse should specify the exact quantity and type of fluids (e.g., "Offer sips of water hourly today," or "Remind the mother to drink 8 oz of water each time she feeds the baby."). Nursing activities for collaborative care problems focus on preventing, monitoring for, and reporting the complication; therefore, they are subdivided into focus assessments and preventive nursing activities. Nursing activities for individualized nursing diagnosis care plans focus on several aspects of care; therefore, they are subdivided into assessments, independent nursing actions, patient/family teaching, and collaborative activities.
- *Rationales.* A rationale is provided for each of the specific nursing activities. Because of space limitations, only basic information is provided. The introductory material for the clinical condition provides further rationale.

EXERCISE ILLUSTRATING HOW TO USE THIS BOOK

A 28-year-old woman who is gravid 6, para 4 at 30 weeks' gestation reports to the emergency department with complaints of vaginal bleeding. The woman states that her provider informed her that she was at risk for bleeding due to low placental attachment noted on an earlier sonogram. This is her first episode of bleeding. She denies pain and says she has saturated one vaginal pad within the past hour. Discharge is bright red.

On assessment the nurse notes that the woman's oral temperature is 98.2°F, heart rate 90 beats per minute, blood pressure is 112/64; and respirations are 24 per minute. Fetal heart rate (FHR) is 140 beats/min with average variability. Uterine contractions (UCs) are absent. She is obviously anxious, tears occasionally, and voices concern about the welfare of her baby.

1. **Identify the appropriate clinical condition or medical diagnosis based on cues from the woman's data.** Many times this will be the admitting diagnosis in the woman's record. In this case, the data support the presence of placenta previa, based on sonographic evidence of low placental attachment and painless, vaginal bleeding at 30 weeks' gestation. You can confirm this by looking up late antepartal bleeding (placenta previa and abruptio placenta) in the table of contents and reading about the etiologies and signs and symptoms of antepartum bleeding on pp. 179 in Chapter 6.

Cues (Data)
- History of low placental attachment: predisposes the woman to bleeding
- Bright red vaginal bleeding: objective indication of placenta previa
- Absence of pain: subjective indication of placenta previa
- Absence of UCs: UCs are absent in 80% of women with vaginal bleeding
- Normal FHR: indicates maternal blood loss rather than fetal compromise
- 30 weeks' gestation: time during which upper and lower uterine segments begin to differentiate and cervix begins to dilate
- Tearing: subjective indication of fear/anxiety
- Expression of concern regarding welfare of fetus: subjective indication of fear

2. **Look in the table of contents for the clinical condition called late antepartum bleeding (placenta previa and abruptio placenta)** The table of contents refers you to pp. 179 in Chapter 6. In Chapter 6, look at the "Collaborative (Standardized) Care" section, beginning on p. 181, for a description of the care that is needed for all women with late

antepartum bleeding as a result of placenta previa. The collaborative problem potential complication of placenta previa: hemorrhage, hypovolemic shock, DIC applies to this woman, as it would to any woman with antepartal vaginal bleeding. Add the focus assessments and preventive nursing activities in this section to the woman's care plan. Individualize them as necessary (e.g., for "Promote nutritional food intake," you should add this particular woman's food preferences).

Follow the same procedure for the rest of the collaborative care plans (potential complications) for late antepartum bleeding (placenta previa and abruptio placentae), because in any woman with antepartum bleeding, including the woman in this exercise, the complications of preterm labor (premature rupture of membranes, fetal hypoxia, anemia, and intrauterine infection) may develop. Therefore, focus assessments and preventive nursing activities from those complications should be added to her care plan. Examples of focus assessments for the woman with placenta previa include:
- Assess for abdominal tenderness, pain, and rigidity
- Assess for visible vaginal bleeding: count or weigh vaginal pads. One gram of pad weight = 1 ml of blood loss
- Assess for UCs
- Assess FHR
  Preventive nursing activities include:
- Institute bed rest, usually with bathroom privileges
- Avoid vaginal and rectal exams

3. **Individualize care for the woman by referring to "Individualized (Nursing Diagnosis) Care Plans" in Chapter 6.** You will select the care plan or plans that best suit this woman's individual needs and add them to her plan of care.
   A. **Nursing Diagnoses.** Identify the nursing diagnoses that are appropriate for this particular woman. This section lists several nursing diagnoses that are commonly seen with acute antepartum bleeding: placenta previa. This woman *does not* have data to support the NDCPs, Interrupted Family Processes,[1] or Acute Pain;[1] therefore, there is no need to include either of these nursing diagnoses in your patient's plan of care. Based on the cues (data) in this case, you should include the following nursing diagnosis in this woman's care plan: Anxiety/Fear[1] related to fear of fetal compromise.
   B. **Goals, Outcomes, and Evaluation Criteria.** For each nursing diagnosis, choose the goals, outcomes, and evaluation criteria that best fit the woman's data and individualize them as

/ continues

I continued

needed. For the nursing diagnosis of Anxiety/Fear[1], you might use the following:

- Displays no physical symptoms of anxiety (e.g., trembling, pallor, or facial tension)
- Concentrates and participates in decision making regarding own care and treatment
- Identifies and uses support persons (e.g., partner, caregivers)

C. **Nursing Activities.** For each nursing diagnosis (for this woman, only Anxiety/Fear[1]), choose the nursing activities most likely to achieve the outcomes you have selected. The *rationale* provided should help you to decide which activities are appropriate. Individualize them as necessary. For this woman's nursing diagnosis of Anxiety/Fear,[1] nursing orders on a care plan might include:

- Instruct on use of relaxation techniques such as slow, purposeful deep breathing, guided imagery, and progressive muscle relaxation.

- Explain all tests and procedures, including sensations likely to be experienced.

Note that the NDCP Anxiety/Fear[1] also refers you to the generic NDCPs for Anxiety)[1] and Fear,[1] on pp. 10 and 15, respectively, in Chapter 2. Therefore you should include appropriate goals and interventions from those generic NDCPs in the care plan for this woman.

D. **Other Nursing Diagnoses.** At the end of the content about some clinical conditions, although not included in the care plan on acute antepartum bleeding (placenta previa and abruptio placenta), you may find a list of additional nursing diagnoses that may accompany that clinical condition but are not so commonly seen. Review this list to determine whether you should add any of these to the care plan. Not all clinical conditions include a list of other nursing diagnoses.

END NOTES

1. Nursing Diagnoses—Definitions and Classification 2009–2011. Copyright © 2009, 2007, 2005, 2003, 2001, 1998, 1996, 1994 by NANDA International. Used by arrangement with Blackwell Publishing Limited, a company of John Wiley & Sons, Inc. In order to make safe and effective judgments using NANDA-I nursing diagnoses it is essential that nurses refer to the definitions and defining characteristics of the diagnoses listed in this work.

2. Bulechek, G. M., Butcher, H. K., Dochterman, J. M. (2008). *Nursing Interventions Classification* (5th ed). St. Louis, MO: Elsevier, by permission.

RESOURCES

American Nurses Association, (2004). *Nursing: Scope and Standard of Practice*. Silver Spring, MD: Author.

REFERENCES

Bulechek, G. M., Butcher, H. K., Dochterman, J. M. (2008). *Nursing Interventions Classification* (5th ed). St. Louis, MO: Elsevier,.

GENERIC CARE PLANS

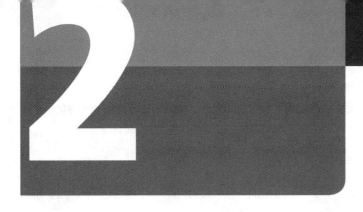

NURSING DIAGNOSIS CARE PLANS (GENERIC)

This chapter contains *generic* care plans for common nursing diagnoses that could apply to a woman with any one of several conditions or medical diagnoses. The nursing activities are appropriate for all women with that particular nursing diagnosis, regardless of the etiology of the nursing diagnosis or the phase of the woman's pregnancy, birth, or postpartum period. For example, when a woman experiences pain, regardless of the cause of the pain, the nurse will perform the activity, assess pain level by using a scale of 1 to 10.

The generic *nursing diagnosis care plans* (NDCPs) are used in conjunction with *collaborative* (standardized) and *individualized* (nursing diagnosis) care plans specified in each topic care plan (e.g., the care plan for late antepartum bleeding). The generic NDCPs include the North American Nursing Diagnosis Association title, related factors (when applicable), and signs and symptoms. Also included are nursing interventions classifications (NICs) and nursing activities and rationales.

Nursing Diagnosis: ACTIVITY INTOLERANCE[1]

This section refers to activity intolerance related to any physiologic or psychologic stressor occurring during pregnancy, labor, birth, or postpartum.

Goals, Outcomes, and Evaluation Criteria

- Woman maintains activity level within usual capabilities, as evidenced by normal heart rate and blood pressure (BP) during activity and absence of fatigue, weakness, and shortness of breath.
- Woman uses energy-conservation techniques.
- Woman verbalizes importance of gradually resuming normal activities.

NIC Interventions[2]

Energy Management (0180)—Regulating energy use to treat or prevent fatigue and optimize function.

Teaching: Prescribed Activity/Exercise (5612)—Preparing a patient to achieve and/or maintain a prescribed level of activity.
Environmental Management (6480)—Manipulation of the patient's surroundings for therapeutic benefit.

Nursing Activities and Rationales

Assessments

- Assess the woman's ability to ambulate and perform self-care activities. Helps determine the extent of the woman's activity intolerance in order to set realistic goals.
- Assess for changes in pulse rate following activity. Heart rate may increase by 20–30 beats/min after activity depending on the amount and type of activity. Increases in excess of 20–30 beats are abnormal and may indicate cardiac compromise and warrant further evaluation.
- Assess for presence of orthostatic changes in blood pressure. A drop in blood pressure upon standing or during activity may be related to fluid volume depletion, infection, or pain. Significant increases or decreases in blood pressure with activity warrant further evaluation.
- Assess for changes in respiratory rate. Activity increases metabolic rate and oxygen consumption, which may increase respiratory rate and cause dyspnea.
- Assess for presence of infection. The presence of fever, increased white blood cell count, or purulent drainage is an indication of infection. Infection is a significant cause of weakness and fatigue due to increased metabolic requirements.
- Assess for abnormal laboratory data. Abnormal laboratory data, including but not limited to liver, renal, and blood chemistry studies, may be indicative of underlying disease or complications.
- Assess the woman's nutritional intake and needs. Women who are inadequately nourished will not have the energy reserves necessary for labor, birth, or self-care and infant care after birth or healing. Identifying nutritional deficits aids with planning appropriate interventions.
- Assess the woman's perception of her activity intolerance. Provides a baseline regarding the woman's awareness of her fatigue and its cause and to guide treatment.
- Assess for emotional stress. Psychologic stress can produce depression, which may result in activity intolerance to the same degree as physiologic stress. Identifying psychologic stressors helps with planning appropriate corrective interventions.
- Assess sleep patterns and adequacy of sleep. Prolonged periods of wakefulness or frequent sleep interruptions disrupt the normal sleep cycle and lead to fatigue and inability to tolerate normal activities. Hormonal changes may alter the woman's ability to fall asleep or stay asleep, which places the pregnant woman at increased risk for fatigue. Pregnant women require more sleep and rest than do nonpregnant women because of increased metabolic needs and higher levels of progesterone.

- Assess emotional status. Psychologic stress can produce depression, which may result in activity intolerance to the same degree as physiologic stress. Identifying psychologic stressors helps with planning appropriate corrective interventions.

Independent Nursing Actions

- Maintain adequate food and fluid intake. Prevents nutritional deficits, protein losses, and cellular dehydration and/or hypovolemia.
- Encourage rest periods after activities such as meals, bathing, caring for infant, or ambulation. Helps prevent overexertion and minimizes oxygen consumption.
- Organize the environment by placing frequently used items within easy reach. Conserves energy and prevents fatigue.
- Encourage the woman to participate in care planning and goal setting. Allows the woman a sense of control over her own care and increases her motivation to reach established goals.
- Assist with care as needed, without promoting dependence. Conserves energy while allowing the woman to remain in control of her situation and care.
- Encourage active range of motion (ROM) and other exercises. Prevents hazards associated with immobility (e.g., pneumonia, muscle weakness or atrophy, constipation, deep vein thrombosis, joint stiffness).
- Encourage a gradual return to normal activities. Prevents fatigue while building endurance.
- Encourage verbalization of feelings about activity limitations. Helps reduce anxiety and enhances coping with situation.

Patient/Family Teaching

- Teach the woman and her family signs of fatigue. *Increases the woman's awareness of when she is becoming fatigued so that she can reduce her activities or take a rest period.*
- Teach the need for assigning priorities to activities. The woman can plan to carry out activities that require the greatest amount of energy early in the day or after rest periods. Low-priority activities can be postponed or omitted when energy levels are too low to carry them out safely.
- Teach the woman to avoid strenuous activities until energy levels return to normal. Prepregnancy activities may not be as well tolerated during pregnancy or after delivery; therefore, the activity level may require modification.
- Teach energy-conserving self-care techniques. Assists woman with conserving energy by minimizing oxygen consumption.

Nursing Diagnosis: ANXIETY[1]

This section refers to anxiety related to any physiologic or psychologic stressor or event, such as a threat or perceived threat to pregnancy or newborn, or lack of knowledge or lack of financial resources.

Goals, Outcomes, and Evaluation Criteria

- Woman is free of signs of anxiety (e.g., trembling, pallor, facial tension).
- Woman participates in decision making regarding her own care and treatment.
- Woman identifies and uses support persons (e.g., partner, caregivers).
- Woman verbalizes a sense of control and/or acceptance of the situation.

NIC Interventions[2]

Anxiety Reduction (5820)—Minimizing apprehension, dread, foreboding, or uneasiness related to an unidentified source of anticipated danger.

Calming Technique (5880)—Reducing anxiety in patient experiencing acute distress.

Coping Enhancement (5230)—Assisting a patient to adapt to perceived stressors, changes, or threats that interfere with meeting life demands and roles.

Emotional Support (5270)—Provision of reassurance, acceptance, and encouragement during times of stress.

Presence (5340)—Being with another, both physically and psychologically, during times of need.

Simple Relaxation Therapy (6040)—Use of techniques to encourage and elicit relaxation for the purpose of decreasing undesirable signs and symptoms such as pain, muscle tension, or anxiety.

Touch (5460)—Providing comfort and communication through purposeful tactile contact.

Nursing Activities and Rationales

Assessments

- Assess verbal and nonverbal indicators of fear/anxiety. Determines the presence and level of anxiety. This information provides a baseline on which to plan nursing interventions and measure their effectiveness. Nonverbal cues may be the first recognized since some patients may not recognize or verbalize their own anxiety. Behavioral and physiologic changes increase in severity as anxiety increases.
- Assess woman's or partner's ability to participate in decision making. Participation enhances the feeling of control; however, it is important not to increase stress by requiring more involvement than the woman can comfortably tolerate.
- Assess level of understanding of the diagnosis, treatment, and prognosis. Teaching begins with an assessment of the woman's level of knowledge so that it can be individualized to her and her partner. Knowledge and understanding decrease fear.
- Assess for physiologic symptoms of anxiety. Anxiety stimulates the autonomic nervous system resulting in these symptoms: increased blood pressure, heart rate, and respirations; heart palpitations; diaphoresis; cold, clammy hands; dizziness and headache; tremors, dry mouth; and nausea.

- Assess the level of anxiety. Anxiety ranges from mild to panic. Mild anxiety may increase alertness and improve ability to comprehend and learn. Moderate anxiety produces periodic inattention, decreased ability to communicate and learn, and a need for direction. Severe anxiety impairs the ability to learn and communicate details. Panic creates distorted perception, inability to learn, and inability to communicate or function.

Independent Nursing Actions

- Provide calm, accepting environment. A peaceful, non-threatening environment encourages the woman to express feelings and fears, recognize anxiety, and identify its causes. Acceptance of feelings validates them, promoting further discussion and exploration of feelings.
- Encourage verbalization of anxieties. Fear of the unknown or fear due to misunderstanding of disease or treatment significantly increases anxiety. Anxiety is reduced when fears are eliminated or reduced.
- Help the woman to identify source of stressors. Helps woman to recognize and resolve anxiety. Sometimes a stressor can be modified or removed; at other times, coping skills may require reinforcement.
- Encourage participation of significant other to the extent possible. The presence of the partner and/or significant individuals increases feelings of security and decreases feelings of fear.
- Encourage the woman to identify and use stress-reducing techniques that have been beneficial in the past. Techniques that have been successful in the past are likely to be successful with any stress-producing event. Women are more likely to use techniques that have proven successful in the past.

Patient/Family Teaching

- Provide time with the woman to explain procedures, offer reassurance, and listen to concerns. Establishing rapport, providing active listening, offering empathy, and explaining procedures demonstrates compassion, reduces fear, and establishes trust.
- Teach relaxation techniques such as slow, purposeful, deep breathing, guided imagery, or progressive muscle relaxation. These techniques are helpful in assisting the woman with retaining control of emotions and decreasing physical symptoms created by anxiety.

Nursing Diagnosis: CONSTIPATION[1]

This section discusses constipation related to pregnancy, inadequate fluid and/or fiber intake, inadequate physical activity, irregular defecation pattern, opioid pain medications.

▐ Goals, Outcomes, and Evaluation Criteria

- Woman reports return to usual bowel pattern.
- Woman passes soft formed stool without laxatives or enemas.
- Woman eats diet rich in fiber.
- Woman drinks adequate amount of daily fluids.
- Woman participates in exercise program within prescribed limitations.

▐ NIC Interventions[2]

Bowel Management (0430)—Establishment and maintenance of regular pattern of bowel elimination.
Constipation/Impaction Management (0450)—Prevention and alleviation of constipation/impaction.
Fluid Management (4120)—Promotion of fluid balance and prevention of complications resulting from abnormal or undesired fluid levels.
Teaching: Individual (5606)—Planning, implementation, and evaluation of a teaching program designed to address a patient's particular needs.

▐ Nursing Activities and Rationales

Assessments

- Assess the woman's normal or usual pattern of bowel elimination. Bowel patterns vary among individuals and may range from one bowel movement each day to one bowel movement every 2 or 3 days. The woman's normal pattern needs to be determined in order to plan corrective interventions.
- Assess dietary intake of fiber. With insufficient fiber in the diet there is little residue available to form the bulk of fecal material.
- Assess intake of fluids. When fluid intake is inadequate, fecal material may lack sufficient fluid content to permit easy passage through the lower intestinal tract.
- Assess activity pattern. When exercise is insufficient, normal peristaltic action may be decreased and muscles of the digestive tract may lose their tone, resulting in constipation and/or fecal impaction.
- Assess current use of prescription, over-the-counter, and herbal remedies. Many medications, such as antidepressants, antacids, analgesics, antihypertensives, and dietary supplements, can cause constipation.
- Assess the woman's use of laxatives or enemas. Prolonged use of laxatives or enemas decreases normal functioning and causes dependency.
- Assess for stress or excessive worry. Excessive stress or worry can depress physical functions so that digestion and elimination are adversely affected.

Independent Nursing Actions

- Provide privacy. Lack of privacy may serve as an inhibitory condition that affects the desire and ability to defecate.

- Assist the woman to the bathroom or up to a bedside commode if feasible. Allows the woman to assume a more normal position for defecation and requires less energy than use of a bedpan.
- Encourage use of natural cathartics when needed (i.e., prunes, prune juice, beans). These foods are high-fiber foods that increase bulk and fluid in the fecal material for easy passage.

Collaborative Activities

- Consult patient's provider for advice on use of stool softener or bulk-forming agent, if necessary. May be necessary until hormone levels return to prepregnant state to establish a regular bowel routine. Stool softeners reduce the surface tension of feces, allowing water to penetrate and soften stool. Bulk-forming agents help to hold water in the bowel and stimulate peristalsis.

Patient/Family Teaching

- Encourage establishment of a regular time for defecation. Without the habit needed to ensure elimination of feces at the same time each day, the desire to defecate may not be strongly felt, resulting in constipation.
- Teach the relationship between fluid intake and bowel elimination, encouraging a daily intake of between 2000 and 3000 ml fluid (8–10 glasses of water or other fluids). Adequate fluid intake is essential to keep fecal material moist enough to permit easy passage through the lower intestinal tract.
- Teach the woman the need for increasing dietary fiber in her diet. Raw fruits and vegetables add fiber and fluid to fecal material. Fiber-containing foods do not break down during digestion. They draw fluid into the intestine as they pass through the bowel, adding bulk and making the passage of stool easier.
- Teach the need for maintaining an exercise program within prescribed parameters. Lack of exercise, periods of decreased mobility, or bed rest contribute to constipation. Exercise facilitates normal peristaltic action and helps maintain muscular tone of the digestive tract.
- Teach how and when to use pharmacologic measures. The continued use of laxatives or enemas causes the intestinal tract to become less responsive to normal physiologic responses and produces dependency on the laxative or enema.

Nursing Diagnosis: DEFICIENT DIVERSIONAL ACTIVITY[1]

This section discusses deficient diversional activity related to psychologic or cognitive barriers (e.g., lack of motivation, depression, embarrassment), forced inactivity (e.g., prolonged, prescribed bed rest or hospitalization), physical barriers to usual recreational activities (e.g., fatigue, pain), and socioeconomic barriers (e.g., financial constraints, lack of support system).

Goals, Outcomes, and Evaluation Criteria

- Woman identifies methods of coping with feelings of depression, anger, or boredom created by physical barriers.
- Woman demonstrates or verbalizes enjoyment in leisure activities.
- Woman demonstrates social involvement as evidenced by interaction with close friends, family members, or work group.
- Woman redirects energy toward interests that are fulfilling.

NIC Interventions[2]

Recreation Therapy (5360)—Purposeful use of recreation to promote relaxation and enhancement of social skills.
Energy Management (180)—Regulating energy use to treat or prevent fatigue and optimize function.
High-Risk Pregnancy Care (6800)—Identification and management of a high-risk pregnancy to promote healthy outcomes for mother and baby.
Pain Management (1400)—Alleviation of pain or a reduction in pain to a level of comfort that is acceptable to the patient.

Nursing Activities and Rationales

Assessments

- Assess physical and mental abilities to participate in recreational activities. What may be interpreted as decreased interest in recreational activity may be a lack of physical ability to participate in activities previously enjoyed. This may be especially true during pregnancy when weight gain and fatigue may prohibit usual physical activities.
- Identify the woman's interests. The woman is more likely to participate in activities that stimulate her interest or in those that she enjoys.
- Monitor emotional, physical, and social responses to diversional activity. Determines the effectiveness of the diversional activity in relieving the woman's boredom or depression and ensures that activities do not produce adverse physical responses such as fatigue.

Independent Nursing Actions

- Encourage socialization with others. All humans need interaction with others. Pregnant women may impose social isolation on themselves because of their size and difficulty maneuvering within the environment; or they may be required to take maternity leave from their job depending on the type of work (e.g., heavy lifting). Lack of stimulation results in boredom and may lead to depression, lowered self-worth, reduced productivity, and even feelings of anger or hostility.
- Provide anticipatory guidance for common experiences that high-risk mothers have during the postpartum period (e.g., exhaustion, depression, disenchantment with

childbearing, marital discord). Women in high-risk pregnancies often feel vulnerable, and birth of a baby often means that significant lifestyle changes are necessary (e.g., sexual, social, recreational, and employment activities). Knowledge in advance of possible emotional or physical encounters can help the individual anticipate changes in physical and mental ability.

- Include the woman in planning the daily routine. Participation in planning daily activities gives the woman a sense of self-control and may stimulate a renewed interest in usual or new activities.

Patient/Family Teaching

- Teach the woman and significant other(s) to plan activities for periods when energy is highest. Fatigue is a common problem during pregnancy and after birth because of hormonal changes, metabolic changes, and physical exertion. Recreational activities as well as activities of daily living should be planned during the morning hours when energy reserves are generally greatest.

Nursing Diagnosis: DEFICIENT KNOWLEDGE[1]

This section refers to deficient knowledge about stages of pregnancy, birth process, complications, procedures, infant care, etc., related to lack of previous experience or exposure, disinterest or lack of motivation to learn, lack of educational resources, misinterpretation of information or reduced cognitive ability, etc.

Goals, Outcomes, and Evaluation Criteria

- Woman identifies the need for additional information regarding pregnancy and birth.
- Woman uses knowledge to make health-promoting lifestyle choices.
- Woman demonstrates healthy behaviors (e.g., adequate nutrition, sleep, rest).
- Woman participates effectively in self-care.
- Woman explains rationale for therapeutic interventions and limitations.
- Woman verbalizes self-care measures to reduce the physical discomforts of pregnancy, delivery, or postpartum period.
- Woman demonstrates understanding of labor and delivery as evidenced by description of birthing options, signs and symptoms of labor, stages and phases of labor and delivery, pain control methods, effective breathing and relaxation techniques, potential complications, and effective pushing techniques during delivery.
- Woman demonstrates adequate breastfeeding as evidenced by early recognition of infant hunger cues, proper technique for attaching infant to breast, signs of adequate milk supply, and nipple evaluation.

- Woman demonstrates understanding of self-care as evidenced by description of physical aspects of care, e.g., episiotomy, perineal, and breast care, fundal massage; identification of appropriate fluid and nutrient intake; rest and exercise; and resumption of sexual activity.

NIC Interventions[2]

Breastfeeding Assistance (1054)—Preparing a new mother to breastfeed her infant.

Lactation Counseling (5244)—Use of an interactive helping process to assist in maintenance of successful breastfeeding.

Parent Education: Infant (5568)—Instruction on nurturing and physical care needed during the first year of life.

Prenatal Care (6960)—Monitoring and management of patient during pregnancy to prevent complications of pregnancy and promote a healthy outcome for both mother and infant.

Postpartal Care (6930)—Monitoring and management of the patient who has recently given birth.

Teaching: Individual (5606)—Planning, implementation, and evaluation of teaching program designed to address a patient's particular needs.

Teaching: Infant Nutrition (5626)—Instruction on nutrition and feeding practices during the first year of life.

Teaching: Infant Safety (5628)—Instruction on safety during first year of life.

Teaching: Prescribed Diet (5614)—Preparing a patient to follow a prescribed diet correctly.

Teaching: Prescribed Medication (5616)—Preparing a patient to take prescribed medications safely and to monitor their effects.

Teaching: Procedure/Treatment (5618)—Preparing a patient to understand and mentally prepare for a prescribed procedure or treatment.

Teaching: Psychomotor Skill (5620)—Preparing a patient to perform a psychomotor skill.

Nursing Activities and Rationales

Assessments

- Assess the woman's current knowledge level and willingness to learn. Avoids overteaching or underteaching, because the nurse's perception of what the woman needs to know may differ from what the woman actually knows or wants to learn. The nurse should not assume that multigravidas are highly knowledgeable because of previous experiences, nor should the nurse assume that the woman has little or no knowledge. If the woman is not willing or able to learn, teaching will be of little benefit. The topics in which women are most interested may not match those of the healthcare provider; thus, it is important to assess the woman's interest rather than make assumptions about essential teaching points.
- Determine the woman's learning style (e.g., visual or auditory). Tailors learning to the individual woman's needs.

- Seek feedback to validate woman's understanding of prescribed treatment(s) and/or procedures and recommendations for self-care. Initial assessment of a woman's knowledge base is essential in planning and revising a teaching plan. Learning does not always result from teaching; therefore, feedback is essential.

Independent Nursing Actions

- Provide anticipatory guidance for self-care throughout pregnancy and the postpartum period. Because of the profound changes that occur during pregnancy, women are generally motivated to learn about their bodies and about healthy behaviors and simply require guidance in learning about self-care. In addition, new parents will be less anxious if they are equipped with adequate knowledge of infant care.

Patient/Family Teaching

- Help woman set realistic learning goals. Realistic goals provide motivation and criteria with which to evaluate learning.
- Involve family and/or support person in teaching. Family or other support persons may reinforce information presented.
- Use a variety of teaching strategies to facilitate learning (e.g., hands-on activities, verbal/written feedback, learner participation and return demonstration). People learn in different ways. Some understand the spoken word better than others; some grasp the meaning in an analogy or story example; others benefit most from direct application of the learned skill. Whatever the method, constructive feedback is essential in the learning process so that correct skills and logical thinking are validated.
- Provide written materials; use pictures to illustrate content. Increases understanding of content; improves retention and recall.
- Provide a quiet, comfortable environment for teaching. Facilitates learning.
- Discuss the importance of learning the content and how it will contribute to positive pregnancy outcomes. Most adult learners are more receptive to learning when they can see the advantage of the information and the immediate benefit to them.
- Keep an open attitude regarding the woman's and family's cultural and spiritual practices. If the woman feels accepted, trust can develop and learning is enhanced.
- Document details of the teaching and learning (e.g., content, written materials provided, woman's verbal responses that indicate learning has occurred). Nursing interventions should be a part of the permanent record. Allows continuity of care and further teaching if needed.

Nursing Diagnosis: FATIGUE[1]

This section discusses fatigue related to sensory overload (e.g., lights, noise, temperature), increased physical exertion, pregnancy (first trimester), electrolyte imbalances, anemia, lack of sleep, infection, extreme stress, and other physiologic and psychologic stressors.

Goals, Outcomes, and Evaluation Criteria

- Woman verbalizes feelings about the effects of fatigue on lifestyle.
- Woman maintains a consistent pattern of sleep and rest.
- Woman establishes priorities for daily activities.
- Woman uses energy-conservation techniques.
- Woman adapts lifestyle to energy level.
- Woman recognizes energy limitations.
- Woman maintains adequate nutrition.

NIC Interventions[2]

Energy Management (0180)—Regulating energy use to treat or prevent fatigue and optimize function.
Sleep Enhancement (1850)—Facilitation of regular sleep/wake cycles.
Simple Massage (1480)—Stimulation of the skin and underlying tissues with varying degrees of hand pressure to decrease pain, produce relaxation, and/or improve circulation.
Support System Enhancement (5440)—Facilitation of support to patient by family, friends, and community.
Mood Management (5220)—Providing for safety, stabilization, recovery, and maintenance of a patient who is experiencing dysfunctional depression or elevated mood.

Nursing Activities and Rationales

Assessments

- Determine causes of fatigue (e.g., pain, inadequate rest, depression). Ensures that all aspects of the problem can be addressed.
- Assess psychologic response to the situation and availability of support system(s). Pregnancy is physically demanding and may cause psychologic stress, which contributes to the woman's fatigue.
- Assess nutritional status and usual food intake. Additional calories and nutrients are needed during pregnancy to accommodate the growing fetus and maternal tissues. If intake is not adequate, calories and nutrients will not be available to provide maternal energy.

Independent Nursing Actions

- Assist the woman with identifying her energy patterns. Determining when the woman has the most and least energy helps her plan and prioritize activities of daily living to accommodate energy levels.
- Explain the purpose of pacing and prioritization. Prioritizing and pacing activities may decrease fatigue.

Patient/Family Teaching

- Teach energy conservation technique. Women may be unaware of simple measures that can be taken to avoid nonessential energy-consuming activities.

- Teach the client how to perform muscle relaxation or other nonpharmacologic forms of sleep inducement. Although rest cannot resolve fatigue caused by conditions that cannot be eliminated (e.g., cancer, chronic anemia), rest and relaxation can help the woman relax (mentally and physically) and replenish her energy supply.
- Teach the woman to recognize signs and symptoms of fatigue that suggest the need to reduce activity. Recognition of fatigue helps the woman know when to decrease activities. Reduction of activity levels in accordance with perceived fatigue levels is imperative to the success of any treatment regimen.

Nursing Diagnosis: FEAR[1]

This section discusses fear related to environmental stimuli or stressors (e.g., hospitalization, invasive procedures), lack of knowledge, language barrier, physical losses (e.g., loss of function, death), maturational changes (e.g., pregnancy, parenthood), etc.

Goals, Outcomes, and Evaluation Criteria

- Woman expresses understanding of risks to the infant.
- Woman seeks information to reduce fear.
- Woman uses relaxation techniques to reduce fear.
- Woman verbalizes satisfaction with symptom control.
- Woman verbalizes a sense of control.
- Woman differentiates between real and imagined threats.

NIC Interventions[2]

Coping Enhancement (5230)—Assisting a patient to adapt to perceived stressors, changes, or threats that interfere with meeting life demands and roles.

Anxiety Reduction (5820)—Minimizing apprehension, dread, foreboding, or uneasiness related to an unidentified source of anticipated danger.

Emotional Support (5270)—Provision of reassurance, acceptance, and encouragement during times of stress.

High-Risk Pregnancy Care (6800)—Identification and management of a high-risk pregnancy to promote healthy outcomes for mother and baby.

Childbirth Preparation (6760)—Providing information and support to facilitate childbirth and to enhance the ability of an individual to develop and perform the role of parent.

Security Enhancement (5380)—Intensifying a patient's sense of physical and psychologic safety.

Nursing Activities and Rationales

Assessments

- Assess the woman's knowledge about labor, delivery, infant care, etc. Assessment serves as a basis for a teaching plan, if one is necessary. Fear may result from misconceptions or lack of knowledge.
- Assess for physical manifestations of fear. Woman may be reluctant to verbalize fears or may be unaware of the fears. Identification of physical manifestations of fear helps the nurse determine the degree of fear and plan appropriate interventions.

Independent Nursing Actions

- Stay with the patient to promote safety and reduce fear. Presence and the assurance of skilled nursing care can diminish fear.
- Create an atmosphere to facilitate trust. Trust is essential to the helping relationship. In the absence of trust, fear or anxiety may escalate in response to the nurse's approach. By conveying a caring attitude and genuine interest in the woman, the nurse can foster the development of trust, which enables the patient to express thoughts and feelings openly.
- Encourage woman to express her fears and concerns. Expressing one's fears often reduces them.
- Encourage expression of factors that magnify feelings of fear (e.g., lifestyle changes, fetal well-being, financial changes, family functioning, and personal safety). A sense of greater self-control and adequacy in confronting danger reduces fear. Awareness of factors that intensify fears increases control and reduces fear when the reality of a situation is confronted.
- Provide diversional activities geared toward the reduction of tension. Activity uses energy and dissipates the physical reaction to fear.
- Encourage the woman to identify and use coping techniques that have been beneficial in the past. Techniques that have been successful in the past are likely to be successful with any new stress-producing event. Women are more likely to use techniques that have proven successful in the past.

Patient/Family Teaching

- Explain procedures and sensations likely to be experienced (e.g., during labor and birth, during amniocentesis). Fear of the unknown is one of the most important contributing factors to anxiety.
- Teach partner measures to comfort the woman during labor (e.g., back rub, back pressure, positioning). Diversional activities can help rechannel the woman's emotional energy and promote comfort, thereby reducing the fear of future pain episodes.
- Instruct in self-care techniques to increase the chance of a healthy outcome (e.g., hydration, nutrition, activity modifications, prenatal care). The degree of danger can be minimized for the high-risk mother and infant by patient compliance. Confronting the danger through self-care reduces fear.

Nursing Diagnosis: IMPAIRED PARENTING[1]

This section applies to impaired parenting related to lack of access to resources, unemployment, poor home environment; unplanned or unwanted pregnancy; unrealistic expectations for self, infant, or partner; poor communication skills; lack of knowledge about parenting skills; physical illness; premature birth, illness, nondesired gender, birth anomaly; disability, depression, history of substance abuse or dependency, etc.

Goals, Outcomes, and Evaluation Criteria

- Parent(s) verbalize positive feelings toward infant/child.
- Parent(s) demonstrate affection and caring toward infant/child.
- Parent(s) participate in family therapy and/or parenting classes.
- Parent(s) verbalize need for assistance.
- Parent(s) collaborate with each other about care of the newborn.

NIC Interventions[2]

Abuse Protection Support: Child (6402)—Identification of high-risk, dependent child relationships and actions to prevent possible or further infliction of physical, sexual, or emotional harm or neglect of basic necessities of life.

Attachment Promotion (6710)—Facilitation of the development of the parent–infant relationship.

Family Integrity Promotion (7104)—Facilitation of the growth of individuals or families who are adding an infant to the family unit.

Family Support (7140)—Promotion of family values, interests, and goals.

Family Therapy (7150)—Assisting family members to move their family toward a more productive way of living.

Parenting Promotion (8300)—Providing parenting information, support, and coordination of comprehensive services to high-risk families.

Risk Identification: Childbearing Family (6612)—Identification of an individual or family likely to experience difficulties in parenting and prioritization of strategies to prevent parenting problems.

Nursing Activities and Rationales

Assessments

- Assess parent's expectations of the newborn during pregnancy. Parents develop an ideal image of their child during pregnancy. How closely the real child resembles the ideal after birth influences the bonding process. If discrepancies in the parent's view of the ideal versus real child are identified early on, corrective actions can be taken to enhance bonding.
- Assess for prolonged labor, woman's fatigue, effect of pain medications, and problems with breastfeeding. These factors can delay the development of initial positive feelings toward the newborn and the mother's ability to provide physical care. If these are identified early, corrective measures can be taken to enhance parent–infant bonding and provide support to the mother for care of the infant.
- Assess for parental behaviors that indicate lack of attachment. Turning away from the infant, refusing to hold the infant, failing to place the infant in family context, handling the infant roughly, indifference to infant's safety needs, viewing the infant as distasteful or ugly are behaviors that may indicate lack of parent–infant attachment. Early recognition of failure to bond helps the nurse plan corrective strategies or refer the parent or parents for counseling or therapy.
- Assess for infant behaviors that negatively affect parent–infant bonding. Negative behaviors may include fussiness, feeding poorly, unresponsiveness to parents, averting gaze. Early recognition of behaviors that demonstrate negative parent–infant bonding helps the nurse plan corrective interventions.
- Assess for adequacy of support systems. Parents may need assistance with the care of the infant. A strong support system, such as grandparents, aunts, or uncles, can provide the parents with rest periods when needed or assistance with adjusting to parenting.

Independent Nursing Actions

- Allow the mother time to rest or sleep after delivery. The woman may be too exhausted to respond to the infant in other than a superficial way.
- Provide an opportunity for parents to hold the infant as soon as possible after birth. Early contact between a mother and her infant may facilitate the attachment process.
- Review maternal history for alcohol or drug abuse. Identifies women or families who are at increased risk for impaired parenting.
- Observe infant care routines related to feeding, bathing, diapering, and so on. Evaluates ease with which parents interact and care for the infant and identifies problems with technique or infant–parent relationship that may require intervention.
- Encourage verbalization of concerns for home care of the infant. Identifies parents' perceptions about the ease or difficulty of caring for their infant. If parents view care of their infant as difficult, they may need assistance or counseling.

Patient/Family Teaching

- Teach parents about available community resources. Parents may be unaware of resources that are available to them and how to obtain those resources when needed.

■ *Collaborative Activities*

- Refer for counseling. Children of parents who are unable or unwilling to care for them because of physical or psychologic problems or disabilities are at increased risk for neglect or abuse. It is essential that these situations be identified and parents referred for counseling or therapy to protect the safety of the child.

■ Nursing Diagnosis: INEFFECTIVE COPING[1]

This section applies to ineffective coping related to depression prior to, during, or after pregnancy; uncertainty in coping ability; inadequate resources (e.g., financial reserves, social support, marital discord); altered pattern(s) of tension release, relaxation, self-care; lack of energy reserves for stress management; child-care stress (e.g., sleeping alterations, feeding problems); insufficient self-confidence and/or perception of control or coping ability; inadequate opportunity to prepare for the stressor (e.g., premature infant); maturational changes (e.g., marriage, parenthood, child-rearing problems), etc.

■ *Goals, Outcomes, and Evaluation Criteria*

- Patient participates in activities of daily living.
- Woman identifies coping strategies that have been effective in dealing with stressors in the past.
- Woman accepts support through the nurse–patient relationship.
- Woman verbalizes strategies and/or behaviors to reduce stress.
- Woman verbalizes plans for either accepting or changing the situation.

■ *NIC Interventions*[2]

Body Image Enhancement (5220)—Improving a patient's conscious and unconscious perceptions and attitudes toward his/her body.

Coping Enhancement (5230)—Assisting a patient to adapt to perceived stressors, changes, or threats that interfere with meeting life demands and roles.

Decision-Making Support (5250)—Providing information and support for a patient who is making a decision regarding health care.

Progressive Muscle Relaxation (5250)—Facilitating the tensing and releasing of successive muscle groups while attending to the resulting differences in sensation.

Sleep Enhancement (1850)—Facilitation of regular sleep/wake cycles.

Support System Enhancement (5440)—Facilitation of support to patient by family, friends, and community.

■ *Nursing Activities and Rationales*

Assessments

- Assess adjustment to changes in body image. Alteration in body image may be an issue for the pregnant woman. Identification of the woman's feelings about herself is necessary in order to plan appropriate interventions.
- Assess perceptions and expectations of the pregnancy, birth process, and parenting. Helps with identification of unrealistic expectations so that they can be clarified or corrected.

Independent Nursing Actions

- Encourage the woman to express her feelings/emotions in response to both experience and thoughts. Dealing with feelings is helpful in identifying and describing emotions, and expressing them in ways that facilitate letting go and dissipating the physical arousal that occurs with stress.
- Explore how the woman has dealt with problems or stressful situations in the past. People tend to use the same coping strategies over and over, whether or not they are effective. Identifying strategies that did not work in the past and developing new coping skills appropriate to the present situation assists the woman in successful adaptation.
- Involve significant other(s) in planning coping strategies. Social support modifies the negative effects of stress and helps women cope. Supporting the woman who is having difficulty coping conveys acceptance and provides a foundation for her as she adjusts to the many changes that are occurring.
- Encourage the woman to realistically describe how her role in the family has changed or will change. The woman may have unrealistic perceptions and self-expectations. A realistic reappraisal of the situation can reduce stress. Assisting the woman with describing her new role in realistic terms is beneficial in developing goals for role achievement.
- Discuss alternative responses to the situation. Effective coping requires successful management of many tasks and therefore requires many different strategies. No single strategy can cope with all stressors or situations.

Patient/Family Teaching

- Provide factual information about the woman's and baby's health status. Valid, factual information provides a basis for the woman to explore feelings and alternative coping strategies.
- Repeat teaching frequently. Stress can prevent the woman from accurately hearing or understanding information. Repetition enhances retention of information and ensures that the woman has the information and understanding necessary to make informed decisions.
- Teach the woman to use relaxation techniques and the importance of balance in work and play. Developing a balance between exercise and relaxation diminishes physiologic arousal to stress and promotes optimal health.

Nursing Diagnosis: INEFFECTIVE PERIPHERAL TISSUE PERFUSION[1]

This section discusses ineffective peripheral tissue perfusion related to factors such as decreased attachment of oxygen to hemoglobin due to altered blood pH, oxygen–carbon dioxide exchange problems, interruption of arterial or venous blood flow, decreased hemoglobin concentration, hypoventilation, hypervolemia, hypovolemia, etc.

Goals, Outcomes, and Evaluation Criteria

- Woman demonstrates tissue perfusion to the extremities as evidenced by normal skin color, warm skin temperature, strong, symmetrical peripheral pulses, brisk capillary refill, and absence of edema.
- Woman identifies factors that compromise circulation to the extremities.
- Woman identifies activities that promote vasodilation.
- Woman initiates measures to maximize circulation.

NIC Interventions[2]

Circulatory Precautions (4070)—Protection of a localized area with limited perfusion.

Circulatory Care: Venous Insufficiency (4066)—Promotion of venous circulation.

Peripheral Sensation Management (2660)—Prevention or minimization of injury or discomfort in the patient with altered sensation.

Positioning (0840)—Deliberative placement of the patient or a body part to promote physiologic and/or psychologic well- being.

Fluid Management (4120)—Promotion of fluid balance and prevention of complications resulting from abnormal or undesired fluid levels.

Nursing Activities and Rationales

Assessments

- Assess peripheral circulation. Changes in peripheral circulation such as weak pulses, edema, poor capillary refill, and pale, cool extremities may indicate abnormal circulation and/or clotting. The legs are common sites for clot formation.
- Assess for signs and symptoms of thrombophlebitis and deep vein thrombosis (e.g., pain, positive Homans' sign, increased skin temperature, redness, edema). Pregnancy increases the risk of thrombophlebitis and deep vein thrombosis because of pressure from the expanding uterus on iliac veins, which is caused by decreased tone of venous smooth muscle, secondary to increased progesterone levels in pregnancy. Early recognition and treatment may prevent serious consequences such as pulmonary embolism.
- Assess position of extremities while sitting, lying, or changing positions. Avoiding pressure on the popliteal area helps prevent venous stasis in the legs and feet. Pressure should be equally distributed along the entire leg.
- Monitor hydration status (e.g., hematocrit, blood urea nitrogen, and intake and output). Early detection of hypovolemia or dehydration can reduce the risk of deep vein thrombosis. Dehydration can raise the platelet count, decrease fibrinolysis, increase clotting factors, or increase the viscosity of the blood, leading to clot formation.

Independent Nursing Actions

- Apply antiembolic stockings as ordered. Antiembolic stockings facilitate blood return from the lower extremities to the heart by placing pressure against peripheral veins.

Patient/Family Teaching

- Teach the importance of preventing venous stasis. Understanding how preventive measures work may increase the woman's cooperation and compliance with treatment routines.
- Teach techniques to promote peripheral circulation and avoid venous congestion (e.g., moderate exercise, early ambulation postpartum, adequate fluid intake). Early ambulation significantly reduces the incidence of thrombophlebitis by promoting venous return, which depends almost entirely on contraction of the calf muscles. Prolonged sitting deactivates the calf-muscle pump, allowing venous pressure to increase. Fluids help maintain adequate blood volume so that formed elements remain in the center of the flow and do not adhere to vein walls.

Nursing Diagnosis: PAIN[1]

This section discusses pain related to pregnancy, complications of pregnancy, labor, birth, or other biological, chemical, physical, psychologic, or spiritual causes.

Goals, Outcomes, and Evaluation Criteria

- Woman uses nonanalgesic relief measures to control pain (e.g., breathing techniques).
- Woman demonstrates relaxation techniques that are effective for achieving individually defined comfort level.
- Woman discusses the advantages and disadvantages of available analgesia/anesthesia alternatives.
- Woman reports pain level at (specify number) or lower, on a scale of 0–10.
- Woman uses analgesics appropriately to control pain.

NIC Interventions[2]

Analgesic Administration (2210)—Use of pharmacologic agents to reduce or eliminate pain.

Anxiety Reduction (5820)—Minimizing apprehension, dread, foreboding, or uneasiness related to an unidentified source of anticipated danger.

Pain Management (1400)—Alleviation of pain or a reduction in pain to a level of comfort that is acceptable to the patient.

▊ *Nursing Activities and Rationales*

Assessments

- Assess the nature of the pain (location, frequency, severity, duration, precipitating factors, relieving factors); use a numbered scale to rate severity. Pain is a subjective experience; must be understood to plan the most effective, yet least intrusive, pain-relief measures.
- Determine the preferred analgesic and/or anesthetic (e.g., epidural), route of administration, and dosage to achieve optimal pain relief. The pharmacologic method of pain relief used is dependent on the woman's special needs and desires, and the benefits versus risks to the mother and baby (e.g., slowing down or stopping uterine contractions). Analgesics administered systemically cross the maternal blood–brain barrier and placenta, resulting in hypnotic effects on both mother and fetus (e.g., neonatal respiratory depression). The nurse can assist the family in making an informed decision by describing the agents being considered, evaluating the mother's willingness to participate in pain relief measures, and assessing the ability of significant other(s) to provide support.
- Assess vital signs and level of consciousness at appropriate intervals and record. Blood pressure, pulse, respirations, and alertness are important indicators of both pain level (e.g., elevated blood pressure, tachycardia, increased respirations, or restlessness) and too much analgesia (e.g., bradycardia, hypotension, and respiratory depression). The fifth vital sign is pain, and it should be assessed frequently to determine the woman's comfort and the need for continued analgesia and to adjust nursing interventions for ongoing comfort.
- Determine any effects the woman's culture and religion may be having on her perception of pain and her pain responses. A pain response (such as crying out) may be acceptable in some cultures but not in others; the nurse must not confuse stoic acceptance with absence of pain. Some religions view pain as a blessing; others as punishment. This would affect the woman's perception of and anxiety about the pain.

Independent Nursing Actions

- Encourage verbalization of fears and concerns. When an individual's basic human needs are met (physical and psychosocial), pain may be reduced. Internal endorphins affect perception of pain, which also is influenced by psychosocial factors such as the woman's expectations, childbirth education, and her interpretation of what is occurring throughout the birthing experience.
- Use therapeutic communication strategies to acknowledge the woman's pain experience and convey acceptance of the woman's response. Women experience different levels of pain in response to the same or similar situations and attach different personal meanings to the painful event(s). The process of acknowledging and validating the woman's pain experience can itself have an analgesic effect by reducing pain perception.
- Control environmental factors that may influence the woman's response to pain (e.g., room noise, lighting, temperature). Extended negative stimuli or any element in the environment that may be causing anxiety can inhibit the release of internal endorphins. Reduction of these morphine-like hormones decreases the woman's pain threshold.
- Provide pain-relief measures before pain becomes severe. Increases the effectiveness of the analgesic.
- Use a positive approach when administering analgesics (e.g., "This will help control your pain."). Decreases anxiety; anxiety increases pain.
- Evaluate the effects of interventions and document. One should not assume that pain-relieving interventions are successful. The nurse can plan future nursing actions on the basis of evaluation of the current plan by assessing the woman's pain status (using pain rating and nonverbal cues) at appropriate intervals. A common reason for unrelieved pain is failure to assess pain and pain relief routinely.

Patient/Family Teaching

- Teach and guide the woman through nonpharmacologic measures to enhance pain control (e.g., simple relaxation therapy, guided imagery). Based on the gate-control theory, noninvasive pain relief techniques help reduce the perception of pain by stimulating large-diameter nerve fibers that carry information such as touch to inhibit pain transmission (analogous to closing the gate).
- Explain all treatments and procedures, including sensations likely to be experienced. The level of endorphins in the body can alter an individual's perception of pain. These morphine-like proteins decrease in the presence of anxiety, tension, and extended negative stimuli. Educating the woman about all procedures, including pain-relief options, helps reduce anxiety and thereby pain associated with anxiety.
- Advise the woman to inform her care provider if her pain is not relieved. Maximum pain relief is the right of every woman. A variety of pain relief measures may need to be tried before finding the most effective one.

▊ Nursing Diagnosis: RISK FOR IMPAIRED PARENT–INFANT/CHILD ATTACHMENT[1]

This section pertains to risk for impaired parent–infant/child attachment related to infant prematurity, illness or a problem that alters parental contact, physical barriers, fear/anxiety, separation of parents and infant/child, inability of parents to meet their own personal needs, substance abuse, etc.

Goals, Outcomes, and Evaluation Criteria

- Parent(s) verbalizes positive feelings toward infant/child.
- Parent(s) exhibits bonding behaviors (e.g., eye contact and *en face* position with newborn; choosing a name during the pregnancy; practicing healthy behaviors during pregnancy; responding to infant cues; holding, touching, stroking, patting, kissing, and smiling at newborn).

NIC Interventions[2]

Attachment Promotion (6710)—Facilitation of the development of the parent–infant relationship.
Parent Education: Infant (5568)—Instruction on nurturing and physical care needed during the first year of life.
Risk Identification: Childbearing Family (6612)—Identification of an individual or family likely to experience difficulties in parenting and prioritization of strategies to prevent parenting problems.

Nursing Activities and Rationales

Assessments

- Assess woman for history of substance abuse. Identifies individuals or families who are at increased risk for parenting alterations. Substance abuse impairs the woman's physical and emotional ability to care for or attach to her infant.
- Assess parent's expectations of newborn during pregnancy. Parents develop an ideal image of their child during pregnancy. How closely the real child resembles the ideal after birth influences the bonding process. If discrepancies in the parent's view of the ideal versus real child are identified early on, corrective actions can be taken to enhance bonding.
- Assess for prolonged labor, fatigue, effect of pain medications, and problems with breastfeeding. These factors can delay the development of initial positive feelings toward the newborn and the mother's ability to provide physical care. If identified early, corrective measures can be taken to enhance parent–infant bonding and provide support to the mother for care of the infant.
- Assess for parental behaviors that reflect lack of attachment. Turning away from the infant; refusing to hold the infant; failing to place the infant in family context; handling the infant roughly; indifference to the infant's safety needs; viewing the infant as distasteful or ugly are behaviors that can negatively affect infant attachment. Early recognition of these behaviors helps the nurse plan corrective strategies and/or refer the parent/parents for counseling or therapy.
- Assess for infant behaviors that negatively affect parent–infant bonding. Negative behaviors may include fussiness,

feeding poorly; unresponsiveness to parents; averting gaze. Attachment requires interaction; if either the infant or a parent does not interact or provide feedback, attachment is delayed. Early recognition of such behaviors helps the nurse plan corrective interventions.
- Assess for adequacy of support systems. Parents may need assistance with the care of the infant. A strong support system, such as grandparents, aunts, or uncles, can provide the parents with rest periods when needed or assistance with adjusting to parenting.

Independent Nursing Actions

- During pregnancy, provide information about normal physical and psychologic changes and fetal development. Use pictures or sonogram to illustrate the appearance of the fetus. Facilitates understanding and helps the woman/parents to see pregnancy as a normal, healthy event rather than an illness; provides motivation for healthy behaviors. Also aids in parent–infant attachment by helping make the fetus a reality for them.
- Allow the mother time to rest or sleep following delivery. The woman may be too exhausted to respond to the infant in other than a superficial way.
- Provide an opportunity for parents to hold the infant as soon as possible after birth. Early interaction and active involvement with the infant foster attachment and promote stronger emotional ties. This is a critically sensitive period during which interactional capabilities are enhanced. This is the best time for bonding.
- Delay instillation of prophylactic antibiotic ophthalmic ointment for 1 hour after birth; allow the parent(s) and infant uninterrupted time together. Allows the infant to open his or her eyes and make eye contact.
- Observe infant care routines (feeding, bathing, diapering, etc.). Evaluates ease with which parents interact and care for the infant to identify problems with technique or infant–parent relationship that may indicate the need for intervention.

Patient/Family Teaching

- Teach parents about available community resources. Parents may be unaware of resources that are available to them and how to obtain those resources when needed.

Collaborative Activities

- Refer for counseling if there are risk factors. Children of parents who are unable or unwilling to care for them due to physical or psychologic problems/disabilities are at increased risk for neglect or abuse. It is essential that these situations be identified and parents referred for counseling or therapy in order to protect the safety of the child.

Nursing Diagnosis: RISK FOR INFECTION[1]

This section pertains to risk for infection related to factors such as stasis of body fluids, chronic conditions (e.g., diabetes mellitus, anemia), perineal wound (e.g., episiotomy or laceration), previous history of urinary tract infection, rupture of amniotic membranes, intrauterine fetal monitoring, cesarean birth, prolonged labor, retained placental fragments, poor nutrition, etc.

Goals, Outcomes, and Evaluation Criteria

- Woman remains free of infection.
- Woman identifies factors that contribute to personal susceptibility to infection.
- Woman follows detection procedures as evidenced by assessing vaginal drainage and/or abdominal wounds, as appropriate.
- Woman demonstrates proper hand-washing technique.
- Woman takes measures to reduce personal risk of infection.

NIC Interventions[2]

Infection Control (6540)—Minimizing the acquisition and transmission of infectious agents.

Infection Protection (6550)—Prevention and early detection of infection in a patient at risk.

Nursing Activities and Rationales

Assessments

- Assess for signs or symptoms of localized or systemic infection (e.g., elevated temperature, increased heart rate, change in drainage/secretions, redness or swelling at episiotomy site, concentrated urine, malaise). Detects the presence of infection early so that treatment interventions can be initiated.
- Assess laboratory values (e.g., complete blood cell count, cultures, urinalysis). Laboratory studies are used to differentiate inflammation from infection. In general, an elevated white blood cell count is a sign of infection. However, the white blood cell count normally increases during labor and may stay elevated during the first few postpartum days in the absence of infection (returns to normal by 7 days postpartum).
- Assess nutritional status. Malnutrition predisposes to infection.
- Assess for recent exposure to diseases (e.g., rubella, sexually transmitted diseases, hepatitis). Identifies risk for infection and anticipates possible interventions should infection occur.

Independent Nursing Actions

- Provide appropriate skin care to edematous areas. Edema decreases circulation in the affected area, which increases the risk for skin breakdown and subsequent risk for infection.
- Maintain standard precautions and careful hand washing. Controls the spread of microorganisms by care providers.
- Promote good nutrition. Malnutrition predisposes to infection.

Patient/Family Teaching

- Explain the importance of correct hand-washing techniques. Pathologic organisms are primarily spread by the hands. Correct hand washing remains the single most important activity for limiting the spread of microorganisms and decreasing the risk for infection.
- Teach the woman and family how to recognize signs and symptoms of infection and when to report them to the healthcare provider. For example, postpartum women should be taught to inspect the episiotomy and/or laceration site for signs of infection using a hand mirror and good lighting. Daily assessment can reduce the risk of a serious infection through early detection. Indicators of localized infection include fever more than 100°F; increased swelling; redness or tenderness in breasts, legs, or incision; green or foamy vaginal drainage; foul-smelling vaginal discharge; and frequency and burning with urination.
- Teach and reinforce appropriate perineal hygiene techniques. Prevents infection. Adequate knowledge regarding self-care is essential to prevention. Careful removal of perineal pads and wiping from front to back once with each tissue helps to avoid contamination of the vaginal area with rectal flora. Pads need to be changed after each urination or defecation. Hands should be washed before and after each pad change.

Nursing Diagnosis: SLEEP DEPRIVATION OR DISTURBED SLEEP PATTERN[1]

This section discusses sleep deprivation or disturbed sleep pattern related to anything that interferes with sleep such as pain, anxiety, depression, urinary urgency, dyspnea, hormonal alterations, loneliness, absence of sleep partner, frequent changes in sleep/wake cycle, medications (e.g., depressants or stimulants), environmental disturbances (e.g., noise, temperature), etc.

Goals, Outcomes, and Evaluation Criteria

- Woman reports relief from symptoms of sleep deprivation.
- Woman identifies measures that will increase rest and sleep.
- Woman identifies factors that contribute to loss of sleep (e.g., pain, reduced physical activity, anxiety).

NIC Interventions[2]

Anxiety Reduction (5820)—Minimizing apprehension, dread, foreboding, or uneasiness related to an unidentified source of anticipated danger.

Progressive Muscle Relaxation (1460)—Facilitating the tensing and releasing of successive muscle groups while attending to the resulting differences in sensation.

Sleep Enhancement (1850)—Facilitation of regular sleep/wake cycles.

Positioning (0840)—Deliberative placement of the patient or a body part to promote physiologic and/or psychologic well-being.

Simple Massage (1480)—Stimulation of the skin and underlying tissues with varying degrees of hand pressure to decrease pain, produce relaxation, and/or improve circulation.

Nursing Activities and Rationales

Assessments

- Assess normal sleep patterns. The amount of sleep a person requires varies with lifestyle, health, and age. A woman's usual sleep pattern serves as a basis for planning adequate sleep time.
- Assess the effect of the woman's current health status and/or medication regimen on patterns of sleep. Sleep patterns during pregnancy are influenced by anxieties of pregnancy and future motherhood, fetal activity, musculoskeletal discomforts, abdominal pressure, and urinary frequency. Awareness of physiologic, emotional, and/or spiritual factors that may be interfering with sleep is necessary for developing a plan to enhance sleep and rest.

Independent Nursing Actions

- Promote the woman's usual bedtime routine (e.g., brushing teeth, reading, bathing). Bedtime rituals help prepare the individual for sleep by promoting mental calmness and physical relaxation.
- Implement comfort measures (e.g., back rub, positioning). Physical discomfort, especially during pregnancy, can directly influence the woman's ability to fall asleep and remain asleep. Comfort measures that enhance muscle relaxation and reduce tension facilitate movement into stage I and II of the sleep cycle in which the woman becomes drowsy, and progressive muscular relaxation occurs with decreasing cerebral activity.
- Decrease external stimuli (noise, lights). External stimuli can hamper the woman's ability to fall asleep or stay asleep.
- Encourage a high-protein snack or glass of milk at bedtime. These foods contain tryptophan, a precursor of serotonin, thought to induce and maintain sleep.

Patient/Family Teaching

- Teach the woman/family about factors that interfere with sleep (e.g., stress, environmental elements such as temperature). Enables the woman to implement lifestyle alterations and prebedtime regimens to enhance sleep.
- Explain the importance of adequate sleep during pregnancy and postpartum periods. Pregnancy involves many physical and emotional stressors that necessitate the need for increased periods of sleep. Sleep is a restorative and recuperative process that facilitates cellular growth, repair of damaged tissues, and rebuilding of new tissues.
- Teach the woman to avoid foods and fluids before bedtime that may interfere with sleep. Stimulants such as caffeine can inhibit the sleep cycle and should be avoided during the 3 to 4 hours just prior to bedtime. Spicy and greasy foods can interfere with sleep by causing indigestion or heartburn.
- Suggest a high-protein snack or glass of milk at bedtime. Certain foods (e.g., milk products, protein foods) contain tryptophan, a precursor of serotonin, thought to induce and maintain sleep.

Nursing Diagnosis: URINARY RETENTION[1]

This section discusses urinary retention related to factors such as obstruction at the bladder outlet (e.g., impacted stool), inadequacy of the detrusor muscle (e.g., loss of voiding reflexes related to anxiety or pain), or impaired innervations (e.g., spinal cord injury), ureterocele (dilation of the distal portion of the ureter), medications, etc.

Goals, Outcomes, and Evaluation Criteria

- Woman empties her bladder with less than 50 ml of residual urine.
- Woman recognizes the urge to void and responds in a timely manner.
- Woman is free of signs and symptoms of urinary tract infection (burning, frequency, urgency, elevated WBC, positive urine culture).
- Woman recognizes and reports symptom onset, frequency, variation, and persistence.

NIC Interventions[2]

Urinary Retention Care (0620)—Assistance in relieving bladder distention.

Perineal Care (1750)—Maintenance of perineal skin integrity and relief of perineal discomfort.

Simple Relaxation Therapy (6040)—Use of techniques to encourage and elicit relaxation for the purpose of decreasing undesirable signs and symptoms such as pain, muscle tension, or anxiety.

Nursing Activities and Rationales

Assessments

- Determine which medications the woman is taking. Some prescribed and over-the-counter medications (e.g., calcium channel blockers and anticholinergics) can cause urinary retention.

- Inspect condition of perineum (e.g., episiotomy in postpartum period). Frequent assessment of the perineal area, e.g., for edema or bruising, provides information about factors contributing to the woman's ability (or inability) to urinate.
- Assess for bladder distention by palpation and percussion. Helps determine the degree of the distention. During the postpartum period, a full bladder may displace the uterine fundus to the right and cause it to rise above the umbilicus.
- Assess for urinary continence, focusing on urinary output, voiding pattern, and preexisting urinary problems. The nurse should measure initial voiding during the postpartum period and assess the height of the fundus before and after subsequent voidings to determine the efficiency of the urinary bladder-emptying process. Voiding less than 200 ml is another important indicator of urinary retention.
- Assess degree of bladder distention by palpation and percussion. Monitors the degree of the distention. In addition to the usual signs and symptoms of a full bladder, during the postpartum period, a full bladder may displace the uterine fundus to the right and cause it to rise above the umbilicus.

Independent Nursing Actions

- Administer pain medication, as appropriate. Perineal lacerations can be very uncomfortable and may cause the postpartum woman to avoid bearing down to urinate; therefore, pain control is important in order to ensure adequate urinary elimination. It should be noted, however, that nonnarcotic analgesics for the postpartum period are preferred for pain relief because opioids can decrease bladder emptying.
- Provide privacy for elimination, and provide enough time for bladder emptying (10 minutes). Most women are socialized to void in private. It is difficult for some women to relax the urinary sphincter unless they are alone.
- Run water or flush the toilet to encourage voiding. Stimulates the reflex bladder.
- Insert urinary catheter, as necessary. Prevents overdistention of the bladder.

Patient/Family Teaching

- Teach the woman the rationale for sitz baths, if used. Sitz baths or a perineal lamp increases circulation and promotes relaxation of surrounding musculature to ease the discomfort caused by episiotomy and/or perineal lacerations. This, in turn, promotes relaxation of the urethral sphincter and subsequent urination.

END NOTES

1. Nursing Diagnoses—Definitions and Classification 2009–2011. Copyright © 2009, 2007, 2005, 2003, 2001, 1998, 1996, 1994 by NANDA International. Used by arrangement with Blackwell Publishing Limited, a company of John Wiley & Sons, Inc. In order to make safe and effective judgments using NANDA-I nursing diagnoses it is essential that nurses refer to the definitions and defining characteristics of the diagnoses listed in this work.
2. Bulechek, G. M., Butcher, H. K., Dochterman, J. M. (2008). *Nursing Interventions Classification* (5th ed). St. Louis, MO: Elsevier, by permission.

RESOURCES

Alexander, L. L., LaRosa, J. H., Bader, H., & Garfield, S. (2007). *New dimensions in women's health* (4th ed.). Sudbury, MA: Jones & Bartlett.

Arenson, J., & Drake, P. (2007). *Maternal and newborn health.* Sudbury, MA: Jones & Bartlett.

Bryanton, J., Gagnon, A. J., Johnston, C., & Hatem, M. (2009). Predictors of women's perceptions of the childbirth experience. *Journal of Obstetric, Gynecologic, & Neonatal Nursing, 37*(1), 24–34.

Hall, P. L., & Wittkowski, A. (2006). An exploration of negative thoughts as a normal phenomenon after childbirth. *Journal of Midwifery and Women's Health, 51*(5), 321–330.

McCance, K. L., Huether, S. E., Brashers, V. L., & Rote, N. S. (2010). *Pathophysiology: The biological basis for disease in adults and children.* St. Louis, MO: Mosby/Elsevier.

Miller, W. B., Sable, M. R., & Csizmadia, A. (2008). Pregnancy wantedness and child attachment security: Is there a relationship? *Maternal & Child Health Journal, 12*(4), 478–487.

Moehler, E., Brunner, R., Wiebel, A., Reck, C., & Resch, F. (2006). Maternal depressive symptoms in the postnatal period are associated with long-term impairment of mother–child bonding. *Archives of Women's Mental Health, 9,* 273–278.

Nilsson, C., & Lundgren, I. (2009). Women's lived experience of fear of childbirth. *Midwifery, 25*(2), e1–e9.

North American Nursing Diagnosis Association (NANDA) International. (2009–2011). *Nursing diagnoses—definitions and classification 2009–2011.* Ames, IA: John Wiley & Sons, Inc., Blackwell Publishing.

Pillitteri, A. (2010). *Maternal & child health nursing: Care of the childbearing & childrearing family.* Philadelphia, PA: Lippincott Williams & Wilkins.

Stein, H. (2007). Patient centered imagery in obstetrics. *International Journal of Childbirth Education, 22*(3), 13–15.

Turner, J. M., Wittkowski, A., & Hare, D. J. (2008). The relationship of maternal mentalization and executive functioning to maternal recognition of infant cues and bonding. *British Journal of Psychology, 99,* 499–512.

Varney, H., Kriebs, J. M., & Gegor, C. L. (2004). *Varney's midwifery.* Sudbury, MA: Jones & Bartlett.

Wittkowski, A., Wieck, A., & Mann, S. (2007). An evaluation of two bonding questionnaires: A comparison of the mother-to-infant bonding scale with the postpartum bonding questionnaire in a sample of primiparous mothers. *Archives of Women's Mental Health, 10,* 171–175.

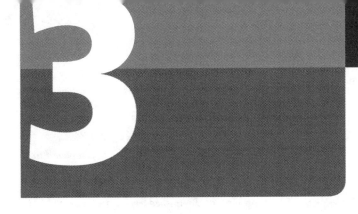

COLLABORATIVE CARE PLANS (GENERIC)

This chapter contains collaborative nursing care plans for common potential complications of various medical diagnoses. As with the nursing care plans in Chapter 2, each care plan applies to any woman with a particular condition or medical diagnosis, such as gestational hypertension. The care plans include a brief description of the potential complication, etiologies and/or risk factors, signs and symptoms, diagnostic studies, a brief overview of medical management, and collaborative (standardized) care for all women with the potential for developing that complication. The nursing activities, which include assessments and preventive nursing actions, apply to all women with the potential for the complication regardless of the medical diagnosis. These care plans are used in conjunction with specific care plans for each condition or disease. Many topics in this book refer to these collaborative care plans.

Potential Complication: ANEMIA

Anemia is characterized by a decreased number of red blood cells (RBCs) and below normal hemoglobin (Hgb) concentration. Anemia results in a reduced oxygen-carrying capacity of the blood, and the heart attempts to compensate by increasing rate and cardiac output. Because this increases the workload of the heart, anemia that occurs with any other complication (e.g., preexisting cardiac disease) may result in congestive heart failure. Anemia is one of the most common conditions affecting pregnant women.

Pathologic anemia must be differentiated from the physiologic anemia of pregnancy, which occurs because the increase in plasma volume (approximately 40–50% greater than prepregnancy levels) exceeds the increase in RBC production. During pregnancy, there is a decrease in normal Hgb (to 12–16 g/dl) and hematocrit (Hct) values (to 37–47%).

Etiologies and Risk Factors

- Dietary iron deficiency (accounts for the majority of the cases of anemia in pregnancy)
- Dietary folic acid deficiency
- Sickle cell hemoglobinopathy
- Thalassemia
- Pregnancy complications with potential for excessive blood loss (e.g., placenta previa)

Signs and Symptoms

- Fatigue, malaise
- Pallor of the skin, sclera, and mucous membranes
- Headache
- Itching and jaundice (while less common, may occur when hemolysis of RBCs occurs)

Diagnostic Studies

- Hgb level: *less than 11 g/dl in first and third trimesters; less than 10.5 g/dl in second trimester*
- Hct value: *less than 35% in first trimester, less than 30% in second trimester, less than 34% in third trimester*
- Microscopic studies: *identifies specific type of anemia*

Medical Management

Medical management varies with the specific type of anemia. In most cases, oral iron supplements (e.g., ferrous sulfate, 30–60 mg/day) are routinely prescribed to prevent iron deficiency anemia.

Nursing Activities and Rationales

Focus Assessments

- Assess Hgb and Hct. Distinguishes between the normal anemia of pregnancy and disease states to determine appropriate interventions. Normal hemodilutional anemia of pregnancy does not require intervention. Hct is an indirect index of the oxygen-carrying capacity of the blood. The Hct reflects the RBC volume.
- Assess for risk factors (see "Etiologies and Risk Factors"). Facilitates prevention and early intervention.
- Assess for symptoms of anemia (e.g., inspect the skin, the sclera, and mucous membranes). Fatigue occurs because the oxygen-carrying capacity of blood is reduced. Pallor occurs because of reduced amounts of hemoglobin and reduced blood flow to the skin. Jaundice occurs when there is an increased concentration of serum bilirubin, which increases when hemolysis of RBCs occurs. Pruritus occurs because of increased serum and skin bile salt concentrations. The sclera and mucous membranes reflect integumentary changes more accurately than the skin, especially in dark-skinned individuals.
- Assess the adequacy of the woman's diet. Determines if diet teaching is needed.

Preventive Nursing Activities

- Teach about foods high in iron and folic acid. Adequate intake of iron and folic acid may help prevent the two common forms of anemia: dietary iron deficiency anemia and dietary folic acid deficiency.

- Teach the correct way to take iron supplements. Milk and milk products need to be avoided at least an hour before and after taking an iron supplement or eating iron-rich foods. Iron binds with calcium in these products, prohibiting complete absorption of the iron. Taking iron with foods and drinks rich in vitamin C (e.g., orange juice) is encouraged because it enhances the effects of iron.

Potential Complication: DISSEMINATED INTRAVASCULAR COAGULATION

Disseminated intravascular coagulation (DIC) is an acute blood-clotting disorder characterized by low levels of fibrinogen, prothrombin, platelets, and factors V and VIII. DIC is always a secondary diagnosis that occurs as a complication of diseases and conditions that cause an imbalance between the body's clotting and lysing functions. The amount of thrombin released exceeds the ability of the body's naturally occurring antithrombins. Widespread and diffuse clot activity occurs in the microcirculation, and clotting factors and platelets are consumed, resulting in a breakdown in clotting activity and generalized hemorrhage. DIC is an emergency situation and requires immediate recognition and treatment.

Etiologies and Risk Factors

- Abruptio placentae (risk factors include abdominal trauma, smoking, premature rupture of membranes [PROM], chronic hypertension, preeclampsia, and cocaine use)
- Hypertensive disorders (preeclampsia, eclampsia)
- Intrauterine fetal death with prolonged retention of the fetus
- Amniotic fluid embolism
- Septic abortion
- HELLP syndrome (hemolysis, elevated liver enzymes, low platelets)
- Septic shock (associated with pyelonephritis during pregnancy)

Signs and Symptoms

- Spontaneous bleeding (e.g., hematuria, oozing from previous puncture sites)
- Tachycardia and hypotension
- Tachypnea and dyspnea
- Diminished or absent bowel sounds
- Small hemorrhages in skin and mucous membranes (e.g., petechiae, ecchymoses)

Diagnostic Studies

- Partial thromboplastin time or activated prothrombin time: *prolonged more than 60 seconds*
- Prothrombin time: *prolonged more than 15 seconds*

- Platelet count: *usually decreased to less than 100,000 µl fibrinogen (less than 150 mg/dl)*
- Fibrin degradations products: *more than 45 µg/ml*
- D-dimer test: *presence of an asymmetrical carbon compound fragment formed in the presence of fibrin split products; positive at less than 1:8 dilution*
- Positive fibrin monomers: *diminished levels of factors V and VIII, fragmentation of RBCs*
- Hgb: *less than 10 g/dl*
- Urine output: *less than 30 ml/hour*
- Elevated blood urea nitrogen: *greater than 25 mg/dl*
- Elevated serum creatinine: *greater than 1.3 mg/dl*
- Clot retraction test: *blood in a plain test tube should normally clot in 10 minutes or less*

Medical Management

Medical management of DIC requires emergency and intensive care to control bleeding and counteract shock. Treatment of the underlying condition(s) (e.g., delivery of a fetus) is essential in order to correct the coagulation problem. However, this care plan focuses on assessment and prevention of DIC, not on treatment. For potential DIC, management is simply to identify and correct risk factors for DIC and perform tests to diagnose it if clinical symptoms that warrant it develop.

Nursing Activities and Rationales

Focus Assessments

- Assess for risk factors (e.g., hypertensive disorders, abdominal trauma, PROM, intrauterine fetal death). All of these events can trigger the acceleration of clotting, resulting in generalized activation of prothrombin and a consequent excess of thrombin, in a chain of sequences that uses large amounts of coagulation factors. Risk factors are routinely assessed at the first prenatal visit.
- Assess for blood pressure (BP) and pulse alterations and compare to prenatal record. Signs of hemorrhage include decreasing BP, increasing pulse rate, and narrowing of pulse pressure. Early detection may prevent serious progression of the abnormal clotting process.
- Observe for diaphoresis. May indicate blood loss and decreasing BP.
- Observe for signs of unusual bleeding. DIC is diagnosed according to clinical findings and laboratory markers. Clinical findings often suggest the need for laboratory tests. Symptoms result from loss of blood volume, decreased organ and peripheral tissue perfusion, and clots in the microcirculation. Signs of abnormal bleeding include spontaneous bleeding from the gums or nose; petechiae around the BP cuff; excessive bleeding from the episiotomy, intravenous line, or injection sites, or from nicks from shaving the abdomen; hematuria; blood in the stool; hemoptysis; cyanotic, cold, mottled fingers and toes; severe muscle, back, abdominal, and chest pain; confusion; dyspnea; and oliguria.

Preventive Nursing Activities

- Teach the importance of prenatal care. Early antepartal care promotes health during pregnancy by managing preexisting medical conditions and facilitating early detection of complications that place the woman at increased risk for DIC.
- Question the woman about current medications, including over-the-counter preparations. Numerous pharmacologic agents can interfere with clotting (e.g., aspirin, nonsteroidal anti-inflammatory drugs, certain diuretic agents, broad-spectrum antibiotics, estrogens, and antihistamines), although these medications do not cause DIC.

Potential Complication: FETAL COMPROMISE (NONREASSURING FETAL HEART RATE TRACING)

Fetal distress or fetal compromise involves evidence that the fetus is in jeopardy (e.g., a change in intensity or frequency of fetal movement or the presence of nonreassuring fetal heart rate [FHR] patterns). Fetal distress is a result of fetal asphyxia in utero, a condition in which hypoxemia (reduction of Po_2), hypercapnia (increase in partial pressure of carbon dioxide [PCO_2]), and respiratory and metabolic acidosis (reduction of blood pH) occur. Any condition that reduces maternal oxygenation or circulation or that reduces fetal-placental exchange (e.g., hypertonic uterine contractions) can cause fetal asphyxia.

▌ *Etiologies and Risk Factors*

- Umbilical cord compression
- Prolapsed cord
- Fetal head compression
- Maternal fever
- Hypertonic uterine contractions (UCs)
- Maternal dehydration
- Uteroplacental insufficiency
- Maternal hypotension or hypertension
- Maternal medication (narcotics)
- Disease states (diabetes mellitus, anemia, cardiac disease, hyperthyroidism, hypertension)
- Abruptio placenta
- Placenta previa

▌ *Signs and Symptoms*

- Persistent nonreassuring FHR patterns
- Tachycardia
- Bradycardia
- Late decelerations
- Decreased or absent variability
- Variable decelerations decreasing to less than 70 beats per minute for longer than 60 seconds
- Fetal scalp pH less than 7.19
- Decrease in or absence of fetal movement once quickening has occurred
- Abrupt, large increase in fetal movement in excess of that generally felt from normal fetus

▌ *Diagnostic Studies*

- Antepartum fetal monitoring (nonstress, contraction stress test). (Refer to the topic, "Antepartum Fetal Monitoring and Other Diagnostic Tests," beginning on p. 60 in Chapter 4.)
- Intrapartum electronic fetal monitoring: *More reliable in identifying the well-oxygenated fetus than the compromised one.*
- Intrapartum fetal scalp stimulation: *Tactile scalp stimulation to evaluate fetal response; FHR acceleration of 15 beats/min for 15 seconds indicates adequate oxygenation and normal acid-base balance; half of infants who do not produce accelerations are in acidosis via scalp blood pH analysis while the other half are in normal acid-base balance (Mattson & Smith, 2010).*
- Vibroacoustic stimulation: *Reassuring response is the same as for fetal scalp stimulation.*
- Fetal scalp blood pH analysis: *Normal scalp pH is greater than or equal to 7.25.*
- Cord blood pH and gases: *Provides information about the fetal acid-base balance and the immediate condition of the newborn after birth.*
- Internal fetal monitoring: *Provides greater accuracy especially with regard to variability, if nonreassuring patterns develop.*

▌ *Medical Management*

Medical management depends on the severity of fetal compromise. Immediate delivery, usually by cesarean birth, is indicated for severe, nonreassuring patterns.

▌ *Nursing Activities and Rationales*

Focus Assessments

- Assess for risk factors for fetal compromise. Identifies those women who have risk factors that may contribute to fetal compromise (see "Etiologies and Risk Factors"). Women with risk factors require more frequent assessment so that preventive measures can be taken and nonreassuring patterns recognized early. Any factor that compromises maternal oxygenation or circulation also affects fetal oxygenation or circulation.
- Assess fetal monitor tracing every 15 minutes throughout the first stage and every 5 minutes throughout the second stage of labor, during and following procedures or activities. Labor, procedures, medications, maternal position, and activities may alter fetal oxygenation, heart rate patterns, and blood flow through the umbilical cord. Careful monitoring allows for early recognition of fetal compromise.
- Assess for nonreassuring patterns (loss of variability, accelerations, decelerations). Nonreassuring patterns may indicate the presence of acid-base imbalance, hypoxia, head

compression, or cord compression. Severe, nonreassuring patterns may indicate the need for immediate delivery in order to save the fetus.

- Assess FHR. Baseline rates less than 100 or greater than 160 beats/min may indicate fetal compromise.
- Assess frequency and duration of uterine contractions. Placental exchange can be compromised when intrauterine pressure exceeds 20 mmHg or contractions are separated by less than 60 seconds, last longer than 90 seconds, or occur more frequently than every 2 minutes.
- Assess maternal vital signs. Identifies fever, hypertension, hypotension, or other factors that increase the risk for fetal compromise.

Preventive Nursing Activities

- Position the woman on her left side avoiding the supine position. Eliminates aortocaval compression, which may compromise placental blood flow by decreasing maternal venous return to the heart and, consequently, cardiac output.
- Maintain oral and/or IV fluid intake. Maternal dehydration and hypovolemia are risk factors for fetal compromise. Maintaining fluid intake increases maternal blood volume and BP, which increases placental perfusion.
- Reposition the woman if cord compression is suspected. Turning the woman from side to side or elevating her hips moves the fetus toward her diaphragm and may help relieve pressure on the cord.
- If fetal distress occurs, discontinue oxytocin if it is being administered. Oxytocin increases the force and duration of uterine contractions, which may result in greater cord compression, fetal head compression, or decreased placental perfusion.
- If fetal distress occurs, administer 100% oxygen. Increases oxygen available to both the woman and the fetus by increasing maternal blood oxygen saturation.
- Teach the woman the need for and benefit of fetal monitoring throughout the labor process. Knowledge alleviates anxiety; anxiety can contribute to fetal compromise.
- Teach the woman how to monitor fetal activity. Decreased or absence of fetal activity once quickening has occurred (at about 20 weeks' gestation) signals fetal distress.

Potential Complication: HEMORRHAGE

Vaginal bleeding may occur any time during pregnancy, but approximately 50% of bleeding during the third trimester is due to placenta previa and abruptio placentae, both of which can result in hemorrhage. Intrapartal hemorrhage can be caused by uterine rupture. Postpartum hemorrhage is most often the result of uterine atony but may also be caused by retained placental fragments, lacerations of the birth canal, uterine inversion, and DIC.

This care plan addresses the care of a woman who is at risk for hemorrhage, regardless of the etiology. Goals and interventions for detecting and preventing hemorrhage caused by specific conditions (e.g., uterine rupture, postpartum hemorrhage) will be found under those topics later in the text.

▋ Etiologies and Risk Factors

- Antepartum hemorrhage: placenta previa, abruptio placentae, ectopic pregnancy
- Intrapartum hemorrhage: uterine atony, uterine rupture, lacerations of the birth canal, DIC
- Postpartum hemorrhage: uterine atony, retained placental fragments, lacerations of the birth canal, DIC

▋ Signs and Symptoms

- Antepartum: Vaginal bleeding or spotting. Suspect placenta previa or placental abruptio whenever there is vaginal bleeding after 20 weeks' gestation. Classically, abdominal pain occurs with abruptio but not with previa; however, this may vary.
- Postpartum: Loss of more than 500 ml blood after vaginal birth or more than 1,000 ml after cesarean birth, or a 10% decrease in Hct between admission for labor and postpartum.
- Decreased blood pressure (BP), increased pulse and respirations, restlessness, thirst, pallor, clammy skin, persistent late decelerations.

▋ Diagnostic Studies

Antepartum

- Speculum exam: Rules out local causes of bleeding; performed if ultrasound reveals a normally implanted placenta; preferably done only after 34 weeks' gestation.
- Transabdominal ultrasound examination: Determines if placenta is attached normally and location of placenta. Ultrasonography can verify placenta previa but cannot always verify abruption. Retroplacental clots may or may not been see with ultrasound.

Other

- Complete blood cell count (CBC): decreased hemoglobin and hematocrit (Hct), possible elevated white blood cell (WBC) count.
- Clotting studies (platelet count, prothrombin time, partial thromboplastin time, fibrinogen, fibrin split products, D-dimer): Rules out clotting abnormality and establishes a baseline for later comparisons.

▋ Medical Management

If hemorrhage occurs, medical management varies with the condition, but in all cases, it will include:

- Intravenous fluid replacement. *Supports blood pressure by expanding intravascular volume.*
- Administration of blood products: Blood, fresh, frozen plasma ,or cryoprecipitate.
- Oxygen therapy.
- Immediate birth may be indicated if hemorrhage is severe and infant is viable.
- Prophylactic antibiotics. *Prevents infection.*

Nursing Activities and Rationales

Focus Assessments

- Assess for visible vaginal bleeding, and count or weigh vaginal pads. Estimates amount of blood loss. One gram of pad weight is equal to 1 ml of blood loss. Excessive blood loss can result in antepartum and postpartum anemia and infection, as well as maternal or fetal death.
- Monitor heart rate, blood pressure, and pulse pressure. Provides information about severity of blood loss and adequacy of fluid replacement. Tachycardia and decreased BP are late signs of blood loss/shock. Narrowing of pulse pressure is a sign of early blood loss. Preexisting hypertension may mask hypotension that occurs with fluid deficit.
- Monitor respirations. Tachypnea is a late sign of blood loss/ shock, but may also be a symptom of pain.
- Assess capillary refill and skin and mucous membrane color. Slow capillary refill and cyanosis are late signs of blood loss. When blood volume decreases, peripheral vasoconstriction shunts blood away from the periphery to the vital organs.
- Monitor CBC (especially Hgb and Hct). Reflects amount and cause of blood loss and adequacy of replacement. Hct greater than 30% is needed for adequate oxygenation.
- Monitor for bleeding from IV site or gums, and for petechiae and hematuria. Indicates coagulation deficiency (e.g., DIC).
- Assess level of consciousness. Reflects decreased circulation of oxygen to the brain, which causes central nervous system irritability.

Preventive Nursing Activities

- Teach the symptoms of hemorrhage and when to call the care provider or go to the hospital. Helps to ensure that the woman will contact the care provider or hospital for timely intervention.
- Provide IV fluid replacement per protocol. IV fluids replace circulating volume lost via bleeding and help to maintain BP and therefore tissue perfusion (e.g., to vital organs) until blood replacement products are available and transfused.
- Type and cross-match per protocol and/or ascertain availability of compatible blood for transfusion. Facilitates rapid delivery and infusion of correct blood product if replacement is needed.

Potential Complication: INFECTION

Acute and chronic diseases, environmental factors, and maturational dynamics all produce conditions favorable for infection. The incidence of infection of the reproductive tract during the postpartum period varies from 1% to 8%. Infection can occur anywhere in the body, but during the antepartum and postpartum periods, the focus is primarily on reproductive tract and urinary tract infections (UTIs).

Etiologies and Risk Factors

During pregnancy and birth, a woman's susceptibility to infection can increase for a variety of reasons, including the following:

- Postpartum period (e.g., inadequate primary defenses such as broken skin, traumatized tissue, stasis of body fluids, change in pH of secretions, postpartum hemorrhage)
- Perineal wound (e.g., episiotomy or laceration)
- Rupture of amniotic membranes
- Intrauterine fetal monitoring
- Lack of normal flora
- Chronic conditions (e.g., diabetes mellitus, anemia)
- Poor nutrition
- Immunosuppression
- History of infections (e.g., urinary tract, mastitis, pneumonia)
- Cesarean delivery
- Prolonged labor
- Retained placental fragments
- Poor personal hygiene habits (e.g., wiping from back to front)

Signs and Symptoms

- Fever and/or chills
- Generalized malaise and anorexia
- Abdominal tenderness or pain
- Abnormally large uterus
- Foul-smelling lochia drainage
- Tender, reddened, and hard breast
- Urinary frequency and/or burning

Diagnostic Studies

- WBC count: *Differentiates between infection and inflammation. A WBC count greater than 18,000/mm³ during the intrapartum or postpartum period indicates infection. The WBC count normally increases during labor and may stay elevated during the first few postpartum days in the absence of infection, but it will return to normal by 7 days postpartum.*
- Cultures (urine, vaginal, blood): *Identifies the presence and type of pathogenic organisms.*
- Urinalysis: *Determines the presence of blood (hematuria), WBCs, casts, and bacteria. Turbid, foul-smelling urine indicates infection.*

Medical Management

Treatment of infections is based on the type, location, and extent of infection. Antibiotic therapy may be initiated after culture and sensitivity studies are completed. Intravenous fluids may be administered if the woman becomes dehydrated from fever. Analgesics may be prescribed for pain management.

Focus Assessments

- Identify factors that place the woman at risk for infection. Recognition of risk factors enhances development of individualized nursing care directed at prevention of complications (e.g., infection).
- Monitor vital signs, especially temperature and pulse. Temperature elevation and chills are often the first signs of endometritis and other reproductive tract infections including mastitis. Tachycardia also is a common sign associated with increased body temperature and metabolic rate.
- Monitor lochia for color and odor (postpartum). Heavy bleeding can predispose the postpartum woman to pelvic infection. Foul-smelling lochia is a sign of infection caused by decomposition of dead bacteria and cells.
- Teach the woman to assess her breasts frequently for signs of mastitis (postpartum). The lactating breast can become infected via fissured or cracked nipples. Detection of early signs and symptoms (e.g., soreness, redness) can help prevent full-blown infection or more serious complications. Mastitis rarely develops during the immediate postpartum period; it usually develops in women who are at least 2 weeks postpartum, at which point women are home and need to know how to assess their own breasts (see "Nursing Care Plan: Postpartum Infection" in Chapter 10).
- Assess for signs and symptoms of UTI. The urinary tract is a common site of infection in women, and even more so during pregnancy and the postpartum period. Because the urinary meatus and anus are in close proximity, Escherichia coli from the rectum can easily spread to the urethra. Other risk factors are increased during the antepartum period, as well. For example, increased progesterone levels cause relaxation of smooth muscles of the kidneys and ureters, leading to urinary stasis.

Preventive Nursing Activities

- Teach proper hand washing, perineal care, and personal hygiene. Prevents introduction of pathogens into the body; prevents transfer of *E. coli* from the anus to the urethral meatus.
- Educate the woman and significant others about signs and symptoms to report (e.g., nausea; vomiting; abdominal distention; burning on urination; painful, reddened breast). Early reporting and subsequent treatment can prevent more severe complications such as peritonitis and septicemia, which can be life threatening.

- Instruct women who breastfeed on correct techniques, breast hygiene, and relief of engorgement. Incorrect breastfeeding can result in fissures; cracked nipples; breast engorgement; and stasis of milk, blood, and lymph, all predisposing factors to infection because they provide a portal of entry for pathogens or cause tissue damage or irritation.
- Teach the woman to void frequently and to avoid carbonated beverages. Frequent emptying of the bladder prevents urinary stasis and subsequent infection. Carbonated drinks alter urinary pH, making it more alkaline, which favors bacterial growth.

▮ Potential Complication: PREMATURE RUPTURE OF MEMBRANES

Premature rupture of membranes (PROM) refers to the rupture of the amniotic sac and loss of amniotic fluid at any time prior to the onset of true labor. Preterm premature rupture of the membranes refers to the rupture of membranes prior to week 37 of gestation. Preterm labor (PTL) and birth are commonly associated with PROM, and the fetus is endangered because of risk for infection and/or premature birth. Also see care plan for Premature Rupture of Membranes in Chapter 6 for further information about this condition.

Etiologies and Risk Factors

- Chorioamnionitis (infection of the membranes that may be subclinical)
- Incompetent cervix
- Weak amniotic sac structure
- Fetal malpresentation
- Fetal abnormality
- Hydramnios
- Vaginal or cervical infection

Signs and Symptoms

- Sudden loss of fluid from the vagina
- Continued leakage of fluid from the vagina

Diagnostic Studies

- Nitrazine paper test: Amniotic fluid is alkaline and causes the paper to turn blue.
- Ferning: Amniotic fluid shows a ferning pattern when placed on a glass slide and examined microscopically.
- Cultures: Detect the presence of infections such as gonorrhea, Chlamydia, or β-Streptococcus.
- Sonogram: Assesses amniotic fluid index.
- WBC count: WBCs greater than $18,000/mm^3$ suggest the presence of infection.

▌ Medical Management

If PROM actually occurs, if the fetus is too young to survive outside the uterus, and PROM does not stimulate labor, the woman is placed on complete bed rest and monitored for indications of infection. If the fetus can survive, labor is usually induced to prevent infection; however, this care plan focuses only on detection and prevention of PROM in women who are at risk for it.

▌ Nursing Interventions and Rationales

Focus Assessments

- Assess for risk factors associated with PROM (see "Etiologies and Risk Factors"). Facilitates early recognition and intervention to minimize the risk to the mother and the fetus from complications.
- Assess for excessive discharge of clear fluid from the vagina. Detects possible rupture of membranes. Amniotic fluid is clear and can be confused with urinary incontinence.
- Assess for vaginal pooling of fluid. Amniotic fluid appears similar to urine but pools in the vagina after membranes have ruptured.
- Test fluid discharge with Nitrazine paper. Differentiates urinary incontinence from PROM.
- Monitor WBC count daily. A WBC count greater than 18,000/mm³ suggests the presence of infection.

Preventive Nursing Activities

- Teach the woman to notify the healthcare provider immediately if symptoms of vaginitis occur. Some forms of vaginitis predispose the woman to PROM.
- Teach the importance of monitoring for and reporting signs of PROM (see "Signs and Symptoms"). Monitoring and reporting do not prevent PROM, but they help to prevent complications should PROM occur. Because PROM represents a threat to both the mother and the fetus, it is important that the woman recognize its occurrence and notify her healthcare provider immediately. The longer the time between PROM and birth of the baby, the higher the risk for fetal and maternal infection.

▌ Potential Complication: PRETERM LABOR

Preterm labor (PTL) is the occurrence of regular UCs accompanied by cervical effacement and dilation between 20 and 37 weeks' gestation. PTL occurs in approximately 9–11% of pregnancies. If UCs and cervical changes are identified early, it is often possible to arrest preterm labor and prevent the birth of a premature infant. Also see the care plan for Preterm Labor and Spontaneous Abortion in Chapter 6 for further information about this topic.

▌ Etiologies and Risk Factors

- History of PTL
- Uterine abnormalities
- Multiple gestation
- Chorioamnionitis
- Polyhydramnios
- PROM
- Placenta previa or abruptio placenta
- Hypertension
- Fetal abnormality
- Malnutrition
- Dehydration
- UTI
- Smoking
- Alcohol or other drug use
- Age older than 40 years
- Age younger than 16 years

▌ Signs and Symptoms

- Uterine contractions
- Complaints of low back pain and/or pelvic pressure
- Cervical changes
- Fetal engagement
- Tachycardia
- Increased vaginal discharge
- Heaviness or aching in the thighs
- Feeling of the baby balling up
- Abdominal pain similar to menstrual cramps
- Diarrhea

▌ Diagnostic Studies

- Fetal fibronectin: Presence of fetal fibronectin in vaginal secretions prior to membrane rupture may indicate impending PTL; test is positive when levels are greater than 0.05 mcg/ml and indicates that birth is likely within 7 to 14 days; conversely, if fetal fibronectin is not present, there is a 98% chance the woman will not go into PTL.
- CBC: Detects the presence of infection, which may be a contributing factor to PTL. A WBC count greater than 18,000 indicates the presence of infection.
- Urinalysis: Detects the presence of WBCs, RBCs, bacteria, and nitrites, which indicate UTI.
- Uterine ultrasound examination: Establishes gestational age, placental location, fetal or uterine abnormalities, presence of multiple gestations, and fetal position.
- Amniotic fluid: Determines lecithin–sphingomyelin ratio to assess fetal lung maturity and provides information about fetal chances for survival or respiratory complications if birth occurs. Amniotic fluid may be cultured to determine if subclinical chorioamnionitis is a cause of PTL. A lecithin–sphingomyelin ratio of 2:1 indicates fetal lung maturity.

Medical Management

- Hospitalization as needed. Allows for frequent assessment and careful monitoring to detect changes and prevent birth if possible.
- Administration of tocolytic drugs. Magnesium sulfate halts labor by decreasing acetylcholine levels, which block neuromuscular transmission; terbutaline (Brethine) inhibits labor by stimulating β-2 adrenergic receptors in uterine smooth muscle; nifedipine (Procardia) inhibits UCs by blocking calcium channels.
- Intravenous fluids. Support circulation, prevent fluid volume deficit, and provide intravenous route for drug therapy.
- Steroid administration. Decreases the risk for respiratory distress syndrome, necrotizing enterocolitis, and intravascular hemorrhage in the neonate.

Nursing Interventions and Rationales

Focus Assessments

- Assess for risk factors associated with PTL (see "Etiologies and Risk Factors"). Allows early recognition and intervention so that labor can be halted, when possible, to allow fetal maturation and to avoid complications that may compromise the mother or fetus.
- Project expected date of birth. Estimates fetal age and viability, factors considered when determining treatment plan.
- Assess quality and timing of UCs. A pattern of contractions lasting more than an hour and occurring as often as every 10 minutes for at least 30 seconds may indicate PTL when accompanied by cervical changes. Preterm UCs without cervical change do not indicate PTL.
- Assess for cervical changes. Effacement, dilation, softening or shortening of the cervix indicates the presence of labor and impending birth. If cervical change occurs in the presence of UCs, it is unlikely that labor can be stopped.
- Assess for abdominal cramping and pain, or lower back pain. These are sometimes associated with PTL.
- Assess for excessive discharge of clear fluid from the vagina. May indicate PROM. Amniotic fluid is clear and can be confused with urinary incontinence. PROM is a common complication of PTL.
- Assess FHR (e.g., nonstress test, contraction stress test). Tachycardia, bradycardia, and decelerations may indicate the presence of fetal distress. Fetal status is a factor in deciding whether to continue the pregnancy.
- Assess maternal vital signs. Elevated temperature and tachycardia may indicate the presence of infection or dehydration, both of which may be contributing factors to PTL.

Preventive Nursing Activities

- Maintain bed rest with the woman in the lateral position and teach the importance of same. Activity may stimulate UCs. The lateral position maximizes uterine blood flow and prevents the fetus from placing pressure on the cervix, which may hasten delivery.

- Teach the importance of drinking adequate fluids and eating a nutritious diet. Poor nutrition and dehydration are risk factors for PTL. Uterine irritability and contractions can occur from dehydration.
- Teach the woman how to palpate for and time uterine contractions. Allows the woman to make an accurate determination of her labor and the need for intervention if she is being cared for at home.
- If risk factors exist or PTL is suspected, advise against intercourse, nipple stimulation, and any activity that produces orgasm. Orgasm involves rhythmic contractions of the uterus. Nipple stimulation and prostaglandins in semen can stimulate UCs even if orgasm does not occur.

Potential Complication: HYPERTENSIVE DISORDERS

Hypertensive disorders (also known as pregnancy-related hypertension and pregnancy-induced hypertension) includes the medical diagnoses of gestational hypertension, preeclampsia (mild and severe), and eclampsia. Women with hypertensive disorders may have mild elevations of BP or severe hypertension with various organ dysfunctions. Eclampsia is defined as preeclampsia with the development of seizures. Also see the care plan on Gestational Hypertension in Chapter 6 for further information on hypertensive disorders.

Etiologies and Risk Factors

- Age older than 40 years or younger than 18 years
- Family history
- Diabetes mellitus
- Multiple gestation
- Chronic hypertension
- Obesity

Signs and Symptoms

Mild Preeclampsia

- BP greater than 140/90 mmHg
- Persistent 1+ to 2+ proteinuria on dipstick

Severe Preeclampsia

- Diastolic BP greater than or equal to 110 mmHg and systolic BP greater than or equal to 160 mmHg on at least two occasions
- Proteinuria greater than or equal to 5 grams of protein in 24 hours
- Oliguria (urine output less than 500 ml in 24 hours)
- Visual disturbances (e.g., blurred vision, spots before eyes)
- Epigastric pain, nausea, and/or vomiting
- Pulmonary edema, dyspnea, moist breath sounds on auscultation, and/or cyanosis

- Elevated liver enzymes
- Thrombocytopenia

Eclampsia

- Signs and symptoms of preeclampsia
- Seizures
- Coma
- Organ dysfunction

Diagnostic Studies

- Urinalysis: Determines presence of proteinuria. 1+ or 2+ protein or more than 300 mg/liter in a 24-hour specimen; for severe preeclampsia, greater than 5 g of protein in a 24-hour specimen.
- Hct: May be reduced because of hemodilution.
- Serial BP readings: BP greater than 140/90 mmHg for mild eclampsia and 160/110 mmHg for severe preeclampsia.

Medical Management

Medical management of gestational hypertensive disorders depends on the severity of the symptoms, gestational age, and the woman's compliance with the medical regimen.

- IV magnesium sulfate. Reduces the risk for seizures.
- Oxytocin. Induces labor when hypertension is severe.
- Activity restriction. In gestations of less than 36 weeks, activity restrictions are often imposed to control symptoms and allow time for the fetus to mature.
- Antihypertensive medications. Reduce and control blood pressure.
- Steroid administration. May be given if delivery seems likely and the woman is at less than 34 weeks' gestation.
- Birth of the infant by induction if cervix is favorable or cesarean if not, if fetus has mature lung profile.

Nursing Interventions and Rationales

Focus Assessments

- Assess for the following: BP, urine protein, decreased urine output, weight gain, facial and/or peripheral edema, changes in neurologic status (e.g., headaches, blurred vision, hyperactive knee jerk, irritability, tinnitus), decreased respirations, lung sounds (for pulmonary edema), and epigastric or right upper quadrant abdominal pain (liver involvement). Early indicators of disease progression and the possible need for increased bed rest and other restrictions. Many of the clinical manifestations of gestational hypertension are a result of vasospasm of the arterioles, e.g., reduced glomerular filtration rate results in protein loss in the urine and reduced urinary output, and sodium and water retention, which in turn contributes to generalized edema.
- Check the availability of resources to help support the high-risk woman in the home environment. Women may have to maintain bed rest at home for several weeks before delivery, which may be taxing on their financial resources. Those lacking in financial and other support systems may need referrals to appropriate community resources.

Preventive Nursing Activities

- Teach the importance of eating a well-balanced diet. Nutritional deficiencies, especially protein and calcium, may contribute to the development of gestational hypertension. However, it has not been proven that a poor diet causes preeclampsia or that dietary changes treat or prevent preeclampsia. A high-protein diet does help replace protein lost in the urine.
- Teach the importance of regular prenatal visits. Helps ensure that patterns that suggest preeclampsia will be detected.
- Teach the need for maintaining prescribed rest and activity levels. Adequate rest increases renal and placental blood flow, which helps reduce BP and edema, and allows the fetus to mature to full gestation if possible.

Potential Complication: URINARY TRACT INFECTION

Urinary tract infection (UTI) refers to symptomatic infections such as cystitis or pyelonephritis as well as asymptomatic bacteriuria (urine containing bacteria). Bacteria can enter the urinary tract from the bloodstream or from the lower urinary tract. *Escherichia coli* is the most common cause of UTIs, which result from introducing the bacteria via contaminated catheters or from ascending infection. UTIs can be serious enough to cause renal damage. UTIs are more common in female patients because of the short length of the urethra. UTIs are especially common during pregnancy, when the urinary structures (renal calices, pelvis, and ureters) begin to dilate at the same time that peristalsis of the ureters decreases. These changes are related to progesterone-like hormones and obstruction from the growing uterus. The result is urinary stasis, which provides an environment conducive for bacterial proliferation. As the uterus continues to enlarge, the bladder becomes displaced, placing it at further risk for infection. Also see care plan for Urinary Tract Infection in Chapter 6 for further information.

Etiologies and Risk Factors

- Pregnancy
- Use of diaphragm and spermicide
- Diabetes mellitus
- Renal abnormalities
- Poor hygiene

Signs and Symptoms

Lower Urinary Tract Infection (Cystitis)

- Tenderness over urinary bladder
- Burning or pain on urination (dysuria)

- Urinary urgency and frequency
- Blood in the urine (hematuria)
- Malaise

Upper Urinary Tract Infection (Pyelonephritis)

- Chills
- Fever
- Unilateral or bilateral flank pain
- Malaise
- Nausea and vomiting
- Appearance of being sick

Diagnostic Studies

- Urinalysis: Presence of more than 100,000 organisms per 1 ml urine indicates microbial overgrowth (infection).
- Urine culture and sensitivity: Identifies causative organism and appropriate antimicrobial agent.
- CT and renal scans: Rules out contributing factors when infections are severe and/or recurrent.
- Urine leukocyte count: Greater than 10 leukocytes/μ indicates injury rather than infection.

Medical Management

Medical management is based on the type of infection and causative organism. Most infections are successfully treated with antimicrobial agents and increased fluid intake.

- Antiseptics. Prohibit microbial growth.
- Analgesics. Reduce pain.

The following care plan, however, focuses on detection and prevention of potential UTIs.

- Cranberry or blueberry juice. May help prevent UTIs in susceptible women because they prevent bacteria from adhering to the bladder wall and change the pH of the urine, producing a hostile environment for bacterial growth.
- Antibiotics. After two documented episodes of pyelonephritis, women are placed on antibiotics for the remainder of their pregnancies to prevent future episodes. Some providers initiate suppressive therapy after only one occurrence of pyelonephritis. Nitrofurantoin (Macrodantin) is the drug most often used for suppressive therapy.

Nursing Interventions and Rationales

Focus Assessments

- Assess for risk factors. Identifies women who are at increased risk for development of UTI so that preventive measures, such as increased fluid intake, can be implemented.
- Assess vital signs. Establishes baseline in women at increased risk for UTIs and identifies signs of UTI (e.g., fever, tachycardia).
- Perform urinalysis. Distinguishes between normal urine and that resulting from injury and infection. Increased bacterial counts support the presence of UTI, whereas increased leukocyte counts support the presence of inflammation or injury.
- Assess for signs/symptoms of UTI. Bladder tenderness, urinary frequency and urgency, and dysuria occur from bacterial irritation of the bladder lining and urethra. Fever, chills, and malaise result from the immune response to infection.

Preventive Nursing Activities

- Encourage increased fluid intake. Fluids flush bacteria out of the urinary system and help prevent ascending infections. Increasing fluid intake is often effective in preventing infections.
- Encourage intake of cranberry or blueberry juice. These juices prevent bacterial adhesion to bladder walls and may reduce the incidence of UTIs. They do not kill bacteria, but produce a hostile environment, reducing bacterial growth.
- Teach the woman to urinate after sexual intercourse. Sexual intercourse may transfer E. coli from the anal area into the urethra and force bacteria colonized at the urethra back up into the bladder. Urinating flushes bacteria out of the bladder and urethra.
- Teach the woman signs and symptoms of UTIs and emphasize the need to report such infections early. Helps ensure early treatment to prevent renal damage and chronic urinary tract infection.
- Teach the importance of finishing the entire course of medication and taking it exactly as prescribed. Prevents drug-resistant strains of bacteria from developing and reduces recurrence of infection.

END NOTES

1. Nursing Diagnoses—Definitions and Classification 2009–2011. Copyright © 2009, 2007, 2005, 2003, 2001, 1998, 1996, 1994 by NANDA International. Used by arrangement with Blackwell Publishing Limited, a company of John Wiley & Sons, Inc. In order to make safe and effective judgments using NANDA-I nursing diagnoses it is essential that nurses refer to the definitions and defining characteristics of the diagnoses listed in this work.
2. Bulechek, G. M., Butcher, H. K., Dochterman, J. M. (2008). *Nursing Interventions Classification* (5th ed). St. Louis, MO: Elsevier, by permission.

REFERENCES

Mattson, S., & Smith, J. E. (2010). *Core curriculum for maternal-newborn nursing* (4th ed.). St. Louis, MO: Saunders/Elsevier.

RESOURCES

Bond, S. (2009). Identifying babies in trouble based on fetal heart rate tracings still a conundrum. *Journal of Midwifery & Women's Health, 2*(54), 159–160.

Centers for Disease Control and Prevention. (2009). *Maternal and infant health research: Preterm birth.* Department of Health and Human

Services. Retrieved from http://www.cdc.gov/reproductivehealth/MaternalInfantHealth/PBP.htm

Chauhan, S. P., Klauser, C. K., Woodring, T. C., Sanderson, M., Magann, E. F., & Morrison, J. C. (2008). Intrapartum nonreassuring fetal heart rate tracing and prediction of adverse outcomes: Interobserver variability. *American Journal of Obstetrics & Gynecology, 6*(199), 623.e1–623.e5.

Dickinson, F., & Soltani, H. (2008). Nitrazine yellow and pre-labour rupture of membranes. *Practising Midwife, 11*(5), 48–52.

Haydon, M. L., Gorenberg, D. M., Nageotte, M. P., Ghamsary, M., Rumney, P. J., Patillo, P., & Garite, T. J. (2006). The effect of maternal oxygen administration on fetal pulse oximetry during labor in fetuses with nonreassuring fetal heart rate patterns. *American Journal of Obstetrics & Gynecology, 3*(195), 735–738.

Lowdermilk, D. L., & Perry, S. E (2007). *Maternity nursing* (7th ed.). St. Louis, MO: Mosby.

McKinney, E. S., James, S. R., Murray, S. S., & Ashwill, J. (2008). *Maternal-child nursing* (3rd ed.). Philadelphia, PA: Saunders.

Pagana, K. D., & Pagana, P. J. (2009). *Diagnostic and laboratory test reference* (9th ed.). St. Louis, MO: Mosby/Elsevier.

Pillitteri, A. (2010). *Maternal & child health nursing* (6th ed.). Philadelphia, PA: Lippincott Williams & Wilkins.

Ross, M. G., & Eden, R. D. (2009). *Preterm labor*. Retrieved from http://emedicine.medscape.com/article/260998-overview

Simpson, K. R. (2008). Intrauterine resuscitation during labor: Should maternal oxygen administration be a first-line measure? *Seminars in Fetal & Neonatal Medicine, 6*(13), 362–367.

ANTEPARTUM CARE

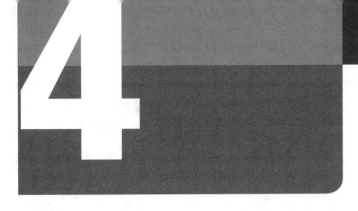

NORMAL PREGNANCY

Jeanne Linhart

NORMAL ANTEPARTUM: FIRST TRIMESTER

The first trimester of pregnancy is one of many physical and emotional maternal changes. Teaching is an important nursing role in caring for normal antepartum women. The core of nursing interventions is essentially the same for all normal antepartum women because it consists of risk assessment, monitoring, prevention, and health promotion activities. Beyond this standardized care, the nurse individualizes care as unique patient needs arise.

Key Nursing Activities

- Screen for risk factors; monitor for complications of pregnancy.
- Encourage healthy behaviors (e.g., nutrition, exercise, rest).
- Continually assess maternal and fetal well-being.
- Treat or teach self-care treatment for minor discomforts of pregnancy.
- Teach signs and symptoms that should be reported to the healthcare provider.

Etiologies and Risk Factors

Maternal physiologic changes in the first trimester are largely in response to the hormones of pregnancy: progesterone, estrogen, human chorionic gonadotropin, and human placental lactogen. These changes are directly linked to most of the common discomforts of pregnancy. There are no etiologies because pregnancy is a normal physiologic event rather than an illness. The idea of risk factors is not appropriate, either, except in the case of high-risk pregnancy.

Signs and Symptoms

The signs and symptoms of pregnancy are categorized as subjective *presumptive* (those changes felt by the woman), *probable* (those changes observed by an examiner but which could be caused by a condition other than pregnancy), and *positive* (those signs that can be attributed only to the presence of the fetus).

Presumptive Signs (Subjective)

- Amenorrhea
- Breast changes: fullness, tingling, heaviness, sensitivity, pigmentation of nipples and areolae
- Fatigue
- Nausea and vomiting
- Urinary frequency
- Quickening (at 16–20 weeks)

Probable Signs (Objective)

- Goodell's sign—Softening of the cervical tip at about week 6
- Chadwick's sign—Bluish coloration of the cervix
- Hegar's sign—Softening and compressibility of the lower uterine segment at about 6 weeks' gestation
- Positive pregnancy test (serum or urine)
- Braxton Hicks contractions (after 16 weeks)
- Ballottement (at 16–28 weeks)

Positive Signs (Objective)

- Fetal movements visible or palpated by examiner
- Fetal heart tones detected by ultrasound or stethoscope
- Visualization of fetus by ultrasound or X-ray

Diagnostic Studies

- The laboratory tests used to confirm/diagnose pregnancy are based on the biologic marker human chorionic gonadotropin. They may be performed on serum or urine; both provide accurate results. Most urine tests require a first-voided morning urine specimen. A wide variety of tests exists; some can be performed at home, while others must be performed in a laboratory.
- Ultrasonography: *Detects presence of fetus, at about 5–6 weeks' gestation.*
- Nuchal translucency: *Performed between 11 and 14 weeks' gestation in women suspected to be at high risk for fetus with Down syndrome or cardiac defects.*

Medical Management

During the first and second trimesters, monthly visits to the care provider are routinely scheduled. Visits are more frequent during the third trimester. In a normal, uncomplicated pregnancy, no medical treatment is necessary. Medical management includes the following:
- Confirming the pregnancy.
- Estimating the date of birth.
- Laboratory tests to detect complications.
- Counseling and treating common discomforts of pregnancy (e.g., constipation, nausea).
- Ongoing monitoring of fetal growth and well-being (e.g., fetal heart rate monitoring, ultrasonography).
- Ongoing monitoring of maternal nutrition and well-being.

- Medications routinely prescribed:
  - ▶ For all women: 30 mg per day of supplemental iron (more if iron deficiency anemia is present).
  - ▶ Prenatal vitamins and a folic acid supplement are prescribed frequently, but not routinely for all pregnant women.

▌ *Collaborative Problems*

The potential complications of pregnancy include all the conditions in Chapters 5 and 6. Examples of other potential complications of pregnancy are hypertensive disorders, premature rupture of membranes, preterm labor, urinary tract infection, abruptio placenta, placenta previa, intrauterine growth retardation, and fetal demise.

COLLABORATIVE (STANDARDIZED) CARE FOR ALL NORMAL FIRST TRIMESTER ANTEPARTUM WOMEN

Perform a comprehensive assessment to identify individual needs for teaching, emotional support, and physical care.

▌ Potential Complication of Pregnancy: GESTATIONAL DIABETES

Refer to topic, "Diabetes Mellitus in Pregnancy," beginning on p. 101 in Chapter 5.

Focus Assessments

- Assess for risk factors, e.g., obesity, chronic hypertension, older than 25 years, gestational diabetes in previous pregnancy, family history of diabetes, previous birth of an infant weighing > 4,000 g, previous unexplained fetal demise. Women with one or more of these risk factors should be screened for gestational diabetes at the first prenatal visit. The 50 g glucose challenge test does not require fasting and need not follow a meal. If blood glucose is ≥ 140 mg/dl, a 3-hour oral glucose tolerance test is performed (Norwitz, Arulkumaran, Symonds, & Fowlie, 2007).

▌ Potential Complications of Pregnancy: PRETERM LABOR, LATE ANTEPARTAL BLEEDING, GESTATIONAL HYPERTENSION, VAGINAL INFECTION AND

TORCH, AND SEXUALLY TRANSMITTED INFECTIONS

Use the care plans in Chapters 5 and 6 to plan care for each of these specific complications. The nursing role, in general, is to:

- Perform a comprehensive prenatal assessment, including a high-risk profile and review of immunization record. Assists with prevention, early recognition, and control of problems and improves maternal condition and fetal outcome.
- Monitor for the signs and symptoms of potential complications. Allows prompt treatment and increases the likelihood of a positive outcome for the pregnancy.
- Teach the woman the signs and symptoms of potential complications. Increases the likelihood of early detection, since the pregnant woman is not hospitalized and routinely sees the healthcare provider only once a month.
- Stress the importance of continuing with prenatal visits. For early detection of complications. Some women may not realize the importance of regular visits to the care provider when they are feeling well and have no problems.
- Provide information about any preventive measures the woman should take (e.g., avoiding caffeine, alcohol, and smoking). Decreases as much as possible the likelihood of complications from factors that are within the woman's control. Not all complications can be prevented.

▌ Nursing Diagnosis: DEFICIENT KNOWLEDGE (PREGNANCY-RELATED CHANGES)[1]

Also refer to generic NDCP, "Deficient Knowledge,[1]" which begins on p. 13 in Chapter 2.

Related Factors: first pregnancy, misinformation (old wives' tales), lack of interest in learning, ambivalence about the pregnancy, unfamiliarity with information resources, cognitive limitations.

▌ *Goals, Outcomes, and Evaluation Criteria*

- Woman differentiates between normal discomforts of pregnancy and signs/symptoms that must be reported to care provider.
- Woman verbalizes understanding of physiologic changes of pregnancy.
- Woman reports using appropriate self-care behaviors to alleviate normal discomforts of pregnancy.

▌ *NIC Interventions*[2]

Learning Facilitation (5520)—Promoting the ability to process and comprehend information.
Prenatal Care (6960)—Monitoring and management of patient during pregnancy to prevent complications of pregnancy and promote a healthy outcome for both mother and infant.

Teaching: Individual (5606)—Planning, implementation, and evaluation of a teaching program designed to address a patient's individual needs.

▌ *Nursing Activities and Rationales*

Assessments and Rationales

- Assess knowledge of physiologic and psychologic changes of pregnancy and beliefs about activities and self-care. Determines teaching needs.
- Inquire about information the woman has obtained from family and friends. Corrects misinformation, if necessary, and reinforces correct information.
- Assess current health promotion behaviors (e.g., diet, exercise, rest). Determines if changes should be made during pregnancy.
- Assess cultural beliefs, perceptions, prescriptions, and proscriptions about pregnancy and childbearing. Prescriptions and proscriptions influence the woman's and partner's emotional responses, dietary practices, activity and rest, and sexual activity. The nurse may need to help the woman to adapt cultural practices to support a healthy regimen during pregnancy.

Independent Nursing Actions

- Insofar as possible, allow cultural prescriptions and proscriptions that the woman believes will achieve a healthy pregnancy if they are not harmful to the pregnancy. For potentially harmful practices, tactfully provide education and propose modifications. For example, in some cultures women believe that witnessing an eclipse of the moon may cause the infant to have a cleft palate. Allowing the woman to do so is not harmful to the woman or pregnancy. Some cultures, however, believe that dental work should not be done because it will cause the baby to have a cleft lip. If the mother needs dental work, the nurse should try to educate her and modify this practice.

Patient/Family Teaching

- Teach the normal physiologic and psychologic changes of pregnancy. Provides a basis for understanding body changes, thereby promoting self-esteem and self-care. Provides motivation for healthy behaviors.
- Discuss fetal development. Helps the woman to visualize what her baby looks like at any given time; promotes maternal–fetal attachment; makes clear the importance of prenatal visits and other measures to support the pregnancy and avoid exposure to teratogens.
- Present information on normal pregnancy sequentially; reinforce earlier teaching; allow time for questions. Allows time for woman to internalize and synthesize information.
- Identify signs/symptoms that may signal complications and that should be reported to the care provider. Most common during first trimester are severe vomiting (hyperemesis gravidarum), chills and fever (infection), burning on urination (urinary tract infection), diarrhea (infection), abdominal cramping (miscarriage, ectopic pregnancy), and vaginal bleeding (miscarriage, ectopic pregnancy). Ensures that complications are promptly identified and treated. The woman may not seek assistance if she mistakes dangerous symptoms for the normal discomforts of pregnancy.
- At subsequent visits, educate regarding danger signals for complications that more commonly occur in second and third trimesters. The woman is likely to be overwhelmed with the amount of new information and will probably not recall information that is presented too far in advance.
- Educate for self-care (e.g., hygiene, nutrition). See "Nursing Diagnosis: Health-Seeking Behaviors,"[1] later.
- Teach self-care measures for the common discomforts of pregnancy. (See Table 4-1. Also see generic NDCPs "Constipation,[1]" "Activity Intolerance,[1]" and "Fatigue,[1]" beginning on pp. 11, 9, and 14, respectively, in this chapter and in Chapter 2.) Most of these symptoms do not require medical treatment. The ability to use effective self-care measures enhances the woman's self-esteem, promotes independence, and reduces anxiety.

▌ Nursing Diagnosis: HEALTH-SEEKING BEHAVIORS[1]

Related Factors: no related factors exist for Health-Seeking Behaviors[1] because this is a wellness diagnosis.

▌ *Goals, Outcomes, and Evaluation Criteria*

- Woman keeps prenatal appointments.
- Woman voices understanding of importance of maintaining optimal health.
- Woman voices understanding of effect of maternal health on the fetus.
- Woman maintains healthy behaviors (e.g., obtains adequate rest, exercises moderately, eats a healthy diet, avoids tobacco and alcohol).
- Woman avoids teratogenic agents (X-rays, sexually transmitted infections, environmental toxins in home or work environment, use of alcohol, nicotine, or other drugs).

▌ *NIC Interventions[2]*

Health Education (5510)—Developing and providing instruction and learning experiences to facilitate voluntary adaptation of behavior conducive to health in individuals, families, groups, or communities.

Prenatal Care (6960)—Monitoring and management of patient during pregnancy to prevent complications of pregnancy and promote a healthy outcome for mother and infant.

Teaching: Individual (5606)—Planning, implementation, and evaluation of a teaching program designed to address a patient's particular needs.

TABLE 4-1 Self-Care Measures for Common Discomforts, First Trimester

Discomfort	Self-care measures
Pain, tingling, tenderness, heaviness in breasts	Wear supportive maternity bra day and night, with pads to absorb discharge. Wash with warm water; keep dry. Breast tenderness is temporary. Avoid excessive nipple manipulation. *Supports enlarging breast tissues.*
Frequency and urgency of urination	Perform Kegel exercises. Empty bladder regularly. Limit fluid intake before bedtime. Wear perineal pad. Avoid caffeine. *Prevents incontinence and nocturia. Caffeine is a diuretic and can increase urinary frequency and urgency even more.*
Tiredness, fatigue	Rest as much as possible. Eat well-balanced diet to prevent anemia. *Anemia contributes to fatigue by decreasing oxygen-carrying capacity of the blood.*
Morning sickness (may occur any time during the day)	Eat dry carbohydrate (e.g., cracker) on awakening and remain in bed until feeling subsides. Alternate dry carbohydrate hourly with fluids (e.g., hot decaffeinated tea or clear coffee, milk) or eat 5 or 6 small meals per day. *Reduces gastric acidity and subsequent stomach discomfort.* Avoid fried, greasy, spicy, odorous, or gas-forming foods. Avoid highly aromatic foods. Do not eat and drink at the same time; take fluids between meals. If possible, have someone else cook. *Decreases nausea and vomiting.*
Excessive salivation	Use mouthwash, chew gum, eat hard candy. *Encourages swallowing of saliva.* Reduce starch intake. *Helps prevent salivation.*
Gingivitis, bleeding, and tenderness of gums	Eat well-balanced diet with adequate protein and fresh fruits and vegetables; brush teeth gently; observe good dental hygiene. Have regular dental checks if not already doing so. *Maintains the integrity of the gingiva and the blood vessels.*
Nasal stuffiness; epistaxis (nosebleed)	Use humidifier or normal saline nose drops or spray. *May increase comfort; nasal congestion is caused by increased estrogen levels and is normal in pregnancy.*
Leukorrhea	Not preventable. Do not douche. Wear perineal pads. Wipe front to back. Contact care provider if pruritus or foul odor occur. Bathe and perform perineal care frequently; do not use talcum powder. *Promotes cleanliness and comfort.*
Mood swings, mixed feelings	Communicate concerns to partner and other support persons. Request referral to support group, if needed. *Ambivalence about the pregnancy is normal during first trimester; some women may need additional support at this time, however.*

▌ *Nursing Activities and Rationales*

Assessments

- Assess level of knowledge regarding health-promoting behaviors in pregnancy. To determine learning needs; woman must have information about health promotion in order to engage in healthy behaviors.
- Monitor nutritional status and weight gain. Indicates progression of the pregnancy, adequacy of nutrition, and absence of complications. Failure to gain sufficient weight is associated with catabolism of maternal tissues and inability to provide for fetal growth. Insufficient weight gain may indicate inadequate nutrition and risk for intrauterine growth retardation (IUGR); excessive gain may indicate the need for diet teaching. (Refer to NDCP, "Risk for Imbalanced Nutrition: Less Than Body Requirements,[1]" in this section, beginning on p. 44.)
- Inquire about exposure to teratogens (e.g., X-rays, sexually transmitted infections, environmental toxins in home or work environment, use of alcohol, nicotine/smoking, or other drugs). Identifies the need for further evaluation and intervention.

- Monitor vital signs. Indicate overall maternal well-being and adaptations associated with pregnancy.
- Monitor fetal heart tones (FHTs). FHTs can be detected as early as 12 weeks' gestation with a Doppler ultrasound device; rate and pattern indicate fetal health status.
- Monitor for complications of pregnancy. (See generic collaborative care plans in Chapter 3 and generic NDCPs in Chapter 2.)
- Assess activity tolerance, work and family responsibilities, and presence of fatigue. To identify any problems with sleep and rest. (See generic NDCPs, "Activity Intolerance[1]" and "Fatigue[1]," which begin on pp. 9 and 14, respectively, in Chapter 2.)
- Inquire about cultural beliefs that may affect prenatal care. The systematic, routine prenatal visits prevalent in the Western biomedical model of care are unfamiliar and even strange to some groups (e.g., for many groups, it is appropriate to see a physician only when ill; pregnancy is considered a normal process, so seeing a physician is considered inappropriate). Even if a woman is familiar with the prenatal care, it may conflict with some of her cultural beliefs and practices.

Patient/Family Teaching

- Instruct about environmental teratogens and their possible effects on the fetus; explore measures for avoiding the harmful environment. The first trimester is a time of organogenesis and is the most vulnerable time for potential damage to the fetus by teratogens. It may be difficult for the woman to avoid teratogens if they are present in her home or work environment.
- Discuss the potential effects on the fetus of certain infections such as TORCH (toxoplasmosis, other, rubella, cytomegalovirus, herpes simplex virus) and HIV. (See "TORCH and Sexually Transmitted Infections," beginning on p. 186 in Chapter 6.)
- Advise to practice safer sex; teach correct use of condoms, if appropriate. Condoms help to prevent STIs, especially HIV. (Refer to "TORCH and Sexually Transmitted Infections," in Chapter 6.)
- Teach harmful effects of alcohol and drug use on fetus, including over-the-counter medications and herbal remedies. These lifestyle choices have damaging effects on the developing fetus.
- Stress the importance of not smoking, if woman uses nicotine/tobacco products. Smoking even as few as 10 cigarettes per day decreases placental circulation and contributes to low birth weight, premature birth, and low Apgar scores at birth. Smoking is also associated with increased risk of abruptio placentae, placenta previa, and fetal death.
- Advise to limit caffeine to < 300 mg per day (about 500–750 ml of coffee). Caffeine causes vasoconstriction of uterine blood vessels and may interfere with cell division in the developing fetus. Consuming > 300 mg per day increases the risk of miscarriage and IUGR.
- Stress the need for good hygiene (e.g., good hand washing, front-to-back perineal care, and voiding after intercourse). Removes and prevents transfer of pathogenic organisms.
- Stress the need to wash hands after contact with cats and advise to not change cat litter boxes. Advise woman to wear gloves while gardening, and advise to cook meat thoroughly. Minimizes the risk for acquiring Toxoplasma gondii and/or Listeria monocytogenes.
- Discuss schedule of office visits during pregnancy. Visits are typically once a month for the first 7 months, every 2 weeks during the 8th month, and every week thereafter until delivery. The woman needs to be aware of visits needed for adequate prenatal care.
- Discuss prenatal testing and the scheduling of testing. The woman will be aware of upcoming tests and her role in preparing for those tests. The importance of timing some tests at specific periods of gestation is also important.
- Advise getting adequate sleep and rest. Offer ideas such as napping at home while preschoolers are sleeping or scheduling rest periods during breaks at work. Adequate rest is necessary in order to meet the metabolic needs created by the growth of maternal and fetal tissues. Although symptoms of fatigue cannot be prevented, they can be minimized if the woman obtains 8 hours of uninterrupted sleep per day, plus one nap. She may need to assign priorities and decrease some outside commitments in order to obtain needed rest.
- Advise frequent bladder emptying (approximately every 2 hours while awake). Fluid intake should never be decreased to prevent urinary frequency. It is important to review safety factors in the home, such as clearing a path to the bathroom and the use of a nightlight since the woman may make several trips to the bathroom at night.
- Remind the woman to avoid food/fluids containing caffeine, to drink warm milk, or eat a light snack at bedtime. Caffeine is a central nervous system stimulant. L-tryptophan in milk may have a sedative effect. Eating a snack may prevent early awakening due to hunger.
- Provide oral and written information on dietary requirements; advise against weight-reduction diets. Sufficient calories and nutrients are needed to achieve fetal growth and development. (See NDCP, "Risk for Imbalanced Nutrition: Less Than Body Requirements,[1]" in this section, beginning on p. 44.)
- Discuss recommendations for activity and exercise; encourage moderate exercise (e.g., swimming, bicycling, pelvic lifting or rocking, modified sit-ups, tailored sitting, and Kegel exercises). Consider cultural norms for physical activity. Such exercises improve muscle tone in preparation for labor and birth, tend to shorten labor, and decrease the need for oxytocin induction. Conversely, strenuous exercise can decrease blood flow to the uterus by 70% and contribute to IUGR and fetal hyperthermia. Many cultural groups encourage pregnant women to be active; however, others believe that any activity is dangerous. This behavior should not be interpreted as laziness or noncompliance.
- Advise that restrictions on activity or travel are generally necessary. In a normal pregnancy, activities do not need to be avoided unless they cause undue fatigue or risk to the fetus. Most airlines, however, require permission from the healthcare provider for the woman to travel by plane during the 9th month of pregnancy.
- Teach measures for preventing constipation. See generic NDCP, "Constipation,[1]" beginning on p. 11 in Chapter 2. Elevated progesterone level relaxes smooth muscle in the gastrointestinal tract, reducing peristalsis and increasing the absorption of water. Oral iron supplements also contribute to constipation.

Collaborative Activities

- Develop positive rapport with the patient. Promotes emotional comfort and security, enhancing open communication.

- Refer to smoking cessation and/or drug dependency treatment program, if needed. Nicotine is a habit-forming drug. Much support is usually needed in order to stop smoking. The same is true for other habituating or addictive drugs.

Nursing Diagnosis: RISK FOR IMBALANCED NUTRITION: LESS THAN BODY REQUIREMENTS[1]

Related Factors: nausea, fatigue, concerns about body appearance (fear of becoming fat), lack of knowledge or misinformation about dietary requirements in pregnancy.

Goals, Outcomes, and Evaluation Criteria

- Woman gains weight appropriate to age and pregnancy trimester.
- Woman consumes a nutritionally adequate diet for body weight, age, and physical activity (prescribed amounts of calories, protein, fats, carbohydrates, vitamins, and minerals).
- Woman maintains normal Hgb (> 11 g/dl) and Hct (> 33%).
- Woman takes prenatal vitamin and iron supplements as prescribed.

NIC Interventions[2]

Nutritional Counseling (4246)—Use of an interactive process focusing on the need for diet modification.
Nutritional Monitoring (1160)—Collection and analysis of patient data to prevent or minimize malnourishment.
Weight Management (1260)—Facilitating maintenance of optimal body weight and percent body fat.

Nursing Activities and Rationales

Assessments

- Assess diet history and current intake. Determines the need for changes in present diet to meet the additional metabolic demands of pregnancy.
- Evaluate current weight, prepregnancy weight, and ideal weight for height (body mass index). Ideal gain for the normal-weight adult woman is 25–35 lb during the pregnancy; women with a low body mass index should gain more than women who have a high body mass index or who are obese. Normal weight gain reduces the risk of low-birth-weight infants. For a normal pregnant woman, only 1–2.5-kg gain is expected during the first trimester.
- Evaluate calorie intake, considering age, prepregnant weight, physical activity level, and the additional calories needed during pregnancy. A normal adult woman does not need to add calories during the first trimester. She should add about 300 kcal/day during the second and third trimesters. A satisfactory weight gain should indicate sufficient caloric intake.

- Monitor the woman's weight. Fluctuations, particularly weight loss, may indicate poor nutritional habits. During the first trimester, growth occurs primarily in maternal tissues.
- Monitor Hgb and Hct. Hgb of < 11 or Hct < 37% (in the first trimester) may indicate iron deficiency anemia in pregnant women. Hgb is essential for normal oxygen-carrying capacity of the blood.
- Monitor urine for acetone, albumin, and glucose. Detects potential complications such as inadequate ingestion of carbohydrates and weight loss. When sufficient calories are not consumed, the body metabolizes fatty tissue for energy, leading to the presence of ketones in the urine.
- Assess the woman's ability to meet her nutritional needs. Financial and cultural issues may interfere with adequate nutrition.
- Assess food preparation techniques. Some cooking methods cause loss of nutrients (e.g., vitamins are lost when vegetables are cooked in a large amount of water; microwaving destroys more folic acid than conventional methods). In addition, undercooking of meats and eggs increases the risk of bacterial and parasitic infections.
- Assess cultural proscriptions and taboos that may affect pregnancy. Such beliefs may conflict with nutritional information given by Western healthcare providers. For example, some groups do not believe in eating meat; this means that the diet may need to be modified in order to obtain adequate amounts of protein. The nurse needs this information in order to be able to offer alternative foods to meet dietary needs.
- Assess for presence of pica. Eating nonfood substances can decrease the woman's appetite for nutritious foods (e.g., eating laundry starch contributes to developing iron deficiency anemia).

Independent Nursing Actions

- Help the woman plan a diet that includes a wide variety of foods, especially fresh foods. Pregnant women have increased metabolic needs for many nutrients, particularly iron and folic acid. Stressing variety is a more positive approach than condemning junk food and is more likely to encourage compliance with a diet containing necessary nutrients. Processed foods contain large amounts of sodium and should be avoided by women with hypertension or peripheral swelling.
- When planning diet with a woman, consider lifestyle influences and food preferences (e.g., for fast food). Increases the likelihood of compliance with the suggested diet.

Patient/Family Teaching

- Provide information about foods needed for appropriate weight gain and nutritional adequacy. Corrects any misconceptions; provides information needed for the woman to manage her own dietary intake. Average daily diet should include 6–11 servings of grain products; 3–5 servings of vegetables; 2–4 servings of fruit; 3 or more servings of milk and milk products; and up to 6 oz (2–3 servings) total of meat, poultry, fish, dry beans, nuts, and eggs.

- Provide information about foods containing protein and the importance of protein to maternal and fetal development. Protein is essential for fetal brain development. Insufficient protein intake, especially during first trimester, is a risk factor for IUGR and may contribute to preeclampsia.
- Instruct about the risks of dieting while pregnant. Inadequate intake may cause insufficient weight gain. Inadequate weight gain indicates a risk for fetal IUGR and maternal complications such as preeclampsia. Weight loss places mother and fetus at risk for acidosis. When calorie intake is not sufficient for energy and growth requirements, body fat is metabolized; ketones are an acidic by-product of lipid metabolism. Adequate calories are also necessary to prevent the body from metabolizing proteins for energy and help ensure adequate iron intake.
- Explain the importance of taking iron supplements (30–60 mg/day of elemental iron) if prescribed. There is an increased need for iron during pregnancy to meet the demands of the enlarging maternal muscle mass and blood volume. It is almost impossible for a woman to ingest enough dietary iron. However, demand for iron is minimal in the first trimester, so a supplement is not usually needed then unless the woman had a nutritional deficit before pregnancy.
- Explain the need for a vitamin and mineral supplement, as needed. Folic acid is essential to fetal development; a supplement of 0.4 mg of folate is often prescribed, as are calcium, zinc, and a multivitamin. Folic acid deficiency contributes to fetal malformation (e.g., neural tube defect), miscarriage, possible placental abruption, and megaloblastic anemia. It is possible to obtain adequate folic acid with a good diet since many U.S.-prepared foods (e.g., cereals) are fortified with folic acid; however, it is frequently prescribed because the effects of a deficiency are so profound. Most organogenesis occurs during the first trimester, so folic acid supplementation must be begun early if it is needed.
- Assess intake of foods that contain zinc. Women who are vegetarian are at increased risk for zinc deficiency, which can result in intrauterine growth restriction, or pre- and post-term labor. They should be advised to increase their intake of root vegetables, leafy vegetables, nuts, and whole grains. The intake of dairy products prevents zinc deficiency in women who use these products.
- Recommend daily intake of 6–8 glasses (1,500–2,000 ml) of fluid, including water, milk, and fruit juices. Fluid is essential for exchange of nutrients and waste products across cell membranes; water is the main substance in amniotic fluid. It aids in maintaining body temperature and preventing constipation and urinary tract infections. Dehydration increases the risk of uterine contractions and preterm labor.
- Also refer to generic NDCP, "Deficient Knowledge," beginning on p. 13 in Chapter 2.

Collaborative Activities

- Refer the woman to Women, Infants, and Children program, Aid to Families with Dependent Children, and/ or state and local food bank or food stamp programs, as appropriate. These programs provide nutrition services for women who qualify. WIC provides vouchers for selected foods for pregnant and lactating women at nutritional risk (e.g., eggs, cheese, milk, juice, and fortified cereals).

INDIVIDUALIZED (NURSING DIAGNOSIS) CARE PLANS

These care plans address unique needs.

Nursing Diagnosis: FATIGUE/ ACTIVITY INTOLERANCE[1]

Use with generic NDCPs, "Activity Intolerance[1]" and "Fatigue,[1]" beginning on pp. 9 and 14, respectively, in Chapter 2.

Related Factors: hormonal and other physiologic changes of pregnancy, increased energy requirements for growth of maternal and fetal tissues; inadequate sleep and rest related to common discomforts of pregnancy (e.g., nocturia, nausea), sedentary lifestyle.

Goals, Outcomes, and Evaluation Criteria

- Woman identifies ways to conserve energy.
- Woman voices feeling of being rested.
- Woman verbalizes understanding of importance of frequent rest periods during pregnancy.
- Woman performs activities of daily living, such as housework, shopping, and preparing meals, without undue fatigue or changes in pulse rate.

Nursing Activities and Rationales

Assessments

- Assess woman's employment requirements and responsibilities (e.g., child care, cleaning) at home. Prolonged standing, heavy lifting, etc. can cause overexertion. Pregnant women need to elevate their feet every 1–2 hours and have frequent rest periods during strenuous work.
- Monitor Hgb level. Detects anemia; fatigue is a symptom of anemia due to decreased oxygen-carrying capacity.

Nursing Actions

- Encourage patient to get 8–10 hours of sleep daily including naps; suggest self-care methods for achieving adequate sleep. Pregnant women require additional sleep/rest due to increased metabolic needs and higher levels of progesterone. (See NDCP, "Health-Seeking Behaviors,[1]" which begins on p. 41 in this chapter.)
- Suggest to significant others that they perform some of the woman's household duties temporarily or suggest to the woman and family that standards for housekeeping, cooking, and so forth, be relaxed during the pregnancy. Fatigue

usually decreases by the second trimester, so the woman may be able to resume her normal role activities then. If the suggestion to relax standards comes from the care provider, the woman is less likely to feel anxious or guilty about what she may perceive as not fulfilling her responsibilities.

Nursing Diagnosis: SEXUAL DYSFUNCTION AND/OR INEFFECTIVE SEXUAL PATTERN[1]

Related Factors: fatigue, breast tenderness, fear of fetal injury or miscarriage, misinformation.

Goals, Outcomes, and Evaluation Criteria

- The couple verbalizes satisfaction with sexual arousal and expression.
- The couple expresses comfort with modifications in sexual expression.

NIC Intervention[2]

Sexual Counseling (5248)—Use of an interactive helping process focusing on the need to make adjustments in sexual practice or to enhance coping with a sexual event/disorder.

Nursing Activities and Rationales

Assessments

- Assess for leukorrhea. Although copious vaginal secretions are normal in pregnancy, their presence may inhibit sexual interest.
- Assess the nature of the couple's relationship. Predicts the couple's ability to cope with alterations in sexuality during the pregnancy. If the relationship has been good, they will likely cope well.
- Assess the couple's level of knowledge about sexuality in general. Misconceptions about sexuality may be compounded by misconceptions about pregnancy. The nurse may need to correct general misinformation before teaching about changes related to pregnancy.
- Identify the concerns of both partners. Facilitates planning of individualized care to meet individual needs.
- Use a broad opening statement to begin assessing sexual activity (e.g., "Many women say they seem to lose interest in sex when they are pregnant."). Broad statements allow the nurse to introduce the subject in a way that allows the woman to discuss it further or let it drop if she is uncomfortable or does not perceive a problem.
- Assess cultural norms and proscriptions for sexual activity. In most cultures, sexual activity is prohibited only near the end of pregnancy; some even prescribe it to keep the birth canal lubricated. However, some cultures require abstinence

throughout pregnancy because intercourse is thought to harm the mother and fetus.

Patient/Family Teaching

- Provide information to clarify misconceptions. Facilitates retention of new information; relieves unrealistic anxieties.
- For leukorrhea, advise washing with mild soap and water; douching is prohibited. To remove excessive secretions. Douching is associated with ascending genital tract infection and air embolism.
- Advise that intercourse need not be restricted unless risk factors (e.g., ruptured membranes, bleeding and spotting, abdominal cramping) develop. Sexual intercourse is not associated with fetal injury in an uncomplicated pregnancy.
- Explain the effect of physiologic changes of pregnancy on sexual desire and expression (e.g., the woman may have diminished desire because of fatigue, nausea, and breast tenderness). Physiologic changes and perceptions about pregnancy may alter responsiveness and spontaneity. This may be difficult for the male partner to understand and may be anxiety producing for the woman. The couple may be relieved to know that these changes are temporary and that sexual desire is often increased during the second trimester.
- Show the couple pictures of variations of coital position. May increase comfort for the woman. For example, some women experience significant breast tenderness in the first trimester, so a position that avoids direct pressure on her breasts could be recommended.
- Suggest alternative methods of sexual expression (e.g., mutual or solitary masturbation) that are acceptable to the couple. Provide reassurance that the methods are healthy. The couple may need reassurance that alternative methods are normal and acceptable. They may feel they need permission to experiment.

Independent Nursing Actions

- Establish a therapeutic relationship. For many people, sexuality is a sensitive topic. A trusting relationship is essential to facilitate the open communication needed to provide assistance.
- Provide privacy; ensure confidentiality; talk to the partners separately, if they prefer, but include both partners as much as possible in order to encourage them to communicate with each other. The partners may be self-conscious about discussing the topic in the presence of others or even with each other. Privacy may be necessary in order to obtain open communication.
- Offer to answer any questions the couple has about sexual functioning. They may be embarrassed to ask questions, even if they are experiencing sexual problems.

Collaborative Activities

- Refer for counseling if sexual problems arise and/or continue. Resolution of sexual issues is important in achieving a positive self-concept. Sex therapy may be needed for couples who have a long-standing sexual dysfunction. When the sexual dysfunction is a symptom of a serious relationship problem, family therapy may be indicated.

Nursing Diagnosis: INTERRUPTED FAMILY PROCESSES[1]

Related Factors: changing roles and responsibilities, inadequate understanding of physical and emotional changes in pregnancy, physical discomforts of pregnancy (e.g., fatigue), ambivalence and labile emotions, changes in the couple's relationship.

Goals, Outcomes, and Evaluation Criteria

- Woman and/or partner express confidence in their ability to manage family problems.
- Woman and/or partner express confidence in their ability to manage and adapt to the physical changes of pregnancy.
- Woman and/or partner communicate effectively.
- Woman and/or partner express feelings and emotions freely.
- Woman and/or partner provide support for each other.
- Woman and/or partner adapt to the developmental transitions of pregnancy.
- Woman and/or partner seek support from extended family and community as needed.
- Woman and/or partner express commitment and loyalty to the family.

NIC Interventions[2]

Family Integrity Promotion (7100)—Promotion of family cohesion and unity.

Family Integrity Promotion: Childbearing Family (7104)— Facilitation of the growth of individuals or families who are adding an infant to the family unit.

Family Process Maintenance (7130)—Minimization of family process disruption effects.

Family Support (7140)—Promotion of family values, interests, and goals.

Nursing Activities and Rationales

Assessments

- Evaluate the woman's relationship with her partner (e.g., observe their interactions if he accompanies her on prenatal visits). Determines his availability and capacity for emotional support; to determine his need for emotional support.
- Assess the woman's (couple's) feelings about the pregnancy. It is normal to feel ambivalent toward the pregnancy because of the changes it will bring to the family (e.g., finances, interruption of professional goals, changes in family roles). However, if these feelings persist, counseling may be needed.

- Identify the couple's (woman's) perceptions of the stressors that pregnancy and childbirth will place on the family. Identifies possible needs for intervention. Pregnancy creates disequilibrium in a family, resulting in the need for members to adapt to new roles and responsibilities.
- Determine how the family has coped with stressors in the past. Evaluates the family's ability to deal positively with the stress of pregnancy and birth. Resources for adapting to stress include family and social support systems, cultural and spiritual beliefs, adequate resources (e.g., time and money), and effective coping mechanisms.
- Assess adequacy of financial resources. In a family with financial problems, pregnancy creates additional stress. If the family does not have insurance, they may not seek prenatal care.
- Assess the availability and involvement of grandparents and other family members. Both the woman and her partner experience family stressors. They may not be able to provide enough support for each other without help from interested family members.
- Assess sibling responses to changes in the family. Even though children may not express negative feelings openly, they may feel insecure about a change in their relationship with their parent(s).
- Explore cultural beliefs about childbearing and parenting. Enables the nurse to provide culturally sensitive care, promote attainment of the maternal role, and enhance the relationship between the woman and her partner.

Independent Nursing Actions

- Reinforce positive coping mechanisms and suggest new ones to replace ineffective coping mechanisms. People tend to use the same coping mechanisms as they have used in the past. They might require help in order to change.
- Encourage the couple to attend childbirth preparation classes. Provide a source of information, peer support, and sharing of problems.
- Encourage grandparents to attend childbirth classes and to participate in the birth, as woman desires. Helps them to feel a part of the pregnancy and birth; promotes their involvement and support.
- Suggest that the partner and baby's siblings come to prenatal visits; have them listen to the fetal heart tones. Makes them perceive the baby as a reality for them and helps them feel involved.

Patient/Family Teaching

- Explain that it is normal to feel ambivalent about pregnancy at first and to be concerned about the ability to manage conflicting role demands. Provides reassurance, relieves anxiety, and increases self-confidence.
- Explain that it is normal for a pregnant woman to experience mood swings. Helps partner to recognize the need to be patient and supportive.

Collaborative Activities

- If financial resources are inadequate, make referrals to community agencies for assistance. Helps ensure that adequate prenatal care is received and that the family can meet basic needs. Woman may be unaware of resources available in her community.
- Refer for psychologic counseling if couple does not achieve acceptance of the pregnancy by the end of the first trimester. The couple may need assistance to work through their ambivalence and accept the pregnancy. They may need help in developing coping and problem-solving skills.

■ *Other Nursing Diagnoses*

Also assess for the following nursing diagnoses, which are frequently present with this condition:

- **Ineffective Role Performance**[1] related to change in family and work roles, fatigue and other discomforts of pregnancy, lack of knowledge, inadequate support system, unrealistic expectations, and/or low self-esteem
- **Constipation**[1] related to decreased peristalsis secondary to effects of progesterone on smooth muscle
- **Risk for Disturbed Body Image**[1] related to sociocultural beliefs and/or lack of preparation for and understanding of body changes
- **Risk for Situational Low Self-Esteem**[1] related to social role changes, unrealistic expectations, and disturbed body image

NORMAL ANTEPARTUM: SECOND TRIMESTER

The second trimester of pregnancy is usually a time of fewer discomforts. Morning sickness and frequent urination subside. The woman begins to show her pregnancy, and the woman experiences quickening. The normal ambivalence about the pregnancy is replaced with commitment to the pregnancy and a growing awareness of the child as a separate being, distinct from herself, and as a person to nurture.

■ *Key Nursing Activities*

- Encourage healthy behaviors (e.g., nutrition, exercise, rest).
- Continue to assess maternal and fetal well-being.
- Treat or teach self-care treatments for minor discomforts of pregnancy.
- Screen for risk factors for complications of pregnancy.
- Teach and reinforce signs and symptoms of complications to report to the healthcare provider.

■ *Etiologies*

In the second trimester, the fetus has completely developed and is growing rapidly. The woman's abdomen enlarges visibly. There are no etiologies because pregnancy is a normal physiologic event, not an illness.

■ *Signs and Symptoms*

Refer to "Normal Antepartum: First Trimester," which begins on p. 39, for a list of presumptive, probable, and positive signs of pregnancy. Some signs and symptoms do not occur until the second trimester.

■ *Diagnostic Studies*

- The tests to diagnose pregnancy are usually performed during the first trimester.
- Tests performed in the second trimester (e.g., sonogram, fetal heart monitoring, amniocentesis) are primarily done to monitor fetal well-being and to detect maternal complications, diabetes mellitus, and hypertensive disorders.
- Maternal serum alpha-fetoprotein level—*screens for neural tube defects (e.g., spina bifida and anencephaly). If alpha-fetoprotein level is abnormal, amniocentesis may be performed to confirm a neural tube defect.*

■ *Medical Management*

During the second trimester, monthly visits to the care provider continue. No medical interventions are needed in a normal, uncomplicated pregnancy. Medical management includes the following:

- Screen for gestational diabetes and hypertensive disorders.
- Continue monitoring of fetal growth and well-being (fundal height and activity, FHR monitoring, ultrasonography).
- Continue monitoring maternal nutrition and well-being (e.g., weight).
- Supplemental iron (30 mg per day) for all women beginning in the second trimester (higher dosage if iron deficiency anemia occurs).
- Prenatal vitamins and a folic acid supplement are frequently prescribed.

■ *Collaborative Problems*

The potential complications of pregnancy include all the conditions in Chapters 5 and 6. Some, such as hypertensive disorders and gestational diabetes, are more likely to occur after the first trimester. Cardiac decompensation, too, is more likely to occur later in pregnancy; however, this is not a complication of a normal pregnancy, but a complication of a high-risk pregnancy.

COLLABORATIVE (STANDARDIZED) CARE FOR ALL NORMAL SECOND TRIMESTER ANTEPARTUM WOMEN

Perform comprehensive assessment to identify individual needs for teaching, emotional support, and physical care.

Potential Complication of Pregnancy: GESTATIONAL DIABETES

Refer to "Diabetes Mellitus in Pregnancy," beginning on p. 101 in Chapter 5.

Focus Assessments

- Perform a glucose challenge test for all women except those at low risk. The most recent practice recommendations are to screen all women for gestational diabetes mellitus through either history and clinical risk factors or testing of blood glucose levels unless the woman is low risk. Low-risk women must meet all of these criteria: not a member of a racial or ethnic group with a high incidence of diabetes (e.g., Hispanic, African, Native American, South Asian, East Asian, Pacific Islander), normal weight prior to pregnancy, no history of abnormal glucose tolerance, no history of poor obstetric outcomes associated with gestational diabetes mellitus, and no known diabetes in first-degree relatives. Screening is usually done between 24 and 28 weeks' gestation. The 50-g glucose challenge test does not require fasting and need not follow a meal. If blood glucose is 140 mg/dl or greater, a 3-hour oral glucose tolerance test is performed (U.S. Preventive Services Task Force, 2008).
- If risk factor assessment was not done previously, assess for risk factors (obesity, chronic hypertension, older than 25 years, gestational diabetes in previous pregnancy, family history of diabetes, previous birth of an infant weighing > 4,000 g, previous unexplained fetal death). Although some risk factors should have been identified at the first prenatal visit, obesity may not develop until the second trimester. Also, some women do not make their first prenatal visit until the second trimester.

Potential Complication of Pregnancy: HYPERTENSIVE DISORDERS

Refer to generic collaborative care plan, "Potential Complication: Hypertensive Disorders," beginning on p. 32 in Chapter 3, and "Hypertensive Disorders of Pregnancy," which begins on p. 170 in Chapter 6.

Potential Complication of Pregnancy: MULTIPLE GESTATION

Refer to "Multifetal Pregnancy," beginning on p. 164 in Chapter 6.

Potential Complication of Pregnancy: URINARY TRACT INFECTION

Refer to generic collaborative care plan, "Potential Complication: Urinary Tract Infection," beginning on p. 33, in Chapter 3, and "Urinary Tract Infections," beginning on p. 195 in Chapter 6.

Nursing Diagnosis: DEFICIENT KNOWLEDGE (PREGNANCY-RELATED CHANGES AND DISCOMFORTS)[1]

Use with generic NDCP, "Deficient Knowledge,[1]" beginning on p. 13 in Chapter 2. Also refer to the NDCP, "Deficient Knowledge (Pregnancy-Related Changes),[1]" in the topic, "Normal Antepartum: First Trimester," beginning on p. 40, in this chapter.

▌ *Nursing Activities and Rationales*

Assessments

- Inquire about any discomforts that have developed since the first trimester. Discomforts during the first trimester are primarily due to hormone changes. Progesterone levels remain elevated throughout pregnancy, and discomforts related to the relatively high estrogen levels in the first trimester resolve in the second trimester. New discomforts may occur, however, especially toward the end of the second trimester.

Patient/Family Teaching

- Reinforce teaching done in the first trimester. Aids in retention of information. Corrects any possible misunderstandings.
- Reinforce the importance of contacting the care provider should signs and symptoms of complications occur. Ensures that complications are promptly identified and treated. Signs/symptoms especially relevant to second and third trimesters include:
  - Persistent, severe vomiting (hyperemesis gravidarum, hypertension, preeclampsia)
  - Sudden discharge of fluid from vagina before 37 weeks (PROM)
  - Vaginal bleeding, severe abdominal pain (miscarriage, placenta previa, abruptio placentae)
  - Chills, fever, burning on urination, diarrhea (infection)
  - Decrease or absence of fetal movements (fetal distress or intrauterine fetal death)
  - Uterine cramping, pressure, or contractions before 37 weeks (preterm labor)
  - Visual disturbances: blurring, double vision, or spots (hypertension, preeclampsia)

- Edema of face, fingers, or sacrum (hypertension, preeclampsia)
- Severe, frequent, or continuous headaches (hypertension, preeclampsia)
- Muscular irritability or convulsions (hypertension, preeclampsia)
- Epigastric pain, severe stomach ache (hypertensive conditions, preeclampsia, abruptio placentae)
- Sudden weight gain of > 2 kg (4.4 lb) per week (preeclampsia)
- Teach self-care measures for the common discomforts of second trimester. Reinforce comfort measures taught in the first trimester. See Table 4-2. The ability to use effective self-care measures enhances self-esteem, promotes independence, and reduces anxiety.

Nursing Diagnosis: HEALTH-SEEKING BEHAVIORS[1]

Refer to the NDCP, "Health-Seeking Behaviors,[1]" in "Normal Antepartum: First Trimester," beginning on p. 41 in this chapter.

▌ *Nursing Activities and Rationales*

Assessments

- Continue monitoring as in the first trimester. Assists in prevention, early recognition, and control of problems; improves maternal condition and fetal outcome.
- Monitor fundal height (measure from superior aspect of the symphysis pubis to the top of the fundus). Between 22 and 34 weeks of gestation, fundal height in centimeters correlates well with weeks of gestation. Increasing fundal height indicates advancing pregnancy and fetal growth; less than normal height may indicate intrauterine growth retardation (IUGR); greater than normal height may indicate multiple pregnancy, hydramnios, or other complications. Size greater or less than expected may indicate wrong dates. An ultrasound may be needed to determine gestational age.

Patient/Family Teaching

- Reinforce teaching done in the first trimester (e.g., regarding teratogens and health promotion behaviors). Repetition reinforces learning.
- Provide information about physical and emotional changes that occur during second trimester. The body continues to

TABLE 4-2 Self-Care Measures for Common Discomforts, Second Trimester

Pruritus (noninflammatory)	Decrease environmental (room) temperature if possible. Take Keri baths. Use distraction. Take tepid baths with sodium bicarbonate or oatmeal added to water. Use lotions and oils, and either change soaps or use less soap. Wear loose clothing. Cut fingernails short. *Cause is unknown. Some of these measures may be soothing to the skin; others help prevent skin irritation.*
Supine hypotension (vena cava syndrome)	Use side-lying position or semisitting position, with knees slightly flexed. Bend from knees, not from waist. Get up slowly after sitting, squatting, or lying down, and sit on edge of bed or assume hands-and-knees posture before arising. *This condition is induced by pressure of the gravid uterus on ascending vena cava, decreasing uteroplacental and renal perfusion. Position change allows improved venous return to the heart.*
Feeling lightheaded and fainting; dizziness, floating sensation, difficulty hearing or focusing attention.	Take deep breaths. Move legs vigorously. Avoid sudden position changes. Avoid warm, crowded areas. Avoid prolonged standing in one position. Avoid hypoglycemia by eating 5–6 small meals per day. Wear support stockings. Sit down and lower head between knees when the feeling occurs. *Condition caused by changes in blood volume and postural hypotension due to pooling of blood in the dependent veins. Most self-care measures aim to improve venous return from the legs.*
Food cravings	Satisfy craving unless it interferes with well-balanced diet. Report very unusual cravings (e.g., clay, laundry starch) to primary care provider. *Ensures adequate diet and that nothing harmful is ingested. Cause of condition is unknown. Culture and geographic area influence craving.*
Heartburn	Avoid fatty and gas-producing foods. *These aggravate heartburn.* Eat small meals, do not overfill stomach, and maintain good posture. *Allows more room for the stomach to function.* Avoid lying down after eating and sleep on a wedge pillow or elevate the head of the bed. *Helps prevent regurgitation of acidic gastric contents into the esophagus.* Chew gum. *Removes bad taste from the mouth.* Sip milk or hot herbal tea. *Dilutes gastric acid.* Do not take antacid unless prescribed by healthcare provider *(antacids can cause constipation, diarrhea, and other side effects).* Avoid baking soda and Alka-Seltzer *(can cause electrolyte imbalance).*
Constipation	See generic NDCP for constipation on pp. 11–12 in Chapter 2. Also see NDCPs, "Risk for Constipation" on pp. 51–52 in "Excess Fluid Volume (Edema), on p. 58 in this section.

change throughout pregnancy, and new sensations are experienced. During the second trimester, the abdomen enlarges visibly, and quickening occurs between 16 and 20 weeks' gestation.

- Provide information about ferrous sulfate supplementation. Iron is usually prescribed beginning in the second trimester. It is needed to help maintain normal Hgb level. Because of the increased demand for iron in pregnancy, it is nearly impossible to ingest enough dietary iron.
- Teach the woman to monitor fetal activity. The mother can usually feel fetal activity at 20 weeks. Movements are frequent, sporadic, and increase with maternal activity. Once it begins, there is an established relationship between decreased fetal activity and fetal death. Absence of fetal activity is usually followed by absence of fetal heart tones (FHTs) within 24 hours. The various methods for assessing fetal activity focus on having the woman keep a fetal movement record (e.g., in the Cardiff Count-to-Ten Method, the woman is instructed to lie on her side, begin counting, and count up to 10 movements; call healthcare provider if < 10 movements in 3 hours, if movements are slowing, if no movements in morning, or if < 3 movements in 8 hours). Monitoring fetal activity is easy and inexpensive.

Collaborative Activities

- Encourage attendance at childbirth preparation classes. Parent education classes provide information and peer support. Most classes are held weekly for several weeks, so the second trimester is a good time to begin attending in order to finish the series before the birth. If parents begin classes in the first trimester, there may be less retention because of the passage of time and because motivation to learn may not be as high early in pregnancy when feelings of ambivalence might be present.

Nursing Diagnosis: RISK FOR CONSTIPATION[1]

Use this section with the generic NDCP, "Constipation,[1]" beginning on p. 11, in Chapter 2.

Related Factors: decreased peristalsis secondary to effects of progesterone on smooth muscle; increased absorption of water from the intestines; inadequate intake of fiber-containing foods; inadequate intake of fluids; taking supplemental iron.

TABLE 4-2 Self-Care Measures for Common Discomforts, Second Trimester

Flatulence, bloating, and belching	Chew foods slowly and well. *Prevents swallowing air.* Avoid fatty and gas-producing foods and avoid large meals. *Prevents delayed emptying.* Exercise. *Increases gastric motility.* Maintain regular bowel habits. *Prevents bloating and flatulence.*
Varicose veins (aching and heaviness in legs and vulva)	Avoid lengthy standing or sitting. Avoid constrictive clothing. Engage in moderate exercise. Rest with legs and hips elevated. Wear support stockings; do not cross legs when sitting. *Improves peripheral circulation by making use of gravity and compression to increase venous return.* For vulvar varicosities, use warm sitz baths. *Relieves swelling and pain.*
Hemorrhoids (varicosities in perianal area)	Avoid lengthy standing or sitting; use warm sitz baths; apply astringent compresses. *Relieves swelling and pain.* Prevent constipation. *Straining at stool creates perineal pressure.* Using lubricated finger, manually reinsert protruding hemorrhoids into rectum. *Relieves pain, facilitates cleansing the area.*
Round ligament pain	Rest. Maintain good body mechanics. Relieve cramping by squatting or bringing knees to chest. Use local heat applications. *These measures may or may not help; reassure the woman that this is a normal phenomenon, to reduce her anxiety.*
Backache, pelvic pressure, joint pain	Use good posture and body mechanics. Avoid fatigue. Wear low-heeled shoes. Sleep on a firm mattress. Apply local heat or ice. Use pelvic rocking and pelvic tilt exercises, rest, back rubs, or lie on the floor and press the back to the floor. *This condition is caused by hormone-induced relaxation of symphyseal and sacroiliac joints. Self-care measures help stabilize the unstable pelvis, strengthen muscles, and induce nonpharmacologic analgesia. If these suggestions do not improve the condition, the woman may need to obtain a special pregnancy girdle that provides extra pelvic support.*
Leg cramps	Have care provider rule out phlebitis. Take adequate dietary calcium or calcium supplements but avoid excessive calcium-containing foods. Avoid chilling extremities. Apply heat to affected muscle. Stretch the affected muscle (e.g., for calf cramp, flex knee and flex foot upward). *This condition is caused by compression of nerves to lower extremities and/or low tissue Ca+ levels. Condition is aggravated by fatigue, poor peripheral circulation, drinking more than 1 qt (1 L) of milk per day, and pointing toes.*

▐ *Nursing Activities and Rationales*

Assessments

- Assess for presence of hemorrhoids. Hemorrhoids are common in pregnancy because venous volume is increased at the same time that peripheral venous stasis is increased. If hemorrhoids cause painful defecation, the woman might postpone evacuation of her bowels. The longer stool remains in the bowels, the more water is absorbed from the stool, allowing hard stool to accumulate in the lower bowel and rectum.

Independent Nursing Actions

- Encourage a program of moderate exercise, such as walking or swimming. Promotes peristalsis. Strenuous exercise, especially if the woman is not accustomed to it, may reduce uteroplacental circulation and cause fetal bradycardia. Long term, it may contribute to intrauterine growth restriction.

Patient/Family Teaching

- Explain the importance of avoiding constipation. Prevents or relieves the discomfort of hemorrhoids.
- Encourage at least 2,000 ml of fluid each day and adding bulk to the diet. Fluid and bulk result in soft stool, which prevents constipation.

▐ Nursing Diagnosis: READINESS FOR ENHANCED PARENTING[1]

Also refer to generic NDCP, "Impaired Parenting,[1]" beginning on p. 16 in Chapter 2; and generic NDCP, "Risk for Impaired Parent-Infant/Child Attachment,[1]" beginning on p. 19 in Chapter 2.

Related Factors: Readiness For Enhanced Parenting [1] is a wellness diagnosis. It refers to the readiness of the caretaker to improve, create, or maintain an environment that promotes optimum growth and development of the child. No related factors are needed in the diagnostic statement.

▐ *Goals, Outcomes, and Evaluation Criteria*

- Woman describes ways in which her role is expected to change with the birth of the baby.
- Woman resolves ambivalence and verbalizes acceptance of the fetus as a separate being, not just a part of her body.
- Woman expresses confidence in her ability to adjust to changing roles.
- Woman exhibits steps in maternal role taking (e.g., seeking opportunities to hold other infants, fantasizing about how the infant will look).
- Woman accomplishes psychologic tasks of pregnancy (e.g., Rubin's seeking safe passage, securing acceptance, learning to give of self, and committing herself to the unknown child).

- Woman seeks information about diet, fetal growth and development and focuses less on her discomforts and more on how she can produce a healthy baby.
- Woman demonstrates positive self-esteem.

▐ *NIC Interventions[2]*

Attachment Promotion (6710)—Facilitation of the development of the parent–infant relationship.

Prenatal Care (6960)—Monitoring and management of a patient during pregnancy to prevent complications of pregnancy and promote a healthy outcome for both mother and infant.

Role Enhancement (5370)—Assisting a patient, significant other, and/or family to improve relationships by clarifying and supplementing specific role behaviors.

▐ *Nursing Activities and Rationales*

Assessments

- Observe for statements demonstrating shift of the woman's focus from self to the fetus (e.g., "Will that hurt my baby?" "Should I be eating more?"). During the second trimester, the fetus normally becomes the woman's major focus. The discomforts of the first trimester have decreased, and her size does not yet cause discomfort as in the third trimester.
- Observe for signs of the woman's concern about ability to protect and provide for the fetus (e.g., selecting exactly the right clothes to wear, expressing fear about world events). Narcissism and introversion are a normal part of second trimester. Some women lose interest in everything except the pregnancy; some become fearful about dangers to the fetus.
- Ask whether the woman ever daydreams about the baby; observe for comments about holding or babysitting other babies. These are steps in maternal role taking. Role-playing involves acting out what mothers do (e.g., holding a friend's baby). Fantasies occur in the mind and allow the woman to safely try out a variety of behaviors (e.g., how she will read to the child).
- Assess for fearful fantasies. Some fantasies may not be positive (e.g., "What if the baby gets sick and I don't realize it? What if the baby cries and I can't stop it?"). In most cases, this will prompt the woman to ask for information or reassurance.
- Assess for attachment behaviors (e.g., has the couple chosen a name for the baby; have they chosen a name for both sexes?). Attachment begins during pregnancy in a normal pregnancy. If it does not occur, there may be problems with bonding after the birth of the baby.

Independent Nursing Actions

- Encourage and stimulate open communication between the woman and her partner. Facilitate discussion of expectations about role changes, as needed. The partners can provide essential support for each other in the parenting role;

open communication allows them to recognize and work out problems in the relationship or the family that may affect parenting.

- Provide an opportunity to view an ultrasound image of the fetus, to note fetal movement, and to hear the FHTs; discuss parents' reactions to these events. Facilitates attachment with the fetus; discussion allows for identifying possible problems; also allows for affirmation of positive expressions of feeling.
- Encourage the partner to participate in labor and birth. Facilitates attachment with the baby; provides support for the mother.
- Guide the woman in visualizing her unborn child if she has not yet had fantasies about the baby. Facilitates making the fetus a reality—separate from her body—thus promoting psychologic development.
- Help the woman to identify strategies needed for managing role changes after the birth of the baby. Provides anticipatory guidance; allows time for the woman to rehearse the role changes before they are actually needed.
- Reinforce healthy behaviors and do not criticize (e.g., praise for eating healthful foods and achieving the desired weight gain; but do not criticize the woman who has not gained enough weight). Promotes self-esteem.

Patient/Family Teaching

- Provide information about infant care, as needed. To relieve fearful fantasies and promote healthy adaptation.
- Discuss fetal responses to stimuli, such as sound, light, and maternal tension; discuss fetal sleep-wake patterns. In the second trimester, women tend to focus on the fetus and how their activities (e.g., eating, sexual activity) affect the fetus. Such information helps the woman to feel a sense of being in control of her baby's well-being.
- Include the partner in care and teaching. Partners often feel more vulnerable during the woman's pregnancy. Anticipatory guidance can help them cope with their concerns.
- Determine whether there is partner or family conflict over cultural, religious, or personal value systems. Such conflict may affect parenting. It may be necessary to refer the couple for professional counseling if they cannot communicate openly and resolve these issues.

Collaborative Activities

- Refer to prenatal and parenting education classes. Provides information, support, and appropriate role models.
- Refer to community agencies for economic and/or social supports as needed. To relieve concerns about finances and the extra expenses caused by adding a member to the family.

INDIVIDUALIZED (NURSING DIAGNOSIS) CARE PLANS

These care plans are designed to address unique patient needs.

Nursing Diagnosis: RISK FOR DISTURBED BODY IMAGE[1]

Related Factors: anatomic and physiologic changes of pregnancy; reactions of others to these changes; cultural or spiritual beliefs about childbearing. This diagnosis refers to the presence of risk factors that predispose to confusion about one's image of one's physical self.

Goals, Outcomes, and Evaluation Criteria

- Woman voices acceptance of appearance.
- Woman voices satisfaction with body appearance.
- Woman maintains cleanliness; dresses appropriately.

NIC Interventions[2]

Body Image Enhancement (5220)—Improving a patient's conscious and unconscious perceptions and attitudes toward her own body.

Nursing Activities and Rationales

Assessments

- Assess the woman's reaction to her body changes. Body changes become noticeable in the second trimester. The woman may be pleased and proud because they represent growth of the fetus. However, some women perceive the changes negatively, believing that they look fat and unattractive. Changes in body function (e.g., altered balance, low backache) also contribute to negative body image. Body image is an important part of self-esteem, which is essential for good parenting.
- Assess educational level and needs. Refer to generic NDCP, "Deficient Knowledge,[1]" beginning on p. 13 in Chapter 2.
- Assess patient's understanding of changes of pregnancy. Determines starting point for patient education and how to proceed with teaching.
- Assess woman's appearance (grooming, clothing, posture, and so forth). An attractive appearance helps preserve a positive self-image and promotes positive reactions from others (e.g., partner).

Independent Nursing Actions

- Stress positive aspects of pregnancy; minimize or explain negative ones. Helps promote a positive attitude.

Patient/Family Teaching

- Provide information about physiologic changes; stress that they are normal and temporary. Provides reassurance. Information may increase understanding and acceptance of changes.

- Assist patient to discuss changes caused by normal pregnancy. Allows woman to verbalize her knowledge of normal physical changes and increases her understanding.
- Use anticipatory guidance to prepare the woman for changes in body image that are predictable. Makes the woman aware of potential changes so that she will know what to expect.
- Include partner and family in teaching and anticipatory guidance and stress importance of partner support. Partner's perceptions and reactions to her body changes can be supportive or harmful to her body image.

Nursing Diagnosis: RISK FOR INEFFECTIVE PERIPHERAL TISSUE PERFUSION SECONDARY TO THROMBOPHLEBITIS[1]

Also refer to generic NDCP for actual "Ineffective Peripheral Tissue Perfusion,[1]" beginning on p. 18 in Chapter 2; and "Thromboembolic Disease," beginning on p. 350, in Chapter 10.

Related Factors: This diagnosis refers to the presence of risk factors that predispose to ineffective tissue perfusion of the extremities such as varicose veins, venous stasis in legs (secondary to relaxation of venous smooth muscle caused by elevated progesterone level), increased blood volume during pregnancy, standing or sitting for prolonged periods with legs in dependent position, wearing constrictive clothing that impedes venous return from the legs, hypovolemia, decreased hemoglobin concentration of the blood, obesity, advanced maternal age, and multiple gestation that contribute to varicosities. Decreased cardiac output can also contribute to venous stasis; however, a woman with decreased cardiac output is not a normal antepartum woman. For that condition, see "Cardiac Disease in Pregnancy," which begins on p. 117 in Chapter 5.

▋ *NIC Interventions[2]*

Circulatory Care: Venous Insufficiency (4066)—Promotion of venous circulation.

▋ *Nursing Activities and Rationales*

Assessments

- Assess for factors that contribute to venous stasis and clot formation (see "Related Factors," preceding). Allow for early intervention and possible prevention of thrombophlebitis. Varicose veins are common in pregnancy.

Patient/Family Teaching

- Encourage the woman to exercise and walk about rather than standing in one position. Promotes venous return by

causing skeletal muscles to contract and compress the veins in the legs.
- Advise the woman to elevate her legs level with her hips when sitting. Uses gravity to promote venous return; prevents pressure in the popliteal area.
- Advise the woman not to cross her legs at the knees when sitting. Prevents pressure on veins.
- Advise drinking at least eight glasses of water per day. Helps prevent hypovolemia, which contributes to venous stasis.

Collaborative Activities

- Refer for treatment of risk factors, as needed (e.g., obesity, varicose veins, decreased hemoglobin). Removes causal factors and prevents venous stasis.

▋ *Other Nursing Diagnoses*

Also assess for the following nursing diagnoses, which are frequently present with this condition.

Anxiety[1] related to (1) physiologic and psychologic changes of pregnancy and (2) unknown outcome

Disturbed Sleep Pattern[1] (or **sleep deprivation**) related to discomforts (e.g., heartburn) and/or anxiety

Ineffective Individual Coping[1] related to unrealistic expectations of pregnancy, prior lack of coping skills, and/or deficient knowledge

Interrupted Family Processes[1] related to (1) changes in family roles secondary to discomforts or complications of pregnancy, (2) the developmental crisis of pregnancy, and (3) strain on family finances

NORMAL ANTEPARTUM: THIRD TRIMESTER

The third trimester of pregnancy is a time of physiologic and psychologic preparation for the birth of the baby and for care of the new infant. Discomforts during this final trimester are related to the enlargement of the fetus and the uterus. The woman may complain of constipation, insomnia, shortness of breath, and urinary frequency.

▋ *Key Nursing Activities*

- Continue to assess maternal and fetal well-being.
- Assess and teach interventions for new discomforts of pregnancy.
- Review signs/symptoms of complications that should be reported to the care provider.
- Teach signs of labor onset and difference between true and false labor.
- Provide information about infant care.
- Plan for discharge after the birth.

Etiologies

There are no etiologies. Pregnancy is a normal physiologic event, not an illness.

Signs and Symptoms

In the third trimester, the fetus has completely developed and is growing rapidly. The abdomen is greatly enlarged. The woman experiences Braxton Hicks contractions and a desire for the pregnancy to end. Refer to "Normal Antepartum: First Trimester," which begins on p. 39, for a list of presumptive, probable, and positive signs of pregnancy—all of which should be in evidence by the third trimester.

Diagnostic Studies

Tests performed in the third trimester are primarily for monitoring fetal well-being and gestational age: They include:

- Fetal heart rate assessment (oxytocin challenge test, nonstress test). *Determines fetal ability to tolerate labor.*
- Amniocentesis. *Determines fetal lung maturity.*
- Sonogram. *Determines fetal size and estimated gestation.*

Medical Management

Visits to the healthcare provider are typically scheduled every 2 weeks during the 8th month and weekly thereafter until the birth. Medical treatment is not needed unless there are discomforts or complications. Medical management for normal third-trimester pregnancy includes the following:

- Screen for gestational diabetes, if indicated.
- Screen for preeclampsia.
- Continue monitoring for other complications of pregnancy (e.g., multiple gestation, placenta previa) and treat as needed.
- Monitor fetal growth and well-being (e.g., sonogram to compare biparietal diameter, femur length, and estimated fetal weight; nonstress or oxytocin challenge test).
- Continue maternal supplemental iron and folic acid.
- Cultures for infections and STIs (including *Trichomonas, Candida,* gonorrhea, herpes simplex type 2, group B *Streptococcus,* and *Chlamydia). Infections may have developed since earlier screenings.*
- Screen for genetic problems (e.g., sickle cell anemia), if not previously done.

Collaborative Problems

The potential complications of pregnancy include all the conditions in Chapters 5 and 6. Some, such as hypertensive conditions and gestational diabetes, are more likely to occur late in pregnancy. Cardiac decompensation, too, is more likely to occur later in pregnancy; however, this is not a complication of a normal pregnancy, but a complication of a high-risk pregnancy. The potential complication infection (vaginal infections and STIs) is especially relevant in the third trimester because of the risk to the fetus if infection is present at the time of birth. Screening may already have been done, but the woman can become infected at any time after the screening.

COLLABORATIVE (STANDARDIZED) CARE FOR ALL NORMAL THIRD TRIMESTER ANTEPARTUM WOMEN

Perform comprehensive assessment to identify individual needs for teaching, emotional support, and physical care.

Potential Complications of Pregnancy (Various)

For assessments and preventive interventions, refer to potential complications of pregnancy in Chapters 5 and 6; and to topics, "Collaborative (Standardized) Care for All Normal First Trimester Antepartum Women" and "Collaborative (Standardized) Care for All Normal Second Trimester Antepartum Women" in this chapter.

Nursing Diagnosis: HEALTH-SEEKING BEHAVIORS (PREPARATION FOR LABOR AND INFANT CARE)[1]

Use with the NDCP, "Health-Seeking Behaviors,[1]" in "Normal Antepartum: First Trimester," beginning on p. 41 in this chapter. Also refer to generic NDCP, "Deficient Knowledge,[1]" beginning on p. 13, in Chapter 2.

Goals, Outcomes, and Evaluation Criteria

- Woman lists the signs of labor.
- Woman differentiates between true and false labor.
- Woman verbalizes understanding of when to come to the birthing unit.
- Woman verbalizes being prepared for labor and birth.

Nursing Activities and Rationales

Assessments

- Continue monitoring wellness as in first and second trimesters. Assists in prevention, early recognition, and control of problems and improves maternal condition and fetal outcome. Although fetus is fully formed in the third trimester, neurologic development and brain growth are still occurring, and fetal iron stores and fat reserves are still being built. Adequate maternal nutrition is essential for these processes.

- Assess level of knowledge regarding signs of labor, location of birthing unit, and so forth. Determines learning needs and allows for individualization of teaching.
- Inquire about preparations that have been made for birth of the baby. If healthy adjustments are being made, the woman/couple will probably have enrolled in parent education/childbirth classes, have purchased equipment and clothing for the infant, and/or made arrangements for going to the birthing unit (e.g., arranged for a babysitter, packed a suitcase). Lack of preparation late in pregnancy may indicate financial, social, or emotional problems.

Patient/Family Teaching

- Review teaching from the second trimester as needed. Aids in recall of information and builds on previous learning.
- Provide information about normal physiologic and psychologic changes of the third trimester (maternal changes, fetal development); use pictures or sonogram to illustrate the appearance of the fetus. Facilitates understanding; helps the woman/couple to see pregnancy as a normal, healthy event rather than an illness; provides motivation for healthy behaviors; and aids in parent–infant attachment by helping make the fetus seem to be a reality for them.
- Teach the premonitory signs of labor, including Braxton Hicks contractions (become more noticeable and even painful), lightening, increased vaginal mucus, bloody show, energy spurt, a 1–3-lb weight loss. These are signs that labor is about to begin; provides opportunity to finalize preparations for labor and birth. These signs occur from a few days to 2–3 weeks before labor begins.
- Provide oral and written information about signs of labor and the difference between true and false labor. Helps ensure that woman/couple will know when to go to the birthing unit. Relieves some of the anxiety that women frequently have about this issue ("How will I know when I am really in labor?"). The woman may fear being embarrassed or disappointed by not being in labor and being sent home. In true labor, uterine contractions (UCs) show a consistent pattern of increasing frequency, intensity, and duration. Walking increases the UCs. Discomfort begins in the lower back, sweeps around to the lower abdomen, and in early labor, feels like menstrual cramps. Progressive dilation and effacement of the cervix occur in true labor. In false labor, UCs are inconsistent in frequency, duration, and intensity. Change in activity decreases or does not affect UCs. Discomfort is felt in abdomen and groin and may be more annoying than truly painful; no change in effacement of dilation of cervix.
- Explain when to call the healthcare provider. The woman should call if there is any question as to whether she is in labor, and she should call if any symptoms of complications occur.
- Explain when to leave for the birth unit, taking into consideration the number and duration of previous labors, distance to the hospital, and type of transportation. Relieves

anxiety and helps the woman/couple feel in control and secure that the birth will not occur at home or on the way to the birthing unit. The woman should go to the hospital when any of these occur: contractions are regular and 5 minutes apart for 1 hour (nullipara) or regular and 10 minutes apart for 1 hour (multipara); membranes rupture, with or without contractions; bright red bleeding occurs; decreased fetal movement occurs; the woman has any feeling that something is wrong.

- Provide information about the stages of labor. Reinforces correct information the woman may already have and relieves anxiety by correcting any misinformation. Allows role rehearsal in advance of labor and birth.
- Assist the woman/couple to write a birth plan, noting cultural, spiritual, and individual preferences. Allows the couple control over their care and enables healthcare personnel to plan in advance to facilitate individualized care. For example, a couple may prefer a female healthcare provider, or they may request the use of only nonpharmacologic pain relief measures.
- Provide oral and written information about infant care and feeding. Written information is important because of the quantity of new information to be learned. This information helps the woman/couple to prepare in advance for parenting (e.g., by buying clothing and supplies, preparing for breastfeeding).

▌Nursing Diagnosis: DEFICIENT KNOWLEDGE (PREGNANCY-RELATED CHANGES AND DISCOMFORTS)[1]

Use with generic NDCP, "Deficient Knowledge,[1]" beginning on p. 13, in Chapter 2. Also refer to the NDCP, "Deficient Knowledge (Pregnancy-Related Changes)[1]" in the topics "Normal Antepartum: First Trimester" and "Normal Antepartum: Second Trimester," beginning on p. 40 and p. 49, respectively.

▌*Nursing Activities and Rationales*

Assessments

- Inquire about any discomforts that have developed since the second trimester. Discomforts in the third trimester are caused primarily by the size of the fetus and encroachment on maternal organs. However, discomforts from previous trimesters may remain or reoccur.

Patient/Family Teaching

- Reinforce teaching that was done in the second trimester. Aids in retention of information.
- Reinforce the importance of contacting the healthcare provider if symptoms of complications occur. See "Normal Antepartum: Second Trimester," beginning on p. 48.

• Teach self-care measures for the common discomforts of the third trimester. Reinforce comfort measures taught in the first trimester (Table 4-3). Enhances self-esteem, promotes independence, and reduces anxiety.

Nursing Diagnosis: RISK FOR INJURY (TO FETUS)[1]

Related Factors: lack of knowledge of symptoms of complications of pregnancy; lack of knowledge of symptoms of other diseases and medical conditions that affect the fetus.

Goals, Outcomes, and Evaluation Criteria

• Woman lists symptoms that require immediate notification of healthcare provider.
• Woman verbalizes understanding of the effects of maternal illness on the fetus.
• Woman will recognize complications that occur and seek treatment promptly.

NIC Interventions[2]

Surveillance: Late Pregnancy (6656)—Purposeful and ongoing acquisition, interpretation, and synthesis of maternal-fetal data for treatment, observation, or admission.

Nursing Activities and Rationales

Assessments

• Continue assessments for complications of pregnancy as in previous trimesters. Although the fetus is fully formed in the third trimester, neurologic development and brain growth are still occurring. Maternal illness can interfere with these processes.

Patient/Family Teaching

• Review teaching from second trimester as needed (e.g., regarding teratogens, infections to avoid). Aids in recall of information and builds on previous learning.
• Reinforce the effects of maternal health and pregnancy complications on the fetus. Although the woman does not need to know in great detail the effects of pregnancy complications, awareness that they can harm the baby may motivate her to have symptoms evaluated if they occur.
• Review the signs and symptoms of complications of pregnancy. Helps to ensure that the woman will recognize reportable symptoms. Especially relevant in the third trimester are epigastric pain, headache, visual disturbances, weight gain of more than 0.5 kg/week, or other symptoms of preeclampsia; absence of fetal movements; symptoms of infection (vaginitis or UTI); vaginal bleeding and/or severe abdominal pain (placenta previa, abruptio placentae). All

TABLE 4-3 Self-Care Measures for Common Discomforts, Third Trimester	
Shortness of breath and dyspnea (occurs in 60% of women)	Practice good posture. Use extra pillows when sleeping. Stop smoking. Avoid overloading stomach. If symptoms do not improve, contact healthcare provider to rule out asthma, emphysema, anemia, or a cardiac complication.
Difficulty sleeping	Use conscious relaxation, back massage, or effleurage. Support body parts with pillows. Take warm shower or drink warm milk before bed.
Nocturia; urinary frequency and urgency	Empty bladder regularly. Do Kegel exercises. Wear perineal pad.
Skin pigmentation, acne, oily skin, itching	Not preventable. Keep skin clean. Oatmeal baths may help itching.
Mood swings, increased anxiety	Recognize that these are normal. Encourage support and communication from partner, family, and significant others.
Gingivitis, bleeding gums	Include protein and fresh fruits and vegetables in diet. Brush teeth gently. Maintain good dental hygiene. See dentist for teeth cleaning.
Nonpitting ankle edema	See NDCP "Excess Fluid Volume (Edema)" on pp. 58 in this care plan.
Perineal pressure and discomfort	Rest and use conscious relaxation techniques to facilitate rest. Maintain good posture. Contact healthcare provider if pain occurs.
Leg cramps	If Homans' sign negative, massage affected muscle or use heat; stretch muscle (e.g., flex foot dorsally for calf cramp). Stand on cold surface. Take an oral supplement of Ca+ carbonate or Ca+ lactate to increase calcium:phosphorus ratio. Take aluminum hydroxide gel (30 ml) with meals to absorb phosphorus. Do not drink more than 1 qt (1 L) of milk per day.
Braxton Hicks contractions	Rest but change positions. Use effleurage. Practice breathing techniques learned in childbirth preparation classes.

of these conditions can harm the fetus. All require prompt evaluation.

- Teach and reinforce the signs and symptoms of preterm labor to all women, not just those considered at risk for preterm labor. Tools for scoring risk will not identify all women who will ultimately go into preterm labor, especially those who are nulliparous. It is crucial that a woman call her healthcare provider and/or go to the birthing unit immediately if she notices signs or symptoms of preterm labor. This information should be included in teaching late in the second trimester (after viability at 23 weeks) and reinforced in the third trimester.

Other Important Nursing Diagnoses

Other diagnoses for all women in the third trimester include:

- Risk for Disturbed Body Image[1]
- Risk for Impaired Peripheral Tissue Perfusion[1]
- Risk for Constipation[1]
- Readiness for Enhanced Parenting[1]

For care plans for these nursing diagnoses, refer to "Normal Antepartum: Second Trimester," beginning on p. 48. It is important to continue these care plans throughout the third trimester.

INDIVIDUALIZED (NURSING DIAGNOSIS) CARE PLANS

Individualized care plans are designed to address unique patient needs.

Nursing Diagnosis: EXCESS FLUID VOLUME (EDEMA)[1]

Related Factors: compromised regulatory mechanisms, excess fluid intake, excess sodium intake.

Goals, Outcomes, and Evaluation Criteria

- Edema remains nonpitting and only in feet and ankles.
- Woman uses comfort measures.
- Woman verbalizes that discomfort is satisfactorily controlled.

NIC Interventions[2]

Fluid Monitoring (4130)—Collection and analysis of patient data to regulate fluid balance.
Surveillance: Late Pregnancy: (6656)—Purposeful and ongoing acquisition, interpretation, and synthesis of maternal-fetal data for treatment, observation, or admission.
Teaching: Disease Process (5602)—Assisting the patient to understand information related to a specific disease process.

Nursing Activities and Rationales

Assessments

- Assess location and extent of edema (pitting edema is when pressure of a finger and thumb leaves a persistent depression). The normal hemodilution that occurs in pregnancy causes a slight decrease in colloid osmotic pressure. Also, near term, the weight of the uterus compresses pelvic veins, delaying venous return, which creates distention and pressure in the veins of the legs and causes fluid to shift to interstitial spaces. Therefore, dependent edema of feet and ankles is normal. However, edema of the face or hands requires further evaluation, as does pitting edema.
- If generalized or pitting edema is present, assess for signs of preeclampsia (2+ proteinuria, BP 140/90 mmHg on at least two occasions 6 hours apart in a woman who was normotensive before pregnancy). Determines if preeclampsia is developing. For further interventions, refer to the generic collaborative care plan "Potential Complication: Hypertensive Disorders," beginning on p. 32 in Chapter 3.

Patient/Family Teaching

- Advise the woman to sleep in a side-lying position. Removes weight of gravid uterus from vena cava and increases venous return. Increases renal blood flow, renal perfusion, and glomerular filtration rate, and mobilizes dependent edema. If edema does not resolve by morning, advise the woman to notify her healthcare provider, because this may indicate a hypertensive disorder or decreased kidney perfusion.
- Teach the woman that it is not necessary to limit fluids or salt/sodium in the diet. Six to eight glasses of fluid per day are needed for biologic processes. Women may mistakenly assume that limiting water will decrease the edema. Inadequate sodium intake can overwork the renin-angiotensin-aldosterone system, causing dehydration and hypovolemia. Women may have heard, incorrectly, that avoiding salt will prevent water retention.
- Encourage the woman to wear support stockings and advise putting them on before getting out of bed in the morning. Compresses tissues and veins, which increases venous return from the legs. Horizontal position removes effects of gravity and mobilizes edema during the night.
- Advise the woman to avoid standing for long periods and walk about periodically when standing. Gravity causes pooling in lower extremities. Activity increases venous return.
- Advise the woman not to cross her legs when sitting. Impedes venous return in popliteal area.
- Teach the woman to rest with the legs elevated several times each day. Makes use of gravity to promote venous return, decreasing pressure in veins and allowing mobilization of interstitial fluid.

Collaborative Activities

- Assess for associated medical problems or complications (e.g., hypertension, cardiac disease, kidney disease). These problems affect kidney function and may contribute to edema.

▌ Nursing Diagnosis: ANXIETY[1]

Use with generic NDCP, "Anxiety,[1]" which begins on p. 10 in Chapter 2.

Related Factors: worries about ability to cope with labor and birth processes; concerns about parenting abilities.

▌ *NIC Interventions[2]*

Childbirth Preparation (6760)—Providing information and support to facilitate childbirth and to enhance the ability of an individual to develop and perform the role of parent.

▌ *Goals, Outcomes, and Evaluation Criteria*

- Woman verbalizes feelings and symptoms.
- Woman reports a decrease in anxious feelings and symptoms.
- Woman demonstrates understanding and realistic expectations of the labor and birth processes.

▌ *Nursing Activities and Rationales*

Assessments

- Assess patient's knowledge of physiologic processes of labor and birth and of procedures associated with labor and birth. Determines patient's need for prenatal education.

Independent Nursing Actions

- Help the woman identify and use appropriate coping strategies such as talking, crying, walking, and keeping busy. Coping strategies reduce fear and anxiety by temporarily helping protect or distance the person from the perceived threat.
- Reassure the woman that labor is different for each woman, and that for the same woman, each of her labors may be different from each other. Helps the woman understand that the unpleasant experiences that she may have heard about from other women will not necessarily happen to her.

Patient/Family Teaching

- Teach about the labor and birth process, as needed. Information reduces fear of the unknown and increases a sense of control and helps to reduce anxiety.
- Explain the pharmacologic and nonpharmacologic comfort measures that can be used during labor. Decreases fears about inability to cope with the pain.

▌ Nursing Diagnosis: INEFFECTIVE BREATHING PATTERNS[1]

Related Factors: crowding of the diaphragm by the fetus and enlarging uterus; medical complications (e.g., anemia, upper respiratory infection, bronchitis, asthma, sinusitis).

▌ *Goals, Outcomes, and Evaluation Criteria*

- Woman demonstrates ease of breathing.
- Woman has an absence of shortness of breath (dyspnea) at rest.
- Woman is free of excessive fatigue.

▌ *NIC Interventions[2]*

Respiratory Monitoring (3350)—Collection and analysis of patient data to ensure airway patency and adequate gas exchange.

▌ *Nursing Activities and Rationales*

Assessment

- Assess rate, rhythm, depth, and effort of respirations. Determines the severity of the problem.
- Assess for fatigue and shortness of breath at rest. Respirations are commonly modified late in pregnancy as the enlarged uterus and fetus decrease the ability of the diaphragm to descend. However, not all women experience serious fatigue or shortness of breath. Shortness of breath during rest may indicate an underlying cardiac or respiratory problem and requires further evaluation.
- Assess for presence of medical problems (e.g., asthma, upper respiratory infection). These exacerbate the normal respiratory changes of pregnancy and should be treated to ensure adequate oxygenation.
- Assess for anxiety. The feeling of shortness of breath is often anxiety producing.

Patient/Family Teaching

- Explain respiratory changes caused by normal pregnancy and reassure the woman that changes are normal and temporary. Relieves anxiety.
- Teach maintaining good posture and sitting up straight. Encourage the use of pillows to create a semi-Fowler's position for sleeping. Makes more room for the diaphragm and for lung expansion.
- Encourage eating smaller, more frequent meals. A full stomach further crowds the diaphragm.
- Advise to avoid smoking and exposure to second- and third-hand smoke. When inspiratory depth is compromised, it is important that the inspired air be rich in oxygen for fetal–placental exchange. Smoking reduces the oxygen available to the fetus.

Nursing Diagnosis: SEXUAL DYSFUNCTION AND/OR INEFFECTIVE SEXUAL PATTERN[1]

Use with the NDCP, "Sexual Dysfunction[1] and/or Ineffective Sexual Pattern,[1]" beginning on p. 46, within the topic, "Normal Antepartum: First Trimester." Many of the interventions are the same, although the related factors may be different in the third trimester than in the first trimester.

Related Factors: fatigue, fear of injury to the woman or the baby, inability to assume customary positions for intercourse, changes in sexual desire (woman or partner), negative body image, emotional and anatomic changes of pregnancy, shortness of breath, painful pelvic ligaments, urinary frequency.

Goals, Outcomes, and Evaluation Criteria

- Woman expresses satisfaction with body appearance.
- Woman and partner adjust to changes in physical appearance.
- Couple expresses satisfaction with sexual arousal and expression.
- Couple expresses comfort with modifications of sexual expression.

NIC Interventions[2]

Prenatal Care (6960)—Monitoring and management of patient during pregnancy to prevent complications of pregnancy and promote a healthy outcome for both mother and infant.

Body Image Enhancement (5220)—Improving a patient's conscious and unconscious perceptions and attitudes toward her body.

Nursing Activities and Rationales

Assessments

- Assess the specific nature of the sexual problem, e.g., lack of desire, discomfort with certain positions, self-consciousness about body appearance. Individualizes interventions to address the cause of the problem.
- Assess cultural norms and proscriptions for sexual activity. In most cultures sexual activity is prohibited only near the end of pregnancy; some even prescribe it to keep the birth canal lubricated. Others, however, require abstinence throughout pregnancy because intercourse is thought to harm the mother and fetus.

Patient/Family Teaching

- Suggest the possibility of maintaining physical contact in ways other than genital intercourse, e.g., kissing, hugging, cuddling, stroking. Helps maintain the couple's warmth and closeness. Although sexual desire may be decreased for one or both partners, the need for physical closeness may still remain.

- Reassure the couple that their feelings are normal and temporary. They may mistakenly believe that reduced sexual desire or performance indicates a lack of love or caring. Some men view the changes of pregnancy as erotic; others begin to view their partner as a mother and must readjust to again think of her as a sex partner.
- Reassure the couple that sexual intercourse will not harm the fetus or the woman, under normal circumstances. In a healthy pregnancy, intercourse will not cause infection or cause the membranes to rupture.
- If the woman has strong uterine contractions after intercourse, advise the use of a condom and avoidance of breast stimulation; if this is not effective, the woman may need to avoid orgasm. Uterine contractions may be due to breast stimulation, which causes the release of oxytocin from the pituitary; the male ejaculate, which contains prostaglandins; or from female orgasm, which normally causes mild uterine contractions.
- Suggest coital positions other than male superior (e.g., side-by-side, female superior, and vaginal rear entry). Prevents pressure on the maternal abdomen and allows better genital-genital access. Also, if the female is flat on her back, the uterus puts pressure on the vena cava, interfering with venous return to the heart, and subsequently with fetoplacental circulation.
- Reinforce that activities that both partners enjoy are acceptable (e.g., oral-genital sex, masturbation, mutual or singly). However, they should not have vaginal penetration after anal penetration. Risk of introducing *E. coli* from the rectum into the vagina.

NURSING CARE PLAN: ANTEPARTUM FETAL MONITORING AND OTHER DIAGNOSTIC TESTS

A variety of antepartal diagnostic and screening tests is used to assess fetal and maternal health status. These procedures include electronic fetal heart monitoring, ultrasonography, amniocentesis, laboratory analysis of maternal blood and urine, and chorionic villus sampling. Some tests are invasive and require a signed consent form; others are noninvasive and essentially risk free. The purpose of this care plan is not to teach the nurse to perform or interpret antepartum tests, but to focus on the care and support of women who are undergoing such tests.

Key Nursing Activities

- Provide information about the purpose and procedure of the test.
- Provide information about the symptoms of complications associated with the test.
- Identify and provide interventions for anxiety.

- Provide for privacy and comfort.
- Prepare the patient, equipment, and supplies for the test.

Etiologies and Risk Factors; Signs and Symptoms

Some diagnostic tests are routinely done at prescribed intervals during pregnancy to monitor fetal well-being and the progress of the pregnancy. Others are done only if fetal or maternal symptoms indicate. Examples of clinical manifestations that indicate the need for tests of maternal or fetal well-being include:

- Lack of fetal movement
- Maternal feeling that something isn't right
- History of preterm labor or birth
- Infections and/or immunodeficiencies
- Maternal disease, such as anemia, heart disease, or lupus
- Multiple gestation
- Pregnancy past 41 weeks of gestation
- Nonreassuring or absent FHTs (i.e., progressive increase or decrease in FHR, late or severe variable decelerations, or absence of FHR variability)
- Less than normal fundal height for gestational age
- Maternal symptoms of pregnancy complications (e.g., elevated blood pressure, generalized edema, premature rupture of membranes, vaginal bleeding, abdominal cramping)

Diagnostic Studies

- **Pelvic measurements**—Occasionally performed at the initial prenatal assessment to determine whether the size and shape of the pelvis are adequate for a vaginal birth.
- **Amniocentesis**—Performed when indicated. It is possible to detect the presence of infection and the presence of meconium in the amniotic fluid. Fetal hypoxia causes increased fetal peristalsis, relaxation of the anal sphincter, and passage of meconium, which stains the amniotic fluid green. Specific tests on amniotic fluid include:
  - ▸ Alpha-fetoprotein—Screens for neural tube defects.
  - ▸ Karyotyping of fetal chromosomes—Screens for genetic problems and fetal abnormalities.
  - ▸ Lecithin-sphingomyelin ratio and presence of phosphatidylglycerol—Assesses fetal lung maturity.
  - ▸ Optical density—Identifies Rh-sensitization.
- **Chorionic villus sampling**—Performed when indicated for first trimester diagnosis of genetic, metabolic, and DNA problems; does not detect neural tube defects.
- **Percutaneous umbilical blood sampling**—Pure fetal blood obtained from umbilical cord while fetus is in utero; used to diagnose hemophilia, hemoglobinopathies, fetal infections, hemolytic disorders, and platelet disorders.
- **Fetoscopy**—Performed when indicated, e.g., when direct observation of the fetus is required, when a sample of fetal blood or skin is needed; aids in diagnosis of conditions such as hemoglobinopathies, coagulation and metabolic disorders,

immunodeficiencies, chromosome abnormalities, Rh isoimmunization, and serious skin defects.

- **Magnetic resonance imaging**—Performed when indicated to identify fetal central nervous system and growth restriction (IUGR) and to evaluate maternal pelvic masses.
- **FHR monitoring**—Performed routinely and when indicated. Correlates the FHR and pattern to UCs or fetal activity. The FHR should not decelerate during UCs; the baseline rate should be 110–160 bpm, and variability (irregular fluctuations in the baseline FHR of ≥ 2 cycles/min) should be present. The following tests make use of the FHR:
  - ▸ **Nonstress test (NST)**—Correlates FHR with fetal activity; a reactive test indicates fetal well-being. The NST does not diagnose hypoxia but suggests absence of hypoxia.
  - ▸ **Contraction stress test or oxytocin challenge test**—Correlates the FHR with UCs to evaluate the respiratory function of the placenta and identify the fetus who is hypoxic or at risk for intrauterine asphyxia. During UCs, blood flow to the intervillous space of the placenta is reduced, decreasing oxygen transport to the fetus. A healthy fetus tolerates this well, but if placental reserve is insufficient, fetal hypoxia occurs along with myocardial depression, which causes a change in FHR and pattern.
  - ▸ **Fetal acoustic stimulation test and vibroacoustic stimulation test**—A modification of the NST, using sound or vibration to stimulate fetal activity.
- **Ultrasonography**—The most commonly used diagnostic procedure; performed routinely and as indicated to estimate gestational age, determine fetal growth (e.g., detect IUGR), detect congenital anomalies, evaluate placental maturity and location, estimate amniotic fluid volume, and evaluate maternal pelvic masses. Specialized tests using ultrasound include:
  - ▸ **Biophysical profile**—Rates five fetal biophysical variables (breathing movement, body movement, tone, amniotic fluid volume, and FHR reactivity) to assess the fetus at risk for intrauterine compromise. Indicated for decreased fetal movement in IUGR, maternal diabetes, preterm labor, postterm labor, and PROM.
  - ▸ **Doppler velocimetry**—Studies blood flow changes in maternal–fetal circulation to assess placental function. Best used when IUGR is suspected or diagnosed. Primarily used for research purposes, but can be used clinically.
  - ▸ **Echocardiography**—Used to examine fetal cardiac structures, ideally between 18 and 22 weeks of gestation.
- **Tests on maternal blood**—Tests on maternal blood include the following: hemoglobin and hematocrit, ABO and Rh typing, complete blood count, tests for syphilis (serologic test, complement fixation test, VDRL [a blood test for syphilis]), maternal serum alpha-fetoprotein, indirect Coombs for women who are Rh negative, 50-g 1-hr glucose screen for diabetes, rubella titer, hepatitis B screen, HIV screen, illicit drug screen, sickle cell screen. Most of these are routinely done; some are done only if the woman wishes (e.g., HIV screen).

- **Tests on maternal vaginal secretions**—Vaginal cultures for Neisseria gonorrhoeae; Pap smear for Chlamydia and group B Streptococcus.
- **Tests on maternal urine**—For presence of protein and glucose (screen for infection, kidney disease, and diabetes).

Medical Management

Medical management includes prescribing, performing, and interpreting the diagnostic procedures.

- Pelvic measurements. Performed by physician, nurse practitioner, midwife, or nurse with special training, using gloved hand and pelvimeter. Pelvic measurements are no longer routinely done.
- Amniocentesis. Sterile procedure requiring consent; guided by an ultrasound, the physician inserts a needle through the maternal abdomen into the uterine cavity to withdraw a sample of amniotic fluid. Local anesthetic may be used.
- Chorionic villus sampling. Sterile procedure; requires consent. Using ultrasound to locate the placenta, uterus, and maternal organs, the physician aspirates a sample of chorionic villi from the edge of the developing placenta. The approach is either through the cervix or the maternal abdomen.
- Percutaneous umbilical blood sampling. The physician inserts a sterile transducer and needle through the maternal abdomen, and fetal blood is aspirated into a syringe. A paralytic agent may be given to prevent fetal movement, and the woman may be lightly sedated.
- Fetoscopy. Guided by ultrasound, the physician makes a small incision through the maternal abdomen, obtains a sample of amniotic fluid, and inserts a fiber-optic endoscope through a cannula to visualize the fetus.
- Magnetic resonance imaging. A noninvasive scanning technique in which the woman is placed in a magnetic field. Magnetic resonance imaging is based on the behavior of hydrogen atoms when placed in a magnetic field and disturbed by radiofrequency signals. Performed by a qualified radiologic technologist.
- FHR monitoring.
  - ▶ Nonstress test (NST). External tocodynamometer is applied to the mother's abdomen to detect uterine or fetal movement; external transducer applied to detect FHR. Can be administered and interpreted by the nurse.
  - ▶ Contraction stress test. External monitor applied as in NST. Intravenous oxytocin or nipple stimulation are used to stimulate three UCs of at least 40 seconds' duration in 10 minutes. Performed by qualified obstetric nurses. Must be done near the labor and birth unit.
  - ▶ Fetal acoustic stimulation test and vibroacoustic stimulation test. See NST.
- Ultrasonography. Use of intermittent high-frequency sound waves to create an image of the fetus. Performed by a physician, nurse, or technician with special training. A transducer is placed on the abdomen or labia majora or inserted into the vagina.
- Tests on maternal blood. Sample drawn from peripheral vein by laboratory technician.

- Tests on maternal vaginal secretions. Samples of vaginal secretions taken by physician or nurse.
- Tests on maternal urine. Clean-catch specimen provided by the patient.

COLLABORATIVE (STANDARDIZED) CARE FOR ALL PATIENTS HAVING FETAL MONITORING AND OTHER DIAGNOSTIC TESTS

Perform comprehensive assessment to identify individual needs for teaching, emotional support, and physical care.

Potential Complications of Amniocentesis: BLEEDING, FETAL INJURY, PERFORATION OF MATERNAL BLADDER OR INTESTINES, INFECTION, PREMATURE LABOR, RH ISOIMMUNIZATION, AND AMNIOTIC FLUID EMBOLISM

Nursing Activities and Rationales

Focus Assessments

- Monitor vital signs after procedure. Detects hemorrhage or amniotic fluid embolism.
- Observe puncture site for bleeding or other drainage. Detects bleeding or leaking of amniotic fluid.
- Obtain FHR before and after procedure. Establishes baseline and evaluates fetal response to procedure.
- Observe and teach patient to observe for UCs after procedure. Detects possible premature labor.

Preventive Nursing Activities

- Use and monitor sterile technique during procedure. Prevents introduction of pathogens.
- If done after 20 weeks, have woman empty her bladder before the procedure. Minimizes the risk for puncture of the urinary bladder.
- Administer Rho(D) immune globulin (RhoGAM) to women with Rh negative blood and who have tested negatively in an indirect Coombs' test. Prevents isoimmunization from fetal blood.
- Instruct the woman to call her healthcare provider if she has any fluid loss, bleeding, fever, abdominal pain, fetal hyperactivity, or decreased fetal activity. Facilitates early treatment

of complications (hemorrhage, infection, premature labor, fetal injury). Incidence of complications is < 1%.

Potential Complications of Chorionic Villus Sampling: MISCARRIAGE, FETAL LIMB REDUCTION DEFECTS, RUPTURE OF MEMBRANES, BLEEDING, INFECTION, RH ISOIMMUNIZATION, AND FAILURE TO OBTAIN TISSUE

Focus Assessments

- Schedule for ultrasound in 2–4 days. Confirms that fetus is still viable.
- Note color and amount of any drainage from the vagina. Detects bleeding.
- Observe the woman for bleeding and/or complaints of cramps and teach her to observe. Detects miscarriage.

Preventive Nursing Activities

- Administer Rho(D) immune globulin to women with Rh negative blood and who have a negative indirect Coombs' test result. Prevents isoimmunization from fetal blood.
- Use and monitor sterile technique during procedure. Prevents introduction of pathogens.
- Instruct the woman to call her healthcare provider if she has any fluid loss, bleeding, fever, or abdominal pain. Facilitates early treatment of complications, e.g., hemorrhage, infection, premature labor.

Potential Complications of Fetoscopy: FETAL HEART RATE ABNORMALITIES, UTERINE CONTRACTIONS, VAGINAL BLEEDING, LOSS OF AMNIOTIC FLUID, AND INFECTION

Focus Assessments

See "Potential Complication of Amniocentesis," preceding.

- Observe abdominal incision for drainage and redness and teach the woman to do the same and report. Detects loss of amniotic fluid, bleeding, and infection.

Potential Complications of Percutaneous Umbilical Blood Sampling: PREMATURE RUPTURE OF MEMBRANES, CHORIOAMNIONITIS, AND FETAL BRADYCARDIA

Focus Assessments

See "Potential Complications of Amniocentesis," preceding.

- Tocolytics and antibiotics are sometimes administered. Prevents UCs and infection, respectively.

Potential Complication of Contraction Stress Test: INDUCTION OF LABOR

Focus Assessments

- Obtain FHR before and after procedure. Establishes baseline and evaluates fetal response to procedure.
- Observe UC pattern and FHR throughout procedure. Detects overstimulation of uterus and/or fetal distress.
- Observe and teach patient to observe for UCs after procedure. Detects possible premature labor.
- After the procedure, discontinue the oxytocin and continue to monitor FHR for 30 more minutes. The body metabolizes oxytocin in about 20–25 minutes.

Preventive Nursing Activities

- Use two-bag (piggyback) intravenous (IV) setup. Allows oxytocin to be discontinued without stopping the maintenance intravenous fluid line if complications develop.
- If uterine contractions become too frequent or if uterus does not relax completely between contractions, stop the oxytocin and notify the physician. Prevents overstimulation of uterus, stimulation of labor, and fetal distress.
- Perform the test in a labor and birth unit, with a physician available. This test may stimulate labor.

INDIVIDUALIZED (NURSING DIAGNOSIS) CARE PLANS

This section includes care plans to address unique patient needs.

Nursing Diagnosis: Anxiety[1]

Use with generic NDCP, "Anxiety,[1]" beginning on p. 10, and generic NDCP, "Deficient Knowledge,[1]" beginning on p. 13, in Chapter 2.

Related Factors: fear of the outcome/prognosis for self and baby; fear of procedures and/or equipment, lack of information about the procedure.

▌ Goals, Outcomes, and Evaluation Criteria

- Woman seeks information regarding procedure.
- Woman identifies several coping strategies.
- Woman demonstrates effective use of coping strategies.
- Woman reports feeling less anxious.
- Woman describes the procedure.
- Woman describes the side effects/warning signs after the procedure.

▌ Nursing Activities and Rationales

Assessments

- Refer to assessments under the collaborative care plans "Potential Complications" of diagnostic tests, e.g., amniocentesis, chorionic villus sampling, fetoscopy, percutaneous umbilical blood sampling, and contraction stress test preceding, p. 62.
- For procedures requiring supine position (e.g., amniocentesis), observe for hypotension, shortness of breath, light-headedness, nausea, and diaphoresis and reposition as needed. In late pregnancy, when the woman is supine, the gravid uterus crowds her lungs, causing shortness of breath. Further, it compresses the vena cava, decreasing venous return to the heart, thereby decreasing cardiac output and causing hypotension. Maternal hypotension causes fetal anoxia.

Independent Nursing Actions

- For invasive procedures (amniocentesis, chorionic villus sampling, fetoscopy, percutaneous umbilical blood sampling) be sure that a consent form has been signed and that informed consent has been obtained. Patients sometimes sign consent forms without reading them or without understanding the explanation that is given them. Ethically and legally, it is informed consent only if the patient understands the procedure and its risks and benefits.
- Act as an advocate if there are questions or concerns that need to be addressed prior to the procedure. Women will sometimes approach the nurse with concerns that they do not express to the primary healthcare provider.
- After the exam, clarify and interpret test results for the woman/couple, as needed. Anxiety may interfere with the woman's/couple's understanding of the explanation provided by the primary healthcare provider; or questions may arise after the primary provider leaves.
- Provide for privacy (e.g., drape for pelvic measurements, lithotomy position, and so forth). Reduces anxiety due to embarrassment and demonstrates respect.

- For amniocentesis, position supine with left lateral tilt, then observe for blood contamination of amniotic fluid. Prevents supine hypotension; many tests are not accurate if the amniotic fluid is contaminated with blood.
- For chorionic villus sampling, be sure that preliminary blood is drawn; have the woman drink water to fill her bladder; place in lithotomy position, if supine, with left lateral tilt. Positions the small uterus for catheter insertion, facilitates visualization of the perineum, and, if abdominal approach is used, prevents supine hypotension.
- For ultrasonography, have the woman drink 1.5 liters of water 2 hours before the exam. If bladder is not full enough on scanning, have her drink 3–4 more glasses and rescan in 30 min. This is not necessary if vaginal approach is used. The woman should have a full bladder for this procedure except when it is being done to localize the placenta before amniocentesis or when a vaginal probe ultrasound is used.

Patient/Family Teaching

- Explain all procedures before they occur. Decreases fear of the unknown.
- Provide factual information concerning the purpose and procedure of the diagnostic test, the sensations the woman will experience, potential complications, and symptoms to report to the healthcare provider after discharge. Because most of these tests are performed on an outpatient basis, the patient must be aware of symptoms of complications. This information is needed for self-care and lessens unrealistic fears and fear of the unknown.
- Be sure the woman/couple is aware of risks and benefits of chorionic villus sampling when performed. One benefit of this test is that early diagnosis is possible, which allows the couple to seek therapeutic abortion if they desire before 14 weeks' gestation.
- Teach the woman/couple to call the healthcare provider if symptoms of complications occur. See collaborative care plans for complications of diagnostic tests, e.g., amniocentesis, chorionic villus sampling, fetoscopy, percutaneous umbilical blood sampling, or contraction stress test preceding on p. 62.

Collaborative Activities

- Refer for counseling when the diagnostic test is being done to screen for genetic abnormalities or for fetal anomalies. Counseling may be needed in order to provide the couple the necessary information for their decision about whether to continue the pregnancy or, in some cases, whether to even have the diagnostic procedure.

END NOTES

1. Nursing Diagnoses—Definitions and Classification 2009–2011. Copyright © 2009, 2007, 2005, 2003, 2001, 1998, 1996, 1994 by NANDA International. Used by arrangement with Blackwell Publishing Limited, a company of John Wiley & Sons, Inc. In order to make safe and effective judgments using NANDA-I nursing diagnoses it is essential that nurses refer to the definitions and defining characteristics of the diagnoses listed in this work.

2. Bulechek, G. M., Butcher, H. K., Dochterman, J. M. (2008). *Nursing Interventions Classification* (5th ed). St. Louis, MO: Elsevier, by permission.

REFERENCES

U.S. Preventive Services Task Force. (2008, May). Screening for gestational diabetes mellitus: U.S. Preventive Services Task Force recommendation statement. *Annals of Internal Medicine, 148*(10), 759–765.

Norwitz, E. R., Arulkumaran, S., Symonds, I. M., & Fowlie, A. (2007). *Oxford American handbook of obstetrics and gynecology.* New York, NY: Oxford University Press.

RESOURCES

Armstrong, M., Caliendo, C., & Roberts, A. (2006). Pregnancy, lactation, and nipple piercings. *Lifelines, 10*(3), 212–217.

Blincoe, A. J. (2007, January). Hypertension in pregnancy: The importance of monitoring. *British Journal of Midwifery, 15*(1), 47–48, 50.

Bulechek, G. M., Butcher, H. K., & Dochterman, J. M. (2008). *Nursing interventions classification (NIC)* (5th ed.). St. Louis, MO: Mosby/ Elsevier.

Clancy, C. (2008). Quitting smoking: Helping patients kick the habit. *Nursing for Women's Health, 12*(4), 282–285.

Davidson, M., London, M., & Ladewig, P. (2008). *Old's maternal newborn nursing and women's health across the lifespan* (8th ed.). Upper Saddle River, NJ: Pearson Prentice Hall.

McKinney, E., James, S., Murray, S., & Ashwill, J. (2009). *Maternal-child nursing* (3rd ed.). St. Louis, MO: Saunders.

Muolland, C., Njoroge, T., Mersereau, P., & Williams, J. (2007, July–August). Comparison of guidelines available in the United States for diagnosis and management of diabetes before, during, and after pregnancy. *Journal of Women's Health, 16*(6), 790–801.

National Center for Complementary and Alternative Medicine (NCCAM). (2007). *What is complementary and alternative medicine (CAM)?* Retrieved from http://nccam.nih.gov/health/whatiscam/

North American Nursing Diagnosis Association (NANDA) International (2009–2011). *Nursing diagnoses—definitions and classification 2009–2011.* Ames, IA: Wiley Blackwell Publishing.

Theroux, R. (2008). Caffeine during pregnancy. *Nursing for Women's Health, 12*(3), 240–242.

U.S. Preventive Services Task Force. (2008, May). Screening for gestational diabetes mellitus: U.S. Preventive Services Task Force recommendation statement. *Annals of Internal Medicine, 148*(10), 759–765.

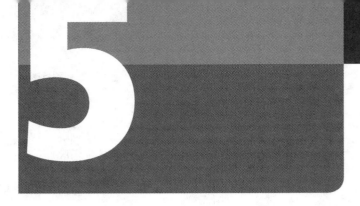

PREGNANCY COMPLICATED BY MEDICAL AND OTHER CONDITIONS

Harriet (Hatsie) Pearson Mallicoat

INFERTILITY

Infertility is a concern impacting quality of life and affecting approximately 10–15% of reproductive age couples (American Society for Reproductive Medicine [ASRM], 2006). *Infertility* refers to the inability to conceive, a prolonged time required for conception, or inability to sustain a pregnancy until birth. Infertility is present when the couple cannot conceive after at least 1 year of unprotected coitus. *Primary* infertility exists when no previous pregnancies have occurred. *Subfertility* is a descriptor for a couple in which both partners have decreased infertility. *Secondary* infertility exists when there has been a previously viable pregnancy but the couple has been unable to conceive during 1 or more years of unprotected intercourse. *Sterility* refers to the absolute inability to conceive or to sustain a pregnancy due to a physical condition such as lack of testes or uterus. The issue of infertility and seeking treatment causes emotional, social, physical, and economic impact for a couple during medical care.

■ Key Nursing Activities

- Assessment and data collection through complete history and physical exam.
- Teach about the ovulation process and therapies for supporting it.
- Explain diagnostic tests and procedures discussing time and rationale for each.
- Approach patient and partner with empathy and sensitive attitude to social, cultural, and spiritual issues involving treatment.
- Teach the woman and her partner about medical therapies and side effects with enough depth that they can seek treatment when necessary.
- Provide emotional support and foster decision making through the difficult infertility process.

■ Etiologies and Risk Factors

Infertility affects between 10% and 15% of couples wishing to conceive. In about 40% of cases, the man is infertile; no known causes or risk factors are present in about 20% of cases. The remainder of cases are due to ovulatory, ovarian, tubal, vaginal, or uterine problems in the female.

Female risk factors include congenital or developmental factors (abnormal formation of external genitals, absence of internal reproductive structures); ovarian factors (primary anovulation, hormonal disorders, amenorrhea after oral contraception, early menopause, increased prolactin levels); tubal/peritoneal factors (decreased motility, absence of fimbriated end of tube, total absence of tube, inflammation of tube or adhesion); uterine factors (tumors, Asherman's syndrome with scarring); and other factors such as endometriosis, sexually transmitted infections (STIs), cervicitis, pelvic inflammatory disease, and exposure to reproductive hazards including vinyl chlorides and alcohol. Also, stress can interrupt the cycle and antisperm antibodies can be formed by the woman against her partner's sperm.

Male risk factors include structural or hormonal disorders (undescended testes, hypospadias, varicocele, damage to testes from mumps, low levels of testosterone hormone); substance abuse (which causes changes and/or decrease in sperm, decrease in libido, impotence, or inability to ejaculate); sexually transmitted infections (cryptorchidism, prostatitis, epididymitis); obstruction or nutritional deficiencies (which disrupt the intricate process of fertility); and other factors involving disorders of endocrine, genetic, and psychologic systems. Workplace hazards or increased heating of the scrotum can also negatively affect sperm.

■ Signs and Symptoms

Subjective: Reported inability to conceive after 1 year of unprotected coitus.

Objective: Presence of one or more risk factors for infertility; absence of uterus, ovaries, tubes in females or testes in males; inability to sustain a viable pregnancy until delivery.

■ Diagnostic Studies

Each partner and the couple combined need evaluation. Tests range from noninvasive to extremely invasive, and sufficient information and preparation with an explanation of the rationale behind the tests needs to be offered to patients. These tests comprise a basic infertility survey, detect ovulation, and assess for immunologic incompatibility and are generally performed on the initial visit. They are done to rule out health problems that may be contributing to infertility. Questionnaires may be completed to evaluate psychologic factors.

Male and Female

- Complete blood cell count (CBC) with sedimentation rate if indicated. Detects or rules out inflammatory conditions that may be contributing to infertility.
- Serology. Determines if syphilis is present.

- Rh factor and blood grouping. Establishes baseline and identifies incompatibilities.
- Urinalysis. Rules out health problems that may be contributing to infertility.
- Chlamydia, gonorrhea testing. Determines presence of STIs.

Female

- Thyroid function. Determines thyroid hormone production as a possible contributing factor to infertility.
- Hormone levels, prolactin, estradiol, luteinizing hormone, progesterone, follicle-stimulating hormone, dehydroepiandrosterone (DHEA), androstenedione, testosterone, 17-hydroxyprogesterone. Determines adequacy because all are important to production of ova.
- Serum plasma progesterone assay. Determines the adequacy of corpus luteum production of progesterone.
- Basal body temperature. Entire cycle is charted. An elevation occurs in response to progesterone; documents ovulation.
- Cervical mucus evaluation (variable timing or ovulation). Evaluates for normal low viscosity, high spinnbarkeit (quality of mucus found near time of ovulation).
- Ultrasound: (ovulation). Detects and/or rules out pelvic abnormalities (uterus, tubes, ovaries) and to screen for follicular collapse if done at ovulation time.
- Hysterosalpingogram (7th–10th day of menstrual cycle). Radio opaque dye instilled into uterus to detect structural abnormalities and determine if fallopian tubes are patent or to determine the need to open them.
- Endometrial biopsy (21st–27th days, late luteal, late secretory phase). Determines endometrial response to progesterone and adequacy of luteal phase.
- Laparoscopy. Determines the presence of abnormalities, adhesions, endometriosis, etc.

Male

- Semen analysis. Evaluates liquefaction, volume, pH, density, count, morphology, motility, white cell count, and ovum penetration test (optional) to establish normal sperm range or identify problems.
- Basic endocrine studies if oligospermia or aspermia are present: hormonal assays, follicle-stimulating hormone, luteinizing hormone, prolactin, testosterone, 17-hydroxycorticoids and 17-ketosteroids, thyroid function; buccal smear and chromosome studies.
- Sperm penetration assay (after 2 days of but no more than 1 week of abstinence). Evaluates ability of sperm to penetrate an egg.
- Testicular biopsy. Determines prognosis and diagnosis in cases of azoospermia or severe oligospermia. When combined with vasography, it evaluates vas deferens and anatomy of testes for abnormalities.

Couple

- Postcoital (Sims-Huhner) test. An examination of postcoital mucus to determine the quality of the mucus and forward motility of sperm. Test is performed after intercourse at the expected time of ovulation or it can be 1–2 days prior to ovulation. The test does not affect a fertilized ovum.
- Sperm immobilization antigen-antibody reaction (variable timing or ovulation). Immunologic test to determine an immune interaction between sperm and cervical mucus.

▌ Medical Management

Management of infertility includes medications, surgical intervention (mentioned under procedures), and assisted reproductive therapies. Much decision making is required of couples since many of the treatments are expensive, and decisions must be made on some issues, such as risks of multiple gestation, need for multifetal reduction, and need for donor oocytes, sperm, embryos, or gestational carrier (surrogate mother) prior to treatment. If conception occurs, whether to or how to tell the child in the future and whether to freeze embryos for later use for another pregnancy are also questions for the couple to answer. Risks and benefits must be weighed since possible risk of long-term effects of medications and treatments on the women, children, and families can occur. Refer to textbooks or other resources for more information.

Medications

- Clomiphene citrate (Clomid): Oral; induces ovulation; treatment of luteal phase problem; common side effects may include visual disturbances, ovarian cysts or enlargement, bloating, nausea and vomiting, headache, hair loss, mood swings, breast tenderness, increased incidence of multiple births, and thick, dry cervical mucus.
- Menotropins (human menopausal gonadotropins; luteinizing hormone, follicle-stimulating hormone [Pergonal]; follitropin alfa [Gonal-F], follitropin beta [genetically engineered]): Intramuscular injection; ovarian follicular growth and maturation; given with human chorionic gonadotropin to induce ovulation. Common side effects include ovarian enlargement, potential hyperstimulation with multiple follicles and bloating (can require hospitalization), local reaction at injection site, multifetal gestations, mood swings, depression, increased incidence of miscarriage, and preterm birth.
- Follitropins (FSH): IM or SQ injection; treats polycystic ovaries; direct action on follicle; common side effects include local irritation, headaches, irritability, depression, fatigue, and edema.
- Human chorionic gonadotropin (Profasi, Ovidrel, Novarel, Pregnyl): Intramuscular or SQ injection; completes oocyte maturation; common side effects include local irritation at injection site, headache, edema, irritability, depression, and fatigue; when taken with gonadotropins, there is risk of ovarian hyperstimulation.
- Gonodotropin-releasing hormone agonists (danazol [oral Danacrine]), nafarelin acetate (nasal), leuprolide acetate (Lupron injection): Nasal spray or injection; treatment of endometriosis or fibroid over a 6-month period; common

side effects include nasal bleeding if nasal spray, irritation at site if injection, menopausal-like symptoms (hot flashes, vaginal dryness), myalgia and arthralgia, headaches, mild reversible bone loss; acne, hirsutism, hoarseness, amenorrhea, fluid retention, and ovarian cysts.

- Progesterone: Oral treatment for luteal phase inadequacy to stimulate endometrium; may be given by suppository; common side effects include breast tenderness, local irritation, and headaches.
- Gonadotropin-releasing hormone agonists (ganirelix acetate, cetrorelix acetate): Subcutaneous injection; controlled ovarian stimulation; common side effects include abdominal pain, headache, vaginal bleeding, and irritation at site of injection.
- Dopamine agonists (Parlodel): Oral; activates dopamine receptors in the pituitary to enhance fertility; common side effects include nausea, vomiting, nasal congestion, headache, dizziness, and decreased blood pressure.

Assisted Reproductive Therapies

- In vitro fertilization-embryo transfer (IVF-ET). The woman's eggs are collected from her ovaries, fertilized with sperm in the lab, and transferred back to her uterus after normal embryo development has occurred; indications are tubal problems, severe male infertility, cervical or immunologic problems.
- Gamete intrafallopian transfer (GIFT). Oocytes are taken from an ovary, placed in a catheter, washed with motile sperm, and immediately transferred back into the woman's tube so fertilization can occur there. The woman must have normal tube patency but the procedure is done for same reasons as IVF-ET.
- Gamete intrafallopian transfer with donor sperm (IVF-ET). The process is the same as gamete intrafallopian transfer but donor sperm is used; indications are the same as for gamete intrafallopian transfer, but it is also done for severe male infertility.
- Zygote intrafallopian transfer. The process is similar to IVF-ET, but ova are replaced in zygote stage. The indications are the same as for gamete intrafallopian transfer.
- Donor oocyte/embryo. Eggs are donated, inseminated, and then transferred into the woman's uterus, which has been hormonally prepped for accepting the embryo. The indications are for early menopause, removal of ovaries or absence of ovaries, autosomal or sex-linked disorders, or lack of fertilization in repeated IVF attempts.
- Gestational carrier (embryo host)/surrogate mother. The couple undertakes an IVF cycle, but the egg is transplanted into other woman's uterus to carry. Surrogacy is when a woman is impregnated with donor sperm from and carries the baby to term for another woman. Indications are an absent uterus, uterus with abnormalities, or medical condition that does not allow carrying of a fetus.
- Intracytoplasmic sperm injection. One sperm is injected into one egg to achieve fertilization with IVF; indications

are male with azoospermia, low sperm count, antisperm antibodies present, or presence of genetic defect.

- Assisted hatching. The zona pellucida is penetrated to create an opening for the dividing embryo to hatch and implant into the uterine wall. Indications are recurrent miscarriage, to improve implantation rate after previous IVF failure, or woman's advanced age.
- Artificial insemination. A man's sperm is used to inseminate his female partner.
- Therapeutic donor insemination. Donor sperm is used to inseminate the female patient.

Surgical Repair or Treatments

- Thyroid replacement if the woman (or man) has hypothyroidism
- Hormone replacement therapy for women with low estrogen levels
- Hydroxyprogesterone supplements for treatment of luteal phase abnormalities
- Treatment of endometriosis if present
- Surgical excision of ovarian tumors or release of tubal obstructions
- Surgical correction of uterine abnormalities such as bicornuate uterus
- Treatment of chronic inflammation or infection (such as from STIs, pelvic inflammatory disease)
- Surgical repair of male varicocele
- Surgical repair of male tubal continuity

▌ *Collaborative Problems*

Potential complications of surgical and/or procedural intervention:

- Infection

COLLABORATIVE (STANDARDIZED) CARE FOR ALL WOMEN WITH INFERTILITY

Perform comprehensive assessment to identify individual needs for teaching, emotional support, and physical care.

▌ Potential Complications of Surgical and/or Procedural Intervention: INFECTION

See generic collaborative care plan, "Potential Complication: Infection," beginning on p. 29 in Chapter 3.

Focus Assessments

- Assess invasive sites/incisions for signs of infection. Check for vaginal bleeding. Warmth, tenderness, swelling, purulent drainage, and erythema are indications of localized

infection. Early recognition allows for early intervention to prevent systemic infection.
- Assess vital signs. Temperature greater than 101°F (38.3°C) indicates the presence of systemic infection. Early recognition and treatment of systemic infection prevents sepsis and septic shock.
- Monitor laboratory data. Elevated white blood cell count indicates localized or systemic infection.
- Assess abdomen for bloating or pain. Some pain can result from air used to displace organs in order to do procedures postoperatively.

Preventive Nursing Activities

- Maintain medical and surgical asepsis. Good hand washing and adherence to sterile technique when indicated reduces the risk for introduction of microorganisms into wounds during surgical procedures or invasive diagnostic testing.
- Encourage the woman to maintain a well-balanced diet. Adequate nutrient intake is essential for tissue healing and a normal immune response.
- Encourage the woman to take adequate fluids. Fluid balance is essential for wound healing.
- Encourage the woman to obtain adequate rest and sleep. Fatigue produces stress, which is associated with increased production of cortisol. Cortisol suppresses normal immunity and increases the risk for development of infection.

INDIVIDUALIZED (NURSING DIAGNOSIS) CARE PLANS

These care plans were designed to address unique patient needs.

Infertility has long-term emotional, psychosocial, and spiritual implications for women who struggle to conceive and who may be unsuccessful in reaching their goal. Because success rates range from 4.6% to 27.3% varying on the age of the woman, the nurse's role is based on a highly specialized knowledge about fertility and reproduction and must be sensitive, supportive, and caring (McCarthy, 2008). Infertile women identified caring behavior in the nurse–patient relationship as nurses being available, providing communication, exhibiting compassion, demonstrating competency, and promoting empowerment (Hershberger & Kavanaugh, 2008).

▮ Nursing Diagnosis: KNOWLEDGE DEFICIENCY[1]

Related Factors: lack of understanding of the reproductive process with regard to conception and causes and treatment of infertility. Use with the generic care plan, "Deficient Knowledge,[1]" beginning on p. 131 in Chapter 2.

▮ Goals, Outcomes, and Evaluation Criteria

- Woman describes reproductive process and factors that negatively affect fertility.
- Woman describes tests and procedures to identify causes of infertility.
- Woman describes possible risk factors of diagnostic testing and treatment regimens.
- Woman describes self-care following diagnostic tests.
- Woman demonstrates signs of self-acceptance (maintains eye contact, smiles, talks about successes).
- Woman describes side effects and self-care measures for prescribed medications (e.g., danazol [Danocrine], clomiphene citrate [Clomid], and other medications mentioned in preceding section).

▮ NIC Interventions[2]

See the generic NDCP, "Deficient Knowledge,[1]" beginning on p. 13 in Chapter 2.

Fertility Preservation (7160)—Providing information, counseling, and treatment that facilitates reproductive health and the ability to conceive.

Reproductive Technology Management (7886)—Assisting a woman through the steps of a complex infertility treatment.

▮ Nursing Activities and Rationales

Assessments

- Assess level of understanding of reproduction and factors that adversely affect fertility and conception and give addition information to fill in gaps. Identifies teaching needs and corrects misconceptions about reproduction or infertility.
- Allow time for questions and processing of information with couple. Facilitates understanding and integration of knowledge.
- Provide information in a supportive manner regarding factors promoting conception, including common factors leading to infertility of either partner. Raises couple's awareness and promotes trust in caregiver.
- Assess the woman's and her partner's interest in alternatives to childbearing and acceptance of types of interventions. Determines if the couple is open to alternatives such as adoption in the event that conception is not possible. Also helps with value clarification as to what procedures and options fit into their value system and they are willing to utilize or not able to undergo due to personal belief system, personal risk, or finances.

Independent Nursing Actions

- Establish a trusting relationship with the woman and her partner. The woman must trust the nurse in order to share personal information, feelings, and concerns.
- Facilitate open communications between the woman and her partner. The ability to discuss and agree upon fertility testing and treatment will facilitate compliance and strengthen partner bonds.

- Encourage verbalization of concerns and fears. Decreases anxiety and allows for identification of needs so that appropriate interventions can be planned.
- Assess cultural, spiritual, and personal values that are also affecting the couple's responses and decision making. An opening to discuss options and the couple's value system will aid in decision making and allow the nurse to establish trust and understanding.

Patient/Family Teaching

- Teach the woman and her partner about normal reproduction and factors that affect fertility. Enhances their knowledge of reproduction as they attempt to conceive, to fill in knowledge gaps and correct misunderstandings about conception and fertility.
- Teach about the purpose, preparation, procedure, and self-care following diagnostic tests for fertility. Provides information about what the woman can expect before, during, and after testing; corrects any misconceptions.
- Teach the importance of maintaining therapeutic medical intervention schedules and timelines. Knowledge of the importance of maintaining treatment protocols may increase compliance and increase the couple's chance for success.
- Teach the actions, timing, and side effects of prescribed medications (e.g., danazol, clomiphene). Provides anticipatory guidance.
- Teach self-care measures of prescribed medications (e.g., danazol, clomiphene). Helps ensure compliance and provides a sense of control in the situation.

Nursing Diagnosis: RISK FOR SITUATIONAL LOW SELF-ESTEEM OR RISK FOR DISBURBED BODY IMAGE[1]

Related Factors: disappointment, loss of biologic fulfillment of becoming a parent, unrealistic expectations, frequent loss of pregnancies, and/or a long period of inability to conceive.

Goals, Outcomes, and Evaluation Criteria

- Woman verbalizes acceptance of self and own limitations; framing experience in realistic terms.
- Woman maintains hygiene and grooming; participates in acts of self-care and nurturing.
- Woman relays pride in successes and accepts failures realistically.

NIC Interventions[2]

Body Image Enhancement (5220)—Improving a patient's conscious and unconscious perceptions and attitudes toward his/her body.

Self-Esteem Enhancement (5400)—Assisting a patient to increase his/her personal judgment of self-worth.

Nursing Activities and Rationales

Assessments

- Assess for factors that contribute to low self-esteem, such as test results or failure to conceive that indicate infertility. Provides a basis for care planning.
- Monitor for negative/positive self-talk. Negative self-talk supports the presence of low self-esteem. Positive self-talk indicates positive self-esteem and may indicate that interventions are effective.
- Assess for feelings of self-blame or punishment. Couples who cannot conceive may have feelings of guilt or think that they caused their infertility. Identifying the existence of those feelings allows the nurse to intervene to correct the couple's misconceptions.
- Assess for blame placed by the partner. Infertility is a couple's problem, but sometimes the unaffected partner blames the infertile partner for the difficulties they're having with conception.
- Facilitate the couple's relationship and communication. Fosters their skills as partners experiencing this treatment and journey together. This will help them grow as a couple and mature whether or not they become parents.

Independent Nursing Actions

- Be attentive, accepting, and respectful of the woman and her partner. Acknowledges the woman's individuality, her depth of concern over her state of fertility/infertility, and communicates acceptance by others.
- Assist the woman to reframe and redefine negative expressions. Promotes positive self-talk, which enhances self-esteem.
- Encourage the woman to meet personal needs (proper hygiene, nutrition, rest), self-nurture, and find ways to make herself feel better. Enhances the woman's ability to look and feel her best, which helps reverse negative body image, withdrawn behavior, and sadness.
- Praise the woman for attainment of goals and improvements in hygiene and grooming. Reinforces desirable behavior and promotes the woman's self-esteem and positive body image.
- Discuss alternatives to childbearing such as surrogacy or adoption if appropriate. Refocuses the woman's attention on what may be possible rather than what is difficult or impossible to achieve. Provides hope for becoming a parent.
- Facilitate grieving process if decision to stay childless is made. Processing the experience will help put it into perspective in the story of her life.

Collaborative Activities

- Refer to a professional counselor for counseling as appropriate. The woman who learns she is infertile may suffer from depression, withdrawn behavior, and altered self-esteem.

Counseling enhances the woman's opportunities for recovery and returning to her usual lifestyle.

Patient/Family Teaching

- Teach the woman esteem-building exercises. Equips the woman with tools necessary for self-improvement.
- Provide information about actions and reflection that will improve self-nurture and self-care with improved self-esteem. Improving the woman's self-worth and body image will positively impact her self-esteem.

Nursing Diagnosis: POWERLESSNESS, RISK FOR[1]

Related Factors: inability to control the situation or prevent what may happen; possible inability to conceive; and the prospect of long-term treatments and expense without achieving desired outcome.

Goals, Outcomes, and Evaluation Criteria

- Woman verbalizes feelings of powerlessness.
- Woman identifies areas that she can and cannot control in her situation.
- Woman participates in the decision-making process regarding selection of testing and assisted reproduction therapies.
- Woman asks questions regarding the therapeutic regimen.
- Woman verbalizes the support she is receiving from her family and friends.

NIC Interventions[2]

Self-Esteem Enhancement (5400)—Assisting a patient to increase his/her personal judgment of self-worth.
Self-Responsibility Facilitation (4480)—Encouraging a patient to assume more responsibility for his or her own behavior.

Nursing Activities and Rationales

Assessments

- Assess the woman's perception of why she (or her partner) is infertile. The woman may blame herself or her partner or feel guilty for something she did or did not do that could have caused her to be infertile. She may feel that there is nothing that can be done to change the situation.
- Assess the knowledge level the woman and partner have regarding infertility, diagnostic tests, medical and surgical management, and possible complications. Increased understanding of infertility, its diagnosis, and treatment will help the woman gain some control of the situation.
- Assess the woman's support systems. The support system is very important to the woman who is facing a potentially long process of tests and treatments with no absolute guarantees for a successful pregnancy. The nurse needs to identify the makeup of the support system and help the woman to recognize who provides her support.

Independent Nursing Actions

- Encourage the partner to be involved in the woman's care. The partner needs to feel he can help in some manner; his involvement is supportive to the woman.
- Encourage the woman and partner to verbalize their feelings, perception of the situation, fears they may have, and the responsibility they have in the process. Verbalization of their feelings, perceptions, fears, and responsibilities is very important to clear up any guilt, self-blame, or misconceptions. Most importantly, the nurse needs to reinforce that the woman and family are not at fault. They need to understand they are not responsible for their infertility and they can help by being compliant with the treatment.

Patient/Family Teaching

- Teach the woman and partner about their responsibilities in regard to management of their infertility. Assists the couple to gain the control they need to participate in the management of their infertility.
- Teach the couple about diagnostic tests and treatments. Increased knowledge decreases fear of the unknown, which decreases stress and allows for increased control of the situation.
- Refer to a professional counselor as needed. Depression can occur with the length of time, energy, and investment into the infertility treatment and struggle to conceive.

Nursing Diagnosis: GRIEVING[1]

Related Factors: actual or perceived loss (inability to conceive; loss of parenthood).

Goals, Outcomes, and Evaluation Criteria

- Woman verbalizes feelings regarding loss (infertility).
- Woman identifies effective and ineffective coping patterns.
- Woman replaces ineffective with effective coping patterns.
- Woman returns to usual role within the family.
- Woman verbalizes comfort with present role within the family.
- Woman verbalizes need for assistance.
- Woman is free of physical signs of grief (inability to sleep or eat, loss of sexual drive, depression).

NIC Interventions[2]

Coping Enhancement (5230)—Assisting a patient to adapt to perceived stressors, changes, or threats that interfere with meeting life demands and roles.
Emotional Support (5270)—Provision of reassurance, acceptance, and encouragement during times of stress.
Family Integrity Promotion (7100)—Promotion of family cohesion and unity.
Grief Work Facilitation (5290)—Assistance with a significant loss.

▌ *Nursing Activities and Rationales*

Assessments

- Assess the degree of distress caused by the diagnosis of infertility. The woman may find it difficult to make decisions or perform self-care when severely distressed over learning that she will not be able to conceive. Determining the degree of distress allows the nurse to plan appropriate interventions.
- Assess for signs of anxiety, fear, or sadness. Psychologic stresses can result in physical changes such as loss of appetite, inability to sleep, or sexual disturbances.
- Assess for feelings of guilt. Determines if the woman (or couple) is blaming herself (or themselves) for their inability to conceive. Self-blame is not an uncommon emotion upon learning about infertility.
- Assess couple's relationship and their family relationships. Determines if the couple's relationship is healthy and/ or strong enough to survive their current situation. If not, interventions can be planned to strengthen the relationship.
- Assess for use of defense mechanisms. Determines if the woman/couple are using unhealthy defense mechanisms that may prolong their grief or interfere with the grief process.
- Assess couple's openness to discussion of alternatives, such as adoption or surrogate pregnancy. Determines if the woman is ready to discuss alternatives to her current situation. Refocusing on other means of obtaining a child may provide hope and help with the grieving process.

Independent Nursing Actions

- Establish trust. The woman is more likely to express her concerns and grief if she trusts the nurse.
- Offer comfort when the woman expresses grief. Grieving persons are especially sensitive to the emotions and sincerity of others. Discussions that produce discomfort for the woman should be avoided until the woman demonstrates readiness by openly communicating her feelings.
- Encourage the woman to postpone decision making while severely stressed. Thinking and decision making are altered by grief and stress. Important decisions should be postponed.
- Encourage expression of sadness over loss. Facilitates the grief process.
- Encourage honest and open communications between the woman and her partner. Prevents the couple from feeling alienated from one another or from blaming one another.
- Reinforce use of constructive defense mechanisms. Mechanisms that are positively reinforced are more likely to be repeated.
- Encourage couple to seek support from others who have also experienced infertility. Persons who have endured the same or similar problems and undergone similar grief can be very helpful to others undergoing the same feelings. It helps

the couple recognize that they are not alone in their feelings.
- Refer for counseling if appropriate. If the couple is unable to express their grief or is paralyzed by their grief, counseling may be appropriate. It is a positive sign when couples are willing to seek assistance in dealing with their grief.

Patient/Family Teaching

- Teach the woman to use constructive defense mechanisms. Strategies such as contact with others, use of distraction, or using quiet time to reflect are constructive and may help the woman cope with her current situation.
- Teach regarding the grieving process as appropriate. Helps the woman understand her emotions and that they are a normal part of the grieving process.
- Teach the woman regarding availability of support groups in her community. The woman may be unaware of the availability of community resources or emotionally unable to seek out such resources.

▌ *Other Nursing Diagnoses*

Also assess for the following nursing diagnoses, which are frequently present, such as:
- Ineffective Individual Coping[1] related to length and stressfulness of treatments and tests.
- Ineffective Sexuality Patterns[1] related to lack of libido secondary to imposed restriction and emotional reactions to infertility and/or testing/treatment.

GENETIC DISORDERS

The study of genetics and genetic disorders has assumed increasing importance because of the Human Genome Project, which began in 1990. The initial mapping sequence was completed in 2000. Since then, genomics and genetic advances have changed nursing implications for prenatal screening and will continue to impact practice.

Standard preconceptual and prenatal care includes assessment of all pregnant women for heritable disorders in order to identify potential problems. Preconceptual genetic screening allows parents the full range of reproductive choices. Because recognition of genetic disorders during pregnancy can be emotionally distressing, the distress must be considered when planning care (Rappaport, 2008).

Genetic disorders may be due to abnormalities of the genes (a segment of DNA) or of the entire chromosome, which are made up of genes. **Chromosomal abnormalities** involve many genes, so they often cause major defects (e.g., Down syndrome, Turner's syndrome). Chromosomal abnormalities can occur in the autosomes or the sex (X, Y) chromosomes and are either *numerical* (e.g., a missing or extra chromosome) or *structural* (e.g., a chromosome has a missing part, adheres to another chromosome, is fragile at a specific site, or the DNA has been rearranged). **Genetic disorders** may be due to *multifactorial* inheritance (caused by an interaction of environmental factors and many genes, e.g., cleft palate, spina bifida, pyloric stenosis, and club foot) or *unifactorial (single) gene inheritance* (an abnormality in a single gene or gene pair).

Patterns of **single gene inheritance** are classified as follows:

- *Autosomal dominant inheritance:* An abnormal gene dominates the normal gene of the pair to produce the disorder/trait. Examples include Huntington's disease, polycystic kidney disease, Marfan syndrome, and achondroplastic dwarfism. Both sexes are equally affected.
- *Autosomal recessive inheritance:* The person must have two abnormal genes in order to have the disorder. That is, both parents must pass on the same abnormal gene in order for the child to be affected. If only one parent passes on the abnormal gene, the child will be a carrier (that is, will be able to pass on the gene to offspring, but will not have the disorder). A carrier state can be undetected until screening is done, often during prenatal care. Most inborn errors of metabolism are in this class. Examples include phenylketonuria, galactosemia, maple syrup urine disease, Tay-Sachs disease, cystic fibrosis, and sickle cell anemia.
- *X-linked dominant:* The abnormal gene is carried on the X chromosome, but because it is the dominant gene, both male and female children are affected by the condition. Since females have two X chromosomes, they are usually affected less often than males. Males transmit the abnormal gene only on the X chromosome to the daughters. Examples include vitamin D–resistant rickets and fragile X syndrome.
- *X-linked recessive:* The abnormal gene is carried on the X chromosome. Therefore, the condition occurs in the male when the abnormal gene is passed on by a carrier mother. There is no male-to-male transmission. Examples include hemophilia, color blindness, and Duchenne muscular dystrophy.
- *Inborn errors of metabolism:* These conditions follow a recessive pattern of inheritance and result in disorder of protein, fat, or carbohydrate metabolism because of absent or defective enzymes.

■ Key Nursing Activities

- Assess for risk factors through detailed family history to determine the possibility of inheritable conditions. Provide guidance through the appropriate testing.
- Teach regarding the disorder and diagnostic or screening test for the disorder, highlighting the difference. A screening test does not give a yes or no answer; it only gives an indication of a problem and the need to do further diagnostic testing that will give answers. Explain that false positives are possible.
- Explain informed consent with proper safeguarding of information.
- Facilitate decision making and emotional support after gaining genetic information; assist with coping with the implications of the test.
- Refer for genetic counseling and follow-up care after counseling.

- Maintain privacy and confidentiality and consistently carry out tasks with respect.

■ Etiologies and Risk Factors

The risk of giving birth to an infant with an inherited disorder is higher in the following situations:

- maternal age of 35 years or older
- parent with known chromosomal abnormality
- delivery of a previous infant with a genetic disorder and/or a congenital anomaly
- previous stillbirth or perinatal loss of unknown cause
- family pedigree documenting an inherited genetic disorder with known ethnic correlation to genetic problems
- maternal metabolic disorder
- significant exposure to radiation, infection, drugs, or chemicals (Perry, Hockenberry, Lowdermilk, Wilson, 2009)

■ Signs and Symptoms

Each genetic disorder is associated with signs and symptoms that may be present at birth or that may be identified later. Specific indication of the disorder is provided by the presence of the abnormal gene on genetic testing.

Signs *during the pregnancy* that indicate increased risk include the following:

- Polyhydramnios
- Oligohydramnios
- Fetal intrauterine growth restriction
- Diminished movement

Signs present *at birth* that indicate increased risk include the following:

- Deviation from expected growth and development milestones
- Development of abnormal characteristics associated with the specific disorder (e.g., protruding tongue, flat nasal bridge, Simian crease, poor muscle tone, low-set ears, abdominal distention, failure to pass meconium)

■ Diagnostic Studies

Genetic evaluation may be done before pregnancy, during pregnancy, or after an infant is born with a disorder.

Preconception and Prenatal Testing

Testing is done to identify parents at risk for transmitting genetic disorders and to diagnose fetal abnormalities prior to or during pregnancy.

- Screening/risk assessment/detailed history. Identifies patients at risk for transmission of a genetic disorder (e.g., family history of hereditary disease/disorders, advanced maternal age).
- Physical examination. Detects signs of inherited disorders.
- Maternal buccal or serum chromosomal and DNA analysis. Determines specific genetic markers.

- Transvaginal ultrasound. Used during the first trimester to determine fetal viability, gestational age, and structural abnormalities. Fetal nuchal translucency screening (fluid at nape of neck) can be indicative of genetic disorder/physical anomalies at 10–14 weeks.
- Level 2 ultrasound. Higher definition ultrasound assesses for fetal growth, development, anatomy, cord vessels and structure, placental position and maturation, and amniotic fluid volume.
- Biophysical profile. Assesses for fetal breathing movements, fetal movement, fetal tone, fetal heart rate, and amniotic fluid volume.
- Alpha-fetoprotein. Usually done as part of triple screen to screen for neural tube defect. Levels are elevated in the presence of an open neural tube defect or open abdominal wall defect. Must be correlated to fetal gestational age and is altered if multifetal pregnancy is present.
- Triple-marker test. Maternal serum tests performed at 16–18 weeks of gestation to measure levels of maternal serum alpha-fetoprotein, unconjugated estriol, and human chorionic gonadotropin; screens for genetic disorders; further tests must be done to diagnose disorders.
- Hemoglobin analyses. Tests for sickle cell and thalassemia anemias.
- Amniocentesis. Performed in early second trimester (15–17 weeks), early (10–15 weeks), for prenatal diagnosis of genetic disorders or congenital anomalies. Amniotic fluid is removed transabdominally with a needle placed in an amniotic fluid sac.
- Chorionic villus sampling and culture. Determines the genetic makeup of the fetus. This is done with an endoscopic needle aspiration of extraplacental villi inserted through the cervix.
- Percutaneous umbilical blood sampling. Tests fetal blood and cells to provide information that is not available through assessment of the amniotic fluid. Blood samples from cord close to placenta are removed with ultrasound guidance. Percutaneous umbilical blood sampling is useful for determining which women are at increased risk of transmitting inherited blood disorders; determines the presence of genetic disorders through chromosome karyotypes; or if the woman is Rh negative and has been sensitized.
- Fetal cell cultures. Detects presences of genetic disorders through chromosome karyotypes.
- Fetal chromosome analysis. Detects chromosome abnormalities through karyotypes.
- Magnetic resonance imaging. Evaluates fetal structure (soft tissue) and growth in selected cases where visualization of fetal detail is critical.

Diagnosis of an Infant With a Birth Defect

A genetic disorder may not be suspected until the infant is born with an anomaly. Tests are performed on the infant to determine whether the anomaly is caused by genetic factors.

- Physical examination, ultrasound, X-ray, echocardiogram. Identifies specific characteristics and structural defects and evaluates organ function and skeletal features.
- DNA and chromosomal analysis. Determines karyotypes and specific genetic markers.
- Tests for inherited metabolic disorders (e.g., cystic fibrosis, phenylketonuria, galactosemia, hypothyroidism). Identifies such disorders early so that treatment can begin early.
- Hemoglobin analysis. Identifies sickle cell disease and related disorders and ABO incompatibility.
- Immunological analysis. Assesses for presence of or exposure to infections.

▌ Medical Management

- Identification of patients at risk for transmission of genetic disorders through pedigree of family documentation and karyotyping of prospective parents.
- Informed consent for all prenatal and postnatal genetic testing.
- Genetic counseling related to risks for fetal transmission of genetic disorders and to outcomes for individuals who have clinical manifestations of or genetic markers linked to a genetic disorder.
- Fetal treatment. When a treatable fetal disorder is identified prenatally (e.g., digitalis for fetal cardiac arrhythmias; galactose-free diet for a mother carrying a fetus with galactosemia).
- Therapeutic abortion. For parents who choose this option for dealing with a genetic disease.
- Counseling regarding childbearing/parenting options and decision making. Couples can decide to conceive or not, to carry the baby to term or not, to prevent pregnancy with tubal ligation or vasectomy, or to conceive using various assistive reproductive techniques (e.g., in vitro fertilization using donor eggs or sperm).

▌ Collaborative Problems

Genetic problems affect 2–3% of living newborns, but because some are delayed in appearance, the number may be higher (Norton, 2008). This care plan focuses on the collaborative problems that result from antepartum diagnostic testing for genetic disorders.

- Potential complications of amniocentesis: fetal injury, infection, fetal loss, amniotic fluid leakage, and bleeding.
- Potential complications of chorionic villus sampling: vaginal bleeding (light spotting to fetal-maternal hemorrhage), spontaneous abortion and fetal loss, chorioamnionitis, oligohydramnios, and rupture of membranes.
- Potential complication of percutaneous umbilical blood sampling: fetal bradycardia, fetal bleeding, infection, cord bleeding, maternal alloimmunization, preterm labor and contractions, maternal thromboembolism.

COLLABORATIVE (STANDARDIZED) CARE PLANS FOR ALL PATIENTS WITH GENETIC DISORDERS

Perform comprehensive assessment to identify individual needs for teaching, emotional support, and physical care.

■ Potential Complication of Amniocentesis: FETAL INJURY OR LOSS, INFECTION, LOSS OF FLUID, OR BLEEDING

Refer to generic collaborative care plans for the following complications: "Fetal Compromise," "Hemorrhage," and "Infection" beginning on pp. 27, 28, and 29, respectively, in Chapter 3. Also refer to "Antepartum Fetal Monitoring and Other Diagnostic Tests," beginning on p. 60 in Chapter 4, for specific care for the woman undergoing amniocentesis.

Focus Assessments

- Perform ultrasound determination of position of placenta, fetal parts, and umbilical cord before performance of amniocentesis. Prevents accidental puncture and injury to the fetus, cord, or placenta.
- Monitor FHR and maternal vital signs before, during, and after amniocentesis. Establishes baseline vitals and determines if variations occur following invasive procedure. Vital signs should remain within these ranges: temperature 97–to 98.8°F, pulse 80–100 beats/min, blood pressure (BP) 100/60–138/88, and respirations 16–22.

Preventive Nursing Activities

- Determine that informed consent was obtained. Establishes that the woman consents to the procedure and understands its related risks, benefits, and expected outcomes. Informed consent protects the patient, nurse, and physician.
- Prepare the puncture site with antibacterial scrub prior to the amniocentesis. Reduces incidence of skin contaminants being introduced into the amniotic sac, which predisposes the woman to infection.
- Teach the woman to report temperature elevation above 101°F (37.8°C) to her physician immediately. May indicate an intrauterine infection. Early reporting of fever will allow for early medical intervention.
- Report any contractions or preterm labor signs to physician. Contractions may lead to preterm labor and may require interventions to avoid early delivery.

■ Potential Complication of Chorionic Villus Sampling: VAGINAL BLEEDING, SPONTANEOUS ABORTION, RUPTURE OF MEMBRANES, INFECTION

Refer to generic collaborative care plans for "Potential Complication: Hemorrhage," "Potential Complication: Premature Rupture of Membranes," and "Potential Complication: Preterm Labor," beginning on pp. 28, 30, and 31, respectively, in Chapter 3. Also refer to "Nursing Care Plan: Preterm Labor and Spontaneous Abortion" and "Nursing Care Plan: Premature Rupture of Membranes," beginning on pp. 197 and 206 in Chapter 6, respectively; and to "Antepartum Fetal Monitoring and Other Diagnostic Tests," beginning on p. 60 in Chapter 4, for care of the woman undergoing chorionic villus sampling.

Focus Assessments

- Assess for excessive vaginal bleeding or leakage of amniotic fluid. Determines the presence of complications. Complications such as fetal loss, rupture of membranes, infection, or bleeding occur in 6 per 10,000 women undergoing chorionic villus sampling (Summers et al., 2007).
- Monitor FHR and maternal vital signs before, during, and for 2 hours after chorionic villus sampling. Establishes baseline and serves as a source for comparison following the procedure.

Preventive Nursing Activities

- Determine that informed consent was obtained. Establishes that the woman consents to the procedure and understands its related risks, benefits, and expected outcomes. Informed consent protects the patient, nurse, and physician.
- Instruct the woman to monitor her temperature for 2–3 days after the procedure and report temperature above 101°F immediately. Increased temperature is a sign of chorioamnionitis, which occurs in 0.5% of patients undergoing chorionic villus sampling.
- Teach the woman to expect some vaginal spotting and to monitor for cramping after procedure. Vaginal spotting is an expected outcome due to disruption of the chorionic villi. Excessive bleeding should be reported, and increased cramping could forewarn of a spontaneous abortion.

Potential Complication of Percutaneous Umbilical Blood Sampling: FETAL HEMORRHAGE AND/OR INJURY, CORD LACERATION, AND THROMBOEMBOLISM

Refer to generic collaborative care plans for Fetal Compromise beginning on p. 27 in Chapter 3. Also refer to "Antepartum Fetal Monitoring and Other Diagnostic Tests," beginning on p. 60 in Chapter 4, for specific care for the woman undergoing amniocentesis.

Focus Assessments

- Monitor fetal heart rate for 2 hours after percutaneous umbilical blood sampling. Determines variations outside FHR baseline in order to verify fetal well-being. Determines whether placenta or blood vessel was punctured and if transfusion might be necessary.
- Monitor puncture site for evidence of bleeding or leakage of amniotic fluid. Amniotic leakage can occur. The site needs to be evaluated for closure so that infection does not occur from an open portal of pathogenic entry.
- Monitor maternal vital signs and for uterine irritability. Elevated temperature and early cramping can be signs of infection. Preterm labor can occur from chorioamnionitis.

Preventive Nursing Activities

- Prepare the woman for ultrasound scanning for percutaneous umbilical blood sampling. Fetal blood sampling and transfusion are performed through the umbilical cord at 1–2 centimeters from its placental insertion site. At this point the cord is well anchored and moves minimally, which decreases the risk of maternal placental blood contamination.
- Determine that informed consent was obtained by the physician. Documentation of informed consent includes the woman's consent to the procedure and verifies that she has been informed of its risks, benefits, and expected outcomes. Informed consent protects the patient, nurse, and physician.
- Instruct the woman to monitor her temperature for 2–3 days after the procedure and report temperature above 101°F (38.3°C). Increased temperature is a sign of chorioamnionitis, which occurs in 0.5% of patients following invasive procedures such as percutaneous umbilical blood sampling.

INDIVIDUALIZED (NURSING DIAGNOSIS) CARE PLANS

This section includes care plans designed to address unique patient needs.

Whether in preparation for testing, during testing, or delivering results and supporting the woman/couple during decision making afterward, the nurse must be mindful of ethics in this delicate situation. The patient has a right to autonomy, nonmaleficence, beneficence, and justice. (Zindler, 2005). In addition, this information needs to be relayed in an objective manner free from bias. Alternatives and counseling to help with decision making should be available and the woman's/couple's preferences should be supported in a nonjudgmental way.

Nursing Diagnosis: ANXIETY[1]

Related Factors: uncertain outcomes of genetic testing and treatments, presence of risk factors (e.g., advanced maternal age, family history), unconscious conflict about essential values/goals of life, situational crisis, threat to self-concept, and guilt.

Refer to generic NDCP, "Anxiety," which begins on p. 10 in Chapter 2.

Goals, Outcomes, and Evaluation Criteria

- Woman seeks information to reduce anxiety.
- Woman verbalizes that she will be able to cope with the results of genetic testing.
- Woman verbalizes understanding of the necessary genetic testing.
- Woman demonstrates positive coping mechanisms throughout genetic testing related to feelings of anxiety.
- Woman uses relaxation techniques to reduce anxiety.

NIC Interventions[2]

Examination Assistance (7680)—Providing assistance to the patient and another healthcare provider during a procedure or exam.
Telephone Consultation (8180)—Eliciting patient's concerns, listening, and providing support, information, or teaching in response to patient's stated concerns, over the telephone.

Nursing Activities and Rationales

Assessments

- Assess for indicators of anxiety. Confusion in thoughts, forgetfulness, impaired attention, difficulty concentrating, and diminished ability to solve problems and make decisions are characteristics of anxiety.

Collaborative Activities

- Refer the woman to community support agencies available for preparation for a child with a genetic disorder. The woman may need support and guidance after she receives the results of her genetic testing that indicate she will have a child with genetic issues. She may be unaware of community resources that are available to her.

Patient/Family Teaching

- Explain the rationale for genetic testing procedures. Gains the woman's cooperation, decreases her anxiety level, and provides her with accurate information for decision making related to the results.
- Explain to the woman that anxiety is normal. Reassures the woman that she is experiencing a normal reaction to her current situation.
- Explain the signs and symptoms of anxiety to the woman. Decreases fear of the unknown and reassures her that what she is experiencing is a normal reaction to anxiety.
- Encourage use of coping strategies such as progressive muscle relaxation, guided imagery, rhythmic breathing, and distraction. These methods have been shown to successfully reduce and manage anxiety.
- Guide the woman through verbalization of what she thinks is going to happen to her and the fetus related to the genetic testing procedure. Provides guidance to the woman in understanding the situation and helps her focus on realistic outcomes.
- Provide the woman with information about the prescribed therapies, community resources, educational programs, support and self-help groups if results are abnormal. Provides information that addresses her physical and psychologic needs. The woman may be unaware of resources available to her.

■ Nursing Diagnosis: DEFICIENT KNOWLEDGE[1]

Related Factors: lack of knowledge and/or experience with genetic testing procedures and outcomes.

Use generic NDCP, "Anxiety,[1]" which begins on p. 10 in Chapter 2.

■ Goals, Outcomes, and Evaluation Criteria

- Woman verbalizes understanding of genetic testing procedure(s), risks, and benefits.
- Woman verbalizes understanding of screening versus diagnostic testing and identifies the disorder the test is focused on.
- Woman verbalizes awareness that further testing may be needed and that decisions may need to be made in a short amount of time.
- Woman describes inherited genetic disorder and its impact on offspring.
- Woman verbalizes expected outcomes of genetic testing.
- Woman verbalizes understanding of information she has received.

■ NIC Interventions[2]

Genetic Counseling (5242)—Use of an interactive helping process focusing on assisting the coping of an individual, family, or group manifesting or at risk for developing or transmitting a birth defect or genetic condition.

Learning Facilitation (5520)—Promoting the ability to process and comprehend information.

Learning Readiness Enhancement (5540)—Improving the ability and willingness to receive information.

Preconception Counseling (5247)—Screening and providing information and support to individuals of childbearing age before pregnancy to promote health and reduce risks.

Support Group (5430)—Use of a group environment to provide emotional support and health-related information for members.

■ Nursing Activities and Rationales

Assessments

- Assess the woman's purpose, perceptions, and goals for genetic counseling. Establishes a baseline of information the woman possesses; determines the accuracy of the information; and determines whether or not her expectations are realistic.
- Assess the quality of family support and coping mechanism available. Determines if family support will be available to assist the woman/couple to cope with information or poor outcomes.

Collaborative Activities

- Provide a referral to a genetic healthcare specialist. Assists the woman with finding current and accurate information on the genetic disorder likely to be experienced by her newborn.
- Refer to providers who will likely be caring for the baby following birth (e.g., pediatric cardiologist or cardiac surgeon) if the fetus has a cardiac defect that will probably be surgically corrected immediately after birth. At times, the woman may be sent to a special center for delivery so that the baby will be born close to the hospital or physician he or she will need immediately after birth. This is especially true if there are a very few centers equipped to care for the baby's condition.

Patient/Family Teaching

- Begin instruction only after the woman demonstrates a readiness to learn. Learning is not likely to occur until after the woman/couple has addressed the feelings about the presence of a genetic disorder that affects the current or future pregnancies.
- Present to the woman/couple that the test being considered is elective and help them with decision making about whether to proceed with testing or not. Some women/couples won't want to seek genetic testing because they have a values system and faith that their child is the child they were meant to have regardless of any genetic defects or disorders.
- Provide information on the transmission risks based upon family history, phenotype, and genotype. Provides the woman/couple with adequate information to make

decisions regarding planning, continuing, or terminating the pregnancy.

- Inform the woman about the genetic disorder, its treatment, and management. It is preferred to tell the woman with her partner so they can begin to process information together. Promotes couple interaction and learning information together to begin to form realistic expectations about the child.
- Present the content in a logical sequence and in a stimulating manner. Presentation from simple to complex assists the woman with mastering the content. Using stimulating approaches helps hold the couple's attention and enhances learning.
- Teach about early fetal development and the effects of personal habits including medication use, teratogens, and self-care. If the woman has an increased risk for delivery of an infant with a congenital anomaly, changes in lifestyle may affect the pregnancy in a positive manner.
- Allow time for questions. Anxiety from hearing an unexpected result can block processing information. The woman/couple needs time to process information and ask questions and receive answers.

Nursing Diagnosis: RISK FOR INTERRUPTED FAMILY PROCESSES[1]

Related Factors: stressors of actual genetic testing results; disruption in the usual functions of the family related to the stress and negative outcomes of genetic testing; the situational crisis created by genetic testing; and the strained family interactions related to the unpredictable or negative outcomes of genetic testing.

▌ Goals, Outcomes, and Evaluation Criteria

- Woman reports comfort with role expectations after the result of genetic testing is known.
- Woman expresses adequate awareness of and contact with professional and social support systems.
- Woman involves family members in decision making regarding outcomes of genetic testing.
- Woman is able to proceed forward and make decisions about the outcome of the pregnancy (termination, continuation).
- Woman adapts to developmental transitions based on outcomes of genetic testing.
- Woman acknowledges existence of condition and its potential to alter family routines.
- Woman participates in anticipatory planning for the new child with a genetic disorder.
- Woman meets physical and psychosocial needs of family members.
- Woman obtains adequate resources to meet the needs of the family members.

- Couple and family work together to promote cohesion and meet goals.

▌ NIC Interventions[2]

Counseling (5240)—Use of an interactive helping process focusing on the needs, problems, or feelings of the woman and significant others to enhance or support coping, problem solving, and interpersonal relationships.

Emotional Support (5270)—Provision of reassurance, acceptance, and encouragement during times of stress.

Family Integrity Promotion (7100)—Promotion of family cohesion and unity.

Family Process Maintenance (7130)—Minimization of family process disruption effects.

Family Support (7140)—Promotion of family values, interests, and goals.

Financial Resource Assistance (7380)—Assisting an individual/family to secure and manage finances to meet healthcare needs.

Normalization Promotion (7200)—Assisting parents and other family members of children with chronic illnesses or disabilities in providing normal life experiences for their children and families.

Role Enhancement (5370)—Assisting a patient, significant other, and/or family to improve relationships by clarifying and supplementing specific role behaviors.

▌ Nursing Activities and Rationales

Assessments

- Assess knowledge base regarding clinical signs and symptoms for child's condition. Determines the woman's knowledge base and establishes need for teaching.
- Assess for family processes and role changes that must occur if the woman/couple is faced with care of an infant with a genetic disorder. Determines the current functioning of the family unit and identifies the initial changes that need to occur so that a plan of action can be devised.
- Assess the family support system's response to the possibility of a genetic disorder before and/or after birth. A strong family support system can provide much needed emotional support when the woman/couple begins to feel hopeless.
- Assess the family for areas of concern, dissatisfaction, and conflict related to decision making for a child with a genetic disorder. Clear identification of the family issues assists the family to begin resolution. Couples who are in newer relationships are at greater risk for future problems due to the stress of a developmental needs child.
- Determine the emotional and psychologic reaction to the infant's genetic condition and its prognosis. Assisting the family to recognize feelings such as anxiety, anger, and sadness will help facilitate their coping and dealing with those feelings in a positive manner.

Independent Nursing Actions

- Support family with grieving process because the initial impact of a genetic disorder is the loss of a dream; the loss of the perfect child that the couple imagined. They must grieve over their loss before they can start planning. Assure them that grief, initial denial, and sorrow are all normal responses to such news.
- Support family with the decision-making process and give information about different options without involving your own judgment. Therapeutic abortion is a choice for some disorders and information should be given as an alternative to the couple's choices.
- Design strategies that will be least disruptive to family functioning if they assume care of the infant with a genetic disorder. Planning provides the family with a realistic picture of the schedule and role changes that will be required to meet family functioning needs.

Patient/Family Teaching

- Teach family members who comprise the woman's support system ways they can help the woman/couple adapt and make decisions about the genetic disorder. A strong family support system can greatly assist the couple with decision making by listening and helping interpret information.
- Teach the couple about the child's genetic condition, treatment requirements, and availability of associated support groups. Accurate and adequate information allows the couple to make informed decisions and helps prepare them for care of a child with a genetic disorder.
- Teach the family how to reset and accomplish goals while caring for an infant with a genetic disorder. Their future goals will need to incorporate the addition of a child with a genetic disorder into the family.

Nursing Diagnosis: SPIRITUAL DISTRESS[1]

Related Factors: conflicting moral, ethical, and religious beliefs regarding genetic testing outcomes and decisions (e.g., whether to have a therapeutic abortion, whether to use contraceptives to prevent pregnancy); situational and maturational losses, current poor relationships, low self-esteem, physical or psychologic stress, and questioning related to life suffering and existence.

Goals, Outcomes, and Evaluation Criteria

- Woman expresses meaning and purpose in life after receiving genetic testing results.
- Woman seeks counsel from clergy and/or leaders from their faith, cultural, or spiritual system to assist with decision making regarding outcomes of genetic testing.

- Woman verbalizes a sense of inner peace, self-control, and trust in decision making related to genetic testing outcomes.

NIC Interventions[2]

Decision-Making Support (5250)—Providing information and support for a patient who is making a decision regarding health care.

Emotional Support (5270)—Provision of reassurance, acceptance, and encouragement during times of stress.

Hope Instillation (5310)—Facilitation of the development of a positive outlook in a given situation.

Spiritual Growth Facilitation (5426)—Facilitation of growth in patient's capacity to identify, connect with, and call upon the source of meaning, purpose, comfort, strength, and hope in his/her life.

Spiritual Support (5420)—Assisting the client to feel balance and connection with a greater power.

Values Clarification (5480)—Assisting another to clarify her/his own values in order to facilitate effective decision making.

Nursing Activities and Rationales

Assessments

- Assess the woman's values and beliefs that will conflict or support decisions regarding genetic testing and outcome decisions. Establishes a baseline understanding of the woman's belief system so that the nurse can support those beliefs while the woman/couple make decisions following genetic testing.
- Assess the woman's feelings regarding the alternatives that conflict with her values, ethics, and/or spiritual beliefs. Verbalization of feelings assists the woman to discuss options and alternatives and provides the nurse with information that will be used in supporting the decisions made by the woman.
- Assess whether the woman has an objective, realistic understanding of the situation. It is important that the woman is well grounded in reality so that she understands the long-term implications of her decisions.
- Determine the woman's usual way of solving a problem when it conflicts with her values, ethics, or spiritual beliefs. Discussing the woman's usual decision-making framework will assist the nurse in providing guidance to continued use of that process.

Collaborative Activities

- Refer the woman to her spiritual care provider for support. Provides additional guidance and support in decision making regarding genetic testing and outcomes.
- Refer the woman for genetic counseling. Assists the woman to gain complete understanding of the ramifications of decisions made regarding the pregnancy and genetic outcomes.

Patient/Family Teaching

- Encourage the woman to seek advice from her primary spiritual caregiver. The primary spiritual caregiver will be able to assist the woman to work through issues and possible decisions that conflict with values, ethics, and/or religious beliefs.
- Maintain a sense of hope when teaching the family about genetic counseling and decision making. The situation needs to be presented realistically, but with hope and positive adaptation emphasized.
- Inform the woman of alternative courses of action based upon her beliefs and values. Assists the woman with understanding that there are choices that may be acceptable and compatible with her belief system.
- Acknowledge the woman's spiritual and cultural background. Demonstrates acceptance and willingness to assist the woman with problem solving, while taking into consideration her belief system.
- Provide information that the woman requests regarding diagnosis, treatment, and prognosis. Providing the woman with accurate information assists her in making informed decisions. The woman demonstrates her readiness to learn when she seeks out information.

Nursing Diagnosis: DECISIONAL CONFLICT[1]

Related Factors: lack of acceptable consequences of alternatives of genetic testing (e.g., whether to continue or terminate pregnancy after a diagnosis of fetal anomaly), multiple or divergent sources or information, unclear personal values or beliefs not providing framework for decision making, lack of experience with making decisions when outcomes are unpredictable.

▌ *Goals, Outcomes, and Evaluation Criteria*

- Woman demonstrates self-direction in decision making.
- Woman uses problem-solving techniques to achieve desired outcomes.
- Woman identifies available professional and family support for achieving desired outcomes.
- Woman exhibits organized thought processes when making decisions.
- Woman identifies alternatives and potential consequences of each alternative.

▌ *NIC Interventions[2]*

Coping Enhancement (5230)—Assisting a patient to adapt to perceived stressors, changes, or threats that interfere with meeting life demands and roles.
Decision-Making Support (5250)—Providing information and support for a patient who is making a decision regarding health care.

Mutual Goal Setting (4410)—Collaborating with a patient to identify and prioritize care goals, then developing a plan for achieving those goals.
Preconception Counseling (5247)—Screening and providing information and support to individuals of childbearing age before pregnancy to promote health and reduce risks.

▌ *Nursing Activities and Rationales*

Assessments

- Assess the woman's psychologic responses to the situation and how her feelings affect her decision-making capabilities. Helps the nurse understand and support the woman throughout the testing and decision-making process.
- Offer information on grief as the loss of a perfect child must be dealt with, and passed through, to begin to take hold and make decisions. The nurse needs to acknowledge the woman's sense of loss and let her know that it is normal to grieve during the process. She also needs to let the woman know that such feelings will continue to occur intermittently. Couples need to be made aware that they may respond differently to their loss. It can be stressful if they do not understand that each individual may process information differently.
- Determine the woman's ability to recognize which decisions need to be made. Assists the nurse with developing strategies to help the woman understand the ramifications of the genetic disorder.

Patient/Family Teaching

- Explain to the members of the woman's support system how they can help in the decision-making process. Allows those who are supportive to play an active role in assisting the woman with decision making.
- Teach the woman how to group the risks and benefits of the situation in order to arrive at the best possible decision for her. Teaching this process allows the woman to visualize the risks and benefits and make an informed decision.
- Support the woman's/couple's decision process and provide a list of ongoing resources. The path of caring for a child who has a genetic disorder is difficult, and community resources and counseling can always be of assistance. Should the couple choose to terminate the pregnancy, they may be in need of counseling to process their decision later, as well as the ongoing sadness or depression that can linger. The nursing implications of caring for the couple embarking on the care of a child with special needs continue throughout the child's life span. Medical and education needs may follow the family always, and a caring nurse will always have an integral role in how the parents navigate the system and their understanding of how they can parent and care for their child and integrate that child into their family.

THE PREGNANT ADOLESCENT

The incidence of teenage pregnancy steadily declined in the United States from 1991 until 2007 but remains higher than that of other industrialized countries. Every year, about 1 million teenagers become pregnant; about half give birth and keep their babies, one third choose to terminate the pregnancy, and about 15% of teenage pregnancies end in miscarriage. Pregnant adolescents are at increased physical, emotional, and social risk. They are unprepared economically, educationally, and psychologically for parenthood because it occurs at a time when both physical development and the developmental tasks of adolescence are still in the process of growth. The younger the adolescent at time of the first pregnancy, the more likely she will have another pregnancy during her teens. Of the girls who become pregnant, over 20% will have a repeat pregnancy (National Campaign, 2009).

▌ *Key Nursing Activities*

- Stress importance of early and consistent prenatal care throughout the pregnancy.
- Identify and support involvement of family members as appropriate and available.
- Facilitate positive communication and problem solving to enhance family processes.
- Provide teaching and care based on the developmental stage of the adolescent.
- Encourage the parents-to-be to attend prenatal and parenting education classes.
- Encourage the girl to continue or return to school; to complete GED; or refer her for career/job counseling.
- Monitor maternal and fetal well-being, with special emphasis on nutrition and maternal and infant safety.
- Assess need for support services (financial or counseling) and refer as appropriate.
- Allow time for communication about options for the pregnancy and desires concerning the outcome for the pregnancy; keeping the baby, relinquishment and adoption, or seeking termination when appropriate.

Developmental assessment must be considered when planning care for the pregnant adolescent because it is an integral part of determining knowledge deficits and planning specific nursing activities to meet individualized care needs.

Overall tasks for this age group are:
- Acceptance of and comfort with one's body image
- Internalization of a sexual identity and role
- Development of a personal value system
- Development of a sense of productivity
- Identification of a life's work
- Achievement of a sense of independence
- Development of an adult identity

Each stage of adolescence has its unique educational challenges and focusing on needs and strengths of that stage will enable the nurse to individualize care of the adolescent's specific needs. They include:

Early adolescent (younger than 15 years). A girl in this group is a concrete thinker who has some degree of discomfort with normal body changes and image. She has minimal ability to foresee consequences of her behavior or visualize her future. She usually has an external locus of control.

Middle adolescent (15–17 years). A girl in this group feels invulnerable and is prone to experimentation with drugs, alcohol, and sex. She seeks independence and relies on peer group for support, information, and suggestions. Pregnancy can alter this normal transition. Operational thought and abstract thinking are present, but she still has difficulty recognizing possible long-term consequences of her behavior.

Late adolescent (17–19 years). A girl in this group thinks abstractly and develops individuality. She is able to anticipate consequences of her behavior, problem solve, and envision being in control.

▌ *Etiologies and Risk Factors*

There is no single cause; it is a complex issue. Adolescent pregnancy and early parenting are risk factors for poor medical, informational, and psychosocial outcomes for parents and their babies. Some of the identified risk factors for teen pregnancy are:
- Lower socioeconomic status
- Poor scholastic achievement
- Poor communication with parent(s)
- Single-parent family
- Having a mother or sister who was a pregnant adolescent
- Early initiation of sexual activity
- Low self-esteem
- Lack of incentive to avoid pregnancy
- Lack of knowledge about or access to contraception
- Drug or alcohol use/abuse (Elfenbein & Felice, 2003; National Campaign, 2009)

Recent birth rate decreases in adolescents have been attributed to fewer teens having sexual intercourse, increased use of contraceptives, and newly available, long-lasting contraceptives.

▌ *Signs and Symptoms*

Signs and symptoms are the same as for any normal pregnancy. See "Normal Antepartum: First Trimester," which begins on p. 39 in Chapter 4. Pregnant teens may not recognize signs as early as adults would and may be in denial of the fact of their pregnancy, which can delay entry into prenatal care.

▌ *Diagnostic Studies*

See "Normal Antepartum: First Trimester," beginning on p. 39, "Normal Antepartum: Second Trimester," p. 48, and "Normal Antepartum: Third Trimester," p. 54, in Chapter 4.

▌ *Medical Management*

Early prenatal care is important; adolescents over age 15 who receive early prenatal care are at no higher risk for complications than women over age 20. See "Normal Antepartum: First Trimester," beginning on

p. 39, "Normal Antepartum: Second Trimester," beginning on p. 48, and "Normal Antepartum: Third Trimester," beginning on p. 54 in Chapter 4.

▌ *Collaborative Problems*

Potential complications of adolescent pregnancy include the following:

- Cephalopelvic disproportion (especially in early adolescence).
- Low-birth-weight infants, intrauterine growth restriction, placental disorders, and prolonged labors. Refer to NDCP for "Risk for Imbalanced Nutrition: Less Than or More Than Body Requirements,[1]" which begins on p. 88 in this chapter.
- Premature birth/preterm labor and delivery.
- Anemia due to increased iron needs of pregnancy and her own growth.
- Preeclampsia or eclampsia.
- Social problems (e.g., child abuse and neglect, single-parent family, lack of education, unemployment, inadequate support system).
- Fetal morbidity from sexually transmitted infections (STIs) and/or substance use (e.g., tobacco, alcohol, other drugs).

COLLABORATIVE (STANDARDIZED) CARE FOR ALL PREGNANT ADOLESCENTS

Perform a comprehensive assessment to identify individual needs for teaching, emotional support, and physical care.

▌ Potential Complications of Adolescent Pregnancy: CEPHALOPELVIC DISPROPORTION

Cephalopelvic disproportion is difficult to predict during pregnancy except in a woman with an unusually and obviously small pelvis. A trial of labor is necessary to see if the baby can descend through the pelvis to be delivered vaginally.

Focus Assessments

- Pelvic measurements: Skeletal immaturity, in adolescents under age 15, creates the risk for pelvic inadequacy. Growth of the pelvis is delayed in comparison to growth in height. If measurements are small, cesarean birth may be necessary. In practice, pelvimetry is rarely used. If cephalopelvic disproportion is suspected during labor, radiographic cephalopelvimetry may be performed.
- Sonogram: Indicates fetal size, position, and lie in relation to maternal pelvis.
- Fundal height: Estimates fetal size. Between 22 and 34 weeks' gestation, with a normal sized fetus, fundal height

in centimeters correlates with weeks of gestation (e.g., at 34 weeks, height would be 34 cm). Uterine fundal height beyond 34 weeks is less accurate and does not correlate to centimeter measurement of same number.

Preventive Nursing Activities

- Stress importance of early and continued prenatal care. Delayed care may be due to pregnancy denial, lack of knowledge about pregnancy, or lack of access to health care due to transportation or insurance. Missed appointments are not unusual for adolescents. Adolescents may not plan ahead for more than a few days and are not likely to understand the importance of prenatal care. Also if the patient is in school or working, she may have schedule conflicts and have difficulty seeing the importance of visits if she feels that everything is progressing normally. Early, consistent prenatal care is essential to good pregnancy outcomes.

▌ Potential Complication of Adolescent Pregnancy: LOW-BIRTH-WEIGHT INFANTS AND INTRAUTERINE GROWTH RESTRICTION

Refer to the NDCP, "Risk for Imbalanced Nutrition: Less Than or More Than Body Requirements,[1]" beginning on p. 88 in this chapter.

▌ Potential Complication of Adolescent Pregnancy: PREMATURE BIRTH

Refer to the generic collaborative care plan, "Potential Complication: Preterm Labor," beginning on p. 31 in Chapter 3.

Focus Assessments

- Inquire about symptoms of preterm labor and fetal movement at each prenatal visit. The goal is to identify preterm labor early in order to keep it from advancing to the point that it no longer responds to medical treatment. Prompt diagnosis is difficult because many of the symptoms are common in normal pregnancy as well.
- Assess for other risk factors for spontaneous preterm labor. Adolescence itself is a risk factor. Adolescents are also more likely to have anemia, poor weight gain, poor nutrition, increased stressors, and can have exposure to sexually transmitted infections, all of which further increase the risk for preterm labor.

Preventive Nursing Activities

- Teach the patient to recognize and report the symptoms of preterm labor: abdominal, back, or pelvic pain; menstrual-like cramps; vaginal spotting or bleeding; increased and/or pink-tinged vaginal discharge; pelvic pressure; diarrhea; and urinary frequency. Ensure that the teen knows what a contraction feels like and discuss its characteristics, since she may be unfamiliar with the information; explain differences between true labor and false labor. Helps ensure that the adolescent understands the significance of the symptoms and the importance of early reporting. Risks of early delivery need to be explained.

Potential Complication of Adolescent Pregnancy: ANEMIA

Refer to generic collaborative care plan, "Potential Complication: Anemia," beginning on p. 25 in Chapter 3, and NDCP for the pregnant adolescent, "Risk for Imbalanced Nutrition: Less Than or More Than Body Requirements,[1]" beginning on p. 88 in this chapter. Iron deficiency anemia is a potential problem for all pregnant women. The adolescent is at increased risk because of her own growth needs, snacking on junk food, being too busy to have real meals, being physically active, or worrying about gaining weight due to body image concerns. It is difficult for many pregnant women to meet all iron needs through diet, and the adolescent's needs are increased due to her own growth needs in addition to the fetus's needs.

Potential Complication of Adolescent Pregnancy: PREECLAMPSIA/ECLAMPSIA

Refer to the generic collaborative care plan "Potential Complications: Hypertensive Disorders," beginning on p. 32 in Chapter 3.

Focus Assessments

- Assess for a gradual increase from prepregnant diastolic BP readings, along with excessive weight gain. The standard definition of preeclampsia is a BP reading of 140/90 mmHg after the 20th week of pregnancy (gestational hypertension) with proteinuria present. Should also assess for accompanying pedal edema, presence of clonus, headaches, visual disturbances, and epigastric pain.

Preventive Nursing Activities

- Stress the need for early and continuing prenatal care. This is vital for early detection and effective management of problems such as preeclampsia. Adolescents are at increased risk for preeclampsia and premature labor.

- Encourage reporting of aforementioned danger signs and symptoms. Facilitates early treatment if problems develop.

Potential Complication of Adolescent Pregnancy: SOCIAL PROBLEMS

Social problems include child abuse and neglect, exposure to violence, having a single-parent family, lack of education, decreased social support, potential of substance abuse, an inadequate support system, and low socioeconomic status.

Focus Assessments

- Assess family situation and support network during first prenatal visit. Determines the amount of support available and the level of involvement the young woman wishes them to have.
- Assess the level of involvement of the baby's father, and the level of involvement desired by the mother. Find out who she considers her support persons and get them engaged in the care process. Many adolescent couples are involved in meaningful relationships, although they might not be married. The father can be an important support person for the young woman and an involved parent-to-be, if he is willing and if she wishes to have him involved. It is not unusual, however, for the adolescent to want her mother as her primary support person during labor.

Preventive Nursing Activities

- If both the adolescent and her mother agree, include the mother in the prenatal care. The younger the adolescent, the more support she needs from her mother in order to commit to a mothering role. Despite the typical conflicts between female adolescents and their mothers, and despite the developmental need to gain autonomy and independence, the pregnant adolescent needs financial and psychologic support in dealing with pregnancy and caring for a new infant. Facilitation of communication during prenatal care can set healthy patterns for later.
- If the pregnant adolescent's partner wishes to be involved and supportive; educate him about pregnancy, childbirth, infant care, and parenting. The partner needs adequate knowledge of the physical and psychologic changes to better understand and have empathy for what his partner is experiencing. Explanation of fetal growth and development can facilitate bonding with the baby and engagement in his partner's prenatal care.
- Refer both the young woman and her partner, if he is involved, to social services for educational and vocational counseling. Many adolescents drop out of school during their pregnancy, and many never complete their education. This further compromises the ability to achieve financial and emotional independence from family and increases the likelihood of a subsequent pregnancy during adolescence.

• Encourage and facilitate prenatal education and parenting education for the pregnant adolescent and support person. Information about growth and development may help prevent child neglect or abuse by helping teenage parents to have more realistic expectations of their infants and appropriate parenting. Classes will help them to learn the skills they need to cope with childbearing and parenting.

Potential Complication of Adolescent Pregnancy: FETAL MORBIDITY FROM SEXUALLY TRANSMITTED INFECTIONS AND/OR SUBSTANCE USE

This complication includes tobacco, alcohol, and other drugs.

Focus Assessments

• Initial prenatal examination should include sexual history (e.g., number of partners, high-risk behaviors for HIV and other STIs, and UTIs). STIs can cause neonatal infections and problems with fetal development. Some STIs (e.g., HIV, herpes, and hepatitis) can be transmitted to the infant during the birth process.

• Initial prenatal examination should include offering HIV testing, cultures for gonorrhea, chlamydia, and evaluation for vaginal infections such as Trichomonas, bacterial vaginosis, and Candida albicans. Observe for herpetic lesions and other STI symptoms throughout the pregnancy. Adolescents have an increased incidence of STIs, which can increase the risk to the fetus. An adolescent's risk for changes to her cells is greater than that of a mature female since her biologic cells are still in a growth phase; thus more harm from a disease process can occur.

• Inquire about and observe for symptoms of use and abuse of tobacco, caffeine, alcohol, and other substances. Teenage mothers are more likely than older pregnant women to use tobacco, alcohol, and other substances. Substance abuse increases the risk of complications of pregnancy and preterm labor, as well as being teratogenic to the fetus.

• Evaluate risk for exposure to violence and use screening to assess potential or experience of domestic abuse. Detects risk to facilitate early intervention if needed.

Preventive Nursing Activities

• Review with the young woman the effects of tobacco, caffeine, drugs (prescription, over the counter, and illicit), and alcohol on her own development as well as that of the baby. Food supplements, herbs, and additives should also be considered for harm to the fetus (e.g., popular energy drinks contain many other unknown substances). Provides information necessary in order for the woman to make lifestyle changes. Adolescents tend to be self-focused, so merely

understanding the effects of substances on the baby may not be enough to motivate her to change. It may be helpful to emphasize the effects of substance use on the adolescent herself as well as the growing fetus.

• Teach and counsel the young woman and partner, if involved, regarding safer sex. Teenagers lack knowledge about STIs and HIV and also believe that they will not acquire them. Many urban myths and inaccurate information also circulate, and the healthcare worker needs to clarify and make sure knowledge is accurate.

• Teach the symptoms of STIs. See rationale immediately preceding.

• Refer the young woman to a smoking cessation or substance abuse program if necessary. Withdrawal from a physically addictive substance poses risks for both mother and fetus; therefore, specialized support and monitoring are needed. Accurate information on how the substance can be harmful is important to plant the desire to change for herself and her child.

INDIVIDUALIZED (NURSING DIAGNOSIS) CARE PLANS

These care plans were designed to address unique patient needs.

It is essential that the nurse develop trust while working with this young, vulnerable population. Nurses can build positive nurse–patient relationships with adolescents and thus foster trust by partnering with them during their pregnancy experience. The partnering process involves engaging the teen, maintaining engagement, working toward mutually derived goals, and disengaging. Specific skills include focusing on the teen and her well-being, remaining nonjudgmental, showing respect, mutual goal setting, affirming the teen's strengths, and building on the teen's support systems (Norris, Howell, Wydeven, & Kunes-Connell, 2009).

Nursing Diagnosis: RISK FOR IMPAIRED PARENTING[1]

Related Factors: lack of knowledge, lack of support between/from significant other(s), ineffective role models, lack of role identity, unrealistic expectations for self, immaturity and less ability to cope with the presence of stressors (e.g., the fact of the pregnancy, the circumstances surrounding the pregnancy, financial pressures). Although Risk for Impaired Parenting[1] is a nursing diagnosis, it is a standardized plan that should be followed for all pregnant adolescents.

Also refer to the diagnosis care plan, "Risk for Interrupted Family Processes,[1]" which begins on p. 79 in this chapter.

Goals, Outcomes, and Evaluation Criteria

Prenatally, the adolescent and/or significant others should:

• Assign specific attributes to the fetus (e.g., "He's so active.") and exhibit behaviors of prenatal bonding.

- Prepare for the baby prior to birth.
- Verbalize positive feelings about having a child and becoming a parent and start making decisions about care (how to feed the baby, planning care for the baby when the mother is back in school).
- Report sufficient help (e.g., time, money, emotional assistance, and so forth) and seek help if needed to be provided by others.
- Build a resource list and network to know where to seek help in the future.

After birth of the infant, the mother and/or significant other will:

- Demonstrate bonding behaviors (also see care plan, "Postpartum Days 1–2," which begins on p. 311 in Chapter 9).
- Demonstrate positive parenting behaviors with confidence.
- State appropriate abilities and behaviors of the newborn.
- Provide appropriate stimulation and nutrition to facilitate the infant's optimum growth and development.

▌ NIC Interventions[2]

Abuse Protection Support: Child (6402)—Identification of high-risk, dependent child relationships and actions to prevent possible or further infliction of physical, sexual, or emotional harm or neglect of basic necessities of life.

Anticipatory Guidance (5210)—Preparation of patient for an anticipated developmental and/or situational crisis.

Attachment Promotion (6710)—Facilitation of the development of the parent–infant relationship.

Coping Enhancement (5230)—Assisting a patient to adapt to perceived stressors, changes, or threats that interfere with meeting life demands and roles.

Family Integrity Promotion (7100)—Promotion of family cohesion and unity.

Parenting Promotion (8300)—Providing parenting information, support, and coordination of comprehensive services to high-risk families.

▌ Nursing Activities and Rationales

Assessments

- Assess the parent(s)' developmental, educational, and economic status. Identifies potential for impaired parenting and the need for interventions prior to delivery. The ability to parent effectively is related to all of these factors. The developmental needs of adolescents interfere with their sensitivity to the needs of the infant, as do stresses from financial pressures and lack of support. Furthermore, lack of emotional maturity contributes to difficulty with communication and problem-solving skills with realistic goals.
- Observe for bonding behaviors during prenatal visits (e.g., speculating about the baby's sex and personality traits, choosing a name). Parent–infant attachment provides the foundation for good parenting. Emotional attachment should begin during the prenatal period. If attachment behaviors are absent, the nurse can intervene to promote attachment before the birth of the baby.

Independent Nursing Actions

- Suggest and provide opportunities if possible for the teen-aged parent(s) to interact with parents and infants who are appropriate role models. Helps adolescents gain realistic information about parenting and infant behaviors. Adolescent parents are, as a rule, less responsive to infant cues and more likely to use punishment; this may be related to their unrealistic expectations of infant behavior.

Collaborative Activities

- Encourage parent(s) to attend prenatal and parenting classes. Helps them acquire parenting skills and learn about infant capabilities and stimulation. Children of adolescent mothers are at a developmental risk because of the adverse social and economic conditions facing the parent(s). These factors can contribute to family instability, poor academic performance, and behavior problems in the offspring.

Patient/Family Teaching

- Provide teaching about the baby and infant care during the last trimester of the pregnancy, preferably, before the birth of the baby. Adolescents are focused on themselves, and at times it is difficult for them to focus on the needs of others. Therefore, the mother may not be as receptive to learn this content until after the baby is born and the mother accepts its reality. Hopefully, as her baby grows and she sees that growth, she will seek information prior to the birth and take it in. If not, the postpartum period will require a huge learning curve with many educational needs about caring for the newborn.
- Provide information about infant development, bathing, and care of a newborn. Use demonstrations and practice. Provides realistic information needed for good parenting. Hands-on practice helps the mother retain information. Return demonstration and time to ask questions after initial teaching will aid in integration of the new knowledge.
- Assess the needs of the adolescent and availability of community programs for continued support and education. Parent as Teachers is a program that guides parents to exhibit healthy behaviors and appropriate guidance with a developing child. A patient does need to enroll early to gain admittance. Anticipation of need and seeking entry can facilitate good parenting.

▌ Nursing Diagnosis: SITUATIONAL LOW SELF-ESTEEM[1]

Related Factors: unanticipated pregnancy, social role changes, physical and developmental changes, feelings of or fear of failure (e.g., school), and rejection by significant others with lack of social support and affirmation.

Goals, Outcomes, and Evaluation Criteria

- Woman describes successes in work, school, and/or personal relationships.
- Woman names several personal strengths.
- Woman accepts positive comments from others.
- Woman functions in roles she perceives as important so she feels worthwhile.
- Woman accepts changing body image as positive and can provide for her baby's growth.

NIC Interventions[2]

Body Image Enhancement (5220)—Improving a patient's conscious and unconscious perceptions and attitudes toward his/her body.

Coping Enhancement (5230)—Assisting a patient to adapt to perceived stressors, changes, or threats that interfere with meeting life demands and roles.

Self-Esteem Enhancement (5400)—Assisting a patient to increase his/her personal judgment of self-worth.

Socialization Enhancement (5100)—Facilitation of another person's ability to interact with others.

Nursing Activities and Rationales

Assessments

- Assess the adolescent's self-perception (including body image). Positive behaviors (excitement over changes, normal weight gain, and baby's movement) or negative tendencies (e.g., expressions of shame, failure to participate in care, negative verbalizations of self, hypersensitivity to criticism) should be noted. Adolescents typically are forming their body image throughout their adolescent period.
- Assess the adolescent's perception of her future (e.g., the outcome of the pregnancy, how she will support the baby and continue her education). She may need assistance in setting realistic goals and outcomes. Low self-esteem may contribute to feelings of hopelessness and negative perceptions of future pregnancy outcomes.
- Assess for changes in relationships with friends, family, and the baby's father that have occurred during the pregnancy. Provide space for dialogue and communication of concerns. Significant others may react with anger, guilt, and shock. Her nonpregnant friends may abandon her. How well the pregnancy is accepted depends, in part, on the circumstances of the pregnancy and whether the mother is in early, middle, or late adolescence.
- Monitor ongoing level of self-esteem (e.g., assess for verbalizations of self-worth, positive or negative self-talk, eye contact, and statements of confidence). Refer to counseling if needed. Determines effectiveness of interventions. Monitor and note changes in self-esteem that occur over a relatively long time span.

Independent Nursing Actions

- Use a caring, nonjudgmental, and accepting approach with the young woman. It is essential to establish trust and feeling of empathy, so the adolescent will be open to receive the information given and feel valued and so she will be motivated to participate in her own care, for herself and her baby.
- Discuss her feelings about her body and the changes that occur with pregnancy; reassure her that changes are normal and part of a healthy pregnancy. As her abdomen enlarges, the adolescent may attempt to control her appearance by dieting. It is important to reassure her that she is not fat and that her body will return to its prepregnant state with some residual changes from having a baby. Information needs to be accurate.
- Assist to identify personal strengths and reinforce strengths she identifies. Helps the adolescent to gain a more positive and realistic view of herself. Reinforcement motivates continuation of the behaviors.
- Avoid teasing and judgment. Support and trust are essential in a caregiving role. Teasing and critical words may damage an already low self-esteem.
- Help the young woman to set realistic goals; praise or otherwise reward any progress toward goal achievement. Successes promote self-esteem. Praise reinforces the behaviors. Always encourage her to do her best for herself and her baby.
- Actively involve the young woman in her care. Gives a sense of participation and responsibility. Adolescents want to be involved in making choices since they are becoming independent and do not want decisions made for them.
- Support decision-making process and guide problem solving when needed. These skills are essential for her to be able to assume responsibility for her newborn as well as for her own life. Adolescents often have not had much experience in problem solving.

Collaborative Activities

- Urge the adolescent to attend prenatal and parent-education classes. Provides information to increase confidence about bodily changes, which is necessary to improve self-esteem; creates opportunities for the young woman to meet others in similar circumstances, giving her a more realistic and perhaps more positive perception of herself and her situation.

Patient/Family Teaching

- Teach the adolescent's parents the importance of their interest and support. Especially for younger adolescents, the parents are highly influential in the development of self-concept.
- Provide help, as needed, with ideas to adjust to her changing body and ways to improve how she feels about her appearance during pregnancy. Adolescents are body conscious; feeling that she appears attractive to others will help her to cope with her changing body.

Nursing Diagnosis: RISK FOR IMBALANCED NUTRITION: LESS THAN OR MORE THAN BODY REQUIREMENTS[1]

Related Factors: lack of information about good nutrition, poor eating habits, potential lack of access to nutritional foods, concern about gaining too much weight, misinformation about the need to limit weight gain in pregnancy, present body weight above or below ideal, intake that does not meet the recommended daily allowance for calories and/or nutrients, and being a young adolescent (fewer than 4 years past menarche).

Goals, Outcomes, and Evaluation Criteria

- Woman gains weight appropriate to her age and gestational age.
- Woman consumes a nutritionally adequate diet (prescribed calories and nutrients for body weight, age, and physical activity).
- Woman maintains normal hemoglobin (greater than 11 g/dl) and hematocrit (greater than 33%).
- Woman takes prenatal vitamin and iron and calcium supplements as prescribed.

NIC Interventions[2]

Nutrition Management (1100)—Assisting with or providing a balanced dietary intake of foods and fluids.
Nutritional Counseling (5246)—Use of an interactive helping process focusing on the need for diet modification.
Nutrition Monitoring (1160)—Collection and analysis of patient data to prevent or minimize malnourishment.
Weight Management (1260)—Facilitating maintenance of optimal body weight and percent body fat.

Nursing Activities and Rationales

Assessments

- Assess current diet history and intake to determine need for addition or alteration in present diet pattern. Body requirements for growth are normally increased during adolescence. The additional metabolic demands of pregnancy along with adolescent growth make proper nutritional intake challenging; may need referral to nutritionist or extra instruction about dietary intake.
- Determine the number of years that have passed since the onset of menstruation. Female adolescents are physiologically mature about 4 years after menarche (linear growth is usually completed by that time). Their nutritional needs are similar to those of other adult women. Young adolescents (fewer than 4 years past menarche) are physiologically and anatomically immature and are likely to be growing. Nutritional needs for these young women are higher, due to the growth needs of both the mother and the fetus.

- Evaluate caloric intake, considering age, pregnancy weight, physical activity level, and the additional calories needed during pregnancy. Nutrient needs can be estimated by using the recommended daily allowance for nonpregnant teenagers and adding the nutrient amounts recommended for all pregnant women. A normal adult woman should add about 400 kcal/day during the second and third trimesters; up to 50 kcal/kg of body weight (23 kcal/lb) is suggested for young, active, growing teens. A satisfactory weight gain should indicate sufficient caloric intake with adequate uterine fundal growth pattern.
- Evaluate current weight, prepregnancy weight, and ideal weight for height (body mass index [BMI]). Ideal gain for the normal-weight adult woman is 25–35 lb; women with a low BMI should gain more than women who have a high BMI. To reduce the risk of low-birth-weight infants, weight gain should be higher for adolescents, at the upper end of the desired range (e.g., as much as 40 lb for a young adolescent with a low BMI or about 7 lb for one with a high BMI). BMI is a guide, and excessive weight loss to meet the range can be unhealthy for overweight teens during pregnancy. Please note that ethnic and athletic body types do not always have good correlation to the BMI.
- Evaluate Hb and Hct at first prenatal visit and at least once more during pregnancy (usually at 28 weeks if normal initially). Iron deficiency anemia is common in the adolescent due to increased nutritional needs associated with personal growth.
- Determine the adolescent's ability to meet her nutritional needs. The adolescent may be inexperienced with grocery shopping and meal preparation and often does not have those roles in the family. Involving the person who prepares food for the family helps ensure the adolescent's nutritional needs will be met.
- Offer nutritionally friendly choices if the adolescent eats out or eats fast food frequently. Helps ensure that the adolescent's nutritional needs will be met.

Independent Nursing Actions

- Help the adolescent to plan a diet that includes a wide variety of foods, especially fresh, healthy, and lightly processed foods. Stressing variety is a more positive approach than condemning junk food and is more likely to encourage compliance with a diet containing necessary nutrients. Teach reading of nutritional labels to educate about foods and those with empty calories.
- When planning diet with adolescent, consider peer, lifestyle, and cultural influences. Increases the likelihood of compliance with the diet. As adolescents become more independent, they make more of their own food choices. They are often influenced by the need for peer acceptance.

Collaborative Activities

- Refer to Women, Infants, and Children (WIC) program and/or the food stamp program. These programs provide nutrition services for women who qualify. WIC provides vouchers for selected foods for pregnant and lactating women at nutritional risk (e.g., eggs, cheese, milk, juice, and fortified cereals).

Patient/Family Teaching

- Include family or support system during all teaching. Ensures that the person involved in shopping for and preparing food gets knowledge needed to support healthy pregnancy for the adolescent.
- Provide information about foods needed for appropriate weight gain and nutritional adequacy. Corrects any misconceptions; provides information needed for adolescent to manage her own dietary intake.
- Provide information about foods containing protein and the importance of protein to maternal and fetal development. Insufficient protein intake, especially during the first trimester, is a risk factor for IUGR and poor fetal brain development, and it may contribute to maternal pregnancy-related hypertension. Individual protein requirements are based on recommended daily allowances for the adolescent's age group, with about 14 g/day added to meet the needs of the pregnancy.
- Instruct about the risks of dieting while pregnant. Inadequate intake may cause insufficient weight gain. Inadequate weight gain indicates a risk for fetal IUGR and maternal complications such as pregnancy-related hypertension. Weight loss places the mother and fetus at risk for acidosis—when caloric intake is not sufficient for energy and growth requirements, body fat is metabolized; ketones are an acidic by-product of lipid metabolism. Adequate calories are necessary to prevent the body from metabolizing proteins for energy as well as to ensure adequate iron intake.
- Explain the importance of taking iron supplements (30–60 mg/day of elemental iron). Iron intake is a major concern with the adolescent diet, both because of the increased need for iron to meet the demands of the enlarging maternal muscle mass and blood volume and the likelihood that the diet will not contain an adequate amount.
- Explain the need for a vitamin and mineral supplement, as needed. Supplemental folic acid is usually suggested, even for adult females. Other nutrients frequently deficient in adolescent diets are calcium, zinc, and vitamins A, D, and B_6.

Nursing Diagnosis: DEFICIENT KNOWLEDGE (FAMILY PLANNING, PREGNANCY PROCESS, SYMPTOMS OF COMPLICATIONS, FUTURE EXPECTATIONS)[1]

Related Factors: incorrect information given by significant others/peers, unfamiliarity with resources for information, inadequate support system, and lack of interest or motivation. Refer to the generic NDCP, "Deficient Knowledge,[1]" which begins on p. 13 in Chapter 2.

▐ *Goals, Outcomes, and Evaluation Criteria*

Adolescent and/or partner (family) will demonstrate/verbalize understanding of:

- Anatomy and physiology of pregnancy.
- Community resources available for support (e.g., education, career planning, and prenatal and infant care classes).
- Signs of impending labor.
- Available methods of birth control.
- Danger signs (e.g., of pregnancy-related hypertension, preterm labor, and premature rupture of membranes [PROM]) that should be reported to the primary care provider.
- Healthy behaviors (e.g., diet, exercise, and safer sex) to promote successful pregnancy outcomes.

▐ *NIC Interventions[2]*

Health System Guidance (7400)—Facilitating a patient's location and use of appropriate health services.
Learning Facilitation (5520)—Promoting the ability to process and comprehend information.
Learning Readiness Enhancement (5540)—Improving the ability and willingness to receive information.
Prenatal Care (6960)—Monitoring and management of the patient during pregnancy to prevent complications of pregnancy and promote a healthy outcome for both mother and infant.
Teaching: Group (5604)—Development, implementation, and evaluation of a patient teaching program for a group of individuals experiencing the same health condition.
Teaching: Individual (5606)—Development, implementation, and evaluation of a teaching program designed to address a patient's particular needs.
Teaching: Safe Sex (5622)—Providing instruction concerning sexual protection during sexual activity.

▐ *Nursing Activities and Rationales*

Assessments

- Determine age and stage of adolescent development. This information is necessary to choose the most effective teaching approach. Adolescents may not be cognitively able to cope with abstractions or inferential problem solving.

Independent Nursing Actions

- Develop a trusting relationship with the young woman. This is essential in motivating the adolescent to learn and to comply with the healthcare regimen. Honesty and respect for the individual promote self-esteem and support the maturation process.
- Stress the importance of ongoing prenatal care and risks to the young woman and her baby. Reinforces that ongoing assessment is crucial, even if the woman feels well. Certain

complications may be avoided or managed early if timely prenatal visits are made.

- Assist the young woman in identifying long-range personal and educational goals. Establishing educational goals may help prevent the adolescent and her infant from being economically dependent on the welfare system and from having a subsequent adolescent pregnancy.

Collaborative Activities

- Refer to prenatal education and parenting classes; refer to adolescent clinic and/or support groups. Education and appropriate social support services are critical in achieving successful outcomes of pregnancy, especially for young adolescents.

Patient/Family Teaching

- Stress the effects of the adolescent's health habits on herself as well as on the fetus. Adolescents tend to be egocentric, so the effect of their actions on a fetus may not be regarded as important to them. Effects on themselves may be better appreciated.
- Orient the teaching to the woman's developmental stage (e.g., for young adolescents, keep teaching simple, direct, and responsive to their immediate needs). Early adolescents tend to be present oriented and concrete thinkers.
- Use a variety of teaching strategies, including audiovisual aids, demonstrations, and games; intersperse teaching with frequent breaks and changes of pace. Typically, teens have a short attention span; they are accustomed to audiovisual information (e.g., from television and computers).
- Present information in small groups with other teens, when possible. Provides peer support and enhances motivation for learning.
- Present information about parenting only at the end of the pregnancy or, preferably, after the infant is born. Adolescents tend to be oriented to the present, so they are generally not ready to learn about parenting skills until the newborn presents as a reality.
- Provide information about the anatomy and physiology of pregnancy and the signs of impending labor. Promotes understanding of body changes and corrects myths and misinformation (e.g., early adolescents may not realize that pregnancy is an outcome of sexual activity); helps the adolescent to differentiate between true and false labor, and know when to call the primary healthcare provider.
- Provide information about normal discomforts of pregnancy, danger signs (e.g., of pregnancy-related hypertension) that should be reported to the primary care provider, and healthy behaviors (e.g., diet, exercise) to promote successful pregnancy outcomes. Refer to care plans for "Normal Antepartum: First Trimester," "Normal Antepartum: Second Trimester," and "Normal Antepartum: Third

Trimester," which begin on pp. 39, 48, and 54, respectively, in Chapter 4.

- Provide information about methods of birth control and safer sex practices. Refer to collaborative care plan for "Potential Complication of Adolescent Pregnancy: Fetal Morbidity From Sexually Transmitted Infections and/or Substance Use," which begins on p. 85 in this chapter.
- Provide information about community resources available for support in continuing the adolescent's education and career planning. Many teen mothers drop out of school during pregnancy, reducing the quality of jobs available to them. Public assistance is often needed, especially in lower socioeconomic groups and when the young woman's family does not support her.

Nursing Diagnosis: INTERRUPTED FAMILY PROCESSES[1]

Related Factors: unexpected and/or unwanted pregnancy; situational or developmental transition and/or crisis; ineffective patterns of communication; negative reaction of family members to the pregnancy; and financial strain on the family.

Goals, Outcomes, and Evaluation Criteria

Family members report:

- Confidence in managing problems.
- Involvement of all members in decision making.
- Receiving help and support from each other.
- Having resources adequate to meet family needs.
  Family members also:
- Express emotions freely.
- Use stress-reduction strategies.
- Express anger and other emotions appropriately.
- Participate in recreational activities together.
- Work together to achieve goals.
- Provide sufficient support for the pregnant adolescent.

NIC Interventions[2]

Developmental Enhancement: Adolescent (8272)—Facilitating optimal physical, cognitive, social, and emotional growth of individuals during the transition from childhood to adulthood.

Family Integrity Promotion: Childbearing Family (7104)— Facilitation of the growth of individuals or families who are adding an infant to the family unit.

Family Planning: Unplanned Pregnancy (6788)—Facilitation of decision making regarding pregnancy outcome.

Family Process Maintenance (7130)—Minimization of family process disruption effects.

Family Support (7140)—Promotion of family values, interests, and goals.

■ *Nursing Activities and Rationales*

Assessments

- Identify the family's cultural values. The family's value system influences how they will respond to the pregnancy. In some cultures, it is common for teenagers to become pregnant; in others it may evoke shame and guilt. Single parenting is also more acceptable in some cultures than others.
- Identify typical family processes (e.g., roles, communication, and decision-making patterns, task assignments). Provides a baseline for evaluating the results of interventions. There may be dysfunctional communication and relationships, or even abuse, in the family unit. Adolescents sometimes become pregnant as a way to rebel against parents or as a way to find love if they do not experience it at home.
- Clearly identify ways in which family processes have been changed or disrupted. Provides information for planning interventions.
- Identify family reactions to the adolescent's pregnancy, and her perceptions of their support; be alert for destructive behaviors. The parents of the pregnant adolescent may have negative feelings and have difficulty being supportive.
- Identify involved members of the family; ask the young woman whom she wishes to be involved and who is most important to her. The father of the baby may or may not wish to assume responsibility, and even if he does, the young woman's parents may be angry and wish to exclude him. The pregnant adolescent will not perceive support to be adequate unless her most important persons are involved. If a parent is involved, the adolescent will be more likely to seek and continue prenatal care.
- Assess the pregnant adolescent's relationship with her mother. The young woman's mother is usually the one who is most involved during the pregnancy and the one who provides help after the baby is born. The mother may think her daughter is too young to assume responsibility and take over too much of the decision making and care of the infant. This can keep the young woman from effectively assuming the mothering role.
- Identify the circumstances surrounding the pregnancy (e.g., baby's father involved, rape, incest). The circumstances of the pregnancy influence the way the family perceives and reacts to the situation. For example, if the pregnancy was a result of rape, incest, or abuse, the family will probably not want the baby's father to be involved.

Independent Nursing Actions

- Facilitate family discussions of the future (e.g., education for the adolescent, care of the baby, adoption, living and financial arrangements). There are likely to be uncertainties and decisions need to be made thoughtfully. If the pregnancy is a crisis situation, family members may respond with strong emotions (e.g., anger, blaming each other). They might need help redirecting and focusing their energies on problem solving, communication skills, and constructive planning.
- Help the parent(s) assess the daughter's needs and assist her in meeting them. Some adolescents become more independent during pregnancy; others become more dependent. Parents can facilitate their daughter's development by understanding how to respond to her needs and foster personal strengths.

Collaborative Activities

- Refer adolescent and significant others for counseling and parenting classes as needed. May help the family with conflict resolution and coping skills, strengthening family relationships.
- Encourage the mother of the teen to be involved if the mother–daughter relationship is positive; update her on current childbearing practices. During labor and birth, the mother of the teen can draw on her own experience to offer reassurance and instill confidence in her daughter. The mother may need updated information in order to not misinform her daughter.
- Include and encourage all family members to enhance integration of the new member. The family unit may be nontraditional, but all need a role to incorporate and facilitate the change that the pregnancy and birth create.

Patient/Family Teaching

- Provide information that is individualized based on needs assessment (e.g., infant care, counseling services, safety needs, integration of baby into family unit, community resources). Helps ensure that adolescent's specific education needs will be met.

PRENATAL SUBSTANCE ABUSE

Substance abuse is the continued use of substances despite related physical, social, or interpersonal problems. Any use of alcohol or illicit drugs during pregnancy is considered substance abuse. Because of the risks to the fetus, women who abuse substances during pregnancy fail to fulfill role responsibilities and may acquire substance-related legal problems. If a pregnant woman uses alcohol or illicit drugs, under law it is considered abuse (American Psychiatric Association [APA], 2000).

The indiscriminate use of illicit substances, tobacco, and alcohol during pregnancy places both the woman and her fetus at risk because substances pass from mother to baby through the placenta. For many who abuse substances, pregnancy is unplanned and may not even be recognized until late in the pregnancy. Prenatal care might not be sought until labor ensues. As a result, prenatal care is inadequate or may be nonexistent, especially if the woman fears legal recourse from medical providers and fears losing custody of the child or criminal prosecution. Personal risk factors, availability of health insurance, access to prenatal care, and the provider's attitude are potential barriers to prenatal care identified in the literature.

Fewer than 10% of pregnant women using drugs will access prenatal care and receive addiction treatment. Prenatal care can serve as a portal to important resources such as counseling, health education, nutrition, parenting skills, and drug treatment.

Illicit drug use during pregnancy is often further compromised by poor nutrition, anemia, and infections. Adverse maternal and infant outcomes can complicate respiratory, cardiovascular, and neurologic systems. Deliveries can be premature or precipitous. Infants are at risk because of impaired mother–infant bonding and poor infant cognitive and motor development (Shieh & Kravitz, 2006).

▌ Key Nursing Activities

- Screen for substance abuse.
- Maintain a nonjudgmental, therapeutic attitude.
- Advocate for access to drug-treatment and harm-reduction measures.
- Promote abstinence and explain risks of continued abuse to mother and fetus.
- Monitor for maternal and fetal complications.

▌ Etiologies and Risk Factors

Women who use illicit drugs, tobacco, and alcohol come from all socioeconomic backgrounds, races, ethnicities, and lifestyles. Half the women between ages 15 and 44 have taken illegal drugs at least once (NIDA, 2006). Also, women, more than men, tend to have a pattern of self-medication and are more likely to combine alcohol and drugs. Substance abuse during pregnancy is estimated to be between 5% and 15%, but self-report is difficult to obtain and inaccurate, thus statistics do not totally representative the scope of the problem. Thus, nurses should consider drug abuse as a possibility when making assessments because the incidence may be as high as 1 in 10 pregnancies.

Chemically dependent women tend to demonstrate a passive response to life and responsibilities, are depressed, have low self-esteem, have difficulty establishing positive intimate relationships, and lack adequate support systems. Substance abuse provides relief for their psychologic distress and loneliness and provides a means, although ineffective, of coping with family difficulties, social relations, work, and life in general. Lower education, adolescence, and lack of employment are risk factors. History of family of origin dysfunction, psychiatric illness, or physical or sexual abuse and violence places the woman at greater risk for using substances to ease her problems.

▌ Substances of Abuse

Most commonly abused substances during pregnancy are alcohol, cocaine/crack, marijuana, phencyclidine, 3,4-Methylenedioxymethamphetamine (Ecstasy), and heroin.

Alcohol is the most commonly used substance. Chronic alcohol use can undermine maternal health and cause fetal alcohol syndrome in the baby. The first trimester is especially a risky time during fetal development, and ill effects are seen from binge drinking or consuming four drinks a week. No amount of use is considered safe during pregnancy.

Cocaine, which is snorted, smoked, or injected, is a stimulant. It can cause uterine irritability and contractions, increase blood pressure, and mimic pregnancy-induced hypertension. Its use is associated with spontaneous first-trimester abortion, abruptio placentae, intrauterine growth restriction, preterm birth, and stillbirth.

Marijuana use is often combined with alcohol and tobacco. Estimated use by pregnant women is 14%, and it is the most commonly used street drug. No teratogenic effects have been identified to date, but it causes increased fine tremors, irritability, startling, and poor habitation to visual stimuli in infants exposed in utero.

Phencyclidine use is associated with overdose or a psychotic response. It is also accompanied by increased blood pressure, hyperthermia, diaphoresis, and possible coma, which compromises the fetus. Evidence of neurobehavioral problems in the newborn have been observed but not well documented.

3,4-Methylenedioxymethamphetamine (*Ecstasy*) has the common side effects of hyperthermia, hyponatremia, and at times, hypertension with heart and kidney failure. Little is known about problems during pregnancy that result from use of Ecstasy.

Heroin is an illicit, addictive, central nervous system depressant and class IV narcotic. Pregnancy is affected by heroin because its use results in poor nutrition, iron deficiency anemia, and pre-eclampsia/eclampsia. Heroin causes an increased rate of breech position, abnormal placenta, abruptio placentae, preterm labor, PROM, and meconium staining. The fetus is at risk for intrauterine growth restriction, withdrawal, and exposure to infections due to maternal lifestyle. Methadone is used in treatment but increases risk to the developing fetus because it crosses the placenta. Prematurity, rapid labor, abruptio placentae, decreased birth weight, and fetal distress are all possible even if the woman is placed in a controlled treatment rehabilitation plan.

Smoking, although not an illicit activity, should be stopped during pregnancy because it is also associated with poor pregnancy outcomes. Many drug users also are cigarette smokers. Low birth weight, placenta previa, abruptio placentae, preterm rupture of membranes, preterm births, and perinatal deaths are linked to smoking more than 10 cigarettes a day.

▌ Signs and Symptoms

Clinical manifestations vary with the substance used, but include the following:

Subjective manifestations: Insomnia, lethargy, increased somnolence, fatigue, increased anxiety, depression, euphoria, apathy, blackouts, nausea, headache, and itching.

Objective manifestations: Alteration of vital signs; fever and sweating; depressed respirations; tachycardia; hypertension or hypotension; cardiac arrhythmias; fetal hyperactivity or decreased fetal movement; fetal bradycardia; bloodshot eyes, conjunctivitis, yellow sclera, constricted or dilated pupils; nystagmus, increased lacrimation; sniffling, inflamed/indurated nasal mucosae, septal erosion, loss of sense of smell; slurred speech; shortness of breath; poor dental hygiene; hepatomegaly, jaundice, or distended neck veins; track marks, scars, cellulitis, or abscesses; drowsiness; impaired attention or memory; tremors; unsteady gait; poor coordination; hyperactivity; hyperactive reflexes; irritability, aggressiveness; poor hygiene, smell on clothing, mood lability; inappropriate affect; delusions; hallucinations; distorted time, spatial relations, and short-term memory; loss of inhibition; seizures; vomiting, diarrhea, weight loss; constipation; social problems (e.g., relationships, job loss).

▐ *Diagnostic Studies*

- Blood alcohol level. Determines present status and severity of problem.
- Substance abuse history and screening (e.g., Michigan Alcoholism Screening Test, Drug Abuse Screening Test), CAGE (acronym for annoyed by criticism, guilty about drinking, and eye-opener drinks), TACE (acronym for tolerance, annoyed by criticism, cut down and eye-opener drinks), and TWEAK (acronym for tolerance, worried, eye-opener, amnesia, and K/cut down): Screens for alcohol use/abuse during pregnancy.
- Routine prenatal blood tests and Pap smear. Further evaluate for additional problems.
- CBC. Assesses overall health, presence of infection, presence of anemia.
- Screening testing for hepatitis B, HIV, group B Streptococcus, and STIs. Often associated with substance abuse and to determine care needed prenatally.
- Blood urea nitrogen, serum creatinine, total protein, albumin-to-globulin ratio. Evaluate renal status.
- Total iron-binding capacity. Evaluates nutritional status, presence of anemia.
- Universal urine toxicology screening. Determines type(s) of drug(s) used and prevents missing drugs that may not be picked up by toxicology screen when history is positive (ACOG Committee of Ethics, 2004).
- Blood alcohol level. Helps determine present status and severity of problem.
- Liver function tests. Determine whether liver damage has occurred.
- Tuberculosis test/chest X-ray. Assess for pneumonia, pulmonary edema, or emboli.
- Serial ultrasound. Assesses fetal size and status; locates placenta.

▐ *Medical Management*

Many of the drugs used to treat substance abuse and decrease withdrawal symptoms are contraindicated in pregnancy because of their teratogenic effects. Disulfiram (Antabuse), for example, cannot be used to treat alcoholism; methadone must be used very cautiously in opioid addiction; and short-acting barbiturates or benzodiazepines used to manage symptoms during alcohol withdrawal are potentially teratogenic and should be avoided if at all possible.

- Detoxification. Hospitalization is necessary. Cold turkey withdrawal poses unacceptable risk to the fetus.
- Methadone treatment. For women who are dependent on opioids such as heroin.
- Monitor for symptoms of medical complications associated with substance abuse.
- Substance abuse counseling and treatment plans.
- Family therapy to avoid relapse.

▐ *Collaborative Problems*

Complications of pregnancy vary with the type and amount of substance used. However, in general, spontaneous abortions are common, as are preterm labor, abruptio placentae, placenta previa, infections, pregnancy-induced hypertension, PROM, polyhydramnios, premature labor, and delivery. Some agents have been found to cause reduced placental blood flow, congenital anomalies (e.g., fetal alcohol syndrome), frequent growth retardation in the fetus, and at times, fetal demise.

Medical complications also vary depending on the drug(s) used. Examples are anemia, hepatitis B and C, tuberculosis, alcoholic hepatitis, pancreatitis, cirrhosis, hypertension, ventricular dysrhythmias, pulmonary disease, intestinal ischemia, phlebitis, urinary tract and vaginal infections, cellulitis, and HIV.

Standardized care for potential complications of prenatal substance abuse is addressed in this chapter using the following nursing diagnosis and collaborative problems:

- Risk for injury (to mother) related to overdose/withdrawal
- Potential complication of maternal substance abuse: injury to fetus (e.g., fetal alcohol syndrome, low birth weight, congenital malformations, and premature birth)

COLLABORATIVE (STANDARDIZED) CARE FOR ALL PATIENTS WITH PRENATAL SUBSTANCE ABUSE

This section discusses individual needs for teaching, emotional support, and physical care.

▐ Nursing Diagnosis: RISK FOR INJURY (TO MOTHER)[1]

Related Factors: substance use, overdose, or withdrawal.

▐ *Goals, Outcomes, and Evaluation Criteria*

- Woman agrees to obtain treatment for chemical dependence.

- Woman attends support and treatment groups.
- Woman describes safety measures for preventing overdose.
- Woman agrees to notify healthcare provider before attempting withdrawal.
- Woman remains free of overdose and relapse.
- Woman maintains a healthy state throughout pregnancy.

◼ NIC Interventions[2]

High-Risk Pregnancy Care (6800)—Identification and management of a high-risk pregnancy to promote healthy outcomes for mother and baby.

Risk Identification (6610)—Analysis of potential risk factors, determination of health risks, and prioritization of risk reduction strategies for an individual or group.

Referral (8100)—Arrangement for services by another care provider or agency.

Surveillance: Safety (6654)—Purposeful and ongoing collection and analysis of information about the patient and the environment for use in promoting and maintaining patient safety.

◼ Nursing Activities and Rationales

Assessments

- Determine the extent of the substance use/abuse (e.g., use the CAGE questionnaire or TACE to screen for alcohol use). Although any use of harmful substances is to be avoided, anticipated problems and interventions will differ depending on whether drug use is occasional and experimental or there is abuse and/or addiction.
- Screen for physical and sexual abuse. Often associated with substance abuse.
- Screen regularly for STIs. Often associated with substance abuse.
- Screen for history of psychiatric illness. Often associated with substance abuse. Dual diagnosis is common and both conditions must be treated for successful recovery.
- Obtain substance use history of the partner if possible. It will be harder for the woman to stop using drugs if she is in an environment where they are used; allows for identifying potential future problems regarding the newborn.
- Monitor temperature (fever). Hyperthermia may occur with methamphetamine or an overdose of phencyclidine.
- Assess pulse (tachycardia, bradycardia). Tachycardia and cardiac problems are associated with cocaine, heroin, methamphetamine, and phencyclidine use.
- Assess respirations (tachypnea, bradypnea). Respiratory compromise is associated with heroin and methamphetamines.
- Monitor blood pressure (hypertension). Hypertension is associated with cocaine and phencyclidine use, heroin withdrawal, and alcohol use.
- Examine eyes and pupils (constricted, dilated). Constriction of the pupils is seen with heroin use; cocaine use and heroin withdrawal are associated with pupil dilation.

- Assess mental status (irritability; aggressiveness; agitation; mood lability; inappropriate affect; delusions; anxiousness, hallucinations; distorted perception of time, spatial relations, and short-term memory; and loss of inhibition). All the drugs of abuse have psychoactive effects. Most cause psychomotor excitation and agitation. Depression and irritability are associated with alcohol withdrawal. Marijuana is associated with distortion of perception of time, spatial relations, and short-term memory and loss of inhibition.
- Assess motor skills (slurred speech, poor coordination, unsteady gait, tremors, nystagmus, hyperactivity, hyperactive reflexes and seizures). Neuromuscular excitation is also manifested as altered motor skills.
- Assess for flushed skin. Sweating and flushing are common with alcohol intoxication and hyperthermia.
- Assess for presence of and identify factors that increase risk for substance abuse. Facilitates initiation of preventive measures and explores areas for intervention and treatment.
- Identify woman's strengths and resources. Empowers the woman to quit using addictive substances.
- Assess interactions with significant others. Evaluates the quality of the interpersonal support available to the woman. She may experience isolation as a result of drug use and/or the disapproval from others because of drug use during pregnancy. Substance-abusing women fear they are viewed as weak willed, sexually promiscuous, and negligent of their children.
- Assess the extent of enabling behaviors by family members. How family members react to her pregnancy and drug use affects the way the woman sees herself and the course of the substance use. Family members often unconsciously become enablers; that is, they help the drug abuser to cover up the consequences of the abuse (e.g., by making excuses, by doing for the woman things she should do for herself). They enable because they want to be helpful, and since they cannot stop the substance abuse or change the destructive behaviors it causes, they cover for the drug abuser.
- Assess for barriers to the woman's obtaining therapy. Assists with substance abuse abstinence. Treatment is long term, and the woman may need transportation, time away from a job, and so forth.
- Determine readiness for change. Enables the nurse to select effective interventions. When the woman is unaware of the need for change, unwilling to change, or discouraged about changing substance use behavior, she is not responsive to change-promoting interventions. As she begins to consider the possibility of change and to form intent to change, she becomes more receptive to strategies designed to bring about behavior changes.
- Assess the woman's spirituality and faith. Faith in a power outside oneself can be empowering and has been shown to be effective in substance recovery, giving those who do have faith another source of support.

- Assess care providers for enabling behaviors and negative feelings about the woman. Staff members may feel anger toward a woman who continues to use substances during her pregnancy and may lack understanding of enabling and codependence; therefore, they may inadvertently use nontherapeutic approaches and be counterproductive in their efforts.

Independent Nursing Actions

- Promote abstinence, reinforce the need for help. Prevents risk to the woman and fetus. As long as the woman is using/abusing drugs, the risk for overdose is present.
- Use a caring, nonjudgmental approach. A moralistic, punitive attitude is likely to elicit a defensive response and be detrimental to recovery.
- Encourage adherence to methadone treatment plan (if the woman is abusing opioids). Eliminates opioid dependency before delivery. Methadone blocks the symptoms of withdrawal from opioids and reduces the craving for street drugs. Methadone crosses the placenta and has been associated with complications such as pregnancy-related hypertension, hepatitis, and placental problems.
- Encourage the woman to continue follow-up prenatal visits. Helps detect drug-related complications (e.g., pregnancy-related hypertension, hepatitis) as early as possible.

Collaborative Activities

- Encourage involvement in support and treatment groups (e.g., Alcoholics Anonymous, Narcotics Anonymous, Women for Sobriety). Facilitates abstinence. Provides contact with others who are managing sobriety and a drug-free life; provides understanding, support, confrontation of denial, and peer pressure for abstinence. Group sharing encourages verbalization and provides opportunity to gain new skills and a sense of community/family within the group. An interdisciplinary model is essential when planning care for the pregnant woman who abuses substances.
- Make appointment with the agency while the woman is in the office/clinic. Passivity and low self-esteem are associated with drug dependence; it may be easier for her to attend meetings than to take the initiative to set them up.
- Involve family members/significant other in treatment. Recovery is more likely to be successful if family members are treated along with the woman. Drug abuse/addiction is a family illness. Family members need help in adjusting to the woman's new behaviors (e.g., abstinence).
- Refer for private addiction counseling, if feasible. There are few drug treatment programs that admit pregnant women. Also, private counseling may be needed initially, especially if the woman is uncomfortable in a group setting.
- Consider referring for acupuncture. A new and promising, but yet unproven, treatment for cocaine abuse.
- Collaborate with advanced practice psychiatric nurses. Enables nurses to deal with their own feelings and provide better care for pregnant women who abuse substances.

Patient/Family Teaching

- Provide the woman and her family with information about the effects of substance use/addiction on the family; provide information about enabling behavior. Knowledge may bring awareness, the first step in the process of change. The woman and her family may not be aware of the nature of addiction and the effects of drugs on the pregnancy/fetus. They may not perceive it as abuse if the woman is using legally obtained drugs.
- Explain the relationship between substance use/abuse and the woman's current health problems. Provides motivation for cessation of substance use.
- Provide information about the effect of drugs on the fetus (e.g., brain damage, fetal malformation). Fear of harm to the baby may motivate the woman to stop using drugs.
- Teach family/significant others (if available) the symptoms of substance use and overdose. Helps ensure that treatment will be given promptly if overdose occurs and to ensure that family members will recognize when the woman is not abstinent.

Potential Complication of Maternal Substance Abuse: INJURY TO FETUS (E.G., FETAL ALCOHOL SYNDROME, LOW BIRTH WEIGHT, CONGENITAL MALFORMATIONS, AND PREMATURE BIRTH)

Focus Assessments

- Assess fetal heart rate (tachycardia, bradycardia, decreased variability). Vasoconstriction and seizures associated with substance abuse decrease uteroplacental blood flow, compromising the fetus. Substances of abuse and their by-products may directly affect the fetus, also.
- Assess fetal movement (may be decreased). Decreased fetal movement is associated with fetal compromise.
- Assess maternal weight gain (may be decreased). Decreased maternal weight gain may be seen as a result of decreased intake and increased metabolism associated with the abused substance.
- Assess maternal fundal height (may be decreased). Decreased fundal height indicates IUGR, which results from the poor nutrition associated with substance abuse.
- Assess biophysical profile (equal to or less than 8). Decreased biophysical profiles are associated with fetal compromise.
- Assess ultrasound (decreased growth, presence of anomalies). Decreased growth from uteroplacental insufficiency

and poor maternal nutrition (IUGR), as well as the presence of anomalies (e.g., fetal alcohol syndrome), can be detected with ultrasound.

- Determine the type(s) of substance(s) being used by the mother. To anticipate more specifically the problems the fetus/newborn may have. For example, prenatal alcohol exposure is the single greatest preventable cause of mental retardation.

Preventive Nursing Activities

- See "Risk for Injury[1] (to Mother)," which begins on p. 94.

INDIVIDUALIZED (NURSING DIAGNOSIS) CARE PLANS

This section includes care plans to address unique patient needs.

▮ Nursing Diagnosis: DYSFUNCTIONAL FAMILY PROCESSES: ALCOHOLISM OR OTHER SUBSTANCE ABUSE[1]

Related Factors: alcohol or other substance abuse, addictive personality, resistance to treatment, unrealistic expectations, poor social supports, inadequate coping skills, lack of problem-solving skills, and codependency issues.

▮ *Goals, Outcomes, and Evaluation Criteria*

- Woman acknowledges the existence of alcoholism within the family.
- Woman recognizes association between role demands, role expectations, family functioning, and alcoholism.
- Woman identifies dysfunctional responses.
- Woman identifies and uses available resources and social supports.
- Woman confronts and constructively manages problems.
- Family members demonstrate support for each other.

▮ *NIC Interventions[2]*

Family Mobilization (7120)—Utilization of family strengths to influence patient's health in a positive direction.
Family Process Maintenance (7130)—Minimization of family process disruption effects.
Family Therapy (7150)—Assisting family members to move their family toward a more productive way of living.
Substance Use Treatment (4510)—Supportive care of patient/family member with physical and psychosocial problems associated with the use of alcohol or drugs.

▮ *Nursing Activities and Rationales*

Assessments

- Identify family strengths, coping mechanisms, and resources. Determines additional assistance that is needed.
- Determine family roles, employment, housing arrangements, financial status, history of domestic violence. Establishes baseline information about family dynamics, potential stressors, and areas for potential change.
- Determine family's willingness and readiness to learn new coping methods. Without acceptance of a need for change, intervention is likely futile.
- Explore how family members have coped with the woman's drug use (e.g., anger, denial, rationalization). Codependent family members need help in learning new coping skills. They struggle with the same feelings of anxiety and low self-worth as the woman.
- Explore willingness and readiness to acknowledge substance abuse problem. Success of treatment often is a reflection of one's acceptance that there is a problem.
- Identify family's level of knowledge about role responsibilities and relationships, alcoholism, recovery process. Determines how to best counsel the family.

Independent Nursing Actions

- Demonstrate empathy and acceptance. Establishes a therapeutic, trusting relationship.
- Use matter-of-fact, nonjudgmental attitude when discussing the woman's addiction. Fosters trust so that the woman will be honest about her drug/alcohol habits. Women often deny or greatly underreport drug/alcohol usage when asked directly about their habits or when they feel they will be judged.
- Encourage the family to verbalize feelings, beliefs, and concerns. Creates an environment for open communication and an opportunity to correct misconceptions or validate feelings.
- Assist the family to problem solve. Helps the family better deal with the present problem and develop lifelong skills.
- Support involvement in therapy and efforts to change behaviors. Reinforces the importance of a family approach to recovery.

Patient/Family Teaching

- Inform the family about community resources (e.g., Alcoholics Anonymous, Narcotics Anonymous) and therapy options. Provides additional information about cessation of substance use and provides additional social support.
- Teach the family positive coping mechanisms and stress management skills. Enhances the family's success.

Nursing Diagnosis: IMBALANCED NUTRITION: LESS THAN BODY REQUIREMENTS[1]

Related Factors: increased metabolism secondary to pregnancy; nonnutrient cravings; and anorexia, nausea, vomiting, and diarrhea secondary to substance abuse.

Goals, Outcomes, and Evaluation Criteria

- Woman demonstrates appropriate weight gain for stage of pregnancy.
- Woman relates nutritional needs during pregnancy.
- Woman reports consumption of a balanced diet.
- Woman avoids further nutritional decline as evidenced by laboratory values within normal limits (iron, albumin, electrolytes), hydration and good skin turgor, moist mucous membranes, urine output and specific gravity within normal limits.

NIC Interventions[2]

Nutrition Management (1100)—Assisting with or providing a balanced dietary intake of foods and fluids.

Nutritional Monitoring (1160)—Collection and analysis of patient data to prevent or minimize malnourishment.

Nursing Activities and Rationales

Assessments

- Monitor dietary intake; encourage the woman to keep an intake diary or use 24-hour recall at visit. Helps determines the adequacy of nutritional content and calories and identify areas of need.
- Assess teeth and oral cavity. Poor dental health and inflamed mucous membranes may make it difficult to eat certain foods. Diet plan may need to be modified. Oral hygiene is linked to fetal health.
- Weigh patient and measure fundal height at each prenatal visit. Determines trends in weight gain and loss and evaluates effectiveness of interventions. Ideal gain for the normal-weight adult woman is 25–35 lb during the pregnancy; women with a low BMI should gain more than women who have a high BMI or who are obese.
- Monitor laboratory values. Detects anemia, malnutrition, or electrolyte imbalances, which are associated with substance abuse and malnutrition.
- Monitor urine output, specific gravity, skin turgor, and oral mucous membranes. Detects adequacy of hydration.

Independent Nursing Actions

- Provides nutritional counseling, emphasizing protein intake. Prevents or corrects nutritional deficits.

- Encourages supplementation with prenatal vitamins, ferrous sulfate, calcium, and folic acid if indicated. Prevents or corrects deficits that may occur during pregnancy due to increased needs.
- Encourage small, frequent meals. Small meals are less overwhelming to the woman who may have difficulty eating or who experiences nausea. Meals throughout the day facilitate ingestion of required nutrients, supply greater energy, and prevent gastric distention, which causes nausea.
- Help to plan a budget for groceries; help the woman to make a food plan, choosing nutritional snacks and foods. Helps ensure that the woman will consume the nutrients she needs. Problem solving and decision making may be impaired due to substance use; the woman may require help with these basic activities.

Collaborative Activities

- Collaborate with the dietician to provide the woman with information about nutrient requirements and resources. Helps ensure the woman eats a well-balanced diet. Dietician has specialized knowledge to enable planning a diet to accommodate the increased nutritional needs of pregnancy and the nutritional deficits caused by substance use.
- Administer prenatal vitamins and iron as ordered. Assists with meeting extra needs associated with pregnancy, corrects nutritional deficits caused by substance use, and prevents anemia.
- Refer to dentist, as needed. Healthy teeth are important to adequate nutrition and maintenance of health. Neglect of dental hygiene is common among those who abuse drugs.

Patient/Family Teaching

- Teach prenatal nutritional needs and the content of an adequate diet, using the *Food Guide Pyramid* (United States Department of Agriculture, 2010). Provides information that facilitates self-care.

Nursing Diagnosis: INEFFECTIVE COPING[1]

Related Factors: lack of self-esteem, ineffective coping mechanisms, an inadequate support system, guilt, and chemical dependency.

Use with generic NDCP, "Ineffective Coping,[1]" beginning on p. 17 in Chapter 2.

Goals, Outcomes, and Evaluation Criteria

- Woman recognizes consequences of decisions.
- Woman identifies and uses available social supports.
- Woman maintains roles and social relationships.

NIC Interventions[2]

Substance Use Prevention (4500)—Prevention of an alcoholic or drug use lifestyle.

Nursing Activities and Rationales

Assessments

- Inquire about current family situation and structures and their impact on the patient's current situation. Establishes a baseline for care planning.
- Identify common stressors and effective coping mechanisms. Ask specific questions to screen for violence. Assists the woman to develop a plan using effective coping mechanisms. Violence can escalate during pregnancy and women who are substance abusers are at increased risk.
- Assess availability and adequacy of supports. Establishes a baseline for care planning; referral to community agencies may be necessary to obtain adequate support.
- Determine barriers that might prevent the use of support systems. Assist in identification of community support networks available. Ensures access to additional support (e.g., the woman may not have transportation).
- Referral for counseling and domestic shelter if needed. Emotional support and physical safety are important during pregnancy.

Independent Nursing Actions

- Provide a nonjudgmental environment. Promotes a trusting and therapeutic relationship. Women often deny or under-report their substance abuse when they feel they are being judged.
- Encourage the woman's involvement in social support groups. Reinforces effective decision-making skills and coping mechanisms. Social support modifies the negative effects of stress.

Collaborative Activities

- Collaborate with substance abuse counselors and therapists in reinforcing and monitoring the use of constructive coping mechanisms. Maintains continuity and reinforces the plan of care.

Patient/Family Teaching

- Instruct the woman regarding effective ways to control anger, to relieve stress and anxiety, and to manage conflict. Helps equip the woman with constructive tools that can be used to cope with stressors.
- Teach relaxation skills such as guided imagery and progressive muscle relaxation. Provides new ways to cope with stress and can be used to help relieve anxiety and tension created by the desire to use.
- Encourage self-care and support her endeavors to change. Positive reinforcement can be helpful in facilitating change.

Nursing Diagnosis: INEFFECTIVE DENIAL[1]

Related Factors: previous ineffective coping skills, process of addiction, inability to accept consequences, inadequate support system, anxiety, and lack of understanding of the action of illicit drugs on pregnancy and the developing fetus. Denial is a defense mechanism to help cope with the stigma, shame, and guilt produced by the substance abuse.

Goals, Outcomes, and Evaluation Criteria

- Woman acknowledges addiction to alcohol/illicit substances.
- Woman verbalizes understanding of adverse effects of substance use on self and fetus.
- Woman verbalizes understanding that substance abuse is causing present social problems.
- Woman abstains from alcohol/illicit substance use.
- Woman demonstrates health-seeking behaviors (e.g., attends support group).

NIC Interventions[2]

Anxiety Reduction (5820)—Minimizing apprehension, dread, foreboding, or uneasiness related to an unidentified source of anticipated danger.

Counseling (5240)—Use of an interactive helping process focusing on the needs, problems, or feelings of the patient and significant others to enhance or support coping, problem solving, and interpersonal relationships.

Nursing Activities and Rationales

Assessments

- Determine the woman's perspective on her pregnancy and her substance use/abuse. Establishes a baseline for care planning.
- Assess understanding of the effects of substance use during pregnancy. Determines what teaching may be needed.
- Assess level of denial. Determines type(s) of interventions needed.
- Determine previous methods of coping, other than substance use. Identifies coping skills upon which to build the plan of care. Denial is the primary defense mechanism used by substance abusers. It prevents the woman from accepting that she has a problem, thereby blocking therapeutic efforts.

Independent Nursing Actions

- Demonstrate empathy, warmth, genuineness, and acceptance. Facilitates a therapeutic relationship that will allow exploration of denial. Confrontation must be done carefully and only after a relationship is established; otherwise, it will increase resistance to change.

- Encourage verbalization of feelings, concerns, and fears. Identifies rational and irrational beliefs; discussion also provides opportunity for the woman to gain insight into the problems that substance use has created for her.
- Assist the woman to identify personal reasons for alcohol/illicit substance use. Facilitates an awareness of why and when substances are used.
- Clearly communicate what is expected of the woman, e.g., attendance at group meetings/therapy sessions. Encourages appropriate health-seeking behaviors. Attending group is an admission of the need for help and the need to stop using drugs.
- Stress that the woman is responsible for her own recovery. The woman must recognize and accept her own responsibility for developing alternative coping behaviors; otherwise, denial will continue. Care provider can provide information and support, but abstinence can come only from the woman.
- Develop a structured plan that incorporates short-term goals for achieving abstinence. Provides measurable opportunities for success. Short-term goals are often easier to meet than long-term goals.
- Encourage replacement of negative behaviors with positive, health-seeking behaviors. Facilitates the transition to health-seeking behaviors.
- Encourage development of relationships with individuals who do not use drugs. Facilitates maintenance of a drug-free lifestyle.
- Acknowledge and reward appropriate behavior; reinforce consequences of denial; give positive feedback when the woman recognizes denial in self and others. Positive feedback enhances self-esteem and reinforces desired behavior.
- Stress to family members the importance of supporting, but not enabling the woman. Family members must recognize enabling and codependent behaviors in order to avoid nontherapeutic approaches with the addicted family member.

Patient/Family Teaching

- Discuss the addiction process and how decision making is influenced. Facilitates the woman's understanding of her disease.
- Provide information about the effects of illicit substances, tobacco, and alcohol on the woman, pregnancy, and the fetus, as applicable. Facilitates the decision-making process. Recognition that substance use is harmful to her fetus may help her to stop denying that drug use is a problem.
- Point out the ways in which substance use has created problems in her life, job, and personal relationships. Awareness of the control the drug has over her life helps to combat the denial.
- Discuss the difference among occasional diversional/experimental drug use and addiction. Provides information needed for insight and recognizing her denial. Substance-abusing women experience much stigma, shame, and guilt, which leads to denial. Helping diminish those feelings may be the first step in breaking down the denial.
- Provide information concerning the kinds and availability of treatment. Facilitates the woman's decision making.

Nursing Diagnosis: INEFFECTIVE HEALTH MAINTENANCE[1]

Related Factors: fear of legal action, inadequate finances, ineffective family coping, lack of understanding about effects of illicit substances on pregnancy and the fetus, and altered decision making related to drug use/abuse.

Goals, Outcomes, and Evaluation Criteria

- Woman verbalizes understanding of healthcare maintenance needs.
- Woman seeks prenatal care and adheres to routine schedule of visits.
- Woman follows recommendations for diet, exercise, and abstinence from illicit substances, tobacco, and alcohol.

NIC Interventions[2]

Health System Guidance (7400)—Facilitating a patient's location and use of appropriate health services.
Self-Responsibility Facilitation (4480)—Encouraging a patient to assume more responsibility for her own behavior.

Nursing Activities and Rationales

Assessments

- Assess mental status, including presence of psychiatric disorders. Women often use alcohol and other drugs to self-treat for depression and anxiety. Dual diagnosis is common, and it is essential to treat both conditions.
- Determine the extent of substance use/abuse and factors that affect use. Establishes the extent to which the substance use/abuse is the cause of failure to keep appointments and so forth. Other factors, such as lack of transportation or insurance, may be involved.
- Determine the woman's understanding of the effects of substance abuse on herself, her pregnancy, and the fetus. Lack of information or of understanding may contribute to ineffective health maintenance. Even though substance use appears to be the obvious etiology, other factors may be involved.
- Identify barriers to obtaining therapy and prenatal care (e.g., lack of child care, transportation, or insurance coverage). Support may be needed in order for the woman to obtain prenatal care and treatment for substance use.
- Monitor the level of responsibility for care displayed by the woman. Evaluates for behaviors consistent with health maintenance and provides effective interventions.

Independent Nursing Actions

- Hold woman accountable for her own actions. Minimizes manipulation and irresponsible behavior.
- Provide time for and encourage discussion of her situation. The woman may have difficulty expressing herself; she may feel indecisive about the pregnancy and/or how she will manage to care for an infant.
- Provide positive feedback when the woman keeps appointments and demonstrates responsible behavior. Reinforces desirable behavior and promotes success.

Collaborative Activities

- Refer to social services for assistance as needed (e.g., transportation, child care). Removes barriers to care.

Patient/Family Teaching

- Provide information about the effects of chemical substances on health, pregnancy, and the fetus. An understanding of the harmful effects of chemical substances may reinforce the need for frequent prenatal visits.
- Inform the woman about care needs during pregnancy (dietary requirements, exercise, activity restrictions) and ways to cope with the discomforts of pregnancy (e.g., meditation, biofeedback, relaxation techniques). Facilitates healthy behaviors during pregnancy. Information can empower her in these areas. When she feels in control of some parts of her life, her self-confidence and self-esteem may increase as well.
- Provide written copies of instructions, appointments made, and visit schedules. Reinforces teaching; anxiety during clinic/office visits may interfere with learning.

Nursing Diagnosis: CHRONIC AND/OR SITUATIONAL LOW SELF-ESTEEM[1]

Related Factors: feelings of helplessness and failure, illicit substance use, failed attempts at abstinence, unrealistic expectations of self, history of abusive relationships, pregnancy-related changes in body image, social role changes related to the pregnancy, behavior inconsistent with values, and failures/rejections.

Goals, Outcomes, and Evaluation Criteria

- Woman verbalizes acceptance of self and own limitations.
- Woman maintains hygiene and grooming.
- Woman relays pride in successful abstinence.

NIC Interventions[2]

Body Image Enhancement (5220)—Improving a patient's conscious and unconscious perceptions and attitudes toward his/her body.

Self-Esteem Enhancement (5400)—Assisting a patient to increase his/her personal judgment of self-worth.

Nursing Activities and Rationales

Assessments

- Identify factors that contribute to poor self-esteem. Establishes a basis for care.
- Monitor negative/positive self-talk. Helps determine extent of problem and success of interventions.

Independent Nursing Actions

- Be attentive, accepting, and respectful of the woman. Acknowledges the woman's individuality and acceptance by others. Spending time with the woman is a way to acknowledge that she is a worthwhile person.
- Assist the woman to reframe and redefine negative expressions. Promotes positive self-talk.
- Encourage expression of feelings such as anger, guilt, and shame. The woman may lack self-respect and may believe the situation is hopeless. Ventilating negative feelings may relieve anxiety and provide the first steps in making change.
- Role model and assist with assertive communication; provide opportunity to practice. Provides a safe environment for practice of new skills. Essential in breaking off relationships with drug users and dealers and in building healthy relationships.
- Encourage to meet personal needs (proper hygiene, nutrition, rest). Helps the woman look and feel her best.
- Praise for attainment of goals and improvements in hygiene and grooming. Reinforces desirable behavior and promotes the woman's self-esteem.
- Assist the woman to make a list of previous accomplishments and positive experiences. When self-esteem is low, the person finds it difficult to remember successes or to view them as successes.

Collaborative Activities

- Refer to a professional counselor for personal and vocational counseling. Enhances the woman's opportunities for self-development and success.

Patient/Family Teaching

- Teach the woman esteem-building exercises. Helps equip the woman with tools for self-improvement. Failure and low self-esteem are commonly associated with drug dependence and abuse.
- Provide information about actions that will improve hygiene and appearance. Improves the woman's self-worth and body image.

Nursing Diagnosis: RISK FOR INFECTION[1]

Related Factors: impaired skin and tissue integrity (cellulitis, thrombosis, and intravenous [IV] drug use), dehydration and malnutrition, anemia, lack of sleep, and method of administration of drugs. Use with generic NDCP, "Risk for Infection,[1]" which begins on p. 21 in Chapter 2.

■ *Goals, Outcomes, and Evaluation Criteria*

- Woman's white blood cell (WBC) count and differential within normal limits.
- STI cultures, hepatitis B, and HIV assays negative.
- Woman abstains from behaviors that place self and fetus at risk for infection.

■ *Nursing Activities and Rationales*

Assessments

- Determine whether the woman engages in risky behaviors (e.g., IV drug use, unprotected sexual intercourse). Establishes a basis for risk.
- Inspect extremities for evidence of track marks, cellulitis, and thrombosis. Determines the integrity of the skin or the presence of manifestations of infection. The intact skin serves as a barrier to infectious microorganisms; breaks in the skin provide a portal of entry.
- Assess for urinary symptoms and/or the presence of foul-smelling, purulent vaginal discharge. Identifies the presence of genitourinary infection.

Independent Nursing Actions

- Encourage the consumption of a well-balanced diet and adequate hydration. Provides the nutrients necessary to prevent anemia and promote cellular repair and regeneration. Poor nutrition is often associated with substance use/abuse.
- Encourage adequate rest and elimination of stress. Enhances immune system functioning.

Collaborative Activities

- Report abnormal laboratory findings to healthcare provider. Facilitates early intervention and prevention of complications related to infection.

Patient/Family Teaching

- Teach the woman about the infectious process and how infections are acquired. Enhances the woman's understanding regarding the transmission of diseases, which may provide motivation for preventive measures.
- Inform the woman that sharing needles and other drug paraphernalia is a way infections may be acquired. Increases the woman's knowledge base in order to prevent the transmission of infections.

DIABETES MELLITUS IN PREGNANCY

Diabetes is a disease involving the inability to create or utilize endogenous insulin for glucose metabolism for the body's energy needs. It may be a preexisting condition, or it may develop during pregnancy as a result of hormone-induced metabolic changes (gestational diabetes). Diabetes is classified as three types according to its etiology by the National Diabetes Data Group Classification.

Type 1 and type 2 diabetes are called *pregestational diabetes* (i.e., the diabetes was present before the pregnancy occurred). Women with *type 1 diabetes* require insulin administration because the islet cells of their pancreas do not secrete insulin due to cellular-mediated autoimmune destruction. Women with *type 2 diabetes* have insulin resistance and may also have impaired insulin secretion; they are typically treated with oral hypoglycemics rather than insulin.

Type 3 (gestational) diabetes is a carbohydrate intolerance that first occurs or is first recognized during pregnancy. Impaired glucose tolerance and impaired fasting glucose are intermediate staging terms for prediabetic states. Impaired glucose tolerance occurs when a 2-hour postprandial blood sugar level is higher than 140 mg/dl but lower than 200 mg/dl. Impaired fasting glucose occurs when a fasting blood sugar level is 100 or higher but lower than 126 mg/dl. These are both associated with syndrome X or metabolic syndrome. Syndrome X is a grouping of signs and symptoms that includes insulin resistance, compensatory hyperinsulinemia, central obesity, high high-density lipoprotein cholesterol, low low-density lipoprotein cholesterol and triglycerides, hypertension, prothrombotic state, and impaired glucose tolerance. This state can also complicate pregnancy.

Pregnancy alterations in glucose metabolism, insulin production, and metabolic homeostasis take place to supply adequate nutrition for both the mother and the growing fetus. Pregnancy is a diabetogenic state that is associated with mild fasting hypoglycemia, postprandial hyperglycemia, and hyperinsulinemia along with some renal changes to allow passage of glucose across the placenta to the developing fetus. These changes allow the fetus to have a continuous supply of glucose. If a woman has preexisting diabetes and becomes pregnant, this state is compounded by glucose metabolism problems. Therefore, a pregnancy complicated by diabetes is considered high risk and requires management to decrease complications. The perinatal mortality rate for well-managed diabetic pregnancies is about the same as for any other pregnancy. The key to a good pregnancy outcome is strict maternal glucose control before conception and careful monitoring during the gestational period.

In uncontrolled diabetes, maternal risks involve increased vascular problems such as retinopathy, nephropathy, and hypertension. The woman is at risk for hyperglycemia, hypoglycemia, and diabetic ketoacidosis. Maternal pregnancy risks can encompass the following:

- Spontaneous abortion
- Preeclampsia
- Preterm labor
- Polyhydramnios or oligohydramnios
- Infection, urinary tract infections, pyelonephritis, chorioamnionitis, and postpartum endometritis
- Diabetic ketoacidosis
- Cesarean or instrumental birth and induction

Fetal and neonatal effects are dependent on the maternal vascular complications and placental insufficiency and evidenced by intrauterine growth restriction and oligohydramnios. The fetus is at risk for the following:

- Congenital defects, especially neural tube defects, congenital cardiac anomalies, gastrointestinal malformations, and renal anomalies
- Macrosomia (large for gestational age) and therefore potentially birth trauma, shoulder dystocia, brachial plexus injuries, facial nerve injuries, and asphyxia
- Intrauterine growth restriction
- Delayed lung maturity
- Unexplained stillbirth

After birth, infants born to diabetic mothers have delayed lung maturity and may have respiratory problems. Also the neonate is at risk for the following:

- Hypoglycemia
- Hypocalcemia
- Hypomagnesemia
- Hyperbilirubinemia and polycythemia
- Cardiomyopathy and anomalies

As a young child, he or she may have learning disabilities and a propensity for obesity and type 2 diabetes.

Key Nursing Activities

- Monitor diabetic control and support the woman in self-management of insulin if she has preexisting or gestational diabetes.
- Assess for glucose metabolism at beginning of pregnancy and at 28 weeks to determine if the woman is acquiring gestational diabetes; if on insulin hemoglobin A1c, every trimester.
- Teach proper diet and encourage exercise during pregnancy.
- Provide information, as needed, for the woman to avoid developing hypoglycemia or hyperglycemia, which can turn into ketoacidosis (in insulin-dependent diabetics) if untreated and how to respond; include the family in teaching.
- Teach symptoms of and need to monitor for maternal complications (e.g., gestational hypertension, renal failure, retinopathy).
- Monitor for fetal size and fetal compromise.

- Be prepared for a difficult labor and birth and/or neonatal complications.

Etiologies and Risk Factors

Type 1 diabetes may be caused by an autoimmune disorder, but the exact cause is unknown. It is defined as immunologic destruction of the pancreas by American Diabetes Association Classification System (ADA, 2010). Specific causes of type 2 diabetes are unknown. It is defined as exhaustion or resistance of the pancreatic cells (ADA, 2010). Risk factors include aging, family history of diabetes, sedentary lifestyle, obesity, hypertension, metabolic syndrome, or previous gestational diabetes. Type 3 (gestational) diabetes is defined as a glucose intolerance that had not previously been present prior to pregnancy (ADA, 2010). Risks for gestational diabetes include obesity, maternal age greater than 25 years, history of recurrent monilial vaginitis, current glycosuria, chronic hypertension, previous large infant (more than 4,000 g), diabetes in a previous pregnancy, family history of type 2 diabetes in a first-degree relative, previous hydramnios, and unexplained fetal death or congenital anomalies. Other factors are ethnic origin of Native American, African American, Asian, Hispanic, or Pacific Islander and having polycystic ovary syndrome.

Another classification system, the White Classification (Mattson & Smith, 2010), rates diabetes from A to D, R, F, RF, G, H, T, and gestation diabetes A1 (controlled by diet and exercise), and A2 (requiring insulin). Classifications are specific to age acquired and vascular changes and neuropathies that are associated with each level. For more information, refer to an obstetrics or maternity care textbook. This care plan will use the ADA classifications.

Signs and Symptoms

Subjective manifestations: olyuria, polydipsia, and polyphagia are the classic symptoms of diabetes. Prior to being diagnosed with diabetes, the woman may also experience symptoms of *hyperglycemia* (e.g., thirst, nausea, abdominal pain, constipation, drowsiness, dim vision, headache) or *hypoglycemia* (irritability, hunger, nervousness, weakness, fatigue, blurred or double vision, dizziness, headache).

Objective manifestations: depend on whether the woman has gestational diabetes, hyperglycemia, or hypoglycemia.

Gestational Diabetes. Elevated blood glucose levels (see "Diagnostic Studies," below).

Hyperglycemia. Flushing; dry skin; vomiting; rapid respirations; weak, rapid pulse; acetone breath; increased urination; urine positive for sugar and acetone; and blood glucose greater than 200 mg/dl.

Hypoglycemia. Pallor, clammy skin, sweating, personality change, shallow respirations, rapid pulse, urine negative for sugar and acetone, and blood glucose 60 mg/dl or less.

If uncontrolled, diabetes can result in an emergency situation, diabetic ketoacidosis (DKA). Without insulin, glucose cannot enter the cells, and the cells starve. The signs and symptoms of

DKA are hyperventilation or Kussmaul respirations, mental lethargy, dehydration, hypotension unless complicated by pregnancy-induced hypertension, abdominal pain, nausea and vomiting, fruity odor to the breath, and ketonuria. The pregnant woman classically presents with abdominal pain, nausea and vomiting, and decreased mentation. If left unchecked, cell starvation will lead to decreased cardiac preload, hypertension, and shock followed by death.

▌ Diagnostic Studies

- Fasting and/or random blood glucose. Fasting blood glucose should be less than 95 mg/dl. Random blood glucose of more than 126 mg/dl on two occasions; assesses recent glucose control and confirm by an oral glucose tolerance test.
- Oral glucose challenge test. More than 130 mg/dl; screens for diabetes but is not diagnostic of diabetes; 50 g of oral glucose or 18 jelly beans as alternative for the challenge. If elevated, do the oral glucose tolerance test. Most care providers screen universally at 24–48 weeks. High-risk patients will be tested during first trimester as well.
- Oral glucose tolerance test. Fasting, more than 95 mg/dl; 1 hour, more than 180 mg/dl; 2 hours, more than 155 mg/dl; 3 hours, more than 140 mg/dl; diagnostic of gestational diabetes if two or more are elevated. A single abnormal value indicates impaired glucose tolerance. Can be a 2- or 3-hour glucose tolerance test.
- Glycosylated hemoglobin A1c. Glucose attaches to hemoglobin a during its 120-day life span value and is dependent on how much glucose is available. Initially and every 2–6 weeks; Hgb-A1c over 7 is associated with increased incidence of congenital anomalies.
- Urine for ketones and glucose. Initially and at each prenatal visit. Assesses glucose control; if blood glucose is elevated, urine glucose and ketones may also be elevated.
- Alpha-fetoprotein testing at 14–18 weeks. With triple testing since diabetics are at risk for open neural tube and ventral wall defects of omphalocele or gastroschisis.

▌ Medical Management

The goals of medical management are to achieve maternal euglycemia (normal blood glucose levels) and detect fetal compromise or maternal complications that necessitate management and possible labor induction. It is desirable to continue the pregnancy to at least 36 weeks and deliver prior to term due to prevent unexplained stillbirths. If maternal conditions such as renal failure, preeclampsia, rapidly worsening retinopathy, or fetal compromise develop, a preterm induction of labor may be essential.

Type 1 Diabetes

- Preconceptual counseling to ensure that blood glucose is well controlled, establish baseline understanding of interaction of diabetes and pregnancy, to evaluate risks and carefully plan pregnancy. Self-management skills should be in place. Evaluation of physical readiness and health of kidneys, eyes, and thyroid should be targeted and all problems corrected before the woman becomes pregnant. Counseling should be offered and stress reduction plans should be in place. To achieve good pregnancy outcome, it is essential that blood glucose be well controlled before conception and during pregnancy; and that a healthy baseline be achieved, stress reduced, and self-management education completed (ADA, 2004).
- Thorough history and documentation of same at beginning of pregnancy if not preconceptually.
- Complete physical and evaluation of blood pressure and check for retinopathy, nephropathies, and coronary artery disease. Lab panel to check A1c and 24-hour urine sample for protein and albumin.
- Adjust insulin according to blood glucose levels with proper diet in place. Maintains euglycemia.
- Use biosynthetic human insulin (e.g., Humulin or Novolin) short and intermediate acting (Lispro, NPH, Lente). Long-acting insulin is not used in pregnancy. It is less likely to cause formation of insulin antibodies, which can cross the placenta and cause fetal weight gain. Insulin pump may be used to avoid multiple injections.
- Proper diabetic diet teaching with specific caloric intake is the cornerstone of therapy to maintain glucose control. Encourage exercise (at least 150 minutes a week) to decrease blood sugar. Approximately 30–35 cal/kg if normal BMI—adjusted if under- or overweight.
- Prenatal vitamins, iron, folic acid. To decrease risk for neural tube defects.
- Blood sugar levels at least two times daily—morning fasting, before lunch and dinner, and at bedtime (all goals are 60–99 mg/dl); 1 hour postprandial (100–129 mg/dl), 2-hour postprandial (90–120 mg/dl); also between 2:00 a.m. and 4:00 a.m. for Somogyi effect; mean daily glucose less than 110 mg/dl and A1c less than 6.0. Tight glucose control will help accommodate fluctuations during pregnancy and improve infant outcome since damage to fetus is due to hyperglycemia (ADA, 2008).
- Fetal surveillance (e.g., alpha-fetoprotein testing, fetal movement, frequent ultrasound, nonstress tests [NSTs], biophysical profile, contraction stress tests, fetal echocardiogram, amniocentesis, Doppler umbilical artery velocimetry). See "Collaborative (Standardized) Care for All Patients With Diabetes Mellitus in Pregnancy," which begins on p. 105 in this chapter. Fetal monitoring testing begins at 32–34 weeks' gestation (ACOG, 2004).
- Schedule frequent prenatal visits, every 1–2 weeks during the first two trimesters, and one or two times per week during the third trimester.
- Monitor for fetal growth, screen for preeclampsia, preterm labor, signs of infection, dehydration, or other problems in addition to glucose control.

- Frequent laboratory tests for maternal status; e.g., for vasculopathies and preeclampsia, ketones and glucose in urine, hemoglobin A1c.
- Behavior therapy if indicated to decrease stress and depression during pregnancy.

During Labor

- Continuous fetal monitoring.
- Blood glucose levels every hour.
- IV therapy (Lactated Ringers solution or Dextrose 5% in Lactated Ringers solution); close intake and output.
- Adjust insulin based on hourly blood glucose levels; insulin infusion can be piggybacked into IV. Intermittent subcutaneous injections also can be used the morning of labor induction.
- Anticipate macrosomia and cephalopelvic disproportion, except in women with a long history of diabetes with vascular changes, who are more likely to have babies with IUGR because they have vascular involvement with their diabetes. If macrosomia is detected, the woman may have a planned cesarean due to fetal size to avoid birth trauma or failure to progress. The trend is to attempt vaginal delivery through induction prior to term.
- Maternal labor support and teaching with inclusion of family members. To decrease fever and increase ability to cope.
- Comfort measures, positional changes, and avoiding supine position. To avoid hypotension syndrome.
- No contraindications for epidural analgesia, spinal anesthesia, or general anesthesia if needed.

During postpartum, there is a significant decrease in insulin needs due to a loss of the antagonistic placental hormones. Medical management includes the following:

- Frequent blood glucose monitoring (every 1–2 hours).
- Adjust insulin based on blood glucose levels.
- Monitor for complications (e.g., preeclampsia, hemorrhage, infection, and thyroid dysfunction).

Type 2 Diabetes

Glyburide (since it does not cross the placenta to the fetus) and metformin are being investigated for control for during pregnancy but are not FDA approved and are restricted to investigational research only.

Care is the same as for type 1 diabetes except for the following:

- Discontinue oral hypoglycemics and institute diet therapy and insulin. Oral hypoglycemics (e.g., tolbutamide) may have teratogenic effects on the fetus. Additionally, insulin requirements fluctuate greatly during pregnancy, and oral dosages cannot be adjusted as finely or as quickly as injectable medications.

During Postpartum

- Discontinue insulin if possible.
- Start oral hypoglycemic.

- Otherwise, same as for type 1 diabetes.

Gestational Diabetes

- Frequent laboratory tests (see type 1 diabetes in preceding section).
- Administer insulin if glucose control cannot be achieved by diet and exercise alone (see type 1 and type 2 diabetes in preceding section). About half of all women with gestational diabetes require insulin at some point in their pregnancy.

During Labor

- Most practitioners opt to deliver diabetic pregnancies prior to 39 weeks' gestation but should only do so if, through amniocentesis, it has been determined that fetal lungs are mature and other complications do not otherwise determine time for birth.
- Continuous fetal monitoring.
- IV therapy and insulin therapy dependent on glycemic control during pregnancy.
- No need to check sugars during labor if blood sugar levels were controlled through diet and exercise during pregnancy; a baseline at admission is all that is needed.
- Intake and output; dip each urine sample for ketones and glucose.
- Assess for hypoglycemia, ketoacidosis, UTI, upper respiratory infection, polyhydramnios, and fetal macrosomia.
- Gestational diabetes is not an indication for cesarean birth unless complications such as macrosomia, preeclampsia, or fetal or maternal complications ensue.

During Postpartum

- Monitor for complications (e.g., preeclampsia, hemorrhage, infection, and thyroid dysfunction).
- Evaluate for type 2 diabetes at 6 weeks postpartum; glucose tolerance screening should be performed 2–4 months after delivery and periodically thereafter. Detection of the 3–5% of women who remain diabetic and need further treatment is imperative. Also about 50% of women with gestational diabetes will eventually develop type 2 diabetes (Gilmartin, Ural, & Repke, 2008).
- Promote postpartum weight loss through breastfeeding, exercising at moderate intensity for 150 minutes or more per week, and continuing a healthy diet.
- Teach and help with breastfeeding to maintain good feeding techniques and promote bonding.
- Discuss proper contraception and aid decision making prior to discharge. Risk and benefits need to be discussed. Oral contraceptives have a risk of clots, and this population is at risk. Progesterone-only methods can affect diabetic control. For a woman who is breastfeeding, some contraceptives containing estrogen will also be a problem. Intrauterine devices can work well but carry a risk of infection. Barrier methods are available. Sterilization is an option if childbearing is complete.

▌ *Collaborative Problems*

Potential complications of diabetes during pregnancy include the following:

- Hyperglycemia, DKA in women with insulin-dependent diabetes.
- Hypoglycemia (insulin shock).
- Maternal vasculopathy (e.g., diabetic retinopathy, nephropathy, coronary artery disease).
- Preeclampsia and eclampsia.
- Infection (e.g., urinary tract infection, pyelonephritis, monilial vaginitis) related to a nutrient-rich medium for bacterial growth secondary to spilling of glucose into the urine, and changes in vaginal pH.
- Difficult labor/birth (e.g., shoulder dystocia, birth trauma, need for cesarean birth).
- Polyhydramnios or oligohydramnios.
- PROM and/or premature labor.
- Congenital anomalies, especially cardiac, central nervous system, and skeletal anomalies; fetal lung immaturity.
- IUGR.
- Miscarriage.
- Sudden, unexplained stillbirth.

Potential complications of diabetes during postpartum include the following:

- Increased risk of postpartum hemorrhage (related to over-distention of the uterus during pregnancy, secondary to hydramnios and large fetal size).
- Increased risk of postpartum infection.
- Neonatal hypoglycemia (caused by neonatal hyperinsulinemia when maternal glucose is no longer available).
- Neonatal respiratory distress syndrome (caused by inadequate production of pulmonary surfactant secondary to prematurity).
- Neonatal hyperbilirubinemia, hypocalcemia, polycythemia, hypomagnesemia/congenital anomalies.

COLLABORATIVE (STANDARDIZED) CARE FOR ALL PATIENTS WITH DIABETES MELLITUS DURING PREGNANCY

Perform comprehensive assessment to identify individual needs for teaching, emotional support, and physical care.

▌ Potential Complications of Diabetes in Pregnancy: MATERNAL HYPERGLYCEMIA, DIABETIC KETOACIDOSIS

Hyperglycemia occurs in women with insulin-dependent diabetes because of ineffective insulin and elevation of hormones that work against insulin moving glucose into cells, resulting in hyperglycemia. The liver tries to respond by pumping more glucose into the system. Fat breaks down to supply energy, resulting in ketone release and metabolic acidosis (including DKA). This problem can be caused by insufficient insulin, excess or the wrong kinds of food, infection, injuries, illness, emotional stress, and insufficient exercise. Hyperglycemia has slow onset over hours or days, the end result of which can be DKA.

Focus Assessments

- Assess respirations (tachypnea) and pulse (tachycardia, weak). Increased findings indicate metabolic acidosis.
- Assess level of consciousness and headache. May have dim vision. Decreased level of consciousness and headache indicate fluid and electrolyte imbalance and cellular dehydration.
- Assess for nausea and vomiting, especially during first trimester. The body may metabolize fats in response to decreased food intake, resulting in ketosis. Abdominal pain is also common.
- Assess for thirst and dehydration. The body loses fluid because of osmotic diuresis, loss of fluid and electrolytes, volume depletion, and cellular dehydration.
- Assess for acetone breath odor. This is caused by breakdown of ketone bodies. When the body cannot utilize glucose, fatty acids are mobilized from fat stores. As they are oxidized in the circulation, ketone bodies are released. Acetone is a simple ketone.
- Assess for flushed, dry skin. Excessive glucose and ketone bodies result in osmotic diuresis, causing cellular dehydration and flushed, dry skin.
- Assess urine for acetone and glucose. When the body cannot utilize glucose, fatty acids are mobilized from fat stores. As they are oxidized in the circulation, ketone bodies are released. Both acetone and glucose are positive with hyperglycemia.
- Assess random blood glucose and also blood level of glycosylated hemoglobin (A1c). These reflect blood glucose level and the need for intervention. A1c indicates glycemic control over the previous 4–6 weeks and provides data for altering the treatment plan and improving glucose control. DKA can occur when blood glucose level exceeds 200 mg/dl.
- Monitor blood glucose to maintain euglycemia values as indicated in medical management (p. 103). Keeping maternal glucose within these ranges decreases the incidence of fetal abnormalities and maternal complications from diabetes.
- Measure fasting blood glucose or random glucose levels during antepartum visits. Establishes need to alter treatment plan; fasting blood glucose should be maintained at 60–100 mg/dl for best pregnancy outcomes.

- Assess weight and encourage exercise unless there are contraindications to activity. Diet, exercise, and insulin are regulated on the basis of weight gain and blood glucose levels.
- Assess for signs and symptoms of infection. Infection requires hospitalization because it can lead quickly to hyperglycemia and ketoacidosis.
- Be especially vigilant for hyperglycemia after the first trimester. Ketoacidosis is more likely to occur during the second and third trimesters because of the increased resistance to insulin and elevated levels of human placental lactogen (an insulin antagonist). Nevertheless, pregnant women are much less likely to have hyperglycemia than hypoglycemia because medical management strives to maintain low normal blood glucose levels. While a blood glucose of 180 is considered high for a pregnant woman, it is not high enough to cause signs and symptoms of hyperglycemia.

Preventive Nursing Activities

- Recognize signs and symptoms of perinatal ketoacidosis and implement emergency measures per facility protocols and/or American College of Obstetricians and Gynecologists and American Diabetes Association guidelines. Emergency care intervention for perinatal ketoacidosis (ACOG, 2005; ADA 2004) includes (1) Hydration: 1 liter of normal saline in 1 hour, then 200–500 ml/hr until 80% of fluid has been replaced and deficit corrected over 24 hours. If hypernatremia is present, 0.35% saline is infused instead of normal saline; (2) Reduction of blood glucose levels with insulin: IV bolus of 10–20 units of regular insulin, then continuous infusion per practitioner's orders; (3) Blood glucose levels: Monitor every 1–2 hours with the goal of 50–70 mg/dl; (4) Ketones with glucose: When serum glucose is 250 mg/dl or lower, decrease insulin infusion by half and change IV line to 5% dextrose. Administer 5–10 g glucose per hour. Once glucose is lower than 150 mg/dl, patient may be fed; (5) Potassium balance: Maintain per practitioner's orders; (6) Bicarbonate: Administered per practitioner's orders until pH is greater than 7.1; (7) Monitoring of arterial blood gases, electrolytes, and ketones: Ongoing; (8) Supportive measures: IV, oxygen, arterial lines, pulse oximetry, urinary catheter, evaluation of kidney function, electrocardiogram, fetal heart monitoring, positioned off vena cava; (9) Infection: Surveillance and prevention; (10) Monitor: Neurologic status, vital signs (hypotension, tachycardia), respiratory status, urine output (for hypovolemia) (Gilbert, 2007).
- Teach signs and symptoms of hyperglycemia. Include support of partner and family in instruction and also in care if patient is unable to do for herself. For self-care and early recognition and correction.
- Teach dietary management and support established diet program determined through nutritionist counseling. Women with gestational diabetes may be able to maintain blood glucose control by carefully balancing diet, exercise, rest, and stressors. The dietary goal is to provide adequate weight gain, prevent ketoacidosis, and stabilize blood glucose levels.
- Teach about blood glucose monitoring and support self-management and planning for maintaining controlled levels. In pregnancy, DKA may occur with blood glucose levels as low as 200 mg/dl (compared with 300–350 mg/dl in the nonpregnant state). Achieving glucose control to minimize fetal risk demands more frequent monitoring than women with type 1 or type 2 diabetes may be accustomed to practicing. Women with gestational diabetes need to learn self-monitoring for the first time.
- Teach insulin administration and have the woman return administration demonstration. Adequate insulin level is the primary factor in ensuring normoglycemia during pregnancy. Insulin requirements change dramatically throughout pregnancy. The woman with type 1 diabetes will need multiple daily injections of mixed insulin instead of her typical one injection per day of intermediate-acting insulin. The woman with type 2 diabetes will need to learn to self-administer injections of insulin instead of taking her usual oral hypoglycemics.
- Teach regarding recommended exercise program. Exercise enhances cellular use of glucose and decreases insulin need, but too much exercise can deplete circulating glucose and cause ketoacidosis. Exercise appears to be safe in women with gestational diabetes.
- Teach risk factors (infection, injury, illness, emotional stress, lack of sufficient exercise, dietary indiscretion). The body reacts to stressors (e.g., infection) by increasing hepatic glucose production and decreasing peripheral glucose use. Stress hormones are released, which impair insulin action and contribute to further elevation of serum glucose.
- Refer to a dietitian to individualize the diet. Even if the woman has had previous nutritional counseling for her diabetes, pregnancy creates special nutritional concerns, so the woman needs in-depth education to incorporate these changes into her usual dietary planning.
- Teach the woman to carry insulin and syringes when away from home. Prevents ketoacidosis in the event symptoms occur.
- Teach the woman to wear an identification bracelet at all times. In case of decreased level of consciousness, caregivers would know quickly how to provide treatment.
- If glucose levels are not controlled, prepare for hospitalization. Maternal hyperglycemia is a key factor in fetal/infant morbidity/mortality. Hospitalization may be necessary to stabilize blood glucose levels. Sustained or frequent hyperglycemia is teratogenic to the fetus during the first trimester and is associated with maternal morbidity (e.g., hydramnios, vaginal infections) as well.
- Prepare for vaginal or surgical birth of fetus if placental aging or insufficiency is detected. The incidence of stillbirth increases when pregnancy is carried to more than 36 weeks' gestation.

Potential Complications of Diabetes in Pregnancy: HYPOGLYCEMIA (INSULIN SHOCK)

Focus Assessments

- Monitor for symptoms of insulin shock (i.e., hunger, sweating, nervousness, weakness, irritability, fatigue, blurred/double vision, dizziness, headache, pallor, clammy skin, shallow respirations, rapid pulse, bad dreams, circumoral numbness). Promotes early detection and prompt correction of the condition. However, mild-to-moderate episodes do not appear to have significant negative effects on fetal well-being.
- Measure blood glucose (60 mg/dl or less). Hypoglycemia is especially likely in women with type 1 diabetes. In early pregnancy, nausea and vomiting may cause a decrease in food intake, low glucose levels, and therefore an excess of circulating insulin.
- Be especially vigilant for hypoglycemia during the first trimester. In early pregnancy, peripheral use of glucose is enhanced at the same time that hepatic breakdown of glycogen is decreased; in addition, food intake may be less because of nausea.

Preventive Nursing Activities

- Teach rule of 15:15 management: if blood sugar is low, take 15 g of fast sugar, wait 15 minutes, check sugar again. If glucose level is greater than 60%, eat a meal to stabilize sugar. If less that 60%, repeat the 15:15 rule (15 g of carbohydrate equals 4 glucose tablets, ½ cup orange juice, 1 cup skim milk, ½ cup regular soda, or five to six hard candies).
- Teach symptoms of hypoglycemia as previously listed. Encourages/enables self-monitoring and early treatment. Pregnant women are much more likely to develop hypoglycemia than hyperglycemia. The goal of therapy is to maintain glucose in a narrow range of 65–130 mg/dl. Many women will experience symptoms of hypoglycemia when their blood glucose is below 65 mg/dl; however, a blood glucose of 130 mg/dl will not produce symptoms of hyperglycemia.
- Teach the woman to carry glucose boosters (e.g., glucagon for use if nauseated, unsweetened fruit juice, soda, hard candies, honey) whenever away from home. Prepares the woman to increase blood glucose level if symptoms occur.
- See "Preventive Nursing Activities" in the preceding care plan, and "Potential Complications of Diabetes in Pregnancy: Maternal Hyperglycemia, Diabetic Ketoacidosis," which begins on p. 105.

Potential Complications of Diabetes in Pregnancy: MATERNAL VASCULOPATHY

This section discusses maternal vasculopathy, which includes diabetic retinopathy, nephropathy, and coronary disease in women with preexisting diabetes.

Focus Assessments

- Obtain baseline electrocardiogram. Determines cardiac status early in pregnancy; evaluates the effects of pregnancy on the heart in the second and third trimesters. Women with coronary artery disease must be managed very carefully in order to achieve good pregnancy outcomes.
- Evaluate for retinopathy in the first trimester; refer to an ophthalmologist if necessary. Detects diabetic retinopathy, which may progress during pregnancy.
- Evaluate for gestational hypertension. Vascular impairment may be caused by diabetes and is made worse by gestational hypertension, a common complication of diabetes in pregnancy.
- Assess baseline and periodic 24-hour urine collection for total protein excretion and creatinine clearance, blood urea nitrogen, and uric acid levels. Provides baseline and ongoing assessment of kidney function. Diabetic nephropathy has a more serious impact on perinatal outcome than any other vasculopathy. It increases the risks of pregnancy-induced hypertension, intrauterine growth restriction, preterm labor, stillbirth, and neonatal death.

Preventive Nursing Activities

- Prevention consists of controlling blood glucose level by means of diet, balanced rest and activity, regulation of stressors, and medication. See previous care plan for "Potential Complications of Diabetes in Pregnancy: Maternal Hyperglycemia, Diabetic Ketoacidosis," which begins on p. 105.

Potential Complication of Diabetes in Pregnancy: PREECLAMPSIA/ECLAMPSIA

Refer to the generic collaborative care plan "Hypertensive Disorders," beginning on p. 32 in Chapter 3.

Focus Assessments

- Measure blood pressure. Detects hypertension (BP greater than 140/90). In women with diabetes, the risk for gestational hypertension is four times greater than normal.
- Assess urine (screen for proteinuria, 1+ to 2+ on dipstick measurement). Proteinuria is a symptom of preeclampsia.

A 24-hour urine collection is a more accurate measure than the dipstick.

- Assess for edema. Edema of the face, hands, or abdomen that is not responsive to 12 hours of bed rest is an early symptom of preeclampsia.
- Assess for weight gain. Edema may be manifested as a weight gain of more than 2 kg in 1 week.
- Assess for subjective symptoms of headache, visual problems, epigastric pain. These are symptoms of preeclampsia.

Preventive Nursing Activities

- Provide blood glucose monitoring and control. Detects increased blood glucose levels so that interventions may be implemented to prevent vascular damage. The highest incidence of preeclampsia occurs in women with preexisting vascular changes related to diabetes. See the previous care plan "Potential Complications of Diabetes in Pregnancy: Maternal Hyperglycemia, Diabetic Ketoacidosis," which begins on p. 105.
- Teach risk factors for gestational hypertension. Facilitates self-monitoring and early treatment.

Potential Complication of Diabetes in Pregnancy: INFECTION

This section discusses infection, including UTIs, pyelonephritis, and monilial vaginitis. Refer to the generic collaborative care plans for "Potential Complication: Infection" and "Potential Complication: Urinary Tract Infection," beginning on pp. 29 and 33, respectively, in Chapter 3. Also see the care plan for Urinary Tract Infections beginning on pp. 195 in Chapter 6.

Focus Assessments

- Assess urine for abnormal color, odor, and presence of leukocytes. These are indicators of UTI.
- Assess for abnormal vaginal discharge and itching (obtain culture, if necessary). These are symptoms of monilial vulvovaginitis.
- Assess for signs/symptoms of ascending UTI/pyelonephritis (temperature 100.4°F, tachycardia, tachypnea, nausea, and vomiting). Infection can lead to hyperglycemia and diabetic ketoacidosis; therefore, hospitalization is indicated if kidney infection develops.

Preventive Nursing Activities

- Teach good hygiene, including front-to-back perineal care. Prevents introduction of pathogens into the urethra.
- Teach other methods for preventing UTIs (e.g., dry genital area with hair dryer on low setting after shower or bath, wear underpants with cotton crotch, do not suppress the urge to

urinate, urinate before and after intercourse). Discourages buildup of moisture, urinary stasis, and bacteria in the genital area.

- Instruct patient to drink 8–12 glasses of water a day. Ensures frequent urination and flushing of the urinary tract. Under the influence of progesterone, the renal pelvis and ureters dilate, resulting in urinary stasis. Stagnant urine, which is also more alkaline in pregnancy, is an excellent medium for growth of microorganisms.
- Control blood glucose level by means of diet, balanced rest and activity, regulation of stressors, and medication. See the previous care plan "Potential Complications of Diabetes in Pregnancy: Maternal Hyperglycemia, Diabetic Ketoacidosis," which begins on p. 105.

Potential Complication of Diabetes in Pregnancy: DIFFICULT LABOR/BIRTH

Difficult labor/birth as a complication of diabetes in pregnancy includes shoulder dystocia, birth trauma, and need for cesarean birth related to large fetal size secondary to fetal hyperinsulinemia.

Focus Assessments

- Assess for weight gain. Diet and insulin are regulated on the basis of weight gain and blood glucose levels to prevent hyperglycemia. The fetus responds to maternal hyperglycemia by secreting more insulin, which acts as a growth hormone.
- Assess fundal height and perform Leopold's maneuvers. Estimates fetal size and position.
- Perform ultrasonography. Part of biophysical profile; estimates fetal weight, amniotic fluid levels, and movement; determines risk for cephalopelvic disproportion. Cesarean birth is often performed when estimated fetal weight is 4,000–4,500 g.
- Perform blood glucose monitoring. Detects hyperglycemia.

Preventive Nursing Activities

- Control blood glucose level by means of diet, balanced rest and activity, regulation of stressors, and medication. See the previous care plan, "Potential Complications of Diabetes in Pregnancy: Maternal Hyperglycemia, Diabetic Ketoacidosis," which begins on p. 105 in this chapter.
- Prepare for complications with birth (shoulder dystocia, cesarean, birth lacerations, postpartum hemorrhage). Macrosomia occurs in 20–25% of diabetic pregnancies, often causing cephalopelvic disproportion and dystocia. Anticipating problems helps ensure positive outcome for mother and neonate. Supportive care should be waiting

for baby in case of abnormalities, hypoglycemia, immature lungs or respiratory distress, etc.

Potential Complication of Diabetes in Pregnancy: HYDRAMNIOS

Focus Assessments

- Assess fundal height measurement at each visit. Provides an indicator of the volume of amniotic fluid in the uterus. Hydramnios occurs in up to 25% of pregnant women with diabetes.
- Perform Leopold's maneuvers. Assesses whether uterine size is due to fetus or amniotic fluid; enables feeling of baby's position and lie.
- Measure random or fasting blood glucose at visits. Assesses glycemic control. Maternal hyperglycemia leads to fetal hyperglycemia, which causes fetal diuresis and contributes to abnormally large amount of amniotic fluid. Serum glucose levels are more accurate than levels obtained using a reflectance meter.
- Assess for maternal dyspnea. Results from upward pressure of the distended uterus on the diaphragm.

Preventive Nursing Activities

- Monitor and control blood glucose level by means of diet, balanced rest and activity, regulation of stressors, and medication. See the previous care plan, "Potential Complications of Diabetes in Pregnancy: Maternal Hyperglycemia, Diabetic Ketoacidosis," beginning on p. 105 in this chapter.

Potential Complications of Diabetes in Pregnancy: LABOR, MISCARRIAGE, AND SUDDEN, UNEXPLAINED STILLBIRTH

Labor, miscarriage, and sudden, unexplained stillbirth are possibly caused by overdistention of the uterus secondary to large fetal size and hydramnios, or related to chronic fetal anoxia. Hyperglycemia can affect the fetus through the transfer of maternal ketonemia to the amniotic fluid and production of a ketotic state in the fetus. Dehydration can alter amniotic fluid function. Maternal hypotension can cause shunting of blood away from the uterus and decrease fetal profusion, causing damaging effects to the fetus. Refer to the generic collaborative care plans for "Potential Complication: Premature Rupture of Membranes" and "Potential Complication: Preterm Labor," beginning on pp. 30 and 31, respectively, in Chapter 3.

Focus Assessments

- Assess for signs and symptoms of miscarriage and/or preterm labor (e.g., uterine contractions, loss of mucus plug, vaginal bleeding, rupture of membranes). PROM and preterm labor may be caused by overdistention of the uterus secondary to large fetal size and hydramnios.
- Assess fetal size (such as by ultrasonography) and hydramnios. Macrosomia occurs in 20–25% of pregnancies in which the mother is diabetic. Hydramnios occurs about 10 times more often in pregnancies complicated by diabetes.
- Monitor fetal activity. Indicates fetal viability.
- Perform an ultrasound. This is used initially and throughout pregnancy. It uses biparietal diameter, abdominal circumference, and femur length to monitor fetal growth, estimate gestational age, and detect abnormalities.
- Perform an NST weekly at 28 –32 weeks, then twice weekly after 32 weeks. Fetal heart rate accelerations in response to fetal activity are a good indicator of placental perfusion and fetal well-being. Activity decreases before changes occur in the fetal heart rate. This will probably be combined in a biophysical profile with sonogram.
- Perform amniocentesis in the third trimester. Tests for phosphatidylglycerol to evaluate fetal lung maturity. Fetal hyperinsulinemia inhibits surfactant production. Steroids may be given to enhance lung maturity if delivery is necessary.
- Perform biophysical profile. Scores fetal well-being based on a combination of NST results, amniotic fluid volume, fetal breathing movements, fetal tone, and fetal activity. A score of 8–10 is reassuring, 4–6 requires further evaluation, and lower than 4 is ominous.

Preventive Nursing Activities

- Maintain euglycemia. See the previous care plan, "Potential Complications of Diabetes in Pregnancy: Maternal Hyperglycemia, Diabetic Ketoacidosis," which begins on p. 105. Be aware that tocolytics such as terbutaline (Brethine) and corticosteroids (e.g., betamethasone) may elevate serum glucose level. In cases of PROM and preterm labor, maternal hyperglycemia causes fetal hyperglycemia; this, in turn, causes hydramnios from fetal diuresis, as well as macrosomia from fetal hyperinsulinism. In cases of early pregnancy, miscarriage may be related to poor glycemic control before conception and during the early weeks of pregnancy. In cases of unexplained stillbirth, this is possibly due to chronic fetal anoxia. Occurs more often in women with vascular disease or poor glycemic control.
- Teach signs and symptoms of miscarriage (first trimester) and preterm labor (second and third trimesters). Promotes early detection and treatment and, possibly, promotes longer gestation.

Potential Complication of Diabetes in Pregnancy: CONGENITAL ANOMALIES

This includes anomalies as a complication of diabetes in pregnancy especially cardiac, central nervous system, and skeletal anomalies. Neural tube abnormalities can occur in diabetics.

Focus Assessments

- Determine duration of preexisting diabetes, existence of vasculopathies, and diabetic control before conception. Helps predict likelihood of fetal mortality and congenital anomalies, which are linked to these phenomena.
- Perform an ultrasound, biophysical profile, and other tests of fetal well-being. Tests for fetal viability, age, size, and oxygenation. Congenital anomalies, occurring in 6–10% of infants born to diabetic women, are the most important cause of perinatal deaths in diabetic pregnancy. Congenital anomalies cause up to 40% of perinatal deaths of infants born to diabetic mothers.
- Perform a fetal echocardiogram (may be done at 18–22 weeks). Cardiac defects are the most common anomalies seen in infants of diabetic mothers. By 18–22 weeks' gestation, the entire heart can be seen on ultrasound, so most anomalies should be identifiable.
- Measure maternal serum alpha-fetoprotein (16–18 weeks). Assesses for open neural tube defects, which are more likely in the presence of diabetes.

Preventive Nursing Activities

- Monitor and control blood glucose level by means of diet, balanced rest and activity, regulation of stressors, and medication. See care plan for "Potential Complications of Diabetes in Pregnancy: Maternal Hyperglycemia, Diabetic Ketoacidosis," which begins on p. 105. The incidence of congenital anomalies, which may be caused by hyperglycemia, hyperketonemia, and hypoglycemia, is related to the severity and duration of the diabetes.
- Teach the woman the importance of taking prenatal vitamins, iron, and folic acid. Supports increased nutritional needs and prevents neural tube defects and anemia.
- Teach the woman about fetal kick counts and review danger signs for preeclampsia, preterm labor, infections, and other possible risks to fetus. Ensures early recognition to facilitate early intervention.

Potential Complication of Diabetes in Pregnancy:

INTRAUTERINE GROWTH RESTRICTION

Intrauterine growth restriction (IUGR) is caused by compromised uteroplacental circulation resulting from maternal vascular disease.

Focus Assessments

- Assess ultrasound. Ultrasound is obtained initially and throughout pregnancy. It uses biparietal diameter and femur length to monitor fetal growth, estimate gestational age, and detect abnormalities.
- Perform an NST weekly at 28–32 weeks, then twice weekly after 32 weeks. FHR accelerations in response to fetal activity are a good indicator of fetal well-being. If uteroplacental circulation is compromised, the fetus may be hypoxic as well as growth restricted. Biophysical profiles usually are indicated.
- Assess fundal height and perform Leopold's maneuvers. Evaluates fetal size, position, and lie.
- Monitor for preeclampsia. IUGR is related to compromised uteroplacental circulation. It becomes more severe in the presence of preeclampsia. See care plan for "Hypertensive Disorders of Pregnancy" on p. 170 in Chapter 6.

Preventive Nursing Activities

- Monitor and control blood glucose level by means of diet, balanced rest and activity, regulation of stressors, and medication. Promote bonding with baby while in utero to begin good parenting interaction and caring. See care plan for "Potential Complications of Diabetes in Pregnancy: Maternal Hyperglycemia, Diabetic Ketoacidosis," which begins on p. 105. IUGR is related to compromised uteroplacental circulation. It becomes more severe in the presence of ketoacidosis.

INDIVIDUALIZED (NURSING DIAGNOSIS) CARE PLANS

This section includes care plans to address unique patient needs.

Nursing Diagnosis: INEFFECTIVE HEALTH MANAGEMENT, SELF[1]

Related Factors: knowledge deficits (e.g., effects of diabetes in pregnancy, self-care), ineffective coping with pregnancy and diabetes, and insufficient resources (e.g., transportation to buy food to follow dietary regimen, money to purchase monitoring supplies).

Goals, Outcomes, and Evaluation Criteria

- Woman will verbalize necessary information about self-monitoring and control of diabetes.
- Woman will verbalize information about the potential effects of diabetes on herself and the fetus.
- Woman states the signs and symptoms of hyperglycemia and hypoglycemia.
- Woman seeks help promptly in the event of complications of diabetes in pregnancy.
- Woman follows recommendations for diet and exercise and verbalizes guidelines.
- Woman demonstrates correct procedure for insulin administration.
- Woman demonstrates correct procedure for glucose monitoring.
- Woman achieves satisfactory glucose control throughout pregnancy.
- Woman seeks help and asks questions when in need.
- Woman demonstrates self-caring and caring for the fetus through good self-management performance.

NIC Interventions[2]

High-Risk Pregnancy Care (6800)—Identification and management of a high-risk pregnancy to promote healthy outcomes for mother and baby.

Mutual Goal Setting (4410)—Collaborating with patient to identify and prioritize care goals, then developing a plan for achieving those goals.

Nutritional Counseling (5246)—Use of an interactive helping process focusing on the need for diet modification.

Referral (8100)—Arrangement for services by another care provider or agency.

Teaching: Disease Process (5602)—Assisting the patient to understand information related to a specific disease process.

Teaching: Prescribed Activity/Exercise (5612)—Preparing a patient to achieve and/or maintain a prescribed level of activity.

Teaching: Prescribed Diet (5614)—Preparing a patient to correctly follow a prescribed diet.

Teaching: Prescribed Medication (5616)—Preparing a patient to safely take prescribed medications and monitor for their effects.

Teaching: Psychomotor Skill (5618)—Preparing a patient to perform a psychomotor skill.

Nursing Activities and Rationales

Assessments

- Assess knowledge of disease process, management, effects on pregnancy and fetus, and potential complications. Provides base for planning teaching interventions. Women must take an active role in diabetes control during pregnancy because of the intense monitoring needed. In order to care for her diabetes on a daily basis, the woman must have an adequate understanding of her disease and the therapeutic regimen.
- Assess support system, including significant others and socioeconomic factors. Any area of stress can precipitate complications, making it difficult to maintain euglycemia.
- Assess emotional status. Determines how the woman is coping with pregnancy superimposed on diabetes. Even a normal pregnancy creates some degree of stress and anxiety; a high-risk pregnancy, even more so.
- Assess coping abilities and capability for managing diabetes. Provides information about the level of responsibility the woman can be expected to assume; aids in establishing realistic goals and effective interventions.
- Assess the woman's food intake and eating habits (using 24-hour recall), her knowledge of basic nutrition, and her perceptions of modifications needed in her diet. Address specific cultural diet habits and help integrate these into her diet plan. The woman's perceptions and level of understanding provide a baseline for teaching and motivating the woman to make needed changes. Make adjustments to fit her regular way of eating and adapting them to her diabetic diet will aid her adherence to the plan.
- Teach the woman to monitor fetal kick count. Primarily a screening technique. If the woman notices a decrease in fetal activity, she should contact the care provider for further evaluation of fetal status.

Independent Nursing Actions

- Encourage the woman to express feelings about health status, fetal well-being, and required lifestyle changes. Demonstrates empathy and supports therapeutic relationship.
- Assist the woman to identify and prioritize goals for needed lifestyle changes (e.g., exercise, diet); assist her to make a plan to meet the goals. Promotes the woman's autonomy and provides motivation for following the therapeutic regimen.
- Set periodic dates for assessing progress toward goals. Provides motivation for change and opportunity to modify the plan as needed.
- Reinforce, encourage, and praise woman for all her efforts to maintain a healthy pregnancy for herself and her baby. Normal pregnancy is difficult for many women, and a woman with diabetes who must do so much disease maintenance needs to be encouraged to continue her regimen.

Collaborative Activities

- Refer to nutritionist for diet planning. The woman with gestational diabetes will not be familiar with a diabetic diet.

Women with type 1 or 2 diabetes may not know about the diet modifications that need to be made because of the special nutritional concerns in pregnancy.

- Encourage the woman to enroll in prenatal classes as early as possible in the pregnancy. Reinforces teaching about pregnancy and childbirth.
- Arrange/participate in multidisciplinary care conferences. Pregnancy complicated by diabetes is considered high risk. A favorable outcome is more likely when a multidisciplinary team manages care (e.g., obstetrician, internist, neonatologist, nurse, nutritionist, and social worker).

Patient/Family Teaching

- Teach illness care. Illness care includes continuing insulin; calling the healthcare provider with symptoms of illness, fever, most recent blood glucose level, urine ketones, and last insulin dose; increasing oral intake of fluids to prevent dehydration; and resting as much as possible. If the woman is unable to reach her healthcare provider and her blood glucose is over 200 mg/dl with positive urine ketones, she should seek emergency treatment at the nearest healthcare facility. Emphasize the importance of not treating herself for this.
- Provide written materials describing diet, exercise, insulin administration, glucose monitoring, effects of diabetes on pregnancy and fetus, and symptoms of complications. It is essential, but difficult, to control diabetes in pregnancy. It is a complex disease, and the woman will need reference materials for details she is unable to recall.
- For women with pregestational (type 1 and type 2) diabetes, educate regarding any changes in diabetic management (e.g., changing the frequency of blood glucose monitoring, changing from oral hypoglycemic agents to insulin). Women with preexisting diabetes will already have established routines for diabetic management; they may not realize the extent to which pregnancy changes the need for and difficulty in controlling blood glucose. Insulin requirements are decreased in the first trimester and then may double or even quadruple by the end of the pregnancy.
- Explain the need to follow a consistent daily schedule—eating, exercising, and taking insulin at the same time each day. This is essential for maintaining tight glucose control.
- Reinforce the need for monitoring blood—rather than urine—glucose during pregnancy. The renal threshold for glucose is lowered in pregnancy, so a small amount of glucose is normally found in the urine of nondiabetic women. Blood glucose is, therefore, more accurate and enables better control.
- Teach the woman the finger-stick procedure for self-monitoring of blood glucose using a reflectance meter (e.g., Glucometer). Have the woman perform return demonstration. Even in women with pregestational diabetes, a thorough assessment of the woman's skill is essential to ensure

accurate monitoring during pregnancy. Daily insulin needs are adjusted on the basis of serum glucose levels. Note that values obtained with a reflectance meter may vary 10–15% from plasma values.

- Reinforce the need to self-monitor serum glucose levels the prescribed number of times a day (e.g., before meals, 2 hours after each meal, at bedtime, in the middle of the night, and at any sign of hyperglycemia or hypoglycemia). Because maternal metabolism, insulin needs, and insulin utilization change greatly during pregnancy, frequent monitoring is necessary to maintain a narrow range of blood glucose (between 60 and 130 mg/dl) in order to ensure positive pregnancy outcomes. Frequent measurement demonstrates to the woman the impact of her diet and exercise on glucose levels, thereby providing motivation to comply with the therapeutic regimen.
- In addition to monitoring blood glucose, reinforce the need for monitoring ketones in the first morning urine, if a meal is missed or delayed, and when illness occurs. Ketonuria indicates that the body is in a starvation state that requires an increase in carbohydrates or adjustment of insulin frequency, dosage, or type. A trace of ketones is not an indication for treatment; however, if ketones appear repeatedly at the same time each day, some diet adjustment may be needed. If the urine contains a large amount of ketones, the woman should contact her healthcare provider immediately.
- Teach home screening for hypoglycemia (i.e., check blood glucose level) and treatment for symptomatic hypoglycemia. If blood glucose is less than 60 mg/dl, the woman should eat or drink 10–15 g of simple carbohydrates (e.g., unsweetened fruit juice, a cup of milk, 1 tablespoon of honey or corn syrup); repeat in 15 minutes if glucose level remains below 60 mg/dl. Simple carbohydrates will quickly elevate the blood glucose level. Only small amounts are used because more will cause the level to increase too much, resulting in hyperglycemia.
- Reinforce diet teaching (e.g., total calories are commonly divided among three meals and two snacks; meals should be eaten on time and never skipped). Food intake should provide 30–35 kcal/kg of present pregnancy weight, which is 2,000–2,500 calories/day for most women. Complex carbohydrates should provide 50–60% of total calories because they provide a more sustained glucose release than simple carbohydrates.
- Remind the woman to eat a bedtime snack with at least 25 g of carbohydrate and some protein. Prevents ketosis during the night.
- Teach potential effects of diabetes on pregnant woman (hydramnios, dystocia, UTI, vaginal infections, preeclampsia, miscarriage, preterm labor) and fetus (macrosomia and related birth trauma, inhibition of lung maturity, IUGR, cardiac dysrhythmias/anomalies, neurologic damage, and neonatal hypoglycemia). Understanding promotes recall

of information and compliance with treatment plan. Also ensures early recognition and treatment of complications.

- Provide information about the need for daily, mild exercise. Women who already have an active lifestyle should continue an exercise program (e.g., brisk walking, swimming). Sedentary women should begin by exercising 3–4 times a week for 15–30 minutes and gradually increase intensity and duration. Exercise need not be vigorous to be beneficial. Regular exercise enhances glucose utilization and decreases insulin need; however, wide fluctuations in physical activity can unfavorably affect glucose control. Exercises that use the upper body are not associated with increased uterine contractions.

- Advise the woman to exercise after meals. This is when blood glucose begins to rise. When insulin is peaking, exercise may cause hypoglycemia; when insulin action is waning, exercise may cause hyperglycemia.

- Women with vasculopathy should exercise only as recommended by the healthcare provider. Such women typically depend completely on exogenous insulin and are at increased risk for wide fluctuations in blood glucose levels and ketoacidosis, which can be made worse by exercise.

- Warn against exercising if glucose exceeds 200 mg/dl. If glucose is elevated, exercise promotes ketoacidosis.

- Teach specifics of insulin administration and dosage to women with gestational diabetes; assess and teach, as needed, those with preexisting diabetes. Adequate insulinization is the primary factor in maintaining normoglycemia in pregnancy. Insulin requirements change dramatically during pregnancy, necessitating frequent adjustments in dosage. Establishes the woman's competence with injections or subcutaneous insulin pump.

- Reinforce prescribed dosage, type, and frequency of insulin, e.g., most women will require two to four injections a day, with a combination of short-, intermediate-, and long-acting insulin. A woman with type 1 diabetes may be accustomed to one injection per day. Multiple daily injections are needed during pregnancy. The woman with type 2 diabetes must switch from oral hypoglycemics to insulin. A mixture of shorter- and longer- acting insulins helps to prevent peaks and valleys in the serum glucose.

- Demonstrate procedures (e.g., blood glucose monitoring and insulin measurement and administration) and have the woman return demonstration. Establishes the woman's comfort and competence with procedures.

- Teach foot care and general skin care (e.g., avoid tight clothing, wear properly fitting shoes or slippers at all times, cut toenails straight across). Diabetic women are at risk for infections and neurologic changes.

- Teach stress management and relaxation techniques. Reduces release of stress hormones, which impair insulin action and contribute to further elevation of serum glucose.

■ Nursing Diagnosis: ANXIETY[1]

Related Factors: threat to maternal and fetal well-being, complexity of self-care regimen, and lifestyle changes. Refer to the generic NDCP, "Anxiety,[1]" beginning on p. 10 in Chapter 2.

■ *Goals, Outcomes, and Evaluation Criteria*

The woman and/or partner or family will:
- Report and demonstrate adequate ability to concentrate.
- Report adequate sleep.
- Report that anxious feelings are tolerable/manageable and increased coping mechanisms are in place.
- Ask for help, as needed.

■ *NIC Interventions[2]*

Anxiety Reduction (5820)—Minimizing apprehension, dread, foreboding, or uneasiness related to an unidentified source of anticipated danger.
Coping Enhancement (5230)—Assisting a patient to adapt to perceived stressors, changes, or threats that interfere with meeting life demands and roles.
Emotional Support (5270)—Provision of reassurance, acceptance, and encouragement during times of stress.

■ *Nursing Activities and Rationales*

Assessments

- Assess the woman's concerns regarding the pregnancy and current situational stressors. Detects any misinformation or issues that may be contributing to anxiety.

Independent Nursing Actions

- Use therapeutic communication to create an open relationship with the woman. Promotes trust and relieves anxiety and creates safe environment for self-expression.

- Assist the woman in recognizing and verbalizing feelings such as anxiety, anger, or sadness. The first step in treating anxiety is to assist the woman to recognize that she is anxious.

- Provide realistic reassurance to the woman and family. Risks do exist and need to be factual. Relieves anxiety. The perinatal mortality rate for well-managed diabetic pregnancies is about the same as for any other pregnancy. Knowing reasons for the work of intense self-management gives reasons to maintain good glucose control and surveillance and adhere to diet and exercise plan.

- Encourage exercise if not contraindicated. Exercise can relieve stress.

- Evaluate access to supplies and information to maintain self-management of diabetes. Having the right tools and education helps one feel empowered to care for oneself.

- Provide contact numbers for members of the multidisciplinary team. It is reassuring to know that problems will be addressed immediately, 24 hours a day.

- Encourage attendance at diabetes classes and support groups. Talking with others in similar situations promotes networking and establishes support.

Patient/Family Teaching

- Discuss the situation with the woman and partner/family, providing factual information about diagnosis, treatment, and prognosis. Helps ensure that emotional reaction is in response to the real, rather than an imagined, situation (some fears may be unrealistic and ungrounded). Knowledge helps to promote a sense of control over the situation.
- Answer questions about health status in an honest manner. Builds trust and reduces anxiety.
- Explain all diagnostic tests and procedures, including sensations likely to be experienced. Knowing what to expect helps the woman/family to better cope.

PRENATAL ANEMIA

Anemia is the most common antepartal complication in the United States, affecting 20–50% of pregnant women. Anemia is characterized by a decreased number of red blood cells (RBCs) and below normal hemoglobin (Hgb) concentration. This results in reduced capacity of the blood to carry oxygen to the vital organs of the mother and the fetus.

During pregnancy, anemia increases the risk for hypertension in adulthood and preterm birth. The need increases in the second half of pregnancy during fetal growth. It can increase maternal mortality by increasing the chance for preeclampsia and decreasing the woman's tolerance to hemorrhage. It increases the risk of puerperal complications (e.g., delayed healing of episiotomy or incision) and infections and decreases the iron available for fetal stores. Fetal risks include low birth weight, prematurity, stillbirth, and neonatal death in women with severe iron deficiency (Hgb less than 6 g/dl).

■ Key Nursing Activities

- Observe for complications of anemia (differentiate between physiologic and inherited disease states).
- Provide dietary teaching.
- Provide teaching about prescribed medications (e.g., iron, folic acid).

■ Etiologies and Risk Factors

- Inadequate intake of iron is the most common cause of prenatal anemia. During pregnancy, increased iron is needed for the increased production of maternal and fetal RBCs. Also, during the third trimester, the fetus stores iron for use during the first 4–6 weeks of life after birth. These maternal/fetal demands approximately double the dietary iron needed by a pregnant woman. The recommended daily allowance for

iron during pregnancy is 27 mg/day; however, the most iron that can reasonably be obtained from the average diet is about 15–18 mg/day. Anemia occurs twice as often in non-Hispanic black women than in non-Hispanic white women. Adolescent pregnant women have the highest prevalence of all races. Low-income women, most of whom are also minority women, have higher rates of iron deficiency anemia. Risk factors also include:
  - ▶ Diet poor in iron-rich foods
  - ▶ Diet poor in iron absorption enhancers with dietary vitamin C
  - ▶ Diet rich in foods that diminish iron absorption (dairy, soy, spinach, coffee, and tea)
  - ▶ Pica (eating nonfood substances)
  - ▶ Gastrointestinal disease
  - ▶ Heavy menses
  - ▶ Short interpregnancy interval
  - ▶ Blood loss at delivery (ACOG, 2008a)
- Folic acid deficiency anemia (megaloblastic anemia) occurs in about 1–4% of pregnant women in the United States. Folic acid needs increase during pregnancy from 50 mcg to 400 mcg per day because of rapid cell multiplication, increased urinary excretion of folic acid, and fetal needs. If the mother is diagnosed with folic acid deficiency, there is a high likelihood that she also will have an iron deficiency. Low folic acid intake is associated with neural tube defects.
- Genetically induced anemia (e.g., sickle cell anemia, thalassemia) may also occur in the pregnant woman. Sickle cell is a recessive inheritable anemia as heterozygous trait or homozygous disease. In the disease state, sickled hemoglobin, when deoxygenated, causes local hypoxia, which can progress to tissue and organ damage, painful vasoocclusive crises, and increased susceptibility to infection. Depending on the extent of the disease, there is an increase in maternal and perinatal morbidity and mortality. Thalassemia is defined by defective alpha or beta globin chains and can range from little or no anemia to anemia with accompanied fertility problems.
- Smoking, living at high altitudes, and adolescent pregnancy all increase the risk for developing prenatal anemia because they increase the quantity of RBCs required by the body.

■ Signs and Symptoms

Subjective: Fatigue, headache, decreased exercise tolerance, anorexia, weakness, malaise, dyspnea, pica, itching.
Objective: Pallor of skin and conjunctiva, edema, inflammation of the lips and tongue (glossitis).

■ Diagnostic Studies

- Hemoglobin. *Fewer than 11 g/dl in the first and third trimesters, and fewer than 10.5 g/dl in the second trimester.*
- Hematocrit. *Lower than 35% in the first trimester, lower than 30% in the second trimester, and lower than 34% in the third trimester.*
- Red cells indices. *Microcytic and hypochromic cells for iron deficiency anemia. Megaloblastic cells for folic acid deficiency.*

- Hgb electrophoresis. *To determine if sickle cell trait or disease is present.*

▎ *Medical Management*

Medical management varies with the specific type of anemia and includes the following:

- Frequent prenatal visits
- Supplemental oral ferrous sulfate or gluconate (iron deficiency)
- Supplemental oral folic acid (folic acid deficiency)
- Diet rich in foods containing iron and folic acid

Sickle cell disease and anemia may have other complications and management plans (for further information refer to an obstetrics textbook).

▎ *Collaborative Problems*

Potential complications of prenatal anemia include the following:

- Infection and delayed wound healing
- Gestational hypertension/preeclampsia
- Postpartum bleeding/depression

COLLABORATIVE (STANDARDIZED) CARE FOR ALL PATIENTS WITH PRENATAL ANEMIA

Perform a comprehensive assessment to identify individual needs for teaching, emotional support, and physical care.

▎ Potential Complication of Prenatal Anemia: INFECTION AND DELAYED WOUND HEALING

Refer to generic collaborative care plan, "Potential Complication: Infection," beginning on p. 29 in Chapter 3.

Focus Assessments

- Assess respirations (tachypnea). May be increased because of reduced oxygen-carrying capacity of the blood.
- Assess temperature (38°C or 100.4°F). Fever is the hallmark of most infections. It is an adaptive host-defense response produced by the effects of pyrogens on the hypothalamus, causing it to regulate body temperature at a higher level than normal in an effort to eliminate pathogens.
- Measure pulse (tachycardia). In the presence of fever, peripheral vasodilation occurs in an adaptive attempt to cool the body. Vasodilation lowers the BP, and the body attempts to adapt by increasing the pulse rate. Fever also increases the metabolic rate, which increases heart rate.
- Evaluate for urinary symptoms and check urinalysis. Detects possible infection; the woman may have asymptomatic urinary tract infection during pregnancy.

- Assess wounds if present (red and warm to the touch, drainage, edema). These classic symptoms are a result of the body's adaptive inflammatory response. They all result from vascular changes and exudate. Swelling occurs as exudate accumulates and also from the presence of prostaglandins and bradykinin. Redness and warmth result from increased blood flow to the area.
- Assess for pain. Symptom of infection that may result from edema or tissue damage.
- Assess for malaise. Infections produce fatigue from fever, increased immune response, and endo- and exotoxins from pathogenic organisms.
- Monitor laboratory data for indications of infection. Leukocytosis: greater than 14,000 in first trimester, greater than 17,000 in second trimester, greater than 14,700 in third trimester. The body responds to the presence of pathogens by increasing the number and types of circulating WBCs.

▎ Potential Complication of Prenatal Anemia: PRETERM LABOR

Use generic collaborative care plan, "Potential Complication: Preterm Labor," beginning on p. 31 in Chapter 3.

INDIVIDUALIZED (NURSING DIAGNOSIS) CARE PLANS

This section includes care plans to address unique patient needs.

▎ Nursing Diagnosis: IMBALANCED NUTRITION: LESS THAN BODY REQUIREMENTS FOR IRON[1]

Related Factors: poor dietary intake; intolerance of iron-rich foods, knowledge deficit of iron-rich foods, nausea and vomiting, and insufficient finances.

▎ *Goals, Outcomes, and Evaluation Criteria*

- Woman reports 15 mg iron intake over a 24-hour diet recall.
- Woman correctly states six foods that she prefers that are rich in iron.
- Woman tolerates prescribed iron intake and compliance to medication schedule.
- Woman has laboratory values within normal limits (Hct more than 35% in the first trimester, more than 30% in second trimester, more than 34% in third trimester; Hgb more than

11 g/dl in the first and third trimesters, more than 10.5 g/dl in the second trimester.

- Woman reports adequate energy levels or improvement from pretreatment.

◼ NIC Interventions[2]

High-Risk Pregnancy Care (6800)—Identification and management of a high-risk pregnancy to promote healthy outcomes for mother and baby.

Nutrition Management (1100)—Assisting with or providing a balanced dietary intake of foods and fluids.

Nutrition Therapy (1120)—Administration of food and fluids to support metabolic processes of a patient who is malnourished or at high risk for becoming malnourished.

Nutritional Counseling (5246)—Use of an interactive helping process focusing on the need for diet modification.

Nutritional Monitoring (1160)—Collection and analysis of patient data to prevent or minimize malnourishment.

◼ Nursing Activities and Rationales

Assessments

- Monitor adequacy of iron intake by use of 24-hour recall. Determines adequacy of iron intake in one 24-hour period.
- Assess knowledge of iron-rich foods and the amount needed for a healthy pregnancy. Determines specific learning needs.
- Monitor motivation of the woman to comply with diet changes. If the woman is not motivated to comply, then further assessment is necessary to determine the reason for noncompliance and plan interventions to increase motivation.
- Assess food preferences and cultural/religious dietary alterations. May affect motivation/compliance with recommendations. Individual and cultural food preferences must be taken into account prior to making recommendations.
- Monitor for frequency of nausea and vomiting. Nausea and vomiting can have a negative impact on intake of iron supplements and iron-rich foods. Iron supplementation may increase nausea.
- Monitor Hgb and Hct levels. Baseline results are an indicator of the severity of anemia. Follow-up results reflect success of iron intake and/or supplementation.
- Monitor woman's perception of energy level using scale of 1 (unable to complete simple task) to 5 (active, able to maintain normal activities without fatigue). Low iron levels lead to fatigue; as iron levels increase, the fatigue level should improve.
- Assess financial ability to purchase proper food. Affects ability to follow dietary recommendations of health provider.

Patient/Family Teaching

- Advise the woman to include lean meats in her diet or to combine nonmeat foods with foods rich in vitamin C. Iron

absorption is higher for animal products than for vegetables. Absorption from nonmeat sources is enhanced by the intake of vitamin C.

- Advise the woman to include dark green, leafy vegetables; eggs; and whole-grain and enriched breads and cereals in her diet; also include dried fruits, legumes, shellfish, and black strap molasses. These are all good sources of iron.

Collaborative Activities

- Consult with dietitian to establish proper iron intake level for specific woman's need and alternate iron-rich foods to meet individual/cultural preferences. Assists with planning for proper iron intake. The amount of iron needed is dependent upon age of the woman and previous iron intake. A dietitian is able to determine specific needs for a particular woman and take cultural/individual food preferences into account when planning a diet.

◼ Nursing Diagnosis: CONSTIPATION[1]

Related Factors: ingestion of iron supplements. Use with generic NDCP, "Constipation,[1]" beginning on p. 11 in Chapter 2.

◼ Nursing Activities and Rationales

Patient/Family Teaching

- Explain that pregnancy increases the risk for constipation and that oral iron medications further increase that risk. Helps the woman understand the importance of preventive measures such as diet, fiber, fluids, and exercise. Black strap molasses is high in iron and may help prevent constipation caused by oral iron.

◼ Nursing Diagnosis: DEFICIENT KNOWLEDGE (OF IRON MEDICATION AND SIDE EFFECTS)[1]

Related Factors: lack of information concerning effects and side effects of iron supplementation. Also refer to generic NDCP, "Deficient Knowledge,[1]" beginning on p. 13 in Chapter 2.

◼ Goals, Outcomes, and Evaluation Criteria

- Woman describes side effects of iron supplementation.
- Woman describes correct administration of medication.
- Woman identifies safe storage of iron supplementation to prevent accidental poisoning of children.

■ NIC Interventions[2]

Teaching: Prescribed Medication (5616)—Preparing a patient to safely take prescribed medications and monitor for their effects.

■ Nursing Activities and Rationales

Patient/Family Teaching

- Teach the woman about the purpose of iron, its role in maternal and fetal health, and the difficulty of obtaining adequate amounts in the diet during pregnancy. Helps increase compliance. Because iron may be irritating to the gastrointestinal tract and may cause constipation, the woman may be tempted to skip doses.
- Teach about the correct administration of iron. Proper timing of administration of iron helps ensure proper absorption. If tolerated, iron should be taken on an empty stomach. However, if nausea occurs, it is acceptable to take iron with food and in smaller doses divided throughout the day. Tea and coffee decrease the absorption of iron and should be avoided. Iron should not be taken within 1 hour after ingesting milk or milk products because iron binds with calcium, which decreases its absorption.
- Teach the woman to take iron with fluid or food rich in vitamin C. Vitamin C increases absorption of iron.
- Teach the woman to take iron with food if she experiences nausea from the iron. Food decreases nausea associated with iron.
- Teach the woman that iron supplementation may lead to constipation. Enables the woman to take preventive measures (e.g., increase fluid and fiber intake).
- Teach the woman to keep iron medications out of the reach of children. Prevents toxicity in children.
- Teach the woman to cook with iron utensils if feasible. Very small amounts of iron leach out into the food from iron utensils.

CARDIAC DISEASE IN PREGNANCY

Cardiac disease is a leading nonobstetric cause of mortality during pregnancy. Congenital pathology or an acquired valvular lesion complicates approximately 1–3% of pregnancies and accounts for 10–15% of maternal mortality. A significant trend in recent years is decreased incidence of valvular disease from rheumatic fever because of increased diagnosis and proper treatment of strep throat in developed countries, although immigrant women are still in danger due to undertreatment. Another trend nurses must keep in mind is that, although most congenital disease is corrected, there is a tendency for American women to postpone childbearing. Age can be an important variable in her heart's ability to maintain function during pregnancy.

Adaptation to the demands of pregnancy requires dramatic cardiovascular changes that most women can adjust to without problems. The woman with cardiac disease is challenged by these changes and becomes at risk for cardiac decompensation and complications that include congestive heart failure, arrhythmias, and stroke. Dynamic cardiovascular changes that occur in a normal pregnancy to accommodate fetal growth and development include:

- Cardiac output, which is determined by heart rate and stroke volume, increases 50% by term. Most increase is during the first trimester, but it peaks at about 20–26 weeks of gestation.
- Heart rate is 10–25% higher in pregnancy than in the prepregnancy state. Heart rate increases to pump the additional blood volume required to sustain growth and development of the fetus.
- Plasma volume increases by 40–50% at term over prepregnancy levels. RBCs increase, in comparison, by only 20–30%. This shift in ratio of plasma volume to RBCs results in physiologic dilution of the blood and can cause physiologic anemia of pregnancy. Pulse is increased by about 10 beats per minute. Inability to adjust can lead to pulmonary congestion or worsening ischemia. Aneurysms can be formed or dissect with increased volume and increased pulse rate.
- Peripheral vasodilation and a corresponding decrease in systemic and pulmonary vascular resistance occur so the circulatory system can accommodate the increased blood volume. Women with left-to-right shunt are at risk for shunt reversal with lower systemic vascular resistance.
- Blood flow to the skin, kidneys, and uterus increases. Colloid osmotic pressure decreases, leading to increased fluid movement from the intravascular space into the interstitial space. Edema is possible and likely.
- After week 24, in a supine position, the woman's uterus can compress the inferior vena cava, causing a 25–30% decrease in cardiac output and supine hypotension syndrome.
- With pregnancy, a hypercoagulability state occurs, which can create problems for mechanical heart valves if atrial fibrillation exists.
- Fetus is at risk for prematurity, low birth weight, intrauterine growth retardation, and preterm birth. The fetus also is at increased risk for congenital heart disease.

■ Key Nursing Activities

Classification of heart risk in relation to function is helpful in guiding care and is done initially to establish baseline and at follow-up visits dependent on type of cardiac disease and level. Nurses must support the patient in creating a lifestyle change that decreases activity and avoids risk of cardiac decompensation. Diagnostic testing will guide therapy throughout the pregnancy.

- *Before pregnancy.* Nurses should be aware of cardiac risks and pregnancy. Preconceptual teaching can be very informative because many women with congenital heart problems are not aware of the increased risk and can use the education to make an informed choice about whether or not to become pregnant. Conditions for which pregnancy is medically contraindicated are: New York Heart Association (NYHA) class greater than II, Eisenmenger's syndrome, severe pulmonary hypertension, severe aortic stenosis, and Marfan syndrome with aortic root dilatation more than 40 mm. Correction of defect is best executed prior to a pregnancy beginning.

- *During pregnancy.* A woman's ability to function can be more important than her diagnosis. Specific activities, especially during the third—most critical—trimester, include:
  - ▶ Promote rest (e.g., bed rest, household help, hospitalization); promote pacing to economize woman's strength and energy.
  - ▶ Monitor conditions that stress the heart, including infections, emotional stress, coexisting conditions such as hypertension, anemia, hyperthyroidism, or obesity. Monitor for and prevent complications of cardiac disease (e.g., cardiac decompensation). If complications are found, contact members of the health team so the client can receive treatment.
  - ▶ Provide education and psychosocial support with assessment of social support and family needs, providing and connecting to network to aid access to community support possibilities.
- *After pregnancy.* Once pregnancy has been established, nursing can continue to educate and assist in promoting health throughout the course of gestation. Nursing activities should focus on promoting and preserving personal health or improving health status to achieve a successful outcome for both mother and baby, and on minimizing stress on the heart, especially between 28 and 32 weeks' gestation.

▌ Etiologies and Risk Factors

- Congenital heart disease is the leading cause of cardiovascular pathology in childbearing women.
- Many of the acquired valvular lesions can be attributed to rheumatic heart disease.
- Other pathologies may result from toxic (e.g., cocaine), metabolic (e.g., diabetes mellitus, thyroid disorders), or infectious (e.g., endocarditis from IV drug abuse) insults.
- Increased maternal age, obesity, atherosclerosis, tobacco abuse, and other traditional causes of coronary artery disease contribute to primary myocardial infarction in pregnancy.
- Renal and pulmonary disorders are also risk factors.

▌ Signs and Symptoms

Nurses are challenged when caring for women with cardiac disease in pregnancy to carefully distinguish abnormalities from the normal, physiologic changes in the cardiovascular system during pregnancy from those that mimic cardiac disease and those that represent clinical cardiac decompensation.

Normal Findings

- Normal objective manifestations: Jugular vein pulsation, displaced left-ventricular apex/apical pulse, persistent S_2 splitting, S_3, systolic murmurs less than grade III/IV, venous hum, sinus dysrhythmia, pulmonary basilar rales, and peripheral edema. These normal changes also may produce expected findings on diagnostic tests, such as electrocardiogram and echocardiography.
- Normal subjective manifestations: Fatigue, chest discomfort, dyspnea, orthopnea, hyperpnea, palpitations, and syncope (vasovagal).

Abnormal Findings

Clinical manifestations are based on the specific cardiac lesion and the functional abnormality produced by the lesion. Abnormal findings that herald cardiac decompensation are as follows:

- Abnormal objective manifestations: Prominent jugular venous distention (greater than 4 cm higher than sternal angle), general or chamber-specific cardiomegaly/heave, loud P_2; wide split of S_2, summation gallop, systolic murmur (greater than grade III/IV), diastolic murmur, significant cyanosis/clubbing, edema (progressive, generalized, and/or facial), peripheral cyanosis. Be particularly alert for irregular, weak, rapid pulse, edema, lung crackles, orthopnea, rapid respirations, moist frequent cough, and cyanosis of lips and nail beds.
- Abnormal subjective manifestations: Fatigue at rest, exertional chest pain, severe or progressive dyspnea, progressive orthopnea, paroxysmal nocturnal dyspnea, dysrhythmia (atrial fibrillation, conduction disorders, tachyarrhythmias), syncope with exertion, cough, hemoptysis. Be particularly alert to mother's complaints of increasing fatigue and difficulty breathing with activities, feeling of smothering, coughing, heart racing, and edema.

▌ Diagnostic Studies

- Electrocardiogram. Done to evaluate ventricular function, valve structure, chamber size, heart wall motion and blood flow. Abnormal findings: Dysrhythmias, ventricular hypertrophy, ST-segment changes, T-wave changes, bundle branch blocks, Q waves.
- Chest X-ray. Assess size of heart and presence of fluid. If X-ray studies are performed, ensure that the woman's abdomen and pelvis are covered with a lead apron. Abnormal findings: Cardiomegaly, pericardial effusion.
- Echocardiogram. Best diagnostic tool for evaluations of suspected cardiac disease. Abnormal findings: Valvular abnormalities, valvular regurgitation, hypokinesis, ventricular dilation, atrial and/or ventricular enlargement, axis deviations, congenital defects, shunting.

- Ejection fraction. Measures the heart's pumping capacity, especially that of the left ventricle.
- Magnetic resonance imaging, radionuclide angiography and computerized tomography scanning.
- Laboratory findings. Significant findings are elevated cardiac enzymes (CPK-MB more than 10–12 U/L), elevated serum glutamic oxaloacetic transaminase greater than 35 U/L, elevated lactate dehydrogenase greater than 45–90 U/L, decreased Po_2 (less than 75 mmHg on room air), increased hematocrit (greater than 48%), decreased hematocrit (lower than 35%), decreased hemoglobin (less than 10 g/dl). Biochemical assays of smooth muscle myosin heavy chain can diagnose cardiovascular disease.
- Cardiac catheterization and aortography. Coronary artery thrombus, atherosclerosis, stenosis, aneurysm, and spasm.
- Ultrasonography. Evaluation of fetal growth and development, placenta placement and grade, cord perfusion, amniotic fluid level. Abnormal finding that can occur with cardiac disease. Fetal growth retardation.

Medical Management

General Management

- Preconceptual, first trimester and repeat evaluation at 8th or 9th month of pregnancy. Determines level of cardiac disease to help guide activity, need for education, need for resources and extra support, and develop a plan for care.
- Admit to hospital 10–14 days prior to due date for controlled rest if NYHA class IV. NYHA classification is used in conjunction with functional capacity, exercise tolerance, degree of cyanosis, medication needs, and history of dysrhythmia to guide team decisions for prenatal approach to pregnant cardiac patient. Pregnant women may change levels as physical demands of pregnancy increase and care needs must change to have a successful outcome. For further information about NYHA functional capacity of cardiac disease, see American Heart Association website at www.americanheart.org/presenter.jhtml?identifier=4569.
- Treatment is aimed at minimizing the cardiac workload while optimizing maternal and fetal tissue perfusion.
- Avoid infections (risk for endocarditis); treat aggressively if they occur and preventively when indicated by disease.
- Reduce maternal physical activity, promote rest and best function possible.
- Limit weight gain (to 15 pounds, or as directed by physician).
- Limit sodium intake to 2–4 g/ day (if indicated).
- Iron supplements (prenatal vitamins), good balanced nutrition.
- β-blockers (for sustained heart rate greater than 90–100 beats/min).
- Digoxin, if clinically indicated, for NYHA class I/II, likely throughout pregnancy for NYHA class III/IV. Refer to American Heart Association website www.americanheart.org/presenter.jhtml?identifier=4569 for classification of functional capacity and objective assessment of cardiac disease.
- Heparin or other anticoagulants throughout pregnancy if the woman has a mechanical heart valve or other condition that increases the risk for clots. Heparin is a large-molecule drug and does not cross the placenta.
- Stool softeners to avoid constipation. Prevent straining; forced expiration against a closed airway, when released, causes blood to rush to the heart and overload the cardiac system.

General Medical Management During Prenatal Care

Antepartum care necessitates collaboration within the multidisciplinary team for the pregnant woman. Members should be from cardiology, obstetrics, anesthesia, pediatrics/neonatology, genetics, nutrition, and nursing. Nurses should be from units where care will be delivered to the woman and her baby. Key decisions made include:

- Timing of the birth, location, and supplies
- Invasive hemodynamic monitoring
- Endocarditis prophylaxis
- Anesthesia method
- Anticoagulation
- Potential problems and risks
- Frequency of prenatal visits
- Decision about need for early admission (Arafah & Baird, 2006, p. 37)

General Management During Labor and Delivery

Labor and delivery place extreme demands on the heart of the pregnant woman. Blood volume (300–500 ml) is displaced with each uterine contraction, which increases cardiac output. The labor and delivery period are critical times for mother and baby who have acute needs for accurate assessments and specialized care to ensure a safe delivery.

- Vaginal delivery is the goal. If cesarean delivery or episiotomy is performed, antibiotic prophylaxis for infective endocarditis is no longer recommended routinely in the absence of infection. If the woman is in the highest risk category (prosthetic cardiac valve, previous infective endocarditis, unrepaired congenital heart disease, or has a prosthetic device or patch), intravenous antibiotics may include ampicillin, cefazolin, ceftriaxone, and clindamycin for cesarean or vaginal delivery (ACOG, 2008b, pp. 1192–1193). Low forceps extraction/vacuum extraction may be used for safety. Limits maternal pushing.
- Withhold heparin if on anticoagulation before delivery. Decreases bleeding risk during birth and postdelivery.

- Supplemental oxygen may be indicated. Oxygen needs will increase during contractions for both mother and fetus.
- Maternal heart monitor, oxygen saturation, and frequent vital sign checks are essential with close monitoring of fetal heart rate and reactivity. Evaluates fetal need for increased oxygen.
- Epidural anesthetic using narcotic for pain control while supporting hemodynamic parameters. Helps prevent tachycardia and reduces workload of heart.
- Place in left lateral semirecumbent position. Reduces hypotension; may need to adjust delivery position to avoid supine hypotension syndrome.
- Intrapartum invasive hemodynamic monitoring for NYHA class III/IV. Monitor intake and output. Ensures avoidance of fluid overload.
- Support mother during labor with comfort measures, teaching, focused breathing, and presence.
- Include family members and give them jobs when feasible. Helps make them feel as though they are part of the team. Family-centered care is a goal.
- Be aware of cardiovascular events such as myocardial infarction, spontaneous coronary artery dissection, and stroke, which are rare but can occur.

General Postpartum Management

- The postpartum period (especially the first 48 hours after birth, up to 72 hrs) is the most common time for the development of congestive heart failure because of increased cardiac output due to autotransfusion from the contracting uterus. Risks for pulmonary edema and hemorrhage exist. Monitor for pulmonary embolus for the 3 days following birth due to fluid shifts. Hemodynamic monitoring is continued until blood pressure and apical and radial pulses return to normal.
- Treatment of congestive heart failure, if indicated, with oxygen, IV digoxin, IV furosemide (Lasix), frequent checking of vital signs, and observation. Auscultate lung fields every 1–4 hours as indicated by recovery and stabilization status.
- Assess for presence of chest pain, shortness of breath, general anxiety, and edema.
- Provide pain relief that is adequate to prevent increased cardiac demands.
- Teach the new mother about her body's changes and her new baby's behavior and needs.
- Facilitate bonding and help the mother take on her new role with the infant. Assist with breastfeeding or initiate pumping to start milk supply early if mother's intent is to breastfeed when able. Make sure if mother is on medications, they are compatible with nursing. Feeding methods may need evaluation dependent on mother's fatigue level.
- If baby is in high-risk nursery, promote early family contact and provide photos and information to mother. Refer to support groups as appropriate.

- Activity restriction may continue for initial weeks postpartum and extra help may be needed at home. Refer to social services for assistance with home care and preparation for discharge.
- Follow up with cardiologist 4–6 weeks postpartum. Postpartum is a high-risk period for stroke, especially for women with cardiac disease and hypertension and for those who smoke. Preeclampsia is also a risk factor.
- Diet to give nurturance for recovery, stress reduction continues for physical return, and treatment of anemia (as in the prenatal period) to maintain iron stores.
- Provide counseling about contraception and exploration of methods that decrease the risk for thromboembolitic event.

Congenital Cardiac Disease

Tetralogy of Fallot

- This condition is usually repaired in childhood and is the most common cyanotic heart disease present in pregnancy. Pregnancy is discouraged if the heart is unrepaired.
- Anticoagulant therapy, oxygen administration, and hemodynamic monitoring during labor and birth.

Eisenmenger's Syndrome

- Most defects are repaired during childhood, greatly reducing the risk during pregnancy; pulmonary hypertension as result of left-to-right shunt with ventricular septal defect.
- Consider termination of pregnancy if mother is in major cardiac risk category.
- Hospitalization and bed rest for hemodynamic instability.
- Anticoagulation therapy, avoid hypotension and increasing pulmonary vascular resistance, continuous oxygen therapy and oxygen saturation over 90%.
- Epidural anesthesia and assisted vaginal delivery preferred.
- Eisenmenger's syndrome may be a contraindication for pregnancy.

Atrial Septal Defect

- Most common congenital defect with small left-to-right shunt; pregnancy is usually well tolerated.
- Avoid hypotension and tachycardia.
- Labor in lateral position, with oxygen and monitoring.
- Epidural and vaginal delivery.
- Surgical closure during pregnancy if complications occur.

Patent Ductus Arteriosus

- Maternal complications depend on size of the ductus if it is unrepaired.
- If there is a large lesion, decrease in systemic vascular resistance can cause reversal and increase mortality risk.
- Avoid hypotension and monitor oxygen.
- Epidural and vaginal delivery.
- Surgical closure during pregnancy if complications occur.

Coarctation of the Aorta

- Relatively uncommon and should be repaired before conception.
- Termination of pregnancy should be considered due to maternal risks.
- Bed rest, if severe, with strict blood pressure control.
- Surgical correction during pregnancy if severe complications occur.
- Epidural and assisted delivery.

Acquired Cardiac Lesions

Mitral Stenosis

- Most common rheumatic valvular lesion in pregnancy
- Avoid hypotension and monitor BP during labor
- Avoid fluid overload; treatment of pulmonary edema with diuretics (no thiazide agents); treatment of tachyarrhythmias with digoxin, β-blockers, chemical or electrical cardioversion
- Anticoagulation to prevent thromboembolism (no warfarin)
- Epidural and assisted delivery

Aortic Stenosis

- Most common valve lesion in the United States, can be congenital or rheumatic
- Physical activity reduced and observe for congestive heart failure or dysrhythmias
- Bed rest, if severe
- Epidural and assisted delivery

Ischemic Cardiac Disease

- Myocardial infarction can occur with the three strongest risk factors being chronic hypertension, diabetes, and advancing maternal age older than 33 years.
- Most frequent in last trimester and postpartum and associated with prematurity and low birth weight of infant.
- If it occurs during pregnancy, attempt to delay delivery for 2–3 weeks.
- Evaluate for thrombophilias and prevent coagulation with heparin if indicated.
- Oxygen and cardiac support.
- Labor in left recumbent position.
- Avoid Valsalva maneuver during pushing.
- Bacterial endocarditis prophylaxis.
- Epidural and assisted delivery.

Peripartum Cardiomyopathy

- Optimize cardiac output; digoxin may be used
- Oxygen administration; left lumbar position
- Pain control essential with assisted delivery

▋ Collaborative Problems

Potential complications of cardiac disease in pregnancy include the following:

- Cardiac decompensation
- Fetal growth retardation (IUGR)/fetal injury
- Preterm delivery

COLLABORATIVE (STANDARDIZED) CARE FOR ALL PATIENTS WITH CARDIAC DISEASE IN PREGNANCY

The primary goal of nursing care for the cardiac patient who is pregnant and her family is focused on the complications that may occur and to reduce potential risks for complications. Perform a comprehensive assessment to identify individual needs for teaching, emotional support, and physical care.

▋ Potential Complication of Cardiac Disease in Pregnancy: CARDIAC DECOMPENSATION

Focus Assessments

- Assess prepregnant cardiac status and for risk factors. Take thorough history and note all medications patient is taking. Preexisting problems are complicated by the increased cardiovascular demands of pregnancy and, therefore, increase the likelihood of cardiac decompensation. For example, risks are greater in older women, those with comorbidities, and those who are obese. Medications can harm the fetus and may need to be changed.
- At each visit, assess heart rate, BP, and pulse for tachycardia and irregularities. Heart rate greater than 110 bpm is a symptom of cardiac decompensation. When the heart cannot maintain sufficient cardiac output, blood pressure falls and the body attempts to compensate by increasing heart rate.
- Assess respirations, e.g., tachypnea greater than 20–34/min, cough, dyspnea, hemoptysis, bibasilar rales. These are symptoms of cardiac decompensation. As left heart failure occurs, blood backs up in the pulmonary circulation, producing pulmonary vascular congestion.
- Assess heart tones and chest pain (murmur that predates pregnancy, diastolic murmur, systolic murmur greater than grade III/IV). Identifies type and extent of cardiac problem.
- Assess mental status; e.g., debilitating fatigue, anxiety. The initial signs may indicate inadequate oxygenation of brain tissue.
- Assess extremities for edema. Assess integument, nail beds, and mucous membranes for cyanosis. Edema is a symptom of right heart failure as pressure rises in the systemic venous circulation. Cyanotic changes indicate inadequate circulation of oxygenated blood to the periphery. This occurs when there is a decrease in peripheral vascular resistance, which causes a worsening of right-to-left shunting.

- Assess Homans' sign. Report signs of thromboembolism such as pain, redness, tenderness, or swelling in the extremities. Homans' sign is indicative of thrombosis.
- Monitor weight gain at each visit. Encourage patient to weigh daily at home. Weight gain should be limited in order to decrease demands on the heart. Also, a weight gain of more than the normal 2–2.5 lb/wk may be due to edema, which could be indicative of cardiac decompensation or a condition such as preeclampsia.
- Assess potassium intake and for symptoms of hypokalemia. Symptoms of hypokalemia include thirst, vertigo, confusion, hypoventilation, muscle weakness, twitching, tetany, and irregular pulse. Decreased potassium levels may be associated with cardiac dysfunction, or they can be an adverse reaction to digitalis.
- Monitor laboratory test results. For example, an increased WBC count is indicative of infection.
- Assess for factors that can increase stress. Refer to high-risk pregnancy support group if available. Stress increases the production of cortisol, which increases heart rate and oxygen demands on the heart.
- At each visit, continue to monitor blood pressure, heart rate, and respiratory rate and compare with prepregnancy baseline. Listen for signs of pulmonary edema such as crackles, changes in heart sounds, cough, and dyspnea. Allows early treatment if decompensation develops.
- Determine the patient's and support persons' understanding of heart disease effects on pregnancy and the pregnancy's effect on the patient's heart. An understanding of the impact of these interactions will aid support of her family for the change in lifestyle and adjustments necessary for the healthiest pregnancy.

Preventive Nursing Activities

- Stress the importance of seeing the primary care provider every 2 weeks in the first half of pregnancy and weekly thereafter. Cardiac decompensation and pregnancy complications can develop rapidly. Frequent assessment is essential. Teach danger signs and evaluate each visit.
- Reclassify the woman (as needed) in terms of the NYHA classification system. As the demands on the heart increase, the woman's status may worsen, especially after blood volume peaks at about 32 weeks' gestation.
- Teach the woman to sleep/rest in the left lateral recumbent position. Promotes venous return to the heart, and therefore leads to adequate cardiac output and blood pressure.
- Assist the woman to plan for additional help with household chores, care of other children. Ensures adequate rest and prevents strain on the heart. Minimum rest requirements include 10 hours' sleep per night; a 30-minute rest period after each meal; no lifting or straining; light housework; and some easy walking.
- Promote good prenatal nutrition. In addition to providing a well-balanced diet high enough in iron, protein, and calories to support the pregnancy, other dietary considerations exist. There is a need for adequate protein and limited sodium in order to prevent fluid retention; a need to ensure adequate potassium; and a need to avoid foods high in vitamin K (e.g., raw, dark green, and leafy vegetables) if taking heparin. A substitute source for folic acid in the diet is also needed.
- Teach measures to prevent, identify, and report signs and symptoms of infection. Prompt medical treatment is essential to prevent cardiac problems. Infection increases the heart rate, can directly spread pathogens to the heart, and can precipitate congestive heart failure.
- Assess lifestyle patterns, emotional status, and the environment of the woman. Explain activity restrictions. Reduction in activity may range from ensuring daily rest periods to complete bed rest (after 30 weeks), depending on the severity of the condition.
- Teach the woman and family about her condition and encourage her to report to the primary care provider subjective symptoms of worsening cardiac condition. This information is needed for self-care and prompt medical intervention. A worsening of the woman's cardiac status may be indicated by decreasing ability to carry out normal activities, increasing dyspnea with or without physical activity, nocturnal dyspnea and other respiratory symptoms, fatigue, cyanosis, and change in pulse rate.
- Instruct the woman to be watchful for signs of thromboembolism such as redness, tenderness, and pain or swelling of the legs and to seek medical care immediately. Ensures early intervention.
- Instruct the woman to avoid constipation by taking in adequate fluids and fiber. Prevents straining with bowel movements.
- Teach relaxation techniques. Reduces emotional stress and decreases blood pressure and pulse.
- Teach the woman to elevate her legs several times a day when sitting. Prolonged dependent position of the feet impairs venous return, causes pooling of blood in the lower extremities, and adds stress to the heart, which must overcome the force of gravity.
- Teach the woman how to apply and care for antithrombotic stockings. Stockings compress the veins in the legs, promoting venous return and reducing venous stasis.
- Discuss and create plan for activities of diversion and enjoyment since the woman will be on rest so much of the day. Decreases the risk for boredom.
- Refer to home health care or specialists as needed. This will keep the woman following activity reduction plan and not tending to overdo.

During Labor

- Position in lateral decubitus position during labor/delivery; do not use stirrups. Administer supplemental oxygen if needed. Facilitates cardiac function. In traditional lithotomy position, the uterus compresses the inferior vena cava, decreasing venous return to the heart and causing a 25–30% decrease in cardiac output. Stirrups create venous compression and impede circulation.

- Carefully monitor fluid intake and output, heart rate and rhythm, blood pressure, and pulse oximetry during labor. In addition to routine assessments for all laboring women, assessments for cardiac decompensation must be made because of the additional burden labor and birth place on the already compromised cardiovascular system. Heart rate should be less than 110 beats/min between uterine contractions; respiratory rate should be less than 24/min. The hypotension commonly associated with anesthesia poses grave maternal risks.
- Minimize pain and anxiety during labor and birth. Narcotic epidural is recommended for pain control and management of labor. Emotional stress and pain tend to increase pulse and BP; they also increase oxygen usage.
- Lower the woman's legs immediately after delivery. Decreases effects of the sudden increase in venous return that results from the contracting uterus.
- Monitor closely after delivery for bleeding and cardiac decompensation during the next critical 2–3 hours. Ensures early detection of complications.

Potential Complication of Cardiac Disease in Pregnancy: FETAL GROWTH RETARDATION/ FETAL INJURY

Focus Assessments

- Starting at about 32 weeks' gestation, assessing NST is generally performed at each clinic visit. Nonreactive NST may indicate fetal hypoxia, which occurs as a result of maternal cardiac decompensation. This may be combined with the biophysical profile for antepartum fetal surveillance and assessment of amniotic fluid levels. The biophysical profile consists of five variables with scoring 0–2 and a cumulative score. Components are fetal breathing and gross body movements, fetal tone, qualitative amniotic fluid volume, and reactive nonstress fetal heart rate. A normal score is 8–10; an equivocal is 6; and an abnormal score is less than 4.
- Assess for decreased amniotic fluid (amniotic fluid index of less than 15 cm between weeks 28 and 40). Associated with IUGR and fetal injury.
- Assess serial ultrasonography. Determines gestational age and size of fetus and detects IUGR and placental grading.
- Monitor fetal movement including FHR patterns and variability with each maternal assessment. Compare with baseline. Abnormal fetal heart rate and response (rate less

than 120 or greater than 160 beats/min, irregular rhythm, decreased or absent variability, late decelerations) are indicators of fetal hypoxia when the maternal heart cannot compensate for fetal needs.

- Monitor vital signs and report deviations from desired parameters. Evaluate for signs of preeclampsia. Maternal BP is maintained above 100/60 mmHg and fetal heart rate is between 120 and 160 beats per minute. Fetal growth is dependent on good placental profusion, and maternal vital signs are indicators of maternal status.
- Monitor fundal height. Determines fetal size and weight; fundal height should correlate with fetal gestation. Growth ultrasounds may be done every 4–6 weeks to assess growth in addition.
- Assess for signs of preeclampsia, elevated BP, proteinuria, visual changes, headaches, edema, and epigastric pain. Ensures early detection of conditions that can affect fetal or maternal well-being.
- Assess for signs of preterm labor, backache, cramping, abdominal pressures, leakage of fluid. Ensures early detection of preterm labor.
- Assess for signs of urinary tract infection or vaginal infection, which can also cause uterine irritability and move into premature labor. Ensures early detection of preterm labor.

Preventive Nursing Activities

- Teach about the effect of cardiac decompensation on placental circulation and fetal tissue perfusion. Provides motivation to participate in treatment plan and adhere to guidelines.
- Teach the correlation between the treatment plan and prevention of cardiac decompensation. Provides motivation to participate in treatment plan and not to disregard potential danger signs.
- Encourage smoking cessation if the woman is a smoker. Smoking further interferes with fetoplacental circulation and contributes to IUGR.
- Teach the woman to identify signs and symptoms of cardiac decompensation. Enables prompt medical treatment. The woman is often the first person to recognize changes that are consistent with cardiac decompensation.
- Beginning at week 24, instruct the woman to use a method to assess daily fetal movement and kick count (e.g., Cardiff or Sandovsky). Teach the woman parameters for contacting her healthcare provider. Reassure the woman that fetal movement is variable in response to fetal sleep cycles and maternal activity. Consistent movement later in pregnancy is one indicator of fetal health. Sudden decreases may indicate fetal jeopardy.
- Teach the mother the importance of fetal activity. Teach the mother to keep a daily fetal movement chart after 24 weeks of gestation since it is an indicator of fetal well-being.

Potential Complication of Cardiac Disease in Pregnancy: PRETERM LABOR

Refer to generic collaborative care plan for "Potential Complication: Preterm Labor," beginning on p. 31 in Chapter 3. Also, refer to "Preterm Labor and Spontaneous Abortion," beginning on p. 197 in Chapter 6.

Focus Assessments

- Assess the home situation for adequate help and support of bed rest. Determines the need for additional assistance to maintain enforced bed rest.

Preventive Nursing Activities

- Instruct the woman on the importance of maintaining prescribed bed rest/activity limitations. Activity may stimulate uterine contractions, in addition to increasing the demands on the heart. Understanding the significance of this may improve compliance with this restriction.
- Teach the woman to recognize and report signs and symptoms of preterm labor. Evaluate each visit. Early treatment may prevent preterm birth. Include information about what a contraction feels like and the importance of reporting signs so treatment can be implemented before the cervix starts dilating.
- Maintain hydration. Dehydration can cause irritability of the uterus and cause blood pressure changes.
- Teach the woman to report symptoms of urinary tract infection. Irritability from infection can cause contractions.

INDIVIDUALIZED (NURSING DIAGNOSIS) CARE PLANS

This section includes care plans to address unique patient needs.

Nursing diagnoses focus on educational needs, assessment of all systems involved, referrals to appropriate team caregivers, and facilitation of patient involvement in all care planning. Anticipatory guidance and decision-making support are essential nursing functions to aid in addressing the wide range of needs for the pregnant woman affected by cardiac disease.

Nursing Diagnosis: ACTVITY INTOLERANCE[1]

Related Factors: decreased cardiac output, hypoxemia, anemia, bed rest, and imbalance between oxygen supply and demand.

■ *Goals, Outcomes, and Evaluation Criteria*

- Woman completes activities of daily living without exacerbation of cardiac disease state (as manifested by absence of or

no reported increase of dyspnea, fatigue, syncope, or chest pain).
- Woman states components of devised daily rest regimen and has some enjoyed leisure activities.
- Woman accepts help with household chores and care of children.
- Woman accepts support from family and community resources as needed.

■ *NIC Interventions[2]*

Energy Management (0180)—Regulating energy use to treat or prevent fatigue and optimize functioning.

Sleep Enhancement (1850)—Facilitation of regular sleep/wake cycles.

Teaching: Prescribed Activity (5612)—Preparing a patient to achieve and/or maintain a prescribed level of activity.

Self-Care Assistance (1800)—Assisting another to perform activities of daily living.

■ *Nursing Activities and Rationales*

Assessments

- Assess functional status according to the NYHA classifications. Assessment of functional status reflects the capacity of the woman to tolerate activity. This enables the nurse to plan interventions that are achievable and safe for the woman based upon the degree of functional impairment.
- Assess support systems available to the woman. By using information about the amount and quality of caregiver support available to the woman, the nurse can determine any deficits in internal support systems (family, friends, older children) and provide referrals to external caregiving sources.
- Assess self-care and home maintenance needs. Determines whether she will need help with these needs or whether her energy reserves are adequate to meet them.
- Evaluate pattern of sleep and rest (number of hours slept per night, number of unplanned awakenings per night and cause, nap times, and length). Patterns of sleep and rest are unique to each individual. Adequate daily rest is essential in pregnancy complicated by heart disease to promote acceptable cardiac output and placental blood flow. Sleep and rest can often be difficult in even a normal pregnancy because of the physical changes of pregnancy. In the woman with cardiac disease, sleep and rest can become even more difficult secondary to orthopnea and paroxysmal nocturnal dyspnea.

Collaborative Activities

- Arrange for assistance as needed with self-care, child care, and housework. Family and /or friends may provide needed assistance if available /able. Outside agencies may be needed if a deficit in support is identified or to provide relief for primary caregivers.

Patient/Family Teaching

- Educate the woman on the need for pacing activities and any prescribed activity restrictions. Prescribed activity will be based on NYHA classifications. Class I and II patients can usually do light housework with no lifting or straining. Class III and IV patients will likely be prescribed bed rest, especially late in pregnancy. Cardiac decompensation and hypoxic fetal injury can occur when activity surpasses the functional ability of the heart.
- Teach the woman the optimal positioning for sleep and rest. The left lateral recumbent position is the preferred position for sleep and rest. This position relieves the pressure of the gravid uterus from the inferior vena cava and promotes venous return. Adequate venous return is an essential component of cardiac output.
- Develop a specific daily rest regimen with the woman; e.g., 10 hours each night in bed and scheduled naps. Adequate rest and pacing of activities conserve energy and promote maternal and fetal well-being. Specifying a plan of action with the woman's input increases likelihood of compliance behaviors.

Other Nursing Diagnoses

Also assess for the following nursing diagnoses, which are frequently present with this condition:

- Ineffective Sexual Pattern[1] related to activity limitation and fatigue.
- Risk for ineffective peripheral tissue perfusion[1] (thromboembolism) related to valvular lesions or diminished venous return.
- Fear[1] related to the effect of cardiac disease on well-being of self and fetus.
- Deficient diversional activity[1] secondary to prescribed bed rest.

HIV IN PREGNANCY

Human immunodeficiency virus (HIV) is a retrovirus that targets and destroys CD4 T helper cells—cells that are essential for acquired immunity. The virus produces a progressive infection that leads to acquired immunodeficiency syndrome (AIDS) with increasing loss of the CD4 cells. AIDS is a progressive, debilitating disease that eventually results in death due to immune system collapse. These viruses are transmitted via blood and body fluids, semen, vaginal secretions, and human milk. HIV infections are caused by HIV-1 or HIV-2 viruses. HIV-1 activity is seen globally. HIV-2 is primarily confined to South Africa. Women may be infected with HIV for many years before developing AIDS.

Women are the fastest growing segment of persons becoming infected with HIV, which mostly occurs from unprotected sexual contact and IV drug use from contaminated needles. This increased incidence of HIV among women has also resulted in increased numbers of infected infants. Hispanic and African American women are disproportionately affected by HIV/AIDS, making up about 78.6% of cases among women, although they represent only 12.6% of the U.S. population (CDC, 2010). Antiviral drug treatments slow transition of HIV to AIDS and have made it possible for HIV-infected women in developed countries to live to raise their children.

HIV vertical transmission can occur from mother to fetus any time during pregnancy, birth, or breastfeeding. Pregnant women with HIV might not know they have the disease. Prenatal screening is vital to ensure that women receive the care they need for a healthy outcome for the newborn. Women with HIV prior to becoming pregnant may not receive adequate prenatal care or have issues with access to care, which may further compromise the health of both the mother and the infant.

Transmission is based on the timing of prenatal care, degree of viremia during pregnancy, access to care, use and adherence to drug therapy, and route of delivery. With appropriate antiviral treatment for the mother during pregnancy, for the exposed infant after delivery and no breastfeeding exposure, HIV transmission to the infant has been decreased to fewer than 2% of infants born to HIV-positive mothers. Proper treatment becomes a global issue for women because developing countries have decreased access to antiviral medications, limited availability of prenatal care, and high dependence on breastfeeding for infant nutrition, which compounds the problem. Stigma of seropositive status hinders pregnant women making the choice to be screened prenatally. If a pregnant woman goes untreated, transmission to the child during pregnancy and birth is about one third, with increased risk of transmission occurring from breastfeeding after delivery. See Table 5-1 for the WHO and CDC stages of HIV infection.

Key Nursing Activities

- Early screening for detection and counseling about indications for testing and HIV risk factors for mother and infant.
- Teaching about management of HIV infection, self-care, and ways of preventing and detecting opportunistic infections.
- Teaching regarding transmission, symptoms of infection, antiviral and other medications, and reinforcement of adherence to prevent drug resistance.
- Monitoring of maternal and fetal well-being during pregnancy, birth, and postpartum.
- Encouraging and teaching for health maintenance and treatment following birth and throughout life span.

Etiologies and Risk Factors

Risk factors for HIV include:

- Multiple sex partners or serial monogamy
- Infected with another sexually transmitted infection
- Personal use of illicit IV drugs or sexual partner with history of illicit IV drug use
- Emigrant from an HIV-endemic area such as Haiti or Africa
- History of employment in sex trade (prostitution)

TABLE 5-1 Comparison of World Health Organization (WHO) And CDC Stages of Human Immunodeficiency Virus (HIV) Infection* By CD4+ T-lymphocyte Count and Percentage of Total Lymphocytes

WHO Stage[†]	WHO T-lymphocyte Count and Percentage[§]	CDC Stage[¶]	CDC T-lymphocyte Count and Percentage
Stage 1 (HIV infection)	CD4+ T-lymphocyte count of ≥ 500 cells/µL	Stage 1 (HIV infection)	CD4+ T-lymphocyte count of ≥ 500 cells/µL or CD4+ T-lymphocyte percentage of ≥ 29
Stage 2 (HIV infection)	CD4+ T-lymphocyte count of 350–499 cells/µL	Stage 2 (HIV infection)	CD4+ T-lymphocyte count of 200–499 cells/µL or CD4+ T-lymphocyte percentage of 14–28
Stage 3 (advanced HIV disease [AHD])	CD4+ T-lymphocyte count of 200–349 cells/µL	Stage 2 (HIV infection)	CD4+ T-lymphocyte of 200–499 cells/µL or CD4+ T-lymphocyte percentage of 14–28
Stage 4 (acquired immunodeficiency syndrome [AIDS])	CD4+ T-lymphocyte count or < 200 cells/µL or CD4+ T-lymphocyte percentage of < 15	Stage 3 (AIDS)	CD4+ T-lymphocyte count of < 200 cells/µL or CD4+ T-lymphocyte percentage of < 14

* For reporting purposes only.
[†] Among adults and children aged ≥ 5 years.
[§] Percentage applicable for stage 4 only.
[¶] Among adults and adolescents (aged ≥ 13 years). CDC also includes a fourth stage, stage unknown; laboratory confirmation of HIV infection but no information on CD4+ T-lymphocyte count or percentage and no information on AIDS-defining conditions.

Source: CDC. (2008, December 5). Comparison of the revised World Health Organization and CDC surveillance case definition and staging systems for HIV infection. *Morbidity and Mortality Weekly Report (MMWR), 57* (RR20, Appendix B), 10–11

- Receipt of a blood transfusion between 1977 and 1985 (Gilbert, 2007)

Heterosexual sex is the number one transmission source for women. The greatest risk for transmission to the fetus is during delivery; more than 60% of transmissions occur during exposure to birth canal secretions and blood. Cesarean delivery is often considered and planned for the mode of delivery of the infant.

Disease progression during pregnancy in the United States and Europe has not been demonstrated in medical studies; however, in developing countries, it is suggested that pregnancy may aid disease progression. Hormonal effects of pregnancy may increase the risk of toxicity of antiretroviral therapy, especially nucleoside reverse transcriptase inhibitors, leading to lactic acidosis and hepatic failure, which has caused maternal deaths. Some signs and symptoms of HIV progression and/or drug side effects are similar to normal signs and symptoms of pregnancy; thus, careful assessment is essential during pregnancy. Some risks associated with HIV-positive women are intrapartal or postpartal hemorrhage; postpartal infection; poor wound healing; and infections of the genitourinary tract.

Signs and Symptoms

Subjective manifestations: Weakness, fatigue, headache, nasal congestion, anorexia, nausea, abdominal pain, myalgia, arthralgia, pharyngitis, photophobia, visual disturbances, changes in sensorium, anxiety, fear, or depression. Women with HIV/AIDS may also express feelings of social isolation, hopelessness, lack of social support, and/or denial.

Objective manifestations: Elevated temperature; tachycardia; dyspnea or hyperventilation; ulceration of oral, anal, or vaginal mucosa; vaginal infection; rash; skin lesions; lymphadenopathy; splenomegaly; vomiting; diarrhea; weight loss; seizures; cognitive changes; peripheral neuropathy; neurologic disorders.

Opportunistic infections: Additional symptoms associated with opportunistic infections include recurrent vaginal infections (candidiasis, bacterial vaginosis, trichomoniasis); ulcerative herpes simplex, condyloma, or syphilis; oral infections such as thrush; cough and shortness of breath, which may indicate pneumonia, mycobacterium, or tuberculosis; floaters and blurring vision (cytomegalovirus); diarrhea (*Salmonella*); skin lesions, which may indicate Kaposi sarcoma (more common in men than women).

Medication side effects: Lactic acidosis and hepatic dysfunction; nausea; vomiting; fatigue; tachycardia; dyspnea or hyperventilation; and abdominal pain. Pregnancy can enhance the side effects of nucleoside analogues, producing a syndrome similar to acute fatty liver of pregnancy. For further information, refer to other resources and textbooks.

Diagnostic Studies

- CBC with differential, platelet count. *Determines the presence or progression of anemia, which is common in HIV, leukocytopenia, and thrombocytopenia.*
- Type, Rh factor, and antibody screen. *Blood type in case of needed transfusion.*
- Rubella titer, HbsAg, tuberculosis screening with purified protein derivative or chest radiograph.
- Immunoglobulin testing. *Determines the presence of antibodies to cytomegalovirus, Toxoplasmosis gondii, hepatitis, and other diseases.*
- Papanicolaou (Pap) smear. *Screens for cervical cancer because of increased incidence of invasive cervical cancers.*
- Gonorrhea, *Chlamydia* cultures, and TORCH (toxoplasmosis, other, rubella, cytomegalovirus, herpes simplex virus) screen, VDRL screen. *Determine the presence of STIs such as gonorrhea, syphilis, or chlamydia, and hepatitis B, C, and D, and herpes.*
- Ultrasonography every trimester. *Screens for IUGR, congenital abnormalities, and placental problems.*
- Urinalysis, blood urea nitrogen, serum creatinine, liver enzymes, total protein, and albumin. *Determines the presence of renal or liver disease.*
- HIV testing: enzyme immunoassay. *Tests for antibodies to the human immunodeficiency virus. Used to determine if a person has been exposed to and produced antibodies to the HIV-1 retrovirus. If positive, must have follow-up testing.*
- Rapid HIV testing sometimes used in labor for rapid indication of seropositivity. *Enables initiation of care prior to delivery to decrease transmission since labor and delivery are critical times for HIV transmission to the infant.*
- Western blot technique follows enzyme immunoassay in secondary screening to confirm a positive result. *Highly specific test for HIV-1 antibodies; used to validate a positive enzyme immunoassay test finding. Another test, immunofluorescence assay, is also a follow-up test for positive confirmation.*
- HIV testing: CD4 cell count. *Measures the extent of immune damage. The normal adult CD4 cell count is 500–1,770 cells/L or between 32% and 62% of total lymphocytes. CD4 cell counts below 200 cells/L or decreased to lower than 14% of total lymphocytes are associated with immune damage, and opportunistic infections are likely to develop. AIDS diagnosis begins at less than 200 CD4 cells/L. Treatment usually begins if there are fewer than 350 CD4 cells/L.*
- HIV testing: plasma HIV RNA levels. *Measures the amount of virus in the serum, which reflects active viral replication. A higher viral burden predicts more rapid disease progression and a higher risk of vertical transmission. Levels are monitored to determine drug treatment responses and serve as guide to disease process, drug management, effectiveness of treatment, and to determine delivery mode. A level below 1,000 copies/ml is associated with low risk for disease progression, and vaginal delivery may be attempted. If a level is above 55,000 copies/ml, a higher risk for disease progression and transmission exists, and antiretroviral treatment will be initiated.*
- Resistance testing of virus for specific medications will be done if acute infection, viral rebound, or persistent viremia exists.

Medical Management

HIV Infection

- Treatment adheres to the same standards of care that apply to all other HIV-infected persons.
- Care is determined by CD4 counts and viral load levels. Medication regimens are prescribed accordingly. Standards of care change quickly. Resources and current treatment recommendations are available at Internet sites such as www.aidsinfo.nih.gov (National Institutes of Health), www.cdcnpin.org/scripts/hiv/index.asp (Centers for Disease Control and Prevention, National Prevention Information Network), and www.who.int/hiv/en/ (World Health Organization). Nursing care advice is found at www.anacnet.org (Association of Nurses in AIDS Care). The Antiretroviral Pregnancy Registry collects nonidentifying information from healthcare providers for documentation of pregnancies managed with antiretrovirals and their maternal and fetal outcomes.
- Antiretroviral combination drug therapy or highly active antiretroviral therapy, a multidrug treatment, is used during pregnancy. Presently, there are three categories of HIV drugs used in pregnancy, including nucleoside, nonnucleoside-analogue reverse transcriptase inhibitors, and protease inhibitors (e.g., ritonavir). Fusion inhibitors, another category of HIV drugs, are not used in pregnancy. A combination of drugs is highly effective in slowing the HIV virus if the drug regimen is available, affordable for the patient, and the drug regimen is followed closely. These drugs prevent the replication of the HIV-1 retrovirus and infection of noninfected cells. Standards of practice change often as new research results become available. Adherence is imperative for avoidance of drug resistance. Common medications used are zidovudine (ZDV, AZT, Retrovir), lamivudine (3TC or Epivir), and nevirapine (NVP, Viramune). FDA regulations must be addressed for safety in pregnancy, and the drug category of the medication needs to be noted. In most pregnancies in the United States, antiretrovirals are used regardless of viral load to prevent transmission of the virus to the fetus.
- Antibiotics. For treatment and prevention of bacterial opportunistic infections or STIs if present.
- Antifungal agents. For treatment of fungal opportunistic infections if present.
- Immunizations for hepatitis A and B, Haemophilus B influenza, pneumococcal infection, and viral influenza.
- Total parenteral nutrition. Treats nutritional deficits and protects both the mother and fetus when disease state has progressed.
- Analgesics. Decreases pain and inflammation resulting from opportunistic infections.

Antepartum Management

- Universal screening of all pregnant women with counseling offered.
- Complete history including menstrual, medical, obstetrical, and social history and habits. Establishes risk factors for opportunistic infections, potential complications, health habits that may pose threats to the woman or fetus, presence of STIs, and current treatments for HIV infection. Many women with HIV are at risk for domestic violence, and early assessment can enable access to community resources for aid.
- Complete physical assessment and evaluation of immunization status. Provides a baseline of data for future comparisons as the pregnancy evolves. Update vaccinations (pneumococcus, influenza, hepatitis A and B, tetanus) as possible during pregnancy to increase immunity.
- Laboratory assessments including CBC, HIV RNA viral load, CD4 cell counts, urinalysis, antibody screen, rubella titer, hepatitis B surface antigen, cervical cultures, and skin tests for toxoplasmosis and tuberculosis. RNA viral level and CD4 count every trimester (refer to diagnostic studies). Establishes the presence of existing infections and serves as a baseline for future comparisons.
- Normal prenatal care guidelines for maternal and fetal surveillance with appropriate assessments, testing, and evaluations. Serial ultrasound testing, NST, biophysical profiles as indicated for high-risk pregnancy even if normal progression in the current pregnancy. Most HIV-positive pregnant women will have normal pregnancies without adverse maternal and fetal morbidity if their HIV viral load is well controlled and with close monitoring. Presence of HIV makes high-risk pregnancy.
- Mental health services if depressive reaction to HIV diagnosis. Depression is common in those with chronic illnesses, those with a new diagnosis such as HIV, from medication side effects, or from increased anxiety. Depression needs to be assessed and treated.
- Substance abuse treatment if needed and appropriate. Discontinuation of substance abuse is imperative for the health of the mother and the growing fetus.

Management During Delivery

- Route of delivery will be determined by provider based on risk of vaginal delivery. Cesarean section will be considered if indicated. Cesarean section delivery is recommended after 34 weeks when HIV RNA levels are greater than 1,000 copies/ml. Cesarean delivery decreases the neonate's exposure to infected maternal blood/secretions and decreases vertical transmission of HIV. Risks to the mother versus benefits to the infant are weighed in the decision-making process.
- Avoidance of all invasive procedures, such as vaginal exams after rupture of membranes, fetal scalp electrode monitoring, fetal scalp sampling, and vacuum extraction. Decreases the risk of HIV-1 transmission via inoculation of virus into fetus.
- The infant must be cleaned of blood/secretions immediately following birth and bathed as soon as possible. Decreases the risk of transmission of HIV-1 to infant. No blood draws or injections until after bath decreases transmission.
- If vaginal delivery, goal is ruptured membranes for fewer than 4 hours prior to delivery. Ruptured membranes for greater than 4 hours is associated with increased transmission of HIV.
- IV zidovudine infusion throughout labor at 2 mg/kg over 1 hour. If cesarean delivery, same regimen at least 3 hours prior to delivery. Antiretroviral therapy during labor and delivery dramatically decreases the transmission of HIV.

Postpartum Management

- Frequent assessments for postpartum bleeding. Anemia is common side effect of HIV disease and drug treatments.
- Assessment for use of protease inhibitors. If patient is taking protease inhibitor, do not administer methylergonovine (Methergine) for bleeding. Protease inhibitors are contraindications for coadministration of *methylergonovine* due to possible coronary vasospasms.
- Monitor for presence of infections (vaginal discharge, incision and episiotomy, urinary symptoms) and promote perineal hygiene. HIV-infected women are at increased risk for infections such as UTIs, delayed wound healing, postpartum endometritis, and vaginitis.
- Breastfeeding discouraged; supportive measures for breast engorgement implemented. Prevents transmission of HIV-1 to the infant via human milk. Because the woman cannot breastfeed, she needs a supportive bra and ice packs for relief of engorgement.
- Comprehensive discharge planning initiated, including follow-up appointment, fertility management, safer sex practice, and importance of universal precautions. Continued care is important to health maintenance for both mother and infant. Contraception and safe-sex practices decrease transmission to others.
- Monitor for signs of clinical depression and referrals when indicated. A woman with HIV is at higher risk for postpartum depression.
- Teach about the importance of adherence to antiretroviral medications and prophylactic drugs against opportunistic infections. Fights progression of disease.

▌ Collaborative Problems

Potential complications of HIV/AIDS include:

- Opportunistic infections (*Pneumocystis jiroveci* pneumonia, *Mycobacterium avium* complex, *Mycobacterium tuberculosis*, candidiasis, coccidioidomycosis, cryptococcosis, histoplasmosis, Kaposi sarcoma, cryptosporidiosis, toxoplasmosis, cytomegalovirus). *This problem is addressed by the NDCP, "Risk for Infection* [1] *(Opportunistic)," following.*

COLLABORATIVE (STANDARDIZED) CARE FOR ALL PREGNANT WOMEN WITH HIV/AIDS

Perform comprehensive assessment to identify individual needs for teaching, emotional support, and physical care.

Nursing Diagnosis: RISK FOR INFECTION (OPPORTUNISTIC)[1]

Related Factors: invasive procedures, rupture of amniotic membranes, malnutrition, environmental exposure to pathogens, inadequate acquired immunity, and inadequate primary and secondary defenses (broken skin and decreased ciliary action).

Although Risk for Infection[1] is a nursing diagnosis, it is standardized care in the sense that the plan should be followed for all pregnant women with HIV/AIDS. Also, use generic NDCP, "Risk for Infection,[1]" beginning on p. 21 in Chapter 2.

Nursing Activities and Rationales

Assessments

- Assess for history of opportunistic infections. Determines the likelihood of woman's developing opportunistic infections during pregnancy or after delivery. The presence of opportunistic infections is evidence of a diminished immune response. HIV-infected women who have had one episode of opportunistic infection are at greater risk for developing later infections.
- Assess for signs/symptoms of infection (e.g., fever, chills, dyspnea, weakness/fatigue, mouth lesions, diarrhea, and dysuria). It may be impossible to prevent opportunistic infections; however, early recognition of infection allows for early treatment and better prognosis.
- Assess for temperature greater that 38.3°C (101°F). Bacterial, fungal, and viral infections produce an inflammatory response leading to increased white blood cell count and fever. Caution: People with AIDS may not run a fever in response to infections because of their impaired immune response.
- Assess respiratory status (e.g., dyspnea, tachypnea, cough, fatigue, weakness, crackles, and hypoxia). These may be symptoms of *Pneumocystis carinii, Mycobacterium avium* or *Mycobacteria tuberculosis*.
- Assess mucous membranes. Redness and painful white patches on oral mucous membranes are a sign of Candida albicans, a painful opportunistic fungal infection that occurs in the mouth, esophagus, and stomach of women who are HIV positive. Candida can also affect the vaginal and anal mucous membranes, producing itching, white patches, drainage, and pain.

- Assess for diarrhea. Opportunistic infections such as cryptosporidiosis cause unrelenting, watery diarrhea, which can lead to malnourishment and fluid and electrolyte imbalances.
- Assess skin for lesions, excoriation, breakdown, cyanosis, and rash. Skin lesions can become excoriated, leaving a portal of entry for other pathogens. Such symptoms may reflect opportunistic infections or drug toxicities.
- Assess weight. The HIV-infected woman may experience fatigue and decreased appetite, which will compromise her own and her fetus's well-being. Weight is a good indicator of nutrient intake adequacy. Weight gain should occur with pregnancy and proper fetal growth.
- Assess for postpartum bleeding, lochia changes, and Hgb/Hct. Anemia increases the risk for infections. Endometritis can occur during postpartum. Early recognition ensures early treatment.
- Assess knowledge of immune deficiency, opportunistic infection, and transmission of HIV virus to her newborn and to others. Provides a baseline to individualize teaching plan and eliminate misconceptions. In order to cope with HIV infection on a daily basis, the woman must have an adequate understanding of her disease and any prescribed therapeutic regimen. However, the woman may have been undergoing treatment for HIV infection, been cared for at home, researched information about HIV/AIDS, or received education from her healthcare provider. Although many women will have accurate information about HIV/AIDS, do not assume that they all understand their condition or how to prevent its spread.
- Assess support system by identifying the person or persons who help her the most during time of need. The woman may not have previously identified a primary support person, especially if she is just learning about her diagnosis of HIV infection. Discussing past crises may help her identify a person or persons she can depend on now.
- Assess mental status (e.g., depression, anxiety, and fear). Poor mental status may result from stress and concerns due to disease process and fear of pregnancy outcome possibilities.
- Assess and monitor the following laboratory data:
  - CBC and differential. *Determines the presence of infection. WBC counts greater than 10,000 cells/mm³ (greater than 14,000 during the intrapartum and early postpartum periods) indicate inflammation or infection. WBC count greater than 30,000 cells/mm³ is a panic value that indicates very serious or overwhelming infection.*
  - CD4 and viral load counts. *Establishes the likelihood of disease progression during pregnancy and used as guide for management.*
- Assist with diagnostic studies, including cultures, bronchoscopy, X-rays, and serum electrolytes. Determines the presence of opportunistic infections and monitors the effectiveness of treatments.

- Monitor fluid and electrolyte status. Candida infections of the mouth may prevent the woman from drinking or eating. Copious water can be lost when diarrhea is present. Both conditions may result in fluid and electrolyte imbalance.

Independent Nursing Actions

- Encourage self-care, including adequate sleep, decreasing stress, avoiding infections, and following dietary recommendations. The woman has increased nutritional needs due to pregnancy and HIV. Following good self-care habits will enhance immune system.
- Observe universal precautions and promote good perineal care. Decreases the risk of transmission of HIV-1 to her infant and to healthcare providers.
- Ensure intake of well-balanced diet and provide supplements if necessary. Prevents weight loss and malnutrition, which increases the HIV-infected woman's risk for opportunistic infections.
- Ensure adequate fluid intake. Prevents hypovolemia and cellular dehydration, which are complications of opportunistic infections such as cryptosporidiosis, or they result from reduced appetite or pain from mouth lesions.
- Ensure adequate rest and periods of uninterrupted sleep. Prevents further fatigue, which is associated with opportunistic infections and malnutrition.
- Encourage the woman to balance exercise with rest. Prevents stress produced by fatigue. Stress is thought to further reduce immune function and increase the likelihood of viral replication and opportunistic infections.
- Use calm, reassuring approach. Maintain a nonjudgmental attitude. Women may have increased fears regarding their risk for infection. This approach helps alleviate anxiety and stress, which may lower their resistance to opportunistic infections or serve as co-factors for triggering viral replication and progressive disease. Nursing care can be impacted by the nurse's own judgments, and all patients deserve the same care.
- Answer questions honestly. Honesty allows for the establishment of trust and allows the woman some control of her disease by being well informed.
- Culture wound drainage, mouth lesions, blood, stool, and urine as needed. Identifies offending organisms so that appropriate antimicrobial therapy, if available, can be initiated.
- Maintain sterility of invasive lines and invasive procedures. Prevents the introduction of pathogens that can readily cause infection in women who are immunodeficient.
- Screen visitors for communicable diseases. Protects the woman who is immunocompromised from sources of new infections.

Collaborative Activities

- Teach about the availability of community resources; make appropriate referrals. The woman may be unaware of resources and AIDS support groups in her community.

- Assess need for supportive services. If HIV has progressed, maternal weakness may impact activities of daily living, and supportive services and networking may be necessary.
- If patient is active substance abuser, provide appropriate referrals for treatment. Drug use can depress immune system and interfere with medication action.

Patient/Family Teaching

- Teach about care of the infant following birth. The mother will need to be informed about continuum of care for the baby and treatment for prevention of transmission and problems with her new infant for reassurance as parent.
- Teach about administration of antiretroviral medications and monitoring for side effects. Promotes understanding of disease and required treatment and adherence and evaluation of side effects and change if needed.
- Teach ways to decrease the risk of transmission of HIV to her infant and others. Avoiding breastfeeding decreases risk of transmission because HIV-1 is found in human milk. Good hand washing and universal precautions must always be used.
- Teach signs/symptoms of disease progression and opportunistic infections, as needed. Understanding her potential for infections and signs and symptoms associated with infections increases the likelihood of early reporting and treatment.
- Teach use of safe sex practices. Prevents the transmission of HIV-1 to noninfected individuals and prevents other STIs from developing in the HIV-infected woman. STIs are more severe in the immune-compromised individual.
- Teach the woman to avoid others if possible when they are ill to avoid becoming ill. When CD4 cell counts are low, the woman is at increased risk for developing common infections such as colds, influenza, Staphylococcus infections, etc. These infections are more serious in immune-compromised individuals.
- Teach ways to reduce her exposure to infections. Good hand-washing techniques; avoiding pet wastes; using disinfectants such as 10% bleach solution to clean household surfaces; thoroughly cooking meats, eggs, and vegetables; and maintaining good personal hygiene will decrease the woman's exposure to potential pathogens and prevent exposing others to HIV.
- Teach the importance of keeping prenatal appointments so that her CD4 cell and viral load counts and complete blood cell count can be monitored. Provides the practitioner with information about the woman's immune system and the likelihood of disease progression. The CBC provides information about Hgb and Hct and the presence of infection or anemia.
- Teach the woman to maintain prescribed antiretroviral drug therapies. Helps prevent replication of the retrovirus and subsequent progression of disease, as well as decreasing the risk of perinatal transmission of HIV; however, drug schedules must be strictly adhered to in order to achieve

drug effectiveness and prevent drug resistance. Women may experience unpleasant side effects from these drugs and avoid taking them routinely. Increased understanding of how the drugs work may increase compliance. Resistance to drug therapy occurs over time; however, adherence to drug schedules is essential.

- Teach the woman to avoid alcohol, drugs, and smoking. Prevents maternal and fetal compromise. Substance use/abuse may be associated with HIV/AIDS. These habits are physical stressors that may exacerbate viral replication and disease progression. In addition, alcohol intake may lead to fetal alcohol syndrome; recreational drugs may produce other birth defects; and smoking increases the risk for neonatal death and low birth weight.

- Provide written materials describing diet, exercise, medications, information on effects of HIV/AIDS on pregnancy and fetus, and symptoms of complications/opportunistic infections. HIV/AIDS is a complex disease, and the woman will need reference material for details she may be unable to later recall.

INDIVIDUALIZED (NURSING DIAGNOSIS) CARE PLANS

This section includes care plans to address unique patient needs.

▌ Nursing Diagnosis: DEFICIENT KNOWLEDGE RELATED TO HIV INFECTION AND DISEASE PROCESS AND POTENTIAL RISK TO SELF AND FETUS[1]

Related Factors: lack of information and knowledge base, risk factors, nutritional needs, how it impacts pregnancy, treatments, and lifelong maintenance needs. Refer to the generic NDCP, "Deficient Knowledge,[1]" beginning on p. 13 in Chapter 2.

▌ *Goals, Outcomes, and Evaluation Criteria*

- Woman verbalizes reason and meaning of HIV antibody testing.
- Woman verbalizes understanding of positive results and its implications for self and fetus.
- Woman verbalizes understanding of further lab testing and procedures.
- Woman uses safe sex practices and ways to prevent transmission of HIV to others.
- Woman verbalizes understanding to rights of privacy and the Health Insurance Portability and Accountability Act regulations.

▌ *Nursing Activities and Rationales*

Assessments

- Assess the woman's understanding of her disease status, its treatment, and her need for follow-up care. Allows nurse to plan for individualized teaching and correct misconceptions about HIV infection and its treatment.

Independent Nursing Actions

- Maintain an open and nonjudgmental attitude and display empathy. Women with HIV are concerned about social stigma and judgments from caregivers about their diagnosis, lifestyle, and behaviors. Nurses' prejudices can get in the way of appropriate care and should be evaluated and avoided since all women deserve that the best guidelines are followed.

- Assure confidentiality because it is the woman's right. Document who has access to the woman's health information in her chart. Provide written copy of the Health Insurance Portability and Accountability Act policy. Confidentiality is a patient's right and a nurse's responsibility.

Patient/Family Teaching

- Provide information prior to and post screening for HIV antibody. It is important to discuss the benefits of early diagnosis, opt-out testing, and confidentiality; discuss that antibodies usually appear by 3 months but may not appear until 6 months after infection with HIV; explain that a person may not have symptoms for many months after infection, so testing is the earliest way to determine if disease is present. Early screening enables treatment early in pregnancy to limit transmission and get best care for pregnancy and fetal outcome.

- Provide information about HIV infection and progression to AIDS. Discuss transmission modes (80% of women get it through heterosexual sex) and the need to make safer sex a routine as part of her lifestyle.

- Discuss high-risk behaviors for HIV transmission and risk to mother and fetus. Pregnant women want to avoid risks to their infants and, if given factual information, will avoid behaviors that will risk their growing fetus.

- Counsel about risks to others and ways to avoid transmission; explain universal precautions. Offer to include family members in the teaching process to integrate information into family process so all will get questions answered. The family is a unit, and risk to and from the members needs to be discussed when considering their help in caring for the HIV-infected woman.

- Counsel about risks of opportunistic infections, how to prevent them, and how to recognize signs and symptoms. Avoidance of infections will avoid stressing the immune system and getting infections against which the body has decreased capacity to fight. Signs and symptoms need to be recognized early to ensure early treatment and prevention of further problems. (See "Nursing Diagnosis: Risk for Infection (Opportunistic),[1]" which begins on p. 128 in this care plan).

- Teach at an appropriate level according to the woman's learning needs, language skill level, and cultural background. Effective learning can best be achieved if teaching meets these criteria. Use a medical interpreter as needed to ensure that proper terms are translated and teaching is understood.
- Provide written information and referral to support groups and appropriate websites. Ongoing information and hard copy of information need to be provided for continued reinforcement and learning.
- Explain all procedures and treatments, and note those procedures that can provide risk to the woman during labor and delivery so she can self-advocate. All patients need to understand self-care and management when they have a chronic disease diagnosis.
- Provide and discuss information on medications including side effects and the need for adherence. Understanding the risk for drug resistance and proper administration of medications will foster adherence.
- Explain signs that need to be immediately reported to provider such as drug side effects, problems with pregnancy, depression, need for support services, etc. Early intervention results in better outcomes.
- Discuss standards of care, guidelines, and resources for treatment for HIV during pregnancy. Emphasize the importance of a healthy diet that supports pregnancy and the immune system (see "Nursing Diagnosis: Imbalanced Nutrition: Less Than Body Requirements,[1]" which begins on this page in this care plan). Patients need to be advised of proper care guidelines and how to avoid transmission of HIV to the baby. If the woman understands that compliance with treatment will dramatically decrease the risk to her baby, she will more likely adhere to treatment. Diet can enhance and support the immune system and is a very important part of self-management with disease.
- Offer emotional support while the infant's infection status is assessed during the postpartum period and teach the mother how to give the infant medication. The normal reaction to stress is anxiety and fear. The mother needs reassurance from her care providers during this time of unknowing while waiting for the results of her infant's HIV status. (See "Infant Exposed to HIV/AIDS," beginning on p. 408 in Chapter 12.)

▌ Nursing Diagnosis: ANXIETY[1]

Related Factors: unknown and unpredictable outcomes for the fetus, self, and family secondary to HIV/AIDS and complications. Also refer to generic NDCP, "Anxiety,[1]" beginning on p. 10 in Chapter 2.

▌ *Nursing Activities and Rationales*

Assessments

- Assess the woman's understanding of HIV/AIDS and its treatment. Allows the nurse to plan for individualized teaching and correct misconceptions about HIV infection and its treatment. Knowledge reduces fear and anxiety.
- Assess the woman's emotional status. Determines how the woman is coping with pregnancy superimposed on HIV/AIDS. The stress of pregnancy and concerns about disease progression or transmission of HIV infection to the fetus increase anxiety.
- Assess support systems. Determines if the woman has adequate support systems or needs to be referred to community resources for medical, emotional, or financial support. Knowing what resources may be available reduces stress, fear, and anxiety.

Independent Nursing Actions

- Establish trust. Women are more likely to discuss their concerns if they trust the person in whom they are confiding.
- Be honest. Attitude should be open and nonjudgmental always. Honesty helps establish trust. Many women with HIV infection are upset by social stigma and others' reaction to their diagnosis. They appreciate the honesty and acceptance of their care providers.
- Encourage the woman to talk about her fears of disease process and the transmission of HIV to her child. Verbalizing fears and concerns often reduces anxiety. It also provides information to the nurse so that supportive interventions can be planned. A woman who is HIV positive but has no opportunistic infections can be reassured that she may have a normal pregnancy without fetal transmission of the disease.
- Encourage use of stress-reducing strategies that have been beneficial in the past. Avoids the negative impact of stress on the immune system and prevents the potential progression of the disease. Strategies that have worked in the past are likely to work in the present. When stress is reduced, the woman can make better decisions. When women are stressed, they tend to hyperventilate, which causes the retention of carbon dioxide and is possibly detrimental to the mother and to fetal well-being.
- Encourage the woman to keep scheduled appointments throughout the pregnancy. Good prenatal care and control of HIV infection and/or AIDS decrease the risk for exacerbated disease or fetal compromise.

▌ Nursing Diagnosis: IMBALANCED NUTRITION: LESS THAN BODY REQUIREMENTS[1]

Related Factors: inability to ingest or digest food; nausea for side effects from drugs; or decreased ability to absorb nutrients due to biologic or psychologic factors.

Goals, Outcomes, and Evaluation Criteria

- Woman accurately describes prescribed diet for pregnancy with added nutrition for HIV needs.
- Woman accurately describes well-balanced diet.
- Woman maintains weight and gains for adequate fetal growth with pregnancy.
- Woman maintains body fluid components and chemical indices within normal limits.

NIC Interventions[2]

Nutrition Management (1100)—Assisting with or providing a balanced dietary intake of foods and fluids.

Nutritional Counseling (5246)—Use of an interactive helping process focusing on the need for diet modification.

Nutritional Monitoring (1160)—Collection and analysis of patient data to prevent or minimize malnourishment.

Weight Gain Assistance (1240)—Facilitating gain of body weight.

Teaching: Prescribed Diet (5614)—Preparing a patient to correctly follow a prescribed diet.

Nursing Activities and Rationales

Assessment

- Assess body weight and monitor weight trends. Establishes a baseline for later comparisons. Weight is a clinical indicator of adequate nutrition and hydration. Weight loss during pregnancy can adversely affect both mother and fetus, and excessive weight loss is an indication for supplements or parenteral nutrition.
- Assess biochemical measures. Establishes a baseline for later comparisons. Chemical studies such as serum albumin, Hgb, Hct, lymphocyte count, total iron-binding capacity, and serum transferrin are good indicators of nutritional adequacy or inadequacy.
- Assess eating patterns and food likes and dislikes. Determines adequacy of food and fluid intake, and personal likes and dislikes help with nutritional planning.
- Assess mucous membranes and skin turgor. Determines adequacy of fluid intake. Dry or sticky mucous membranes and loss of skin turgor are indications of fluid deficits.
- Assess for physical or psychosocial barriers to eating. Determines if the woman has physical problems such as pain, nausea, or weakness that interfere with her ability to obtain, prepare, or take in foods or fluids. Determines if psychosocial problems such as fear, anxiety, or lack of financial resources are preventing the woman from eating. When obstacles to eating or drinking are identified, interventions can be planned to eliminate them.
- Measure intake and output. Identifies fluid excesses or deficits so that corrective actions can be initiated. Normally, fluid output should approximate fluid intake.
- Assess for signs and symptoms of nutritional deficit. The HIV-infected pregnant woman is prone to anemia and zinc and vitamin A deficiencies (associated with increased infant mortality). Also, infection prevents nutrients from being absorbed. See "Prenatal Anemia," beginning on p. 114 in this chapter.

Independent Nursing Actions

- Encourage six small meals per day. Small meals are less overwhelming to the woman who may have difficulty eating or who might be experiencing nausea. Meals throughout the day supply greater energy and prevent gastric distention, which causes nausea.
- Encourage adherence to vitamin, iron, and calcium supplementation during pregnancy. Maintain adequate nutrition.
- Referral to a nutritionist as appropriate. The pregnant woman has increased nutritional needs secondary to HIV and may need additional support with planning to meet nutritional needs.

Patient/Family Teaching

- Teach about unique diet requirements to support the immune system. Diet should include adequate protein. Protein deficiency can cause depression of cell-mediated immunity, complement, and phagocytes. Diet should include balanced intake of polyunsaturated fatty acids and vitamin E because a high intake can depress the humoral and cell-mediated immunity. Zinc and vitamin A are needed for overall growth and development of immune cells. Adequate pyridoxine, pantothenic acid, and folic acid are necessary for general cell synthesis.
- Teach the woman to eat small, frequent, highly nutritional meals if she is having nausea and vomiting and side effects from medications or pregnancy. Maintains nutrition.
- Teach the need for maintaining nutrient and fluid intake to prevent weight loss. Knowledge of the need to eat and drink in order to maintain a healthy pregnancy may serve as incentive to take in adequate food and fluids.
- Teach the woman to eat high-calorie, protein-rich, and high-carbohydrate foods. Provides adequate calories for mother and fetus, to aid in healing and prevent wasting or loss of fetal well-being.
- Teach to maintain accurate records of weekly weights between prenatal visits. Provides information about weight trends so that corrective measures can be taken if the woman begins to lose weight excessively or not gain weight as needed as the pregnancy progresses.
- Teach proper food handling for food safety. Undercooked foods and too old and not properly stored foods can cause illness.

Nursing Diagnosis: ACTIVITY INTOLERANCE[1]

Related Factors: HIV and pregnancy, especially in women in whom additional medical complications or advanced disease exists. See generic NDCP, "Activity Intolerance,[1]" which begins on p. 9 in Chapter 2. Also refer to textbooks for nursing care of patients with advancing HIV and AIDS.

▌ *Nursing Activities and Rationales*

Assessments

- Assess severity of the woman's fatigue. Establishes a baseline for later comparison in order to evaluate effectiveness of interventions. Fatigue is one of the earliest indications of HIV infection, which is compounded by pregnancy.
- Assess ability to perform activities of daily living. Determines the degree of assistance the woman will need so that appropriate interventions can be planned.

Independent Nursing Actions

- Assure the woman that it is okay and even desirable to rest when feeling fatigued. Some women may feel guilty about taking time out to rest. Assuring her that rest is needed to conserve her energy, for the well-being of her infant, and to maintain her immunity may increase her likelihood of resting before she becomes overly fatigued.
- Explore ways to decrease the woman's fatigue. Modifying the woman's activities will conserve her energy.
- Encourage the woman to prioritize activities, letting go of nonessential tasks. Conserves energy. By omitting nonessential tasks, she is likely to have enough energy to complete those tasks that are essential to her and her baby's well-being.

Patient/Family Teaching

- Teach the need for balancing activities with rest. Excessive activity or inadequate rest will increase fatigue, which can contribute to disease progression and threaten the well-being of the fetus.
- Teach the woman the necessity for at least 8 hours of uninterrupted sleep when possible. Uninterrupted sleep allows for tissue healing and restoration of energy, which may decrease daytime fatigue.
- Teach strategies for energy conservation. Modifying, delegating, and pacing activities throughout the day are strategies that conserve energy and allow a balance between rest and activity.
- Refer to community networks and encourage family networking to help with increased demands of care. Additional resources will aid at times of stress and decrease the woman's physical demands.

▌ *Other Nursing Diagnoses*

In addition to the aforementioned diagnoses, also assess for the following nursing diagnoses, which are frequently present with this condition.

- Compromised Family Coping[1] related to the implications of a positive HIV test in one of the family members.

- Grieving[1] related to perceived decreased quality of life for self and fetus.

SURGICAL PROCEDURES

In the United States, approximately 50,000 women per year have nonobstetric surgery performed during pregnancy. Even though most deliver a healthy newborn at term, complications can occur, such as preterm labor and birth, low birth weight for gestational age, and risk for spontaneous abortion, which is about 8% during the first trimester and 6.6% in the second trimester. The most common first trimester procedure is a laparoscopy (32%). Throughout the second and third trimesters, the most frequent surgical intervention is an appendectomy. These are followed by surgeries for intestinal obstruction, gynecologic problems, and cholecystitis, in descending order (James, Steer, Weiner, & Gonik, 2006). Optimal timing of a surgical intervention is during the second trimester when risk of spontaneous abortion and teratogenicity have passed (first trimester) and before the gravid uterus is at highest risk for preterm labor (third trimester).

Fetal risks are possible due to effects of maternal disease and/or treatments, possible teratogenicity from anesthetic medications, intraoperative decrease in uteroplacental blood flow, and early delivery (Mattson & Smith, 2010). Nurses treat two patients when the pregnant patient enters the operating room.

▌ *Key Nursing Activities*

- Obtain and review maternal physical and history including review of pregnancy course and gestational age of fetus and laboratory test results.
- Record and monitor baseline vital signs, pain level, and FHR.
- Provide information to patient and family about surgical procedures.
- Provide emotional support, especially when surgery is unplanned, reassuring her that she and her baby will be well cared for.
- Involve the partner in the experience to the extent possible.
- Prepare for surgery (e.g., proper identification and allergy bracelet, insert IV, insert indwelling catheter, perform abdominal skin prep, antacid prior to surgery).
- Use and monitor medical and surgical asepsis.
- Monitor woman and fetus prior to, during, and after procedure.
- Position the woman to prevent venacaval compression after 20 weeks' gestation, place in left lateral position or wedge to tilt uterus and displace its weight.

▌ *Risk Factors and Etiologies*

- Nongynecologic conditions include appendicitis, acute cholecystitis, intestinal obstruction, trauma with visceral injury, ruptured aneurysm, maternal cardiac or neurologic conditions, and tumor removals.

- Gynecologic surgeries include cervical incompetence, removal of an ovarian cyst, uterine myoma, reproductive tumor or mass removal, and torsion of fallopian tubes.
- Intrauterine fetal surgery as an intervention for certain prenatal congenital defects.
- Trauma with or without need for surgery occurs in approximately 8% of pregnant women and increases in frequency as pregnancy progresses. Depending on the severity of the incident, trauma can be a precarious situation for the fetus because fetal well-being depends on maternal well-being. Some pregnant women are also targets of physical violence with the gravid uterus sometimes being the focus or at risk due to the size of pregnant woman's abdomen. Trauma is the leading nonobstetric cause of maternal death resulting from head injury or hemorrhagic shock. Fetal death is due to maternal incident or placental injury and abruption.

Signs and Symptoms

Subjective: Nonobstetric conditions requiring surgical intervention vary according to the medical condition. For example, with cholecystitis, the pain will be stabbing, steady, and midepigastric radiating to the right upper quadrant of the abdomen, right flank area, or right shoulder. With appendicitis, the symptoms in the pregnant woman may or may not be consistent with those observed in the nonpregnant woman. The pregnant woman might have radiation of pain to right flank rather than right lower quadrant pain due to gravid uterus. Pain may or may not be present in gynecologic conditions requiring surgery.

Objective: Signs and symptoms are condition specific but may be masked by pregnancy.

- ▶ *Cholecystitis:* Vomiting, rebound tenderness, rigidity; fourfold increase in serum amylase levels, a twofold increase in serum alkaline phosphatase, and an increase in the WBC count from 15,000 to 20,000 mm³. Leukocytosis is a normal response seen in pregnancy, making some diagnoses more difficult.
- ▶ *Appendicitis:* Elevated WBC count with a differential count of greater than 80% polymorphonuclear leukocytes (shift to the left); pyuria because of the proximity of the appendix to the ureter or renal pelvis.
- ▶ *Ovarian or uterine masses:* Masses documented through ultrasound examinations.
- ▶ *Incompetent cervix:* Progressive cervical dilatation during the second trimester.

Diagnostic Studies

- Ultrasonography. Establishes the size, age, position, and viability of the fetus and placenta position and function; detects amniotic fluid level.
- Fetal monitoring. Determines effect of surgery and anesthesia on the fetus, heart rate, variability, and its relationship to fetal movement and uterine activity; placenta condition.

- Perioperative laboratory evaluation, including CBC, urinalysis, type and cross for potential transfusion. Establishes database for future comparisons and identifies potential contraindications to surgery.
- Electrocardiogram. Establishes the presence of preexisting cardiac or pulmonary disease; documents baseline to serve as reference point if changes occur.

Medical Management

Perioperative and Intraoperative Management

- Anesthetic management. Local or regional anesthetics are useful for cervical cerclage. General anesthesia is used with abdominal procedures.
- Informed consent. This includes risks to both the patient and the fetus. All procedures require informed consent by patient or family member if patient cannot sign. The provider obtains informed consent and the nurse verifies that consent has been obtained.
- Preoperative antacid or antiemetic agent. Enhances gastric emptying, increases motility, and decreases gastric acidity.
- Left displacement of the uterus after 20 weeks' gestation during the operation and during the acute care stay. Left displacement of uterus prevents supine hypotensive syndrome.
- Preoperative, intraoperative, and postoperative FHR monitoring. Detects fetal distress and preterm labor and documents fetal viability and well-being.
- Tocolytic agents such as magnesium sulfate, terbutaline (Brethine), nifedipine (Nifidine), and indomethacin can be used between 24 and 34 weeks' gestation if patients exhibit signs of preterm labor.
- Intravenous (IV) fluids of Ringer's lactate or normal saline, started with a 16- or 18-gauge intravenous catheter. Fluid maintenance is essential during preoperative, intraoperative, and postoperative status. Accessible IV line also ensures route for administration of emergency medications if needed.
- Monitoring of maternal oxygen saturation to confirm that it is being maintained at normal level. Fetal oxygenation is dependent on maternal oxygen intake.
- Foley catheterization, depending on the type of surgical intervention. Indwelling urinary catheter is placed to drain urine during surgery to decrease bladder size, which will also prevent irritation of the uterus.
- Abdominal skin preparation. Prevents introduction of microorganisms via incision.

Postoperative Management

Focus is on normal postoperative care and should be individualized in relation to the surgery that was done. All postoperative patients need:

- Vital signs, FHR, and temperature evaluation at routine intervals as prescribed by hospital policy.

- Analgesics for pain control and assessment of pain at regular intervals. Pain must be assessed and treated promptly to decrease the need for pain medications.
- Restoration and maintenance of fluid balance.
- Early ambulation. Prevents thromboembolism and prevents constipation.
- Advancement of diet as tolerated and encouragement of fluids. Flushes medications out of system, prevents urinary tract infection, and maintains hydration.
- Discontinuation of indwelling catheter if placed for surgery. Decreases risk for bladder infection.
- IV antibiotics if at risk for or development of wound infection.

COLLABORATIVE (STANDARDIZED) CARE FOR ALL PREGNANT WOMEN UNDERGOING SURGICAL PROCEDURES

This section discusses individual needs for teaching, emotional support, and physical care.

Potential Complication of Surgery: INFECTION

See generic care plan, "Potential Complication: Infection," beginning on p. 29 in Chapter 3.

Focus Assessments

All assessments for the woman at risk for infection because of cesarean birth are applicable to the patient undergoing a surgical procedure during pregnancy. See the care plan for "Cesarean Birth," beginning on p. 277 in Chapter 8.

- Assess FHR before the surgical intervention for 20 minutes to establish a baseline. If fetus in over 34 weeks' gestation, normal stress test evaluations apply. Evidence of fetal well-being should be present, which includes FHR between 110 and 160 beats/min, average long-term variability, accelerations with fetal movement, and absence of late or severe variable decelerations, tachycardia (which may indicate infection in the fetus), or decreased variability. Assessment of the fetus should be continued throughout the surgical procedure, during the time while the FHR pattern returns to the preoperative pattern, and until the maternal anesthetic and analgesic have worn off.
- Check prenatal record for risk factors. Identifies factors that increase the risk for infection, such as anemia (Hgb less than 11 mg/dl and Hct less than 33%), diabetes, obesity, malnutrition, and respiratory problems (e.g., asthma, smoking).
- Check dressing and drains. Determines the presence of bleeding, excessive blood accumulation, or purulent drainage. Excessive bleeding can lead to shock or impede healing, which increases the risk for infection. Purulent drainage is a sign of infection.
- Monitor lung sounds. Decreased sounds, crackles, or rhonchi may indicate infection in the lungs.

Preventive Nursing Activities

See the topic, "Cesarean Birth," which begins on p. 277 in Chapter 8. Refer also to the generic NDCP "Risk for Infection,[1]" beginning on p. 21 in Chapter 2, and the generic collaborative care plan "Potential Complication: Infection," beginning on p. 29 in Chapter 3.

- Keep prescribed antibiotics on schedule. Maintains consistent blood levels of antibiotics to ensure eradication of pathogens.
- Evaluate for effectiveness of antibiotics and any adverse effect on the fetus. Absence of signs and symptoms of infection indicate that the antibiotic is effective. Changes in FHT or activity may indicate adverse effect of antibiotics on fetus and must be reported.
- Assess for uterine activity. A change in uterine activity can indicate postoperative UTI or early labor due to dehydration, pain, incision, etc.

Potential Complication of Surgery: HEMORRHAGE

See the generic collaborative care plan "Potential Complication: Hemorrhage" beginning on p. 28 in Chapter 3. Also see the collaborative care plan, "Potential Complication: Hemorrhage," in the topic "Cesarean Birth," which begins on p. 278 in Chapter 8.

Focus Assessments

- Monitor fetal well-being postoperatively. If close to term, assess for reactivity. If not, reactivity requirements do not apply. For mature fetus, monitor FHR externally for 20 minutes prior to the surgical intervention to establish a baseline and compare with postoperative findings. Rate should be between 110 and 160 beats/min; average long-term variability; accelerations with fetal movement; and absence of late or severe variable decelerations, tachycardia, or bradycardia (which may indicate hypovolemia in the fetus), or decreased variability. Assessments continue until the FHR pattern returns to the preoperative pattern and the maternal anesthetic and analgesic have worn off.
- Monitor for bleeding. Incisions, drains, and vaginal drainage must be monitored for bright red or excessive bleeding.

Preventive Nursing Activities

- Review operating room documents. Determines blood loss during the surgical procedure to assist with planning for needed interventions.

Potential Complication of Surgery and Anesthesia: FETAL DEMISE

Refer to the generic collaborative care plan "Potential Complication: Fetal Compromise (Nonreassuring Fetal Heart Rate)," beginning on p. 27 in Chapter 3.

Focus Assessments

- Assess fetal movement. Absence of fetal movement per mother's report may indicate fetal demise related to trauma, lack of oxygen, or anesthesia during surgery.
- Assess maternal vital signs, especially blood pressure. Determines the woman's response to general anesthetics or sympathetic blocking agents used for spinal or epidural anesthesia. Hypotension causes decreased uteroplacental perfusion, which may lead to intrauterine fetal asphyxia and death.
- Monitor maternal pulse oximetry. Determines maternal oxygen saturation. Decreased maternal oxygenation affects the amount of oxygen circulating to the fetus. Fetal hypoperfusion may lead to intrauterine fetal death.

Potential Complication of Surgery and Anesthesia: PRETERM LABOR

Refer to the generic collaborative care plan "Potential Complication: Preterm Labor," beginning on p. 31 in Chapter 3.

Focus Assessments

- Palpate uterus for contractions and observe monitor tracing for activity of uterus. Determines if surgical procedure caused uterine irritability and contractions.
- Maintain continuous FHR and UC monitoring. Determines effects of surgery on the fetus and uterus.

Preventive Nursing Activities

- Position the woman in a side-lying position, preferably left lateral. Prevents supine hypotension syndrome.
- Prepare to administer ordered tocolytic agent. Stops preterm labor. Administer IV piggyback bolus of magnesium sulfate ($MgSO_4$) 4–6 g over 20–30 minutes, or terbutaline (Brethine) 0.25–0.50 mg subcutaneous. $MgSO_4$ is a smooth-muscle relaxant that causes blockage of neuromuscular transmission of nerve impulses to the uterine muscle. Terbutaline is a beta-adrenergic agonist that causes uterine muscle relaxation.
- Administer indomethacin (prostaglandin synthetase inhibitor) as ordered to halt preterm labor. The initial dose is 50–100 mg by mouth or by rectal suppository followed by 25–50 every 4–6 hours.

- Administer nifedipine (Nifidine) as ordered to halt preterm labor. Nifedipine is a calcium channel blocker that blocks the flow of calcium ions and decreases smooth muscle activation. Initial loading dose is 20 mg by mouth followed by an additional 20 mg by mouth after 30 minutes. If contractions continue, 20 mg may be given orally every 3 to 8 hours until the maximum dose of 160 mg/day for 48 to 72 hours (Ross & Eden, 2010). Follow provider's order for administration protocol.

INDIVIDUALIZED (NURSING DIAGNOSIS) CARE PLANS

The individualized care plans are designed to address unique patient needs.

Nursing Diagnosis: ANXIETY/ FEAR[1]

Related Factors: previous fetal loss experiences; the woman's lack of understanding of the implications and expected outcomes of her condition; and inability of the woman to cope with her fear in an adaptive manner.

Depending on the type of surgery, urgency of surgery, and age of fetus, anxiety and fear can be varied. Any pregnant woman will have concerns for herself and her fetus, which will elevate anxiety with the approaching surgery. If she is in pain and ill, this can also affect her anxiety level.

Goals, Outcomes, and Evaluation Criteria

- Woman verbalizes concerns and/or fears.
- Woman maintains a sense of purpose despite fear and assists with coping mechanism.
- Woman and family participate in plan of care whenever possible.
- Woman uses relaxation techniques to reduce fear.
- Woman maintains role performance before, during, and after surgical procedure.
- Woman receives support from family members following surgery in return to normal state of health.

NIC Interventions[2]

Anxiety Reduction (5820)—Minimizing apprehension, dread, foreboding, or uneasiness related to an unidentified source of unanticipated danger.
Coping Enhancement (5230)—Assisting a patient to adapt to perceived stressors, changes, or threats that interfere with life demands and roles.
Decision-Making Support (5250)—Providing information and support for a patient who is making a decision regarding health care.

Emotional Support (5270)—Provision of reassurance, acceptance, and encouragement during times of stress.

Presence (5340)—Being with another, both physically and psychologically, during times of need.

Security Enhancement (5380)—Intensifying a patient's sense of physical and psychologic safety.

Support System Enhancement (5440)—Facilitation of support to patient by family, friends, and community.

Nursing Activities and Rationales

Assessments

- Assess for self-reported symptoms of fear. Reports of apprehension, increased tension, decreased self-assurance, dread, terror, panic, and feelings of being scared are symptoms that indicate the presence of fear.
- Assess for behavioral signs of fear and anxiety. The sympathetic response to fear and anxiety produces restlessness, glancing about, difficulty maintaining eye-to-eye contact, feelings of inadequacy, worry, and apprehension.
- Assess for cognitive characteristics of fear and anxiety. Confusion, forgetfulness, impaired attention, difficulty concentrating, and diminished ability to problem solve and make decisions are indicators of fear and anxiety.

Independent Nursing Actions

- Guide the woman through verbalization of what she thinks is going to happen to her and the fetus related to the surgical procedure. Provides guidance to the client in understanding the situation and realistic outcomes.
- Encourage woman to verbalize a realistic description of the surgery and expected outcomes. Fear is decreased when the woman is able to verbalize the procedure to be performed and the expected outcomes accurately.
- Attend to primary physical needs and give feedback as to the status of the baby. Conserves the woman's energy so that she is able to concentrate on her emotional status and facilitates trust. Fatigue increases stress and contributes to fear and anxiety.
- Maintain pain control through regular assessment and treatment. Fear is increased in the presence of pain.
- Identify coping strategies such as progressive muscle relaxation, guided imagery, rhythmic breathing, and distraction. These methods have been shown to be successful in reducing and managing anxiety, especially when they have been effective stress reducers in the past. Also, decreasing anxiety by the relaxation response also decreases the sensation of fear.

Collaborative Activities

- Refer to support groups or community agencies as needed and appropriate. Provides follow-up resources for the woman after discharge from the hospital. The woman may not be aware of community resources or support groups that are available to her.

Patient/Family Teaching

- Provide factual information concerning diagnosis, surgical intervention, and prognosis in both written and verbal forms. Sharing information with the patient assists in reducing fears because the woman will have a better idea of what to expect and reduces fear of the unknown. Because listening abilities are impaired in the woman experiencing fear, information is provided in written form so that the woman will have a reference when her fear is controlled.
- Inform the woman of alternative views or solutions, as applicable. Providing the patient with choices allows the patient to have control when making decisions. Women experiencing fear frequently feel powerless.
- Explain to the patient that fear and anxiety are normal. Provides reassurance that she is not behaving in an inappropriate or abnormal manner.
- Explain the signs and symptoms of anxiety. Helps the woman understand why she is experiencing physical symptoms and reduces her fear of the unknown.

Nursing Diagnosis: IMPAIRED HOME MAINTENANCE[1]

Related Factors: interruption of usual functioning in the home; overtaxed family members who are assuming additional duties due to hospitalization of the pregnant patient; lack of necessary resources and assistance to maintain an orderly home environment.

Goals, Outcomes, and Evaluation Criteria

- Woman verbalizes knowledge about available resources for postoperative follow-up care.
- Woman verbalizes how to access support systems.
- Family members perform expected roles.
- Family members obtain adequate resources to meet needs.
- Family members are involved in problem solving and conflict resolution.
- Woman demonstrates positive self-esteem.
- Woman performs activities of daily living according to postoperative plan of care.

NIC Interventions[2]

Discharge Planning (7370)—Preparation for moving a patient from one level of care to another within or outside the current healthcare agency.

Family Support (7140)—Promotion of family, values, interests, and goals.

Home Maintenance Assistance (7180)—Helping the patient/family to maintain the home as a clean, safe, and pleasant place to live.

Nursing Activities and Rationales

Assessments

- Assess readiness for discharge and discharge learning needs. Provides information about the woman's ability to return to her home environment and function in a safe manner. Provides base for development of discharge plans and promotes individualized teaching.
- Assess the woman's home maintenance requirements. Determines if follow-up care arrangements need to be provided so that equipment or supplies will be present in the home at discharge and the home environment is such that it will not impede the woman's/family's ability to maintain usual roles and tasks.
- Assess the woman's psychologic response to her situation. Determines if there are psychologic barriers (as well as physical barriers) that may prevent the woman from managing self-care at home following surgery.
- Assess adequacy of support systems in and outside of family. The woman may need assistance from her family, friends, or community support systems. Knowledge of who and what are available to the woman and her family will make the transition to home less stressful. Educate patient's family as to reasonable expectations of her recovery and that she needs time to heal prior to returning to regular activities.

Collaborative Activities

- Arrange for postdischarge evaluation, as appropriate. Follow-up assessment of the patient and the fetus confirms attainment of discharge goals and outcomes or helps identify problems that need to be addressed.
- Arrange for caregiver support, as needed. Facilitates the provision of adequate care delivery to the patient postdischarge.
- Coordinate referrals as needed. Facilitates continuity and consistency in delivery of care after discharge.

Patient/Family Teaching

- Teach the woman and family members ways to simply practice home management, housework, shopping, and so forth, and repeat this information frequently. It should not be assumed that the woman knows how to provide her own home care. Information needs to be provided in a clear and understandable manner; women who are recovering from surgery and receiving pain medication may require several teaching sessions to remember all the information needed about home care.
- Answer all questions of family members and reinforce learning. Asking questions is an indication that the woman/family is ready to learn. Positive outcomes are more likely when the woman has an accurate understanding of her condition and possible limitations on activity after leaving the hospital.
- Inform the woman and her family regarding community resources for postoperative care, as needed. Ensures that the woman can access community resources. Knowing that resources are available and can be accessed if needed may lower the woman's stress and better prepare her for home care.

Other Nursing Diagnoses

Assess for the following nursing diagnoses, which are also frequently present:
- Deficient Knowledge[1] related to first-time experiences of surgical procedure during pregnancy.
- Acute Pain[1] related to surgical procedure with incision secondary to patient verbalizations of pain.

END NOTES

1. Nursing Diagnoses—Definitions and Classification 2009–2011. Copyright © 2009, 2007, 2005, 2003, 2001, 1998, 1996, 1994 by NANDA International. Used by arrangement with Blackwell Publishing Limited, a company of John Wiley & Sons, Inc. In order to make safe and effective judgments using NANDA-I nursing diagnoses it is essential that nurses refer to the definitions and defining characteristics of the diagnoses listed in this work.
2. Bulechek, G. M., Butcher, H. K., Dochterman, J. M. (2008). *Nursing Interventions Classification* (5th ed). St. Louis, MO: Elsevier, by permission.

REFERENCES

American College of Obstetricians and Gynecologists. (2004). *Prenatal and perinatal human immunodeficiency virus testing: Expanded recommendations. Committee Opinion No. 304.* Washington, DC: Author.

American College of Obstetricians and Gynecologists. (2005). Pregestational diabetes mellitus, ACOG Practice Bulletin, No. 60. *Obstetrics & Gynecology, 105,* 675–682.

American College of Obstetricians and Gynecologists. (2008a). ACOG Practice Bulletin Number 95: Anemia in pregnancy. *Obstetrics and Gynecology, 112,* 201–207. doi:10.1097/AOG.0b013e3181809c0d

American College of Obstetricians and Gynecologists. (2008b). Committee Opinion No. 421: Antibiotic prophylaxis for infective endocarditis. *Obstetrics & Gynecology, 112,* 1193–1194.

American College of Obstetricians and Gynecologists Committee of Ethics. (2004). ACOG Committee Opinion, No. 294. At-risk drinking and illicit drug use: Ethical issues in obstetric and gynecologic practice. *Obstetrics and Gynecology, 103,* 1021–1031.

American Diabetes Association. (2004). Position statement: Preconception care of women with diabetes. *Diabetes Care, 27*(Supplement 1), S76–S78.

American Diabetes Association. (2008). Consensus statement. Managing preexisting diabetes for pregnancy: Summary of evidence and consensus recommendations for care. *Diabetes Care, 31,* 1060–1079.

American Diabetes Association. (2010). Standards of medical care in diabetes: *Diabetes Care, 33*(Supplement 1). Retrieved from http://care.diabetesjournals.org/content/33/Supplement_1/S11.full.pdf+html Doi:10.2337:dc 10-S011

American Psychiatric Association. (2000). *Diagnostic and statistical manual of mental disorders* (4th ed., rev.). Washington, DC: Author.

American Society of Reproductive Medicine (ASRM). (2006). Frequently asked questions about infertility. Retrieved from http://www.asrm.org

Arafeh, J. M. R., & Baird, S. M. (2006). Cardiac disease in pregnancy. *Critical Care Nursing Quarterly, 29*, 32–52.

Centers for Disease Control and Prevention. (2010). HIV surveillance in women. Department of Health and Human Services. Retrieved from http://www.cdc.gov/hiv/topics/surveillance/resources/slides/women/

Elfenbein, D. S., & Felice, M. E. (2003). Adolescent pregnancy. *Pediatric Clinics of North America, 50*, 781–800.

Gilbert, E. S. (2007). *Manual of high risk pregnancy & delivery* (4th ed.). St. Louis, MO: Mosby.

Gilmartin, A. H., Ural, S., & Repke, J. T. (2008). Gestational diabetes mellitus. *Reviews in Obstetrics & Gynecology, 1*, 129–134.

Hershberger, P. E., & Kavanaugh, K. (2008). Enhancing pregnant, donor oocyte recipient women's health in the infertility clinic and beyond: A phenomenological investigation of caring behaviour. *Journal of Clinical Nursing, 17*, 2820–2828.

James, D. K., Steer, P. J., Weiner, C. P., & Gonik, B. (2006). *High risk pregnancy: Management options.* Philadelphia, PA: Saunders.

Mattson, S., & Smith, J. E. (2010). *Core curriculum for maternal-newborn nursing* (4th ed.). Philadelphia, PA: W.B. Saunders.

McCarthy, M. P. (2008). Women's lived experience of infertility after unsuccessful medical intervention. *Journal of Midwifery and Women's Health, 53*, 319–324.

National Campaign to Prevent Teen and Unplanned Pregnancy. (2009). *National campaign analysis: Preliminary 2007 teen birth data.* Retrieved from http://www.thenationalcampaign.org/resources/birthdata/analysis.aspx

National Institute on Drug Abuse (NIDA). (2006, May 30). *Facts about women and drug abuse.* National Institutes of Health/U.S. Department of Health and Human Services. Retrieved from http://www.drugabuse.gov/WomenDrugs/Women-DrugAbuse.html

Norris, J., Howell, E., Wydeven, M., & Kunes-Connell, M. (2009). Working with teens and babies at risk: The power of partnering. *Maternal Child Nursing, 34*, 308–315.

Norton, M. E. (2008). Genetic screening and counseling. *Current Opinion in Obstetrics and Gynecology, 20*, 157–163.

Perry, S. E., Hockenberry, M. J., Lowdermilk, D. L., & Wilson, D. (2009). *Maternal child nursing care* (4th ed.). St. Louis, MO: Mosby.

Rappaport, V. (2008). Prenatal diagnosis and genetic screening: Integration into prenatal care. *Obstetric and Gynecological Clinics of North America, 35*, 435–458.

Ross, M. G. & Eden, R. D. (2010). Preterm labor. eMedicine from WebMD. Retrieved from http://emedicine.medscape.com/article/260998-overview

Shieh, C., & Kravitz, M. (2006). Severity of drug use, initiation of prenatal care, and maternal-fetal attachment in pregnant marijuana and cocaine/heroin users. *Journal of Obstetrical Gynecological Neonatal Nursing, 35*, 499–508.

Summers, A. M., Langlois, S., Wyatt, P., & Wilson, R. D. (2007, February 29). Prenatal screening for fetal aneuploidy. *Journal Obstetrics and Gynaecology Canada, 29*(2), 146–179.

United States Department of Agriculture. (2010, May). Food Guide Pyramid. Retrieved from http://www.mypyramid.gov/index.html

Zindler, L. (2005). Ethical decision making in first trimester pregnancy screening. *Journal of Perinatal Neonatal Nursing, 19*, 122–131.

RESOURCES

American College of Obstetricians and Gynecologists. (2001). ACOG Practice Bulletin No. 30. Clinical management: Guidelines for obstetrician-gynecologists gestational diabetes. *Obstetrics & Gynecology, 19*, 525–538.

American College of Obstetricians and Gynecologists. (2009). Postpartum screening for abnormal glucose tolerance in women who had gestational diabetes mellitus. ACOG Committee Opinion, No. 435. *Obstetrics & Gynecology, 6*, 1419–1421.

American Diabetes Association. (2010a). *Medical management of pregnancy complicated by diabetes* (2nd ed.). Alexandria, VA: The Association.

Black, M. M., Bentley, M. E., Papas, M. A., Oberlander, S., Teti, L. O., McNary, S., & O'Connell, M. (2006). Trial of a home-based mentoring program delaying second births among adolescent mothers: A randomized, controlled trial. *Pediatrics, 118*, 1087–1099.

Boonstra, H. (2009). Advocates call for a new approach after the era of "abstinence-only" sex education. *Guttmacher Policy Review, 12*(1), 6–11.

Bulechek, G. M., Butcher, H. K., Dochterman, J. M. (2008). *Nursing interventions classification* (5th ed.). St. Louis, MO: Elsevier.

Chang, S. N., & Mu, P. F. (2007). Infertile couples' experience of family stress while women are hospitalized for ovarian hyperstimulation syndrome during infertility treatment. *Journal of Clinical Nursing, 17*, 531–538.

Christensen, C. (2008). Management of chemical dependence in pregnancy. *Clinical Obstetrics and Gynecology, 51*, 445–455.

Cooper, J., & Grossman, J. (2008). Teaching about cardiac emergencies: Implications for maternal/child nurse educators. *Journal for Nurses in Staff Development, 24*, 162–167.

Cunningham, F. G., Leveno, K., Bloom, S., Hauth, J., Rouse, D., & Spong, K. (2009). *Williams obstetrics* (22nd ed.). New York, NY: McGraw-Hill.

Dobbenga-Rhodes, Y. A., & Prive, A. M. (2006). Assessment and evaluation of the woman with cardiac disease during pregnancy. *Journal of Perinatal Neonatal Nursing, 20*, 295–302.

Fessler, K. B. (2003). Social outcomes of early childbearing: Important considerations for the provision of clinical care. *Journal of Midwifery Womens Health, 48*, 178–185.

Giles, M. (2009). HIV and pregnancy: Screening and management update. *Current Opinion in Obstetrics and Gynecology, 21*, 131–135.

Harris, G. D., & White, R. D. (2005). Diabetes management and exercise in pregnant patients with diabetes. *Clinical Diabetes, 23*, 165–168.

Helderson, M. M., Gundeson, E. P., & Ferrara, A. (2010). Gestation weight gain and risk of gestational diabetes mellitus. *Obstetrics & Gynecology, 115*, 597–604.

Johnson, M., Maas, M., & Moorhead, S. (2007). *Nursing outcomes classification (NOC)* (5th ed.). St. Louis, MO: Mosby.

Jorde, L. B., Carey, J. C., & Bamshad, M. J. (2009). *Medical genetics* (4th ed.). St. Louis, MO: Mosby.

Kamel, R. M. (2010). Management of the infertile couple: An evidence-based protocol. *Reproductive Biology and Endocrinology, 8*, 21–33. doi:10.1186/1477-7827-8-21

Kilpatick, K., & Purden, M. (2007). Using reflective nursing practice to improve care of women with congenital heart disease considering pregnancy. *Maternal Child Nursing, 32,* 140–147.

Kirby, D., Lepore, G., & Ryan, J. (2007, November). Sexual risk and protective factors national campaign to prevent teen pregnancy. Retrieved from http://www.thenationalcampaign.org/ea2007/protective_factors_FULL.pdf

Kriebs, J. M. (2006). Changing the paradigm: HIV in pregnancy. *Journal of Perinatal Neonatal Nursing, 20,* 71–73.

Kuczkowski, K. M. (2007). The effects of drug abuse on pregnancy. *Current Opinions in Obstetrics and Gynecology, 19,* 578–585.

Lachat, M. F., Scott, C. A., & Relf, M. V. (2006). HIV and pregnancy: Considerations for nursing practice. *Maternal Child Nursing, 4,* 233–240.

Lashley, F. (2005). *Clinical genetics in nursing practice* (3rd ed.). New York, NY: Springer.

Lowdermilk, D. L., & Perry, S. E. (2007). *Maternity and women's health care* (9th ed.). St. Louis, MO: Mosby.

Mason, M. C. (2009). Hard to conceive. *Nursing Standard, 23,* 22–24.

McCaffey, M. P., Keith, T. L., & Lazear, J. L. (2009). Diabetic crisis in pregnancy: A case report. *Journal of Perinatal Neonatal Nursing, 23,* 131–140.

Mitchell, A., Mittelstaedt, M. E., & Wagner, C. (2005). A survey of nurses who practice in infertility settings. *Journal of Obstetrical Gynecological and Neonatal Nursing, 34,* 561–568.

Montgomery, K. S. (2003a). Nursing care for pregnant adolescents. *Journal of Obstetrical Gynecological and Neonatal Nursing, 32,* 249–257.

Montgomery, K. S. (2003b). Nutrition and HIV-positive pregnancy. *Journal of Perinatal Education, 12,* 42–47.

National Institute on Drug Abuse (NIDA). (2009, May). *Prenatal exposure to drugs of abuse.* National Institutes of Health/U.S. Department of Health and Human Services. Retrieved from http://www.drugabuse.gov/tib/prenatal.html

Perkins, J., Dunn, J. P., & Jagasia, S. M. (2007). Perspectives in gestational diabetes mellitus: A review of screening, diagnosis, and treatment. *Clinical Diabetes, 25,* 57–61.

Pillitteri, A. (2010). *Maternal & child health nursing care of the childbearing family* (6th ed.). Philadelphia, PA: Lippincott.

Porteous, J. (2008). Oh, by the way, the patient is pregnant! *Canadian Operating Room Nursing Journal, 35,* 35–42.

Public Health Service Task Force. (2006). *Recommendations for use of antiretroviral drugs in pregnant HIV-1-infected women for maternal health and interventions to reduce perinatal HIV-1-transmission in the United States.* Washington, DC: Author.

Rayburn, W. F. (2007). Maternal and fetal effects from substance use. *Clinics in Perinatology, 34,* 559–571.

Schneiderman, E. (2010). Gestational diabetes: An overview of a growing concern for women. *Journal of Infusion Nursing, 33,* 48–54.

Serlin, D. C., & Lash, R. W. (2009). Diagnosis and management of gestational diabetes mellitus. *American Family Physician, 80,* 57–62.

Shaver, S. M., & Shaver, D. C. (2005). Perioperative assessment of the obstetric patient undergoing abdominal surgery. *Journal of PeriAnesthesia Nursing, 20,* 160–166.

Sifakis, S., & Pharmakides, G. (2000). Anemia in pregnancy. *Annals of New York Academic Science, 900,* 125–136.

Strandberg-Larsen, K., Gronboek, M., Andersen, A. N., Andersen, P. K., & Olsen, J. (2009). Alcohol drinking pattern during pregnancy and risk of infant mortality. *Epidemiology, 20,* 884–891.

Tyer-Viola, L. A. (2007). Obstetric nurses' attitudes and nursing care intentions regarding care of HIV-positive pregnant women. *Journal of Obstetrical, Gynecological, and Neonatal Nursing, 36,* 398–409.

Williams, J. K. (1998). Genetic testing: Implications for professional nursing. *Journal of Professional Nursing, 14,* 184–188.

Windslow, B. T., Voorhees, K. I., & Pehl, K. A. (2007). Methamphetamine abuse. *American Family Physician, 76,* 1175–1176.

World Health Organization. (2007). *WHO case definitions of HIV for surveillance and revised clinical staging and immunological classification of HIV-related disease in adults and children.* Retrieved from http://www.who.int/hiv/pub/guidelines/HIVstaging150307.pdf

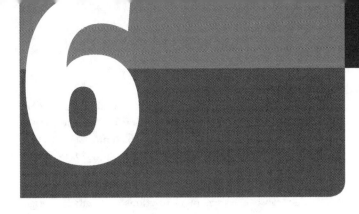

GESTATIONAL COMPLICATIONS

Harriet (Hatsie) Pearson Mallicoat

HYPEREMESIS GRAVIDARUM

Nausea and vomiting affect approximately 50–70% of all pregnant women. They normally start around 4–6 weeks' gestation, peak at 12 weeks, and resolve by week 20. Only a small percentage of these women develop hyperemesis gravidarum (HG). HG is a complication of pregnancy that is characterized by persistent, uncontrollable nausea and vomiting that begins in the first trimester and extends beyond the 20th week of pregnancy. It results in 5% or greater loss of prepregnant weight and dehydration. HG must be excluded from other complicating diagnoses and requires medical intervention.

Severe HG may lead to acid-base imbalances, electrolyte imbalances, ketonuria, hypokalemia, and weight loss compromising pregnancy outcome. If it continues without treatment, it can negatively affect maternal and fetal well-being by causing conditions such as intrauterine growth retardation (IUGR), low birth weight, or death. Adverse outcomes are related to the amount of (or lack of) weight gain during pregnancy.

Women whose pregnancies are impacted by high-risk complications such as HG are at risk during their transition to the mothering role. Nurses need to be aware of the need to support the transition to mothering the infant and foster that life transition during pregnancy and postpartum. With the lack of energy and the fatigue that accompany HG, the taking in of information for the role transition may be lacking, and opportunity and effectiveness of childbirth education may be limited. Education about parenting may need to be delayed until after birth with intensive assistance and teaching at that time to aid the woman in adopting the mothering role. This should be a consideration during the postpartum period (Meighan & Wood, 2005).

■ Key Nursing Activities

- Assessment of signs and symptoms, documentation, and evaluation to differentiate from other possible conditions.

- Differentiate nausea and vomiting from HG.
- Monitor for complications of HG and review laboratory data for evidence of indications of complications.
- Provide information to woman about condition, treatments, collaborative interventions, and risks to mother and fetus.
- Teach self-care measures and self-management.

■ Etiologies and Risk Factors

The exact cause of HG is unknown; however, several theories exist concerning the etiology. They include:

- *Endocrine theory.* The cause may be high levels of human chorionic gonadotropin (hCG), estrogen, and progesterone during the pregnancy. These increased hormones may impact gastric musculature, resulting in regurgitation of duodenal content back into the stomach, causing nausea and vomiting. Abnormal increased levels of thyroid hormones and hCG can also cause excessive nausea and vomiting.
- *Psychosomatic theory.* This theory suggests that psychologic or psychogenic stress may increase the symptoms. Conversion reaction, somatization disorders, and eating disorders have been considered in research.
- *Metabolic theory.* Vitamin B complex and protein deficiency, high fat intake, lower liver function, immunologic factors, presence of *Helicobacter pylori*, and elevated amylase levels have been implicated.

Pregnancy-Related Risk Factors

Pregnancy-related risk factors include pregnancy at a young age; first pregnancy; obesity with high fat intake; nausea and vomiting with previous pregnancies; history of intolerance of oral contraceptives; multiple gestation; preeclampsia; gestational trophoblastic disease; genetic abnormalities; female sex of the fetus; and hydrops fetalis.

Preexisting Disease Risk Factors

Advanced diabetes, anorexia nervosa and bulimia, gastrointestinal diseases such as peptic ulcers and *H. pylori*, and history of motion sickness, allergies, liver and kidney disease, thyroid conditions, or migraines have all been discussed in the literature as possible preexisting disease risk factors. Habits such as smoking, food aversions, high-fat or nutritionally poor diets (low B complex and protein) have also been identified as risks. The condition can occur in families and is more common in nonwhites than whites and more common in non-Hispanics than Hispanics.

■ Signs and Symptoms

Subjective. Complaints of nausea, dizziness, severe weakness, and fatigue.

Objective. Vomiting, inability to hold down fluids, weight loss of 5% or greater over prepregnancy weight, pallor, dry tongue, dehydration (decreased blood pressure, increased heart rate, increased temperature, and decreased urine output).

Diagnostic Studies

- Complete blood count. Increased red blood cells and hematocrit indicates hemoconcentration, which is associated with inadequate fluid intake or excess fluid loss.
- Urinalysis. Urine specific gravity > 1.025. Indicates urinary concentration, which is associated with inadequate fluid intake or excessive fluid loss (e.g., by vomiting).
- Urine ketones. Ketones are produced when fat is broken down to provide energy in the absence of adequate intake.
- Serum chemistries. Azotemia (increased blood urea nitrogen [BUN] and serum creatinine) occurs with salt and water depletion. Serum creatinine increases in response to changes in kidney function due to dehydrations. Hyponatremia (low sodium) and hypokalemia (low potassium) also occur from dehydration. Hyponatremia less than 120 mmol/L can cause confusion, seizures, and respiratory arrest. Hypokalemia can cause cardiac symptoms.
- Obstetric ultrasound. Evaluates pregnancy; rules out hydatidiform mole and multiple gestation, and evaluates fetal growth for normal or retardation and amniotic fluid volume/amniotic fluid index (AFI). Serial ultrasounds compare growth pattern in presence of maternal weight loss.
- Liver enzymes. Increased aspartate aminotransferase (AST) and alanine aminotransferase (ALT) indicate that dehydration is occurring; reversible with intravenous hydration.
- Thyroid and parathyroid levels. May need to be monitored because a biochemical hyperthyroidism can coexist with HG.

Medical Management

Rehydration and Vitamin Supplementation

- Intravenous (IV) therapy. Corrects hypovolemia and electrolyte imbalances.
- Antiemetic drugs (e.g., phenothiazines, metoclopramide, droperidol, ondansetron). Relieve or control nausea and vomiting.
- Parenteral or enteral nutrition. Prevents weight loss and negative nitrogen balance.
- Thiamine supplements orally or intravenous. Replacement to avoid Wernicke's encephalopathy, which, if unchecked, can lead to Korsakoff's psychosis and death. B_{12} and B_6 deficits can cause peripheral neuropathy and anemia.
- Implement protocol to prevent deep venous thrombosis.
- Assessment of weight gain and comparison to prepregnant weight.
- Monitoring of labs for evaluation of condition.
- Fetal surveillance in conjunction with high-risk pregnancy condition.

Medications

- Metoclopramide hydrochloride (Reglan) by mouth/intramuscularly (IM)/intravenously (IV). Antiemetic decreases nausea and vomiting response; helps food move through the GI tract; counteracts progesterone's effect. Observe for extrapyramidal reactions in high doses and tardive dyskinesia with long-term dosing. Common side effects are drowsiness, agitation, seizures (decreases seizure threshold), hallucinations, lactation, constipation, and diarrhea.
- Promethazine (Phenergan) by mouth/IM/IV/rectal. Antiemetic. Side effects are sedation, blurred vision, fatigue, ringing in the ears, nervousness, insomnia, and tremors. Can cause extrapyramidal reactions and anticholinergic effects (blurred vision and dry mouth).
- Proclorperazine (Compazine) by mouth/IM/IV/rectal. Antiemetic. Can cause central nervous system (CNS) effects such as blurred vision, fatigue, ringing in the ears, nervousness, insomnia, and tremors. Can also cause heart palpitations, seizures, dry mouth, constipation, and urinary retention.
- Ondansetron (Zofran) by mouth/IM/IV. Local reaction at site of injection can occur. Common side effects are headache, fever, constipation and diarrhea, extrapyramidal reactions, and cardiac side effects of rapid heart rate, dizziness, feeling faint, and chest pain.
- Doxylamine (Unisom) by mouth. Antihistamine, combined with B_6. May cause increased sedation.

Collaborative Problems

Serious maternal complications of HG, which are beyond the scope of this care plan book but which should be considered, are: Wernicke's encephalopathy (caused by thiamine deficiency), central pontine myelinolysis (neurologic complication of rapid return to normal sodium levels), catheter-related thromboembolism, and lactic acidosis.

Other potential complications of hyperemesis gravidarum include:

- Fluid and electrolyte imbalance with potential for metabolic alkalosis.
- IUGR and low-birth-weight infant.

COLLABORATIVE (STANDARDIZED) CARE FOR ALL WOMEN WITH HYPEREMESIS GRAVIDARUM

Perform a comprehensive assessment to identify individual needs for teaching, emotional support, and physical care.

Potential Complication for Hyperemesis Gravidarum: FLUID AND ELECTROLYTE IMBALANCE: METABOLIC ALKALOSIS

Focus Assessments

- Measure weight daily. Assesses for further weight loss, stabilization, or further nutritional deficiency.

- Assess vital signs. Heart rate increases in response to fluid deficits and to accommodate for metabolic needs. Blood pressure (BP) is decreased in response to inadequate fluid volume and cellular dehydration. Temperature increases in response to cellular dehydration.
- Assess skin turgor, mucous membranes, and urine specific gravity. Establishes the presence of hypovolemia and cellular dehydration.
- Measure intake and output (I and O). Determines adequacy and effectiveness of interventions. Fluid output should approximate fluid intake when fluid balance is restored.
- Monitor serum electrolytes. Electrolyte status not only indicates the presence of nutritional deficiency, but also provides information about the effectiveness of interventions to restore fluid and nutritional balance.
- Assess fundal height measurement and fetal heart tones and assist with periodic fetal ultrasounds. Determines fetal growth and well-being.
- Assess reflexes, level of consciousness and cognition, monitor change in status, and notify provider if present. Determines changes in CNS status from dehydration. Severe hypovolemia and cellular dehydration can progress to shock, which is manifested by mental confusion, coma, and death if not corrected. Signs and symptoms of Wernicke's encephalitis are double or blurred vision, nystagmus, disorientation, delusions, uncoordinated movements, and gait ataxia. Signs and symptoms of central pontine myelinolysis are confusion, horizontal gaze paralysis, spastic quadriplegia, and delirium that can cause brain damage and death.
- Monitor for complications of vascular access. Routine evaluation of IV site can prevent problems that can occur from occlusion, air embolus, and infection.

Preventive Nursing Activities

- Maintain IV fluid and electrolyte replacements. Ensures adequate fluid and electrolyte replacement without producing fluid volume overload or increased electrolyte imbalance.
- Administer antiemetics as ordered. Controls nausea and vomiting. Monitor for side effects and notify provider as needed.
- Advance diet slowly. Increases tolerance to food and fluid and restores hydration and fluid balance.
- Teach measures to minimize nausea and vomiting. See the following nursing diagnosis care plans for "Imbalanced Nutrition: Less Than Body Requirements[1]" and "Nausea and/or Vomiting."
- Maintain enteral or parenteral feedings as prescribed. Supports maternal and fetal nutrition while the woman is unable to intake food or fluids.
- Teach patient and family about all interventions and be supportive during recovery and treatment. Facilitates the woman's understanding of what is occurring and the reasons behind the interventions.

INDIVIDUALIZED (NURSING DIAGNOSIS) CARE PLANS

The care plans in this section were designed to address unique patient needs.

Nursing Diagnosis: IMBALANCED NUTRITION: LESS THAN BODY REQUIREMENTS[1]

Related Factors: inadequate dietary intake, nausea, and vomiting.

Goals, Outcomes, and Evaluation Criteria

- Woman reports that daily weight has stabilized or increased.
- Woman reports ability to tolerate food and fluids and ability to maintain daily intake adequate to meet needs for self and fetus.
- Woman reports adequate energy level and ability to care for self.
- Woman reports absence of nausea and vomiting.
- Laboratory values within normal limits, including hematocrit (Hct) and hemoglobin (Hgb), blood glucose, serum potassium (K+), and serum sodium (Na+).

NIC Interventions[2]

Nutrition Management (1100)—Assisting with or providing a balanced dietary intake of foods and fluids.

Nutrition Therapy (1120)—Administration of food and fluids to support metabolic processes of a patient who is malnourished or at high risk for becoming malnourished.

Nutritional Monitoring (1160)—Collection and analysis of patient data to prevent or minimize malnourishment.

Total Parenteral Nutrition Administration (1200)—Preparation and delivery of nutrients intravenously and monitoring of patient responsiveness.

Nursing Activities and Rationales

Assessments

- Monitor food and fluid intake, intake and output documentation. Determines extent of nutritional/fluid deficiency and determines the effectiveness of therapy. Comparing needed nutrients with the woman's intake will provide an indication of nutritional deficiencies. When intravenous line is in place, intake and output must always be recorded to help establish fluid balance.
- Monitor weight daily by using the same scale, at the same time of day, and with the same type of clothing. Weight loss is an indicator of nutritional/fluid deficiency. Weight gain is used to determine the effectiveness of therapy. Weighing under similar circumstances (scale, clothing, time) ensures accuracy of measurements.

- Monitor for signs of nutritional deficiency. Dry, thinning hair; dry, flaky skin; swelling and bleeding of gums; and reduced energy level reflect nutrient deficiencies.
- Monitor lab values and notify provider if abnormal findings noted. Vigilance is essential to facilitate corrective actions in a timely manner to maximize maternal well-being and fetal growth.
- Monitor for indications of drug side effects (antiemetics). Some women experience adverse reactions to antiemetics. Noting side effects early allows for implementation of corrective actions.
- Assess fetal status by Doppler and document fetal heart rate. Documents fetal well-being when woman is hospitalized.

Independent Nursing Actions

For nursing actions to control nausea, refer to the nursing diagnosis care plan "Nausea and/or Vomiting," which begins on p. 147 in this care plan.

- Assist with developing a dietary plan that provides necessary nutrients and takes into consideration the woman's cultural/religious needs and personal food preferences. Positively affects the woman's motivation to eat, which may aid in preventing nutritional deficits for the woman and fetus.
- Encourage family to bring in home-cooked foods if the woman desires. Helps increase nutritional intake and helps allow the woman some control of her diet.
- Encourage small meals (six meals a day). Increases tolerance for food. Choosing high-caloric, high nutrient value in a small amount of food will provide better nutrition and will be better tolerated.
- Maintain pleasant environment in hospital, help regulate visitor traffic, and allow for privacy. Facilitates eating, provides time with family, and provides pleasing area in which to eat that is free of clutter, old dishes, trash, and odors. Offer oral hygiene and personal care support, which also facilitate eating.

Collaborative Activities

- Determine the need for enteral feedings or total parenteral nutrition supplementation. If emesis continues, alternate methods are needed to provide for the nutritional needs of the fetus. Fetal well-being depends on maternal nutrition. Alternative feeding may be administered at home with home health nurse visits or in hospital.
- Collaborate with dietitian to determine calorie and nutrient amounts needed and to determine woman's food preferences. Nutritional needs are increased during pregnancy to provide for growth and development of the fetus. A dietitian may be able to recommend high-calorie foods that will be tolerated by the woman. Food likes and dislikes, culture, and availability of certain foods must all be taken into consideration when planning diet.

Patient/Family Teaching

- Teach about foods that are high in nutrition and essential to diet. Reinforce what nutritionist has discussed. Vomiting causes loss of potassium. The body does not conserve potassium well, so dietary intake is necessary. Protein and calcium foods are necessary not only for maternal health but also for growth and development of the fetus.
- Teach the woman to avoid the intake of greasy or highly seasoned foods. Prevents gastric irritation, nausea, and delayed stomach emptying, which can increase nausea.
- Teach about calorie-dense foods with high nutritive value. Because the woman has limited intake, all foods that are eaten need to be value added.
- Teach the woman to avoid fluids during meals, but drink at least 100 ml between meals. Fluids during a meal fill up the small amount of stomach space and decrease food intake. However, hydration is important, so encouraging drinking between meals is important to maintain hydration.
- Teach the woman to sit up for 2 hours after eating. Allows gravity to keep food down and avoids gastric reflux.
- Teach family ways to assist the woman so that she receives adequate rest. The woman may need additional help if she is going home so that she can get the rest that she requires. The family may need help in determining how they can help the woman gain the rest that she needs.
- Perform discharge teaching. Teaching should include information about the effects of HG on the mother and fetus; signs and symptoms to report to the care provider; information about the treatment plan; the need for adequate rest, small frequent meals, and oral hydration; measures to avoid nausea and vomiting; medication dosages and schedules and potential side effects; danger signs that need to be reported; and referrals to community resources.

▮ Nursing Diagnosis: ANXIETY/ FEAR[1]

Related Factors: an actual threat to the woman and her fetus, fear of pregnancy outcome, and concerns about her ability to fulfill usual roles. Refer to the generic care plans for "Anxiety[1]" and "Fear,[1]" which begin on pp. 10 and 15, respectively, in Chapter 2.

▮ *Goals, Outcomes, and Evaluation Criteria*

- Woman lists two coping strategies that can be used to decrease fear and anxiety.
- Woman reports decreased physical symptoms of stress.
- Woman reports increase in comfort and ability to self-regulate.

▮ *NIC Interventions[2]*

Anxiety Reduction (5820)—Minimizing apprehension, dread, foreboding, or uneasiness related to an identified source of anticipated danger.

Emotional Support (5270)—Provision of reassurance, acceptance, and encouragement during times of stress.

Presence (5340)—Being with another, both physically and psychologically, during times of need.

Simple Relaxation Therapy (6040)—Use of techniques to encourage and elicit relaxation for the purpose of decreasing undesirable signs and symptoms such as pain, muscle tension, or anxiety.

▌ *Nursing Activities and Rationales*

Assessments

- Assess the woman's perception of the situation. The woman's perception of the situation may or may not be accurate. Regardless of its accuracy, it will affect how she deals with the stressor. Correcting misconceptions helps decrease the level of fear/anxiety.
- Assess support systems available to the woman. A caring support system can help decrease the level of fear/anxiety.

Independent Nursing Actions

- Administer back massage as appropriate. Massage induces relaxation, decreases feelings of isolation, and demonstrates a caring attitude.

Collaborative Activities

- Administer medication as needed. Decreases severe anxiety when nondrug remedies are ineffective. Anxiety and the resulting stress response may increase nausea and vomiting.
- Refer to spiritual leader or counseling as needed. Provides assistance and caring. The woman may have specific cultural or religious needs that can be best addressed by her spiritual leader. If a spiritual leader is not available or she doesn't have one, a referral for counseling may be appropriate.

Patient/Family Teaching

- Teach relaxation techniques if needed. Relaxation aids the woman in developing an internal locus of control, thus reducing anxiety. If the woman is severely stressed, it may be difficult for her to learn new relaxation techniques.
- Teach to monitor for fetal movement. The woman may be anxious about the possibility of fetal loss. Fetal movement may be reassuring to her.

▌ Nursing Diagnosis: NAUSEA AND/OR VOMITING[1]

Related Factors: hormonal changes with pregnancy.

▌ *Goals, Outcomes, and Evaluation Criteria*

- Woman reports satisfaction with control of nausea and vomiting.

- Woman reports a decrease in the frequency and intensity of nausea and vomiting.
- Woman reports ways to cope with and control symptoms, as well as self-care strategies.
- Woman is able to maintain adequate weight gain and fetal growth with decreased incidence of symptoms.

▌ *NIC Interventions[2]*

Acupressure (1320)—Application of firm, sustained pressure to special points on the body to decrease pain, produce relaxation, and prevent or reduce nausea.

Medication Administration (2300)—Preparing, giving, and evaluating the effectiveness of prescription and nonprescription drugs.

Medication Management (2380)—Facilitation of safe and effective use of prescription and over-the-counter drugs.

Nausea Management (1450)—Prevention and alleviation of nausea.

Vomiting Management (1570)—Prevention and alleviation of vomiting.

▌ *Nursing Activities and Rationales*

Assessments

- Assess history and perform complete physical examination. Evaluates condition and adjustment to pregnancy. If nausea and vomiting exist, other conditions must be assessed for and recognized so that treatment to correct problems can be initiated. If nausea and vomiting begin after 9 weeks of pregnancy, they may be from other causes rather than normal physiology of pregnant state.
- Assess nausea for frequency, duration, and precipitating factors. Determines severity of nausea and establishes baseline. Severe nausea will compromise food intake and prevent the fetus from receiving the nutritional support it needs for growth and development. Sensitivity to certain smells and taste, exposure to noxious or toxic substances in environment, motion, or other environmental cues specific to the woman can all be triggers.
- Assess severity of nausea. Establishes method for evaluation of effectiveness of treatment. Nausea is subjective, thus, self-report is essential, but rating can give objective measurement for baseline and rating improvement or decline. A modified Rhodes scoring system using these three questions can be helpful: (1) In the last 12 hours, for how long have you felt nauseated or sick to your stomach? (1 = not at all to 5 = more than 6 hours); (2) In the last 12 hours, how many times have you vomited or thrown up? (1 = none to 5 = 7 or more times); (3) In the last 12 hours, how many times have you had retching or had dry heaves without bringing anything up? (1 = none to 5 = 7 or more times). A total number of 6 or less is considered mild nausea and vomiting; 7 to 12 is moderate; 13 or more is severe (Koren, Boskovic, Hard, Maltepe, Navioz, & Einarson, 2002).

- Assess impact of nausea on quality of life. Establishes severity of problem and its impact on woman's life. Also promotes open communication between nurse and woman and assists her with initiating problem solving.
- Assess for modifiable factors that may contribute to nausea. Determines if controllable factors, such as odors or foods, are precipitating the woman's nausea, so they can be removed or modified.
- Assess for measures that have been successful for controlling nausea in the past. Measures that have been successful for controlling nausea in the past may be successful in the current situation and should be attempted.
- Assess for need of antiemetic medication. Medication can be used to control nausea in some women when nonpharmacologic methods have not been effective in controlling or eliminating nausea.
- Assess for therapeutic effect of the antiemetic medication. By comparing the woman's rating of her nausea before being medicated and at peak reaction time of medication, the effectiveness of the medication can be accurately evaluated.
- Assess for therapeutic effect of nonpharmacologic techniques used by the woman. Techniques such as relaxation, comfort measures, and acupressure may be effective in decreasing nausea.
- Assess for use of home remedies or over-the-counter medications the woman may have used. Home remedies, herbs, or over-the-counter medications may interact with other medications prescribed. Such measures should be used during pregnancy only with the knowledge of the healthcare provider.
- Assess diet history and fluid intake; a 24-hour recall is helpful. Inadequate fluid intake is probably due to nausea and provides an indicator of the severity of the nausea.

Independent Nursing Actions

- Encourage the intake of small, frequent meals. Prevents overdistention of the stomach, which can precipitate nausea and vomiting. Frequent meals maintain blood glucose levels, which also helps prevent nausea.
- Teach the woman to avoid greasy or highly seasoned foods. Dry, bland foods should be eaten when advancing the diet. Prevents nausea from gastric irritation. Fatty foods are more difficult to digest and remain in the stomach longer than carbohydrate foods. BRAT diet—bananas, rice, applesauce, and toast—is helpful.
- Encourage the intake of herbal teas such as ginger, raspberry, or chamomile. Provides a soothing effect that decreases nausea. Research supports the use of ginger as a natural antiemetic. Ginger ale can also be used, but the content should be verified because concentrations of ginger vary.
- Suggest the use of lemon and peppermint. Some women find that lemon in water, peppermint gum, or teas are helpful in reducing nausea.
- Offer preferred food and fluids every 2 hours while the woman is awake. Decreasing the amount of food in the

stomach prevents gastric distention, which helps decrease nausea.
- Encourage the woman to eat a protein snack before going to bed. A protein snack will prevent dips in blood sugar throughout the night, which may contribute to morning nausea.
- Suggest the intake of cold food. Cold foods may be helpful because they have less odor and may be easier to swallow.
- Alter the environment to create a relaxing atmosphere (e.g., remove uneaten food, prevent odors, decrease noise). Decreasing external stimuli may help decrease nausea during mealtimes.
- Promote adequate rest. Adequate rest promotes relaxation that can decrease nausea.
- Maintain clear liquid diet or nothing by mouth status until nausea is decreased. Advance diet slowly. Clear liquids are easily absorbed and leave little residue; therefore, they contribute less to the feeling of nausea. Liquids such as Coca-Cola Classic and ginger ale can aid in reducing nausea in some women. Nothing by mouth status may be necessary, but only if fluid status is being supported by infusion of IV fluids.
- Provide physical comfort, including oral hygiene and personal care, preferred room temperature, cool cloths to forehead, and clean, dry clothes. Promotes comfort and relaxation, which may decrease the feeling of nausea.

Collaborative Activities

- Obtain order for antiemetic medication if needed. Medications may help decrease nausea in some women when nonpharmacologic measures have not been effective.
- Refer to healthcare provider for pharmacologic methods of nausea control. Vitamin B_6 supplements and doxylamine (Unisom) may be suggested by healthcare provider.
- Refer for complementary therapy as appropriate. Acupuncture, like acupressure, can be a complementary therapy of assistance.
- Refer for nutritional counseling if needed. The woman and her family may need additional support with meal planning.

Patient/Family Teaching

- Teach regarding use and safety of prescribed and over-the-counter medications during pregnancy. Ensures that the woman understands that mediations may have an effect on the fetus. Herbal medications can interact with prescribed medications, which may adversely affect both the woman and fetus.
- Teach relaxation techniques. Relaxation through music, breathing exercises, positive imagery, and stillness may decrease the feeling of nausea.
- Suggest appropriate lifestyle changes. Lifestyle changes such as avoiding triggers; avoiding noise and commotion, places that are too warm, smells, and smoke; brushing teeth after meals instead of when awakening; slow movements, lying

down when nauseated, and decreasing activity; decreasing stress; and being aware of effects such as too much activity increasing nausea can all be helpful. Taking vitamins at night, avoiding them for a while, or substituting two children's chewable vitamins can also be helpful in reducing nausea.

- Teach acupressure techniques if appropriate. Acupressure has been demonstrated to reduce nausea in some women. Sea bands are bracelets that press on an acupressure site on one's wrist to decrease nausea.
- Teach the woman to avoid eating and drinking at the same time. The woman should drink liquids only at one small meal; then in 2–3 hours, when the next small meal is attempted, eat only solid foods.

Nursing Diagnosis: IMPAIRED HOME MAINTENANCE[1]

Related Factors: situations such as inadequate support systems, insufficient finances, lack of knowledge, nausea, or hospitalization.

Goals, Outcomes, and Evaluation Criteria

- Woman reports availability of family member(s) or other support.
- Woman reports strategies for role changes among family members.
- Woman reports family's ability to perform activities needed for home to function, such as shopping, household needs, meals, housework, and laundry.
- Woman verbalizes understanding of home care and any prescribed treatments or restrictions.

NIC Interventions[2]

Discharge Planning (7370)—Preparation for moving a patient from one level of care to another within or outside the current healthcare agency.

Family Support (7140)—Promotion of family values, interests, and goals.

Home Maintenance Assistance (7180)—Helping the patient/family to maintain the home as a clean, safe, and pleasant place to live.

Nursing Activities and Rationales

Assessments

- Assess ability to carry out home responsibilities. Determines the degree and type of assistance that may be needed by the woman when she returns home.
- Assess understanding of discharge plans and home care. Determines information needed for the woman to return to her home environment safely and provide for her own needs and those of any dependent children.

- Assess the degree of family and community support available. Determines the woman's available resources. Referrals may be needed if the woman does not have adequate family resources or support systems.

Independent Nursing Actions

- Listen to concerns, feelings, and questions about care at home. Opens communication and provides outlet for emotions and concerns.
- Involve woman and family in deciding home assistance requirements. Empowers the woman and family and allows them a sense of control over their current situation.

Collaborative Activities

- Offer information about sources for financial assistance if arrangements for home healthcare are needed. Women from some cultures will not discuss financial resources with nonfamily members. When offered information concerning resources available, the family receives the information and is provided the opportunity to seek more information if needed.
- Collaborate with agencies and family to plan for continuing care for the woman at home. Providing names of support agencies to the family may help decrease the stress associated with returning to the home setting by decreasing the workload on the family.
- Coordinate referrals among home healthcare providers. Coordinating care decreases stress and confusion as the woman returns to the home setting.

ECTOPIC PREGNANCY

An ectopic pregnancy develops when the fertilized ovum implants outside the uterine cavity. It is an obstetric emergency. Ectopic pregnancies are classified according to the implantation site, with approximately 95% occurring in the fallopian tubes, 5% occurring in the abdominal cavity, 0.3% on the cervix, and 0.5% on the ovary itself. They occur in about 2% of all pregnancies in the United States.

Ectopic pregnancy is responsible for 10% of maternal mortality and is a leading cause of infertility. About 25–70% of women can conceive after treatment for ectopic pregnancy, but of those, 28% will experience another ectopic pregnancy. Rates are increasing due to the increased incidence of sexually transmitted infections (STIs), improved treatment of pelvic inflammatory disease, increased number of tubal sterilizations, and surgical reversal of tubal sterilizations. Approximately 5–25% of abdominal pregnancies can produce a live infant, but deformity rates are as high as 40%.

Women at high risk for ectopic pregnancy should be identified and treated early, before hemorrhage or shock occurs. Prevention is the key to managing ectopic pregnancy. Early detection demands a high level of suspicion for this condition. New diagnostic techniques have allowed better detection, reducing mortality rate by 90%.

■ Key Nursing Activities

- Provide information about condition, symptoms, and the need for immediate care should symptoms arise. Involve partner and family since they may be the ones helping the woman seek care, because this can be an emergent situation.
- Assess family's anxiety over maternal well-being because pregnancy-related deaths can be caused by ectopic pregnancy.
- When diagnosed, teach about condition and treatment alternatives.
- Monitor for hemorrhage and shock.
- Administer analgesics when needed for pain control.
- Provide emotional support for loss of pregnancy and grieving.
- Assess family's level of coping strategies and resources.
- Assess patient's and family guilt over the situation.
- Provide postoperative care and support; include significant other in process.

■ Etiologies and Risk Factors

Conditions that lead to blockage or decreased motility of the fallopian tubes contribute to ectopic pregnancy.

High risks: History of tubal surgeries; sterilization; previous ectopic pregnancy; exposure to diethylstilbestrol in utero; use of intrauterine device; and known tubal pathology.

Moderate risks: Primary infertility and assisted reproduction techniques; previous genital infections; and multiple sex partners.

Low risks: Previous pelvic surgery; smoking; early age of intercourse; and douching. Ectopic implantation has also been associated with altered estrogen and high levels of progesterone, which alters egg motility, and ovulation stimulating drug use.

■ Signs and Symptoms

Clinical manifestations differ with the gestational age of the embryo in an ectopic pregnancy and the site of the implantation, e.g., the fallopian tube, which can rupture. The three classic symptoms are delayed menses, abdominal pain, and abnormal vaginal bleeding (spotting) that occur at 6–8 weeks after the last normal menstrual period.

Early Signs and Symptoms

Subjective. Abdominal pain first noted to be dull, one-sided, in lower quadrant followed by sharp, colicky pain progressing to diffuse, constant severe lower abdominal pain and generalized tenderness.

Objective. There may be absence of common signs of early pregnancy, despite positive pregnancy test. About 20% of women will have a palpable pelvic mass and urinary frequency. Early pelvic exam will show cervical motion tenderness, uterine displacement from an enlarging adnexal mass, and abdominal tenderness on palpation.

Tubal Rupture or Impending Rupture

Subjective. Abdominal pain (unilateral, bilateral, or diffuse; may be sudden and acute), referred shoulder or neck pain, or rectal pain, dizziness or fainting, occasional nausea.

Objective. Afebrile initially, vomiting may follow nausea; maternal blood pressure will stay normal until rupture, then signs of shock.

Progressive Worsening of Condition

Objective. Low-grade temperature (37.2–37.8°C, 99.0–100.0°F), signs of shock (tachycardia and decreased BP after rupture), syncope, dark red or brown vaginal bleeding, adnexal mass or fullness, soft uterus and cervix, increasing cervical motion tenderness on vaginal exam may be present. Cullen's sign (ecchymosis around umbilicus) may develop in undiagnosed ruptured intraabdominal ectopic pregnancy due to hematoperitoneum.

■ Diagnostic Studies

- Pregnancy test. Detects pregnancy.
- Quantitative β-hCG (repeat in 48 hours if low). Indicates low or falling levels and fetal loss regardless of location; should be doubling in 48 hours if fetus is viable for first 8 weeks after conception; may follow a negative pregnancy test if pregnancy is still suspected.
- Transvaginal ultrasound (if pregnancy is greater than 6 weeks). Reveals ectopic mass or a uterine sac.
- Progesterone level. A level of 25 ng/ml is normal. Any value less than 11 ng/ml may be associated with failed pregnancy, but it does not differentiate between a failed intrauterine pregnancy and an ectopic pregnancy.
- White blood cell (WBC) count. May be elevated from inflammation.
- Red blood cell (RBC) count, Hgb, Hct. Decreased with rupture due to bleeding and anemia.
- Type and cross with Rh-antibody status. Blood may be required in the event of hemorrhage or surgery. Woman may be a candidate for Rho(D) immune globulin treatment (RhoGAM).
- Liver and renal function tests. Determines liver and kidney function if the woman is undergoing methotrexate treatment to end early ectopic pregnancy or to prevent growth of fetal cells.
- Laparoscopic salpingostomy. Performed to remove embryo in ectopic pregnancy; is possible prior to rupture of fallopian tube.
- Laparotomy with salpingectomy or salping-oophorectomy. Performed in advanced ectopic pregnancy. Visualizes extrauterine pregnancy and ruptured fallopian tube and to remove and repair.

■ Medical Management

Medical management may be surgical removal of the embryo in an ectopic pregnancy, repair or removal of the tube, and control of bleeding. Nonsurgical care of ectopic pregnancy involves methotrexate alone or as an adjunct to surgery. Nonsurgical care is provided if the woman is hemodynamically stable and has a small ectopic sac with nonviable fetus and low serum hCG levels. The woman must have normal liver and kidney function, no evidence of peptic ulcer disease, ulcerative colitis, leukopenia, thrombocytopenia, or AIDS.

- Methotrexate dosing. Single-dose or multiple-dose intramuscular injections of methotrexate for nonsurgical management: Destroys trophoblastic tissue when the ectopic mass is unruptured and measures 3–5 cm by ultrasound.
- Intramuscular leucovorin. Reduces side effects of methotrexate in multiple-dose method.
- Weekly monitoring of β-hCG until undetectable (when methotrexate is used). Ensures that there is no remaining viable trophoblastic tissue.
- Monitoring of blood count, platelet count, renal function, and liver enzymes (when methotrexate is used). In high doses, methotrexate can cause bone marrow suppression and hepatotoxicity.
- Follow up weekly while on methotrexate. For measurement of β-hCG and vaginal ultrasound.

▌*Collaborative Problems*

Potential Complications of Ectopic Pregnancy

- Hemorrhage
- Paralytic ileus
- Anemia
- Infection
- Rh sensitization (needs Rho(D) immune globulin treatment if Rh negative after procedures)

COLLABORATIVE (STANDARDIZED) CARE FOR ALL WOMEN WITH ECTOPIC PREGNANCY

Perform a comprehensive assessment to identify individual needs for teaching, emotional support, and physical care. See the generic collaborative care plan "Potential Complication: Hemorrhage," which begins on p. 28 in Chapter 3.

▌Potential Complication of Ectopic Pregnancy: HEMORRHAGE

Focus Assessments

- Assess vital signs (VSs), including pulse, respirations, and BP. Helps to identify hidden bleeding into peritoneum.

VSs may remain within normal limits (WNL) initially. With decreased intravascular volume, the BP drops, the pulse pressure narrows, and the heart rate and respirations increase to compensate for the low BP. Because most of the bleeding is internal, evaluation of VSs is critical. For women receiving methotrexate therapy in lieu of surgical intervention, VSs are essential in determining whether abdominal pain is from successful methotrexate therapy or from a rupturing ectopic pregnancy. If the woman experiences orthostatic tachycardia, hypotension, or falling Hct, a ruptured tube should be suspected, and surgery will be needed.

- Assess for visible bleeding (amount and character). After the death of the embryo in the tube, the decidual tissue breaks down, causing vaginal spotting.
- Assess for low abdominal pressure, abdominal pain, or shoulder pain. After death of the embryo, the placenta slowly separates and blood collects in the cul-de-sac. Pressure on the phrenic nerve causes referred shoulder pain. Pressure and pain usually precede tubal rupture and massive bleeding.
- Monitor for severe indigestion (heartburn). Tubal rupture sometimes manifests as bad indigestion or heartburn caused by nerve irritation where there are large amounts of blood in the abdomen.
- Assess for sudden, severe pain. Severe pain usually occurs with rupture of the tube. Hypovolemic shock can occur rapidly when blood is lost into the peritoneal cavity. Transient, colicky abdominal pain is also common in women receiving methotrexate therapy in lieu of surgery. It usually occurs 3–7 days after initiation of the therapy and lasts 4–12 hours. In these women, VSs and laboratory tests are vital in determining the cause of pain.
- Obtain a urine specimen and assess urine specific gravity. A high specific gravity is an indicator of fluid volume deficit. As blood is lost, the kidneys conserve water and sodium in an attempt to stabilize blood pressure; thus urine is concentrated and decreased in volume.

Preventive Nursing Activities

- Strive for early recognition of bleeding. This allows for intervention to begin before tubal rupture and massive bleeding occur.
- Teach the woman on methotrexate to avoid gas-producing foods (e.g., cabbage, onions). Prevents confounding diagnosis. Gas pain from these foods may be mistaken for the tubal rupture.
- Insert indwelling urinary catheter. Allows for easier monitoring of urine output in the presence of heavy bleeding. Urine output is a good indicator of fluid volume deficit and reversal of hypovolemia.

Potential Complication of Ectopic Pregnancy: ANEMIA

See the generic collaborative care plan "Potential Complication: Anemia," beginning on p. 25 in Chapter 3.

Focus Assessments

- Assess for low Hgb and RBC counts. The number of circulating erythrocytes decreases as a result of bleeding; consequently the amount of Hgb is inadequate, and the oxygen-carrying capacity of the blood is reduced.
- Administer iron supplements as prescribed. Iron is an essential component in the synthesis of Hgb.
- Administer transfusion of prescribed blood product if indicated. Replaces blood volume and cells to replenish those that are lost from the body.

Potential Complication of Ectopic Pregnancy: INFECTION

See the generic collaborative care plan, "Potential Complication: Infection," which begins on p. 29 in Chapter 3.

Focus Assessments

- Assess for elevated temperature. As a result of the infecting organism or the woman's own inflammatory and immune responses, body temperature is regulated at a higher level than normal. Fever is a protective mechanism to rid the body of pathogenic organisms.
- Assess for abdominal pain. Blood in the peritoneal cavity produces inflammation of the peritoneum, which causes swelling. It is observed as distention, and it causes pain.
- Assess for WBCs more than 10,000 and neutrophil shift to left. Leukocytes are produced in response to pathogens. The percentage of specific white cells produces shifts (changes) depending on the type of infecting organism.

Preventive Nursing Activities

- Teach the woman signs and symptoms of infection. For early detection and treatment. With significant blood loss, innate host resistance mechanisms are impaired (e.g., phagocytes and antibodies are lost), predisposing the woman to infection. Observe for fever and chills and abdominal tenderness.
- Administer antibiotics as prescribed. This is prophylactic to prevent infection.
- Maintain medical and surgical asepsis. Prevents cross-contamination and introduction of pathogens.

Potential Complication of Ectopic Pregnancy: RH SENSITIZATION

Rh immune globulin is administered to suppress the immune response in nonsensitized women with Rh-negative blood who receive Rh-positive blood cells because of fetomaternal hemorrhage, transfusion, or accident. Injection is indicated routinely at 20–30 weeks' gestation, following birth, miscarriage, termination, abdominal trauma, ectopic pregnancy, amniocentesis, version, or chorionic villus sampling.

Focus Assessments

- Assess Rh factor. All Rh-negative women receive Rho(D) immunoglobulin to prevent sensitization, if the conceptus is of unknown or positive Rh. This is a preventive measure because the effects of isoimmunization can put the next pregnancy at risk. Rh immune globulin promotes lyses of fetal Rh-positive blood cells before the mother forms her own antibodies against them. Rho(D) immune globulin treatment is always given as a precaution, even when the rupture occurs early in pregnancy.
- Teach the woman about Rh sensitization and the necessity to make caregivers aware of Rh-negative status when one is pregnant or receiving blood products. Stress the importance of keeping a record of receiving the Rho(D) immune globulin treatment. Patient needs to be aware of the need to avoid Rh isosensitization.

Preventive Nursing Activities

- Administer Rho(D) immune globulin treatment soon after rupture or event. Must be within 72 hours after rupture/surgery. Prevents isoimmunization and damage to future fetuses.
- Administer microdose for first trimester miscarriage or abortion, ectopic pregnancy, chorionic villus sampling. Full dose is not indicated.
- Verify that the woman is Rh negative and has not been sensitized. If already sensitized, Rho(D) immune globulin treatment will not be effective.
- Discuss the medication prior to injecting. The medication is made from human plasma and is a consideration if the woman is a Jehovah's Witness or of other value system that objects to human products.

Potential Complications of Ectopic Pregnancy: INFERTILITY OR RECURRENT ECTOPIC PREGNANCY

Focus Assessments

- Assess woman's/family's level of knowledge. Determines woman's understanding of future pregnancies so that appropriate teaching can be implemented. If one tube has been damaged or removed, there is a greater risk of recurrence. In addition, tuboplasty does not guarantee future fertility.

Preventive Nursing Activities

- Teach/review signs of ectopic implantation. Facilitates early detection in subsequent pregnancies. The woman is at increased risk since she has already had one ectopic pregnancy.
- Teach methods of contraception, as needed. Contraception should be used for at least three menstrual cycles to allow time for recovery. An intrauterine device may contribute to ectopic pregnancy.
- Teach the woman to treat genital infections, STIs, and pelvic inflammatory disease promptly. These infections can predispose to ectopic pregnancy by causing scarring of fallopian tubes.

INDIVIDUALIZED (NURSING DIAGNOSIS) CARE PLANS

This section includes care plans to address unique patient needs.

Nursing Diagnosis: ACUTE PAIN[1]

Related Factors: pressure of blood collecting in the cul-de-sac, referred shoulder pain, rupture of a fallopian tube, and collection of blood in the peritoneal cavity. Refer to the generic NDCP, "Pain,[1]" on p. 185 in Chapter 2. Also see NDCP for Acute Pain[1] in the topic "Late Antepartum Bleeding" on p. 186 in this chapter.

Goals, Outcomes, and Evaluation Criteria

- Woman expresses satisfaction with pain control (e.g., less than 3 on a scale of 1 to 10).
- Woman demonstrates ability to concentrate on and participate in decisions about own care.
- Woman exhibits no physical signs of pain (e.g., facial expression, restlessness, changes in VSs, moaning).

NIC Interventions[2]

Analgesic Administration (2210)—Use of pharmacologic agents to reduce or eliminate pain.

Anxiety Reduction (5820)—Minimizing apprehension, dread, foreboding, or uneasiness related to an unidentified source of anticipated danger.

Environmental Management: Comfort (6482)—Manipulation of the patient's surroundings for promotion of optimal comfort.

Pain Management (1400)—Alleviation of pain or a reduction in pain to a level of comfort that is acceptable to the patient.

Therapeutic Touch (5465)—Attuning to the universal healing field, seeking to act as an instrument for healing influence, and using the natural sensitivity of the hands to gently focus and direct the intervention process.

Nursing Activities and Rationales

Assessments

- Determine nature, severity, and location of pain using a 1–10 scale. Facilitates planning appropriate interventions, e.g., nonpharmacologic measures and analgesics. Documentation before and after establishes effectiveness of pain control measures.

Independent Nursing Actions

- Offer comfort measures to control pain and anxiety, such as positioning, warm packs, massage, changing lighting in room, soft music, washing face, touch, presence. These are distracters from pain. They can change and decrease the intensity of the pain cycle.

Collaborative Activities

- For severe pain, administer analgesics per order or protocol. This will usually be done as part of preparation for surgery. Narcotics alter the transmission and perception of pain impulses in the CNS.
- If the woman is being treated medically with methotrexate, she should take nothing stronger than ibuprofen for pain. In this situation, care must be taken not to confuse the pain from methotrexate effects with the pain that occurs upon tubal rupture. If the pain cannot be controlled adequately with ibuprofen, the woman should contact her healthcare provider immediately. She needs clear self-care instructions if she is going home with medications.

Patient/Family Teaching

- Explain all procedures and answer questions about the diagnosis and prognosis. Anxiety increases the perception of pain, while information may decrease anxiety.

- Teach the woman about actions of methotrexate and other necessary instructions that need to be followed while on the medication. Increases the woman's understanding about the drug, such as the need to discontinue folic acid, to avoid sun and strenuous activities, and to place nothing in her vagina during treatment.
- Inform the woman of side effects of methotrexate treatment. Stomatitis and conjunctivitis are common; rare effects are pleuritis, gastritis, dermatitis, alopecia, enteritis, increased liver enzymes, and bone marrow suppression, all of which produce or increase pain.
- Advise the woman to report to healthcare provider immediately if she develops colicky abdominal pain or severe abdominal pain. This may indicate impending or actual tubal rupture. May be admitted to the hospital for observation when this pain occurs while on methotrexate therapy; ensures that immediate treatment is implemented if pain is caused by tubal rupture.

Nursing Diagnosis: FEAR[1]

Related Factors: seriousness of maternal condition, sudden onset of acute pain, and threat to future fertility. Refer to the generic NDCP, "Fear,[1]" which begins on p. 15 in Chapter 2.

Goals, Outcomes, and Evaluation Criteria

- Woman concentrates and participates in decision making regarding own care and treatment.
- Woman identifies and uses support person (e.g., partner, caregivers).
- Woman verbalizes acceptance of situation.
- Woman uses relaxation to reduce fear.

NIC Interventions[2]

Calming Technique (5880)—Reducing anxiety in patient experiencing acute distress.
Emotional Support (5270)—Provision of reassurance, acceptance, and encouragement during times of stress.
Presence (5340)—Being with another, both physically and psychologically, during times of need.
Security Enhancement (5380)—Intensifying a patient's sense of physical and psychologic safety.
Simple Relaxation Therapy (6040)—Use of techniques to encourage and elicit relaxation for the purpose of decreasing undesirable signs and symptoms such as pain, muscle tension, or anxiety.
Touch (5460)—Providing comfort and communication through purposeful tactile contact.

Nursing Activities and Rationales

Independent Nursing Actions

- Remain with the woman, but do not expect interaction or decision making in times of acute stress (e.g., just before surgery, during periods of acute pain, when initially receiving the diagnosis of ectopic pregnancy). Promotes safety and reduces fear; if the woman is overwhelmed with stimuli, talking may add even more stress. A high level of anxiety interferes with the woman's ability to communicate and make decisions.
- Be supportive of the woman's response during treatment process and nonjudgmental in caring for the woman. Support should be focused on the patient and family and not on the cause or potential guilt. Nurses should not let their own personal value systems get in the way of caring for their patients.
- Prepare the woman for surgery or treatments in a calm manner. Emergency and unplanned medical treatments can create anxiety and fear of risks and outcomes.

Patient/Family Teaching

- Teach the woman's partner/family about the condition even if the woman is too ill to take it in. It may be necessary to defer teaching until the woman has recovered from surgery and pain is controlled. Teaching the family prior to surgery will help reinforce teaching if the woman is unable to process information. It is important to repeat information after surgery and when pain has been controlled. She will be more receptive to learning when her attention returns to self-care and self-management needs.
- Explain all diagnostic tests and treatments and reasons for each in understandable terms. The woman and partner/family cannot make choices for themselves if they do not understand what those choices entail. They may not understand advanced treatment options and need to have them explained in terms they understand.
- Answer all questions and be factual with answers. Conveys accurate information.

For other nursing activities, see the NDCP for "Anxiety/Fear,[1]" beginning on p. 184 in the topic "Late Antepartum Bleeding" in this chapter.

Nursing Diagnosis: GRIEVING[1]

Related Factors: the loss of a fetus with rupture of fallopian tube or surgery; and possible infertility after tubal rupture.

Goals, Outcomes, and Evaluation Criteria

- Woman identifies and uses effective coping strategies.
- Woman seeks professional help as needed.
- Woman and partner express and share feelings freely with each other.
- Woman and partner express the reality of their loss.
- Woman and partner verbalize acceptance of their loss.
- Woman progresses through the stages of grief and verbalizes that all stages will not progress at the same pace.
- Woman expresses optimism about the future.

▌ NIC Interventions[2]

Active Listening (4920)—Attending closely to and attaching significance to a patient's verbal and nonverbal messages.

Emotional Support (5270)—Provision of reassurance, acceptance, and encouragement during times of stress.

Grief Work Facilitation (5290)—Assistance with the resolution of a significant loss.

Hope Instillation (5310)—Facilitation of the development of a positive outlook in a given situation.

Presence (5340)—Being with another, both physically and psychologically, during times of need.

Spiritual Support (5420)—Assisting the patient to feel balance and connection with a greater power.

Support System Enhancement (5440)—Facilitation of support to patient by family, friends, and community.

▌ Nursing Activities and Rationales

Assessments

- Observe for expressions of guilt, anger, and tearfulness. Identifying level of fear/anxiety facilitates choice of interventions.
- Be aware of body language and of the pitch and inflection of the voice. The woman/family need to have confidence that the nurse is in control of the situation. Nonverbal behaviors can reflect anxiety that is not revealed by the nurse's words.
- Assess availability of support system (e.g., extended family, financial support). Both partners will be grieving; therefore, support from extended family and friends may be needed to facilitate adjustment and adaptation.
- Assess for depression. Depression is potential problem following loss.

Independent Nursing Actions

- Encourage the woman/family to express feelings of grief in ways that are comfortable for them. Facilitates open communication; feelings must be expressed to be resolved.
- Encourage the woman to express feelings of anxiety, anger, or sadness. Facilitates open communications; feelings must be expressed to be resolved. Anger, anxiety, and sadness are common feelings when tubal pregnancy occurs.
- Provide support appropriate to the phase of grieving (e.g., denial, anger, bargaining, and acceptance). Teach family about differences in genders and how they grieve. Helps the woman/family to move through the stages of grieving and successfully resolve the grief.
- Be sensitive to cultural and spiritual needs and practices (e.g., facilitate use of prayer and other religious rituals). The ways in which people express grief may be quite different. Knowing cultural and spiritual practices allows for individualizing care to meet the patient's needs.
- Use touch to communicate concern, as appropriate. Helps to reduce anxiety by promoting a feeling of safety and trust. Touch can be reassuring and can communicate caring.

- Explain to friends and family how they can help. Family members may wish to help, but may need coaching as to the specific details. They may be hesitant because they see the nurse as the expert or because they are afraid of hurting the woman.

Collaborative Activities

- Obtain spiritual advisor of the woman's choice. The woman and family may have spiritual needs that the nurse is not prepared to meet and they may have ongoing support needs.
- Refer for counseling or to support groups as needed. Counseling and group activities with others who have had similar experiences (e.g., fetal loss) may help the couple work through the grief process.

Patient/Family Teaching

- Provide realistic information about the possibility of future pregnancies and recurrence of an ectopic pregnancy. Clarifies any misinformation; helps to alleviate guilt; facilitates adaptation.
- Teach phases of the grieving process. Helps maintain self-esteem by helping the couple to realize that their feelings are normal.
- Point out that the pregnancy could not have developed normally and mother's life was at risk. Surgery or medication was necessary to preserve maternal life.

RECURRENT PREGNANCY LOSS (CERVICAL INSUFFICIENCY)

Recurrent pregnancy loss can be due to a chromosomal disorder, uterine anomalies, endocrine factors, antiphospholipid syndrome, or cervical insufficiency. Normally, cervical change does not occur until after 37 weeks' gestation. Cervical insufficiency (formerly known as cervical incompetence) refers to painless dilation of the cervix during the second trimester or early third trimester that can result in loss of the fetus and preterm birth. With increasing dilation and effacement, premature rupture of membranes can occur, increasing fetal morbidity and mortality. Cervical dilation can happen with each pregnancy, and the woman may have more than one fetal loss before the diagnosis is made.

Diagnosis of cervical insufficiency is made after recurrence of painless dilation or thinning (effacement) of the cervix without contractions, bleeding, infection, premature rupture of membranes or fetal anomalies, and shortening cervical length measured by ultrasound. Usually birth occurs earlier in the pregnancy each time if interventions are not instituted. Treatment usually involves cerclage, a procedure that involves placement of purse-string suture around the cervix to reinforce it. Cerclage is indicated by history, ultrasound diagnosis, physical examination, or a combination of the three. The string is snipped prior to labor when pregnancy reaches full-term gestation if preterm labor does not occur earlier. Research is being conducted on the use of a pessary for support rather than surgical cerclage.

Key Nursing Activities

- Prepare the woman for diagnostic procedures and cerclage.
- Teach regarding treatments for early cervical dilation.
- Offer emotional support for anxiety from repeated fetus losses.

Etiologies and Risk Factors

- Previous second or third trimester cervical dilation or fetal loss.
- Previous history of insufficient cervix or preterm birth.
- Cervical laceration with previous childbirth.
- Cervical conization or cervical biopsy.
- Exposure to diethylstilbestrol in utero; congenital structural anomalies.
- Previous extensive cervical dilation (e.g., second-trimester terminations).
- Infectious diseases.
- Multiple gestations can increase stress on cervix but are not considered a cause.

Signs and Symptoms

Subjective. Verbalization of increased pressure in pelvic area, backache, or feeling like fetus has dropped into the pelvis. Dilation is usually painless, and contractions, if present, are not perceived.

Objective. Premature dilation of the cervix from the internal os outward, second or third trimester fetal loss, increased vaginal discharge or bloody show as the cervix dilates, short cervical length, or cervix funneling with bulging membranes. Contractions may be detected by palpation and uterine monitoring. Ultrasound confirmation of cervical length less than 25 mm. Normal cervical length is greater than 35 mm.

Diagnostic Studies

- Transvaginal ultrasound. Performed early in the second trimester to detect short cervical length or signs of cervical funneling.
- Serial transvaginal ultrasonography. Monitors for cervical changes over time.
- Obstetrical ultrasonography. Determines gestational age, position of fetus and number, placental placement and grading, amniotic fluid volume index, presence of funneling and fetal anomalies, cervical length, and internal os dilation.
- Vaginal examinations with sterile speculum and gentle digital exams. Determines cervical effacement and dilatation, bulging membranes, and fetal station. Avoidance of digital exams to avoid increased dilatation of cervix; occasional gentle digital exam is done to assess dilatation, effacement, position, and consistency. State of the membranes is evaluated. Funneling may be noted, which is bulging of the amniotic membranes through the cervical os.
- Vaginal cultures and wet preps. Rules out infection.
- Urinalysis. Evaluates for urinary tract infections, which can cause uterine irritability and preterm contractions.
- Complete blood count. Rules out infection and possibility of chorioamnionitis; elevation of white blood cells denotes presence of infection.

Medical Management

- Increased frequency of office or clinic visits above established norms.
- Conservative management includes bed rest (no heavy lifting and no coitus, progesterone, anti-inflammatory drugs, and antibiotics).
- Tocolysis added to bed rest and hydration if uterine contractions (UCs) occur and continue.
- Cervical cerclage (Shirodkar or McDonald procedure). Procedure to stabilize the cervix by placing a purse string suture. If amniotic membranes are intact, there is no bleeding, and the cervix is not dilated too much (cm determined by physician), cervical cerclage may be performed as treatment or prophylaxis. Cerclage will not be done if fetal death or anomalies are present. Cerclage is elective (prophylactic at 11–15 weeks' gestation), urgent, or emergent according to time of procedure. Suture is removed at about 37 weeks or left in and cesarean section performed. It may be left in place if future pregnancies are planned. Risks include premature rupture of membranes (PROM), preterm labor, and chorioamnionitis. Prevents the cervix from dilating, thus preventing premature birth.

Collaborative Problems

Potential complication of cervical insufficiency:

- Premature birth

Potential complications of diagnostic and treatment procedures:

- Infection
- Contractions
- Bleeding

COLLABORATIVE (STANDARDIZED) CARE FOR ALL WOMEN WITH CERVICAL INSUFFICIENCY

This section includes care plans designed to identify individual needs for teaching, emotional support, and physical care.

Potential Complication: PRETERM BIRTH

Focus Assessments

- Perform a comprehensive physical, psychosocial, and cultural assessment. Identifies individual and family needs for education, emotional support, and physical care.

- Obtain baseline monitor strip of fetal heart rate (FHR) and pattern of uterine activity. Establishes contractions if present and fetal well-being.
- Assess for bulging, ruptured, or intact amniotic membranes. If membranes are bulging, the woman may require total bed rest or Trendelenburg positioning. If membranes are intact and not bulging, they are normal for that stage of pregnancy.
- Assess for infection by taking vaginal cultures and conducting urinalysis. Determines presence of infection. Vaginal cultures are done for bacterial vaginosis, group B streptococcus (GBS), chlamydia, and gonorrhea.
- Assist with preoperative and postoperative care. Care includes monitoring fetal status and presence of contractions after placement of cerclage suture. Some uterine irritability from suturing may be noted. Postoperative care lasts 24–48 hours.
- Assess for signs of infection or vaginal bleeding. Signs of infection include fever, chills, tender abdomen, and purulent vaginal discharge. Vaginal bleeding that is increasing rather than decreasing needs to be reported. Some postcerclage spotting is normal.
- Monitor for signs associated with tocolytic drugs. Tocolytics increase the cardiovascular workload, which can result in pulmonary edema. Indomethacin is treatment of choice for cerclage but can cause nausea. Fetal monitoring with amniotic fluid surveillance and fetal endocardiogram may be indicated with its use. Beta sympathomimetics can increase cardiac output and should not be administered if maternal apical rate is greater than 120 beats/min. For further information, see "Preterm Labor and Spontaneous Abortion" and "Ectopic Pregnancy," which begin on pp. 197 and 151, respectively, in this chapter, for discussions on the use of magnesium sulfate, nifedipine, and other tocolytics.

Preventive Nursing Activities

- Use Trendelenburg position with bed rest if the woman has bulging membranes or there is a descending presenting fetal head or other body part. May help prevent further cervical dilation by decreasing pressure on the amniotic membranes and cervix.
- Identify support person and have that person stay with the woman. Presence of the partner or primary support person may help decrease anxiety and fear.
- Encourage verbalization of fears and anxiety. Allows the nurse to understand and address specific concerns and fears. Verbal expression of concerns may reduce fears.
- Explain interventions before and during care; explain the risks and benefits of a cerclage. Reduces fear of the unknown. Information is essential for informed consent prior to procedure. A cerclage suture is placed early during the second trimester. Risks for the procedure include infection, cervical injury, displacement of suture, bleeding, PROM, or preterm labor and delivery. The benefit is the possibility of continuation of pregnancy and later gestational age even if preterm labor occurs.
- Teach regarding the need for activity restrictions and limitations, adequate hydration, and refraining from sexual intercourse. These restrictions prevent stimulation of uterine contractions and help prevent cervical dilatation. Intercourse can cause uterine irritability and introduce postcerclage infection. The woman is advised against standing over 90 minutes, heavy lifting, and inserting anything into her vagina. She needs to be taught to report signs of preterm labor, rupture of membranes, and signs of infection immediately.
- Teach about tocolytics if prescribed. The woman may go home on tocolytics, and she needs to understand the risks and benefits of these medications and any side effects that need to be reported. Some women may have home health nurse visits for fetal monitoring while they are on bed rest.

Nursing Diagnosis: RISK FOR INFECTION[1]

Related Factors: invasive procedures to prevent premature birth, to perform cerclage, and/or during premature labor and birth. Refer to the generic NDCP, "Risk for Infection,[1]" beginning on p. 21 in Chapter 2, and the generic comprehensive care plan, "Potential Complication: Infection," which begins on p. 29 in Chapter 3.

Goals, Outcomes, and Evaluation Criteria

- Woman remains free of infection (normal temperature, WBC count and differential values WNL, normal vaginal secretions, clear yellow urine with no pain or burning upon urination).
- Woman promptly verbalizes signs and symptoms that require attention to the healthcare provider.
- Woman promptly reports changes in health status to the healthcare provider.
- Woman adheres to the healthcare plan to decrease her risks for infection.

Nursing Activities and Rationales

Assessments

- Monitor laboratory test results and report abnormal findings to the healthcare provider. Abnormal tests may indicate infection and must be reported immediately to facilitate prompt treatment. During labor, the WBC count increases and remains increased in the postpartum period, thus, findings on the differential provide more valuable data. Serial measurement of the WBC count demonstrates patterns indicative of infection and response to treatment.

Patient/Family Teaching

- Teach signs and symptoms of infection and the need to report abnormal findings to the healthcare provider. Some infections may not become apparent until several days after an invasive procedure when the woman and family are at home.

- Teach the woman to drink six to eight glasses of water a day. Hydration helps prevent infection by diluting the urine and helping prevent urinary stasis. The elevated progesterone level in pregnancy causes dilation of the renal pelvis and ureters, predisposing to urinary stasis, thereby creating a favorable environment for pathogen growth.
- Teach the woman to turn, cough, and deep breathe while on bed rest in the hospital or at home. Facilitates the exchange of oxygen and carbon dioxide by promoting lung expansion. Also helps to prevent stasis of fluid in the lungs, which creates an environment favorable for growth of pathogens.
- Teach regarding pre- and postprocedural care. Decreases fears and increases the likelihood of compliance with necessary procedures and care.
- Maintain side-lying position. Prevents pressure from uterus on abdominal blood vessels and hypotension.
- Encourage daily fetal movement counting. Fetal daily movement counting is helpful to monitor fetal well-being and may serve as positive reinforcement and reassurance for the mother.

Collaborative Activities

- Obtain vaginal, urine, or blood cultures as ordered. Invasive procedures can introduce pathogens and place the woman at increased risk for infection. Pyelonephritis has been shown to cause premature labor.
- Administer antibiotics, as ordered, after assessing for allergies, actions, side effects, and nursing implications. Prophylactic antibiotics may be ordered. The first dose may be given on call for the cerclage. Antibiotics need to be administered on time to maintain a therapeutic blood level. In some instances, the physician may order antibiotics before a culture and sensitivity report has been received. Culture and sensitivity reports must be monitored to ascertain whether the pathogen is sensitive to the antibiotic.
- Administer IV fluids as ordered. Hydration prevents stasis of body fluids and decreases the risk for infection. Hydrated cells are more resistant to pathogens.
- Teach the woman how to assess for signs of infection. The woman is at higher risk for infection with the cerclage suture in place. She will need to monitor periodically for fever and foul-smelling vaginal secretions, which are signs of infection.
- Encourage contact with the healthcare provider's office to discuss her condition as needed. Addresses the woman's questions and concerns, decreases her fear and anxiety, and increases her compliance with her treatment plan and necessary restrictions.

INDIVIDUALIZED (NURSING DIAGNOSIS) CARE PLANS

This section includes care plans designed to address unique patient needs.

Nursing Diagnosis: ANXIETY[1]

Related Factors: possible fetal loss, inability to carry a fetus to term and have a viable fetus, having a premature baby with multiple problems, and inability to fulfill the maternal role in her family. See the generic NDCP, "Anxiety,[1]" which begins on p. 10 in Chapter 2.

Nursing Diagnosis: RISK FOR COMPLICATED GRIEVING[1]

Related Factors: possible loss of a normal pregnancy progression, possible loss of the fetus, premature birth, complications with a premature newborn, and loss of the normal labor process.

See the NDCP, "Grieving,[1]" which begins on p. 154 in the topic "Ectopic Pregnancy" in this chapter.

Goals, Outcomes, and Evaluation Criteria

- Woman expresses feelings about her potential losses to her significant other, support person, or healthcare providers.
- Woman exhibits no signs of depression or withdrawal.

NIC Interventions[2]

Coping Enhancement (5230)—Assisting a client to adapt to perceived stressors, changes, or threats that interfere with meeting life demands and roles.

Emotional Support (5270)—Provision of reassurance, acceptance, and encouragement during times of stress.

Nursing Activities and Rationales

Assessments

- Identify the stage of grieving. Determines the presence of normal/abnormal grieving pattern and plans interventions specific to the particular stage.
- Assess for previous fetal loss experiences. Because cervical insufficiency may not be identified until the second or third pregnancy, it is possible the woman and family have already experienced a loss. This can intensify grieving when faced with the same situation again.

Patient/Family Teaching

- Teach about ultrasonography and other diagnostic tests. Understanding helps to reduce fear and anxiety. Seeing the fetus on ultrasound may be reassuring to the mother.
- Teach regarding plans for labor and delivery. Education reduces fear of the unknown and helps the woman and family to actively participate as much as possible. Active participation provides the mother and family a way to help maintain this pregnancy to a positive outcome.

Nursing Diagnosis: DEFICIENT KNOWLEDGE[1]

Related Factors: the effects of insufficient cervix on oneself, the pregnancy, and the fetus; and regarding the treatments and expected outcome. See the generic NDCP, "Deficient Knowledge,[1]" beginning on p. 13 in Chapter 2.

Goals, Outcomes, and Evaluation Criteria

- Woman verbalizes the meaning of cervical insufficiency.
- Woman verbalizes the treatment plan and states intention to comply with plan of treatment.

NIC Interventions[2]

Anticipatory Guidance (5210)—Preparation of patient for an anticipated developmental and/or situational crisis.
Teaching: Prescribed Activity/Exercise (5612)—Preparing a patient to achieve and/or maintain a prescribed level of activity.

Nursing Activities and Rationales

Assessments

- Assess knowledge about cervical insufficiency and risks of the condition. The woman may lack knowledge regarding cervical insufficiency, or to the other extreme, be very familiar with the condition, depending on her experiences.
- Assess knowledge about cervical cerclage and/or labor and birth. The woman's knowledge level directs the teaching plan. Reinforce that if she is in labor, she must go to the hospital and have the cerclage suture removed to prevent cervical lacerations.

Patient/Family Teaching

- Teach about cervical insufficiency and effect on mother, pregnancy, and fetus; and about treatment options. Increases the woman's understanding of her condition, its possible effects on her pregnancy, and available options.
- Answer questions and reinforce teaching. Include partner/family in teaching. Explain cervical cerclage placement if that is part of the plan. A woman who is physically or emotionally stressed may not be able to retain all the information given initially. Teaching must be reinforced frequently and questions answered honestly. Including the partner/family or other support person(s) is imperative in family-centered care and allows the woman additional support in a stressful situation.
- Teach signs and symptoms of cervical change and importance of reporting to care provider. The usual signs and symptoms of labor may not occur with an insufficient cervix. The woman may have UCs without feeling them, and the cervix may dilate without her awareness of it happening. She needs to know how to palpate and time UCs. She also needs to be aware of other signs that labor may be occurring, such as backache, increasing pelvic pressure, increased vaginal discharge, and leakage of fluid or bloody show.
- Daily fetal movement counts. Self-monitoring the fetal movements will help mother note fetal well-being and keep record for medical personnel. If fetal activity slows, the woman must report to her care provider. This may indicate a change in status, and prompt evaluation is necessary.

GESTATIONAL TROPHOBLASTIC DISEASE (HYDATIDIFORM MOLE)

Gestational trophoblastic disease (GTD) is a term describing a spectrum of disorders arising from placental trophoblasts. This includes hydatidiform mole, invasive mole, and choriocarcinoma. A hydatidiform mole is the most common of the GTD disorders, occurring in about 1 of every 1,500 pregnancies in the United States. With this disorder, the mechanism controlling the trophoblastic tissue is deficient, causing the chorionic villi to develop abnormally into fluid-filled, grapelike clusters. This anomalous growth contains a nonviable embryo that implants in the uterus. It continues to grow and may invade the myometrium (invasive mole) and produce tumor growth or gestational trophoblastic neoplasia (GTN). GTN is recognized as the most curable of all gynecologic cancers.

The significance of GTD for the woman is multifaceted. She must deal not only with the loss of the pregnancy but also with the possibility of developing gestational choriocarcinoma. Treatment and follow-up care focus on assessment for this specific type of cancer. Metastasis occurs most often to the lungs, vagina, liver, and brain. Chemotherapy is required when neoplasm or choriocarcinoma occur. After molar pregnancy, a woman requires follow-up surveillance and postponement of another pregnancy for a year.

Key Nursing Activities

- Teach the importance of follow-up care.
- Teach the importance of pregnancy prevention for 1 year.
- Teach and monitor for the signs and symptoms of complications.
- Provide emotional support for grieving about the lost pregnancy.
- Provide emotional support and information during diagnostic process for possible cancer.

Etiologies and Risk Factors

A hydatidiform mole is believed to occur when chromosomal abnormalities are present in the ovum and/or sperm. As a result, there is an abnormal growth in the placental trophoblasts; a fetus may or may not develop. A formation of fluid-filled, grapelike clusters grows large enough to fill the uterus. These clusters grow rapidly so that the uterus appears large for the gestational age of the fetus. Continued bleeding after evacuation of a hydatidiform mole is suggestive of gestational trophoblastic neoplasia.

Risk Factors

Risk factors for GTD are not well understood. Theories are ovular defect, stress, or nutritional deficiency, especially carotene and protein. The condition has been associated with infertility, previous molar pregnancy, history of spontaneous abortion, oral contraceptives, and low economic status. Maternal age older than 35 or 40 years may be a factor or there may be an abnormal genetic predisposition. Risk is slightly increased in women under the age of 20 years.

Signs and Symptoms

Complete Mole

Signs of a complete mole are absence of embryo or fetus and amniotic sac, generalized areas of abnormal chorionic villi, diploid karyotype that is present from two sperm-fertilizing ovum with no genetic material. Approximately 20% of women with complete molar pregnancies develop a neoplasm requiring more treatment.

Subjective. Excessive nausea (from increased levels of hCG), fatigue, malaise, anorexia from anemia.

Objective. Brownish vaginal bleeding from the 4th week through the second trimester (from weakened uterine wall), uterine enlargement greater than expected for gestation, bilateral ovarian enlargement (from elevated hCG) absence of a fetal heart tone in the presence of signs and symptoms of a pregnancy. Other signs rarely seen due to early diagnosis: vaginal passage of vesicles or grapelike structures, anemia, possible symptoms of preeclampsia if the molar pregnancy continues into the second trimester, respiratory distress related to a trophoblastic pulmonary embolus, especially after molar evacuation, coagulopathy (disseminated intravascular coagulation [DIC]). Uterine involution after evaluation is also common.

Incomplete Mole

Signs and symptoms of an incomplete mole are absence of embryo or fetus and amniotic sac and multiple congenital anomalies. Localized areas of abnormal chorionic villi are present—usually a triploid karyotype with one set from one normal ovum and two sperm. Approximately 5% of women with incomplete mole develop a neoplasm.

Objective. Signs of an incomplete or missed abortion, irregular vaginal bleeding, no fetal heart rate, uterus that is small for the estimated delivery date. Diagnosis commonly occurs in the first trimester due to abnormal bleeding. Lutein cysts occur on the ovaries in 15–20% of cases. In rare cases, a woman has a twin pregnancy with one viable fetus and one molar pregnancy; but it is very high-risk to

the mother and fetus if the woman chooses to continue the pregnancy. A fetus that coexists in this condition may have chromosomal anomalies and growth restriction.

Diagnostic Studies

- hCG level greater than 100,000 mIU/ml. Markedly elevated.
- Maternal serum α-fetoprotein. Low.
- Hgb and Hct. Decreased.
- Urinalysis. Proteinuria.
- Transvaginal ultrasound. After 6–8 weeks' gestation; may reveal characteristic molar pattern (snowstorm); fails to reveal amniotic sac or fetus.
- Fetal heart tones. Absent.
- Histology. Grapelike, vesicular tissue confirms diagnosis of GTD.

Medical Management

- Immediate evacuation of the mole by suction evacuation and curettage. Ensures complete removal. Procedure has associated risk of uterine perforation, hemorrhage, infections, and respiratory insufficiency. If the woman is no longer interested in childbearing, hysterectomy may be performed.
- Oxytocin infusion. Stimulates myometrial contractions to thicken uterine wall and decrease risk of perforation. Also controls bleeding during procedure and postpartum bleeding after evacuation of the mole. Initiated at the beginning of surgery, but not before surgery because of increased risk for trophoblastic embolization.
- Hysterectomy. Woman's age, parity, and predisposition to uterine rupture may warrant hysterectomy. Considered when women have completed childbearing.
- RhoD immune globulin for Rh-negative women who are not sensitized. Prevents antibody formation and injury to fetus in future pregnancy.
- Follow-up care:
  - ▶ Pregnancy prevention for 1 year with the use of barrier techniques; oral contraceptives or systemic hormonal contraceptives after hCG levels have returned to normal. Elevated hCG levels in pregnancy confuse the diagnosis of malignant tumor. Pregnancy is not considered safe until 1 year after the event.
  - ▶ Measurement of serum hCG levels every 2 weeks until normal and then monthly. Monitors for malignant trophoblastic tumor.
  - ▶ Chemotherapy if choriocarcinoma develops. Methotrexate and dactinomycin are the treatments of choice. Approximately 20% of women need to take chemotherapy as part of their treatment. Additional care is required if the woman has metastatic disease.
- Pelvic ultrasound in subsequent pregnancies and serum hCG levels 6 weeks after the birth. Because the woman is at higher risk for developing another molar pregnancy (1%).

▌ *Collaborative Problems*

Potential maternal complications of gestational trophoblastic disease include the following:

- Choriocarcinoma of the trophoblastic tissue
- Infection
- DIC
- Anemia
- Pulmonary embolism
- Preeclampsia
- Hyperthyroidism
- Intrauterine infection or sepsis
- Uterine rupture
- Rupture of ovarian cysts
- Hyperemesis gravidarum
- Emotional trauma
- GTN
- Trophoblastic embolization

Potential complications of evacuation of molar pregnancy include the following:

- Hemorrhage
- Pulmonary embolism
- Uterine perforation

COLLABORATIVE (STANDARDIZED) CARE FOR ALL WOMEN WITH GESTATIONAL TROPHOBLASTIC DISEASE

Perform a comprehensive assessment to identify individual needs for teaching, emotional support, and physical care.

▌ Potential Complication of Gestational Trophoblastic Disease: CHORIOCARCINOMA OF THE TROPHOBLASTIC TISSUE

Focus Assessments

- Assess for continued bleeding after evacuation of a hydatidiform mole. The most suggestive symptom of gestational trophoblastic neoplasia (GTN). GTN refers to persistent trophoblastic tissue that is presumed to be malignant.
- Assess for abdominal pain and uterine and ovarian enlargement. These are clinical signs of GTN.
- Assess for cachexia, weight loss, pyrexia, cough, hemoptysis, dependent edema, bone pain, and skin changes. These signs and symptoms suggest metastatic choriocarcinoma.
- Assess for diagnostic indicators of choriocarcinoma:

  - Complete blood count, platelet count, clotting studies, blood type, and antibody screen. Establish baseline value and detect infection (elevated white count), clotting disorder, anemia, and need for Rho(D) immune globulin treatment.
  - Renal and liver function tests. Detect metastasis and increases in enzymes due to tissue damage.
  - Pelvic ultrasonography. Confirms evacuation of mole and evaluates uterine lining for presence of tumors or abnormal growth.
  - Chest radiograph. Detects metastasis to the lungs.
  - Human chorionic gonadotropin levels (pretreatment, weekly until normal, and then monthly for 1 year). Human chorionic gonadotropin is a sensitive marker produced by the tumor, so it can be used to monitor the need for and the effectiveness of chemotherapy. Increasing or plateauing hCG levels after evacuation of a molar pregnancy are diagnostic of GTN.
  - Serum granulocyte macrophage colony-stimulating factor. A normal SIL-2R assay rules out the presence of choriocarcinoma.
  - Computed tomography scans of the lungs and brain (if diagnosed with choriocarcinoma). Determines the extent of disease.
  - Assess for cough and bloody sputum. Detects metastasis. Lungs are affected by metastasis in 75% of cases of choriocarcinoma.
  - Assess mental status. Metastasis can affect the brain, causing alterations in mentation and behavior.
  - Assess psychosocial status. The woman is dealing with loss of pregnancy, potential for cancer, surgery and/ or chemotherapy, and delay of future pregnancy, all of which are stress producing.
- Assess compliance with follow-up and birth control use. The increased hCG resulting from pregnancy confuses diagnosis of malignancy.

Preventive Nursing Actions

- Teach the importance of follow-up care, for monitoring hCG levels, and for signs of malignancy. Human chorionic gonadotropin levels should progressively decrease. Measurable amounts should not be in the urine 8 weeks after evacuation of the mole. About 5% of molar pregnancies progress to choriocarcinoma with rapid and widespread metastasis. If it does develop, it will be graded, and treatment will be determined by extent of disease.
- Assess for factors that may prevent weekly/monthly blood testing. Ensures compliance with the follow-up plan.
- Teach importance of pregnancy prevention for 1 year. The increased hCG from pregnancy may confuse diagnosis of malignancy; a second pregnancy is likely to be molar.
- Instruct on and monitor compliance with the proper use of the chosen type of birth control; oral contraceptives are the

preferred method. Reinforce and answer all questions about the need to use birth control; reinforce risk of pregnancy.

- Offer emotional support and promote open communications. This is a very stressful time and the woman has a difficult diagnosis. Couples may need additional support through counseling.
- Act as liaison to other support systems and resources. If the woman is positive for cancer she will need collaboration through many types of medical and supportive care while on chemotherapy.

Potential Complication of GTD: ANEMIA

Refer to the generic collaborative care plan, "Potential Complication: Anemia," which begins on p. 25 in Chapter 3. If anemia occurs, refer to "Prenatal Anemia," which begins on p. 114 in Chapter 5.

Potential Complication of GTD: DISSEMINATED INTRAVASCULAR COAGULATION

Refer to the generic collaborative care plan, "Potential Complication: Disseminated Intravascular Coagulation," which begins on pp. 26 in Chapter 3, and to the following collaborative care plan, "Potential Complication of GTD and/or Evacuation of Molar Pregnancy: Hemorrhage," next.

Potential Complication of GTD and/or Evacuation of Molar Pregnancy: HEMORRHAGE

Refer to the generic collaborative care plan, "Potential Complication: Hemorrhage," beginning on p. 28 in Chapter 3.

Focus Assessments

- Save all fluid and tissue passed before evacuation. Aids in differentiating hydatidiform mole from spontaneous abortion, the most common cause of bleeding in the first trimester.
- Palpate and assess uterine fundus for involution and monitor vaginal bleeding postevacuation. Detects uterine contraction and facilitates corrective action if fundus is not firm. The uterine muscle needs to clamp down so the uterine lining will not continue to bleed. Pad counts are important to determine increased or decreased pattern of bleeding.

- Monitor urinary output for amounts less than 30 ml/hr. If bleeding occurs, compensatory mechanisms shunt blood away from the kidneys to the heart and brain, resulting in decreased renal perfusion and subsequent decreased urine output.
- Monitor vital signs and for cold, clammy skin. Symptoms of impending hypovolemic shock. When blood loss occurs, compensatory mechanisms cause peripheral vasoconstriction in an attempt to shunt blood away from the periphery to support circulation to the heart and brain.
- Monitor clotting studies, Hgb and Hct levels, assessing for a decrease over previous levels. Identifies anemia resulting from blood loss; detects clotting abnormalities because the woman is at risk for DIC.

Preventive Nursing Activities

- Establish IV line with large-bore needle. For rapid infusion of blood or volume expanders if needed.
- Restrict activities. Prevents tissue demand for oxygen; prevents injury.
- Ensure cross-match has been performed. Compatible blood should be available before beginning the evacuation procedure. May be needed for transfusion if hemoglobin and hematocrit are too low or to treat hemorrhage.
- Administer oxytocin to aid in uterine involution. Uterus needs to clamp down to deter bleeding.
- Administer Rho(D) immune globulin treatment if Rh negative. Needed to prevent isosensitization.

Potential Complication of Evacuation of the Mole: PULMONARY EMBOLISM

Focus Assessments

- Assess respiratory system (dyspnea, tachypnea, pleuritic pain, cough, hemoptysis, rales, syncope). These are manifestations of pulmonary embolism (occlusion or infarction of the pulmonary circulation). Pulmonary embolism is a life-threatening condition that requires immediate medical intervention.
- Assess cardiovascular system (tachycardia, hypotension). Occlusion of the pulmonary circulation causes hypoxic vasoconstriction and pulmonary edema, thereby decreasing pulmonary–cardiac circulation and, subsequently, cardiac output.
- Assess integument (peripheral or central cyanosis). Cyanosis is related to hypoxia.
- Assess for fever higher than 37°C (98.6°F). Indicates inflammation due to infarction from the thrombus.
- Note results of diagnostic studies, including perfusion and ventilation scans; complete blood cell count (CBC), electrolytes, enzymes, and arterial blood gases;

chest radiograph; and electrocardiogram and angiogram. Identifies changes in pulmonary circulation, presence of leukocytosis, hypoxemia, infarcted or consolidated areas, and pleural effusion.

- Monitor for deep vein thrombosis (check Homan's sign, inspect for redness or heat over the lower extremities). A portion of a peripheral clot can break off and circulate to the lungs. However, in molar pregnancy, pulmonary embolism usually results from entry of trophoblastic tissue into the circulation after evacuation of a significantly enlarged uterus, rather than from peripheral thrombosis.

Preventive Nursing Activities

- If activities are restricted, encourage the woman to change positions frequently and perform active range of motion. Promotes circulation and prevents venous stasis, which predisposes to venous thrombus formation.
- Maintain proper hydration. Prevents hemoconcentration, which increases the risk for venous stasis.

Potential Complication of GTD and Evacuation of Molar Pregnancy: INFECTION

Use with the generic NDCP, "Risk for Infection,[1]" beginning on p. 21 in Chapter 2 and the generic collaborative care plan, "Potential Complication: Infection," beginning on p. 29 in Chapter 3.

Focus Assessments

- Assess culture and sensitivity of vaginal drainage as needed. Bacterial growth is a diagnostic indicator of infection. Sensitivity provides information for choosing the most effective antibiotic.
- Monitor vital signs and for elevation of temperature with increased heart rate. Detects infection. Patient could have lowering of blood pressure, chills and fever, body aches, and tender abdomen, all of which may indicate infection.

Preventive Nursing Activities

- Identify other risk factors for infections. To begin specific interventions to minimize risk as much as possible. Malnutrition, compromised immune system, and IV drug use, for example, add to the existing risk of infection. Special interventions are needed when special risks exist.

INDIVIDUALIZED (NURSING DIAGNOSIS) CARE PLANS

The care plans in this section were developed to address unique patient needs.

Nursing Diagnosis: GRIEVING[1]

Related Factors: loss of pregnancy, potential loss of fertility, or protracted postoperative treatment regimen.

Goals, Outcomes, and Evaluation Criteria

- Woman verbalizes reality and acceptance of loss.
- Woman identifies problems with the grieving process (e.g., problems sleeping, eating) and seeks appropriate help.

NIC Interventions[2]

Grief Work Facilitation: Perinatal Death (5294)—Assistance with the resolution of a perinatal loss.
Grief Work Facilitation (5290)—Assistance with the resolution of a significant loss.

Nursing Activities and Rationales

Assessments

- Assess the significance of the loss to the woman and family. One factor affecting loss and grief responses is the significance of the loss to the woman. Significance depends on the perceptions of the person experiencing the loss. For example, the significance of a lost pregnancy differs depending on whether the pregnancy was wanted or unwanted.
- Encourage and monitor expressions of feelings concerning the loss of the pregnancy. By use of verbal and nonverbal cues, the nurse can assess the degree of sadness or feelings of guilt and can determine readiness to discuss feelings. The woman and her family need the opportunity to express feelings in a nonjudgmental environment to start working through the grief process.
- Identify the stage of grief being expressed (e.g., denial, anger, bargaining, depression, acceptance). Enables the nurse to choose specific communication techniques that will be helpful for the woman and her family. The woman and family are dealing with pregnancy loss and the potential of a serious diagnosis.

Collaborative Activities

- Assess for signs of depression and consult with appropriate healthcare team member if needed. Depression due to the grieving process may require long-term counseling from psychiatrist or mental health counselor.
- Consult the woman's spiritual leader about baptizing the products of conception if the woman/family wishes. Some religions consider the products of conception a living being and in need of baptism.

Patient/Family Teaching

- Provide information about GTD, treatments, and follow-up care, and discuss the possibility of future pregnancies.

Information may relieve guilt feelings and promote decision making and future adaptation.

- Point out that this was not a normal pregnancy and would not have resulted in a healthy baby. There may not even be a recognizable fetus growing, and there is nothing to be gained (and much to lose) by allowing the pregnancy to continue. Allowing the pregnancy to continue places the woman at risk for hemorrhage and gestational choriocarcinoma. There is no possibility of continuing the pregnancy or giving birth to a viable infant.

Nursing Diagnosis: FEAR[1]

Related Factors: unknown or uncertain outcome; inexperience with evacuation procedures; threat of malignancy, metastases, or death; threat of changes in body functions with surgery and possible chemotherapy. Use with the generic NDCPs, "Anxiety[1]" and "Fear,[1]" which begin on pp. 10 and 15, respectively, in Chapter 2.

Goals, Outcomes, and Evaluation Criteria

- Woman reports physical and psychologic well-being.
- Woman identifies effective coping patterns.

NIC Interventions[2]

Counseling (5240)—Use of an interactive helping process focusing on the needs, problems, or feelings of the patient and significant others to enhance or support coping, problem solving, and interpersonal relationships.

Decision-Making Support (5250)—Providing information and support for a patient who is making a decision regarding health care.

Nursing Activities and Rationales

Assessments

- Assess the woman's understanding of the situation. Assists with formulation of the teaching plan and enables the nurse to correct misinformation that may be contributing to the woman's fear/anxiety.
- Monitor verbal and nonverbal responses. This will be an indicator of the degree of understanding and anxiety. By first identifying the degree of anxiety, the nurse can then establish a plan of care.
- Assess the impact of the woman's situation on her roles and relationships. Enables the planning of appropriate interventions to prevent breakdown of the family structure and help the family adapt in a realistic manner.
- Assess the need for support systems and spiritual resources. A high level of anxiety may require assistance from several sources.

Independent Nursing Actions

- Encourage the use of spiritual resources of the woman's choosing. Helps the woman to identify inner strengths that can foster relaxation and calmness.
- Serve as liaison between the woman and other healthcare providers. Provides the woman with one person to call for information, thus decreasing confusion and anxiety.

Collaborative Activities

- Refer to healthcare provider for medication to reduce anxiety as appropriate. Short-term use of antianxiety medications can assist the woman to deal with daily concerns when nonpharmacologic methods are not successful.
- Refer to social services if financial or emotional assistance is needed for follow-up care. Lack of financial assistance may prevent follow-up care necessary for prevention of metastases. The woman may worry about money and about her prognosis if she cannot afford treatment.

Patient/Family Teaching

- Provide factual information about follow-up appointments, procedures done at each appointment, and implications for future pregnancies. Accurate information about what to expect with appointments and procedures will help reduce anxiety and increase compliance. After hCG levels are normal for about 1 year, the probability for recurrence of a mole is only about 2%, so the woman can anticipate a favorable pregnancy outcome in the future.
- Provide information on signs and symptoms of metastasis that need to be reported to the healthcare provider. Confronting the danger through self-care provides control and reduces fear.
- Instruct the woman on the use of relaxation techniques and self-care techniques as needed. These techniques can help decrease anxiety and enhance decision-making ability.
- Reinforce information provided by other healthcare team members as needed. Anxiety may interfere with the ability to recall information. Reinforcement provides further assurance so that the woman may be more inclined to accept the information.

MULTIFETAL PREGNANCY

Multifetal (multiple-gestation) pregnancy occurs naturally in about 3% of the pregnancies in the United States. It is more common today, occurring in about 19% of pregnancies, because of increased use of ovulation-stimulating drugs to induce conception and other assisted technologies. Fertility management in a pregnancy increases the odds of twins to about 25–30% and triplets to about 5%.

About two thirds of twins are due to fertilization of two eggs (dizygotic, fraternal twins), while the remainder occurs from splitting of one fertilized egg (monozygotic, identical twins). This differentiation is important because morbidity and mortality are different for dizygotic and monozygotic twin pregnancies.

One in about 8,100 pregnancies results in triplets. Pregnancies consisting of more than three fetuses are extremely rare. Fetal loss in twin pregnancies is about triple the rate for singleton gestations; about 75% of twin pregnancies are lost before the end of the first trimester. This care plan focuses on twin gestation.

Key Nursing Activities

- Nutritional counseling
- Monitoring for complications related to multiple gestation
- Teaching regarding high-risk pregnancy
- Promoting optimal weight gain
- Providing emotional support
- Offering parent education and support in transition of parents with multiples

Etiologies and Risk Factors

Twins are more likely in pregnancies with a family history of twins (dizygotic) and with use of ovulation-stimulating drugs. Only 50% of twins diagnosed in the first trimester end with a healthy pregnancy outcome and two live infants.

First-trimester loss may be due to:

- environmental factors.
- infections.
- trophoblast dysfunction.
- poor embryo quality.
- lower concentration of placentally produced substances.

Second-trimester losses may be due to:

- congenital anomalies.
- growth restriction.
- chromosomal abnormalities.
- cervical insufficiency.
- twin-to-twin transfusion syndrome in monochorionic placenta.

Increased risk exists for preterm birth, intrauterine growth restriction, gestational hypertension, and antepartum and postpartum hemorrhage.

Signs and Symptoms

Subjective. Reported history of risk factors (see previous discussion); increased nausea and vomiting due to increased hormones of early pregnancy.

Objective. Rapid uterine enlargement, fundal height exceeds norm for weeks of gestation, more than one heartbeat or asynchronous fetal heartbeats, more than one heart tracing on electrocardiography, more than one fetus present on ultrasound examination, palpation of more than one fetus (Leopold's maneuver), hydramnios.

Diagnostic Studies

- Ultrasonography. Identifies the presence of more than one fetus.
- Electrocardiogram. Identifies the presence of more than one fetal heartbeat.
- β-Human chorionic gonadotropin (hCG). Levels elevated in the presence of more than one fetus.
- Maternal serum α-fetoprotein. Levels elevated in the presence of more than one fetus.

Medical Management

- Assessment for pregnancy complications such as bleeding and possible spontaneous abortion, congenital anomalies, maternal anemia, twin-to-twin transfusion syndrome, placental and cord abnormalities, preterm labor (PTL), intrauterine growth restriction, hypertension, hydramnios, and intrauterine fetal demise.
- More frequent visits to care provider. Every 2 weeks in second trimester and weekly thereafter.
- Nutritional counseling. Iron, vitamin, and micronutrient supplementation.
- Diagnostic techniques. Ultrasound examination to determine placenta sites, state of membranes, amniotic fluid, fetal heartbeats, cord vessels and insertion, congenital anomalies, discordant growth patterns, estimation of fetal weight, and amniocentesis.
- Antepartum surveillance. Nonstress testing, amniotic fluid index, contraction stress testing, and biophysical profiles.

Collaborative Problems

Potential complications of multiple gestation (hydramnios) include the following:

- Anemia
- Hypertension
- Congenital anomalies
- Preterm labor

COLLABORATIVE (STANDARDIZED) CARE FOR ALL WOMEN WITH MULTIPLE GESTATION

Perform comprehensive assessment to identify individual needs for teaching, emotional support, and physical care. For general antepartum care, refer to Chapter 4, *Normal Pregnancy*, beginning on p. 39.

Potential Complication of Multiple Gestation: HYDRAMNIOS

In multifetal pregnancy, hydramnios may occur as a result of increased renal perfusion from cross-vessel anastomosis of monozygotic twins.

Focus Assessments

- Assess ultrasonography results. Determines the presence of excessive amniotic fluid; greater than 2 L of amniotic fluid is associated with fetal gastrointestinal abnormalities, neural tube disorders, multiple gestations, and twin-to-twin transfusion syndrome. Ultrasonography is also used to identify monochorionic twins (i.e., two embryos with two separate amnions and one chorion). This is important because monochorionic twins require more intensive surveillance and earlier birth (e.g., a monochorionic placenta may have a vascular anastomosis that leads to twin-to-twin transfusion syndrome, with resulting fetal mortality).
- Assess fundal height for rapid and/or excessive uterine growth. Detects the presence of excessive amniotic fluid. Keep in mind that the presence of multiple fetuses produces greater than expected fundal height, even without hydramnios.

Potential Complication of Multiple Gestation: ANEMIA

See the generic collaborative care plan, "Potential Complication: Anemia," which begins on p. 25 in Chapter 3. Also refer to "Prenatal Anemia," which begins on p. 114 in Chapter 5. Anemia is more common in multiple gestations because of the greater demand for iron produced by the additional fetus or fetuses.

Focus Assessments

- Assess caloric intake. Determines adequacy of intake to support growth and development of more than one fetus.
- Assess for the presence of nausea and vomiting. When severe nausea and vomiting are present, anemia may develop despite the intake of multiple-vitamin and iron therapy.

Potential Complication of Multiple Gestation: HYPERTENSION

See the generic collaborative care plan, "Potential Complication: Hypertensive Disorders," which begins on p. 32 in Chapter 3, and "Hypertensive Disorders of Pregnancy," which begins on p. 170 in this chapter.

Potential Complications of Multiple Gestation: PRETERM LABOR AND POTENTIAL PRETERM BIRTH

Preterm birth is a risk because of uterine dysfunction due to an overstretched myometrium (from the presence of more than one fetus and possibly from hydramnios). Preterm birth is 5.9 times more likely in twins than in singletons. See the generic collaborative care plan, "Potential Complication: Preterm Labor," which begins on p. 31 in Chapter 3, and "Preterm Labor and Spontaneous Abortion," which begins on p. 197 in this chapter.

Preventive Nursing Activities

- Schedule more frequent visits to the healthcare provider, with vaginal exams during the third trimester. Enables frequent assessment for cervical changes (e.g., lengthening, effacement, dilation, bulging membranes).
- Encourage lifestyle modifications (e.g., avoid standing for prolonged periods, avoid working more than 40 hours a week, take work leave if at all possible). Prolonged standing may be a high-risk factor for preterm labor.

INDIVIDUALIZED (NURSING DIAGNOSIS) CARE PLANS

The care plans in this section should be used to address unique patient needs.

Nursing Diagnosis: IMBALANCED NUTRITION: LESS THAN BODY REQUIREMENTS[1]

Related Factors: insufficient intake of nutrients to meet metabolic needs of the mother and fetuses; nausea and vomiting.

Goals, Outcomes, and Evaluation Criteria

- Woman accurately describes dietary intake required for multifetal pregnancy.
- Woman accurately describes well-balanced diet.
- Woman maintains weight for stage of pregnancy.
- Woman maintains body fluid components and chemical indices within normal limits.

NIC Interventions[2]

Nutrition Management (1100)—Assisting with or providing a balanced dietary intake of foods and fluids.

Nutritional Counseling (5246)—Use of an interactive helping process focusing on the need for diet modification.

Nutritional Monitoring (1160)—Collection and analysis of patient data to prevent or minimize malnourishment.

Teaching: Prescribed Diet (5614)—Preparing a patient to correctly follow a prescribed diet.

Weight Gain Assistance (1240)—Facilitating gain of body weight.

▌ *Nursing Activities and Rationales*

Assessments

- Assess body weight and monitor weight trends. Establishes a baseline for later comparisons. Weight is a clinical indicator of adequate nutrition and hydration. Nutritional demands are increased when there is more than one fetus. Institute of Medicine guidelines for weight gain during twin pregnancy are now related to body mass index prepregnant weight. Normal-weight women should have 17–25 kg (37–54 lb) weight gain, overweight women, 14–23 kg gain (31–50 lb), and obese women, 11–19 kg weight gain (25–42 lb) (Rasmussen & Yaktine, 2009). This translates for normal-weight women to a 3,000–3,500 calorie diet/175 g protein/350 g carbohydrates/156 g fat. Underweight women need 4,000 calories/200 g protein/400 g carbohydrates/178 g fat. Overweight women need 3,250 calories/163 g protein /350 g carbohydrates/144 g fat. Obese women need 2,700–3,000 calories/150 g protein/300 g carbohydrates/133 g fat. The American Dietetic Association recommends three dairy, three protein, three vegetable, two fruit, and six grain servings daily (Kaiser & Allen, 2008). Pregnant women must gain at least 37 pounds. The recommendation is that 20% of calories come from protein, 40% from carbohydrate, and 40% from fat to promote the best pregnancy outcome.
- Assess biochemical measures. Establishes a baseline for later comparisons. Chemical studies such as serum albumin, Hgb, Hct, lymphocyte count, total iron binding capacity, and serum transferrin are good indicators of nutritional adequacy. If the woman is anemic, encourage iron-rich foods, iron supplement intake, and black strap molasses.
- Assess diet for calcium, antioxidants, zinc, magnesium, omega-3 fatty acids, folic acid.
  - Calcium intake. The pregnant woman needs 200–300 mg/d more than a nonpregnant woman. Calcium supplements of 1,000–1,300 mg daily plus diet high in calcium and vitamin D are encouraged.
  - Antioxidants. Vitamin C and E are thought to reduce the risk of preeclampsia and preterm births. Supplementation of 1,000 mg of vitamin C and 400 micrograms of vitamin E are recommended.
  - Zinc and magnesium. Prevents formation of free radicals. Deficiency may be associated with fetal neurologic malformations and growth restriction during late pregnancy; deficiency may also be associated with impaired brain function and behavior abnormalities. Supplementation may reduce preeclampsia and preterm

birth. Daily zinc intake is recommended at 12–40 mg, and daily magnesium intake should be 350–460 mg and up to 1,000 mg daily for twin pregnancy.
  - Omega-3 fatty acids. Twins tend to have lower levels in their vascular systems, indicating inadequate dietary supply; thus, supplementation could be helpful. Intake of 300–500 mg per day is recommended through diet and purified supplements without mercury.
- Assess eating patterns and food likes and dislikes. Determines adequacy of nutrient and fluid intake and personal likes and dislikes, which helps with nutritional planning.
- Assess for physical or psychosocial barriers to eating. Determines if the woman has physical problems such as pain, nausea, or weakness that interfere with her ability to obtain, prepare, or take in foods or fluids. Also determines if psychosocial problems such as fear or anxiety or lack of financial resources are preventing her from eating. When obstacles to eating or drinking are identified, interventions can be planned to eliminate them. The woman should be referred to the Women, Infants, and Children program if she is eligible to assist with healthy eating.

Independent Nursing Actions

- Encourage six small meals per day. Small meals are less overwhelming to the woman who may have nausea or difficulty eating, or whose stomach may be crowded by the enlarged uterus. Meals throughout the day supply greater energy and prevent gastric distention, which causes nausea. This will prevent the hypoglycemia that can cause nausea common in the imposed starvation mode of pregnancy.

Collaborative Activities

- Refer for nutritional counseling. Nutrition consultation is needed in the first trimester to improve outcome of pregnancy. The pattern of weight gain is as important as the total weight gain. The increase in the third trimester weight after 28 weeks should be the greatest. Twin birth weight gains should increase by 65 g (by 20 weeks), 37 g (20–28 weeks), and 15 g (28 weeks to birth), respectively, per kilogram per week of maternal weight gain (Luke, 2005). Special and ongoing interventions may be needed to ensure that the woman gains greater weight than is required for a singleton birth.

Patient/Family Teaching

- Teach the need for maintaining nutrient and fluid intake to meet growth requirements for more than one fetus and to prevent weight loss. This knowledge may serve as incentive to take in adequate food and fluids.
- Teach to eat high-calorie, protein-rich, and carbohydrate foods. Ensures the intake of adequate calories and nutrients for mother and more than one fetus.
- Teach to maintain accurate records of weekly weights between perinatal visits. Provides information about

weight trends so that corrective measures can be taken if the woman begins to lose weight or not gain sufficient weight as the pregnancy progresses.

Nursing Diagnosis: DISCOMFORT (E.G., SHORTNESS OF BREATH, DYSPNEA ON EXERTION, BACKACHE, PEDAL EDEMA)[1]

Related Factors: increased size of the uterus, which encroaches on lungs, viscera, and pelvic circulation. The woman may have heartburn due to increased uterine size and pressure.

Refer to the NDCPs "Deficient Knowledge: Pregnancy-Related Changes,[1]" for "Normal Antepartum: First Trimester," "Normal Antepartum: Second Trimester," and "Normal Antepartum: Third Trimester"; those topics begin on p. 40, p. 49, and p. 56, respectively, in Chapter 4.

Goals, Outcomes, and Evaluation Criteria

- Woman reports satisfaction with comfort measures.
- Woman reports use of effective coping measures.
- Woman modifies activities to increase comfort.
- Woman performs self-care management for discomforts that occur.
- Woman differentiates between common discomforts and signs that are cause for concern.

NIC Interventions[2]

Coping Enhancement (5230)—Assisting a patient to adapt to perceived stressors, changes, or threats that interfere with meeting life demands and roles.

Environmental Management: Comfort (6482)—Manipulation of the patient's surroundings for promotion of optimal comfort.

Positioning (0840)—Deliberative placement of the patient or a body part to promote physiologic and/or psychologic well-being.

Progressive Muscle Relaxation (1460)—Facilitating the tensing and relaxing of successive muscle groups while attending to the resulting differences in sensation.

Nursing Activities and Rationales

Assessments

- Identify specific discomforts (e.g., shortness of breath, dyspnea on exertion, backache, pedal edema). Facilitates planning of individualized, effective interventions.
- Assess for complications of pregnancy. Women with multiple gestations are at increased risk for complications because of increased uterine size, increased workload

placed on the mother, increased nutritional needs, and so on. Complications may increase the woman's discomfort or cause acute pain.

- Assess for psychologic concerns and stressors. The woman may have fear regarding her high-risk pregnancy, loss of the fetuses, and/or her ability to care for more than one infant. Identifying specific fears and concerns will guide planned interventions. Fear and anxiety can contribute to her feelings of discomfort.
- Assess sleep pattern. Determines if the woman is receiving adequate sleep and to help identify the need for changing sleep patterns. Adequate sleep is important for growing twins.
- Assess all maternal complaints out of the range of normal. All maternal complaints need to be taken seriously and assessed if out of the normal range. Education about what to expect in a high-risk pregnancy is an essential role for the nurse.

Independent Nursing Actions

- Reassure the woman that some increased discomfort is a normal part of pregnancy and does not necessarily indicate the presence of complication. Reduces fear and anxiety about discomfort. Fear and anxiety contribute to discomfort. Always be vigilant about answering questions. Do anticipatory assessment for potential problems all the time, teaching the woman about common discomforts vs. risks.
- Teach the difference between normal symptoms and those that are danger signs that need to be reported. Ensures that abnormal findings will be reported early so that interventions can be implemented. Teaching should include the difference between false labor and preterm labor; danger signs of preeclampsia; how to count fetal movements for each baby; and the need to contact the provider if fetal movements decrease.
- Teach warning signs for twin-to-twin transfusion syndrome if monochorionic (one placenta) pregnancy and the need to report signs to provider. Facilitates rapid intervention. Warning signs for twin-to-twin transfusion syndrome are rapid uterine growth, unexplained weight gain (7 lbs in 1 week), dyspnea, premature contractions, sudden increase in fatigue, and sudden increase in pressure of the back or abdomen.
- Teach the woman about maternal mirror syndrome and need to report signs to provider. Maternal mirror syndrome can occur with twin-to-twin transfusion syndrome. The mother exhibits preeclampsia-like symptoms that reflect what is occurring with the compromised twin. Signs include vomiting, hypertension, peripheral edema, proteinuria, and pulmonary edema. The nurse needs to evaluate all symptoms and not dismiss them as simply pregnancy related.

Patient/Family Teaching

- Explain the need for additional rest/sleep. Fatigue contributes to discomfort. When the woman is well rested, she is better able to withstand the physical and psychologic demands of a multifetal pregnancy.

- Teach regarding use of modified upright position or lateral position to maximize comfort. Reduces the pressure of the uterus on the diaphragm, increases the area for lung expansion, and promotes comfort. The lateral position relieves pressure on other organs and maximizes blood flow to the uterus.
- Teach the woman to place a pillow between her knees when resting/sleeping. Increases comfort by supporting the legs and may help relieve back pain associated with enlarged uterus.
- Teach progressive relaxation techniques and/or guided imagery. Facilitates muscle relaxation, reduces discomfort, and enhances sleep/rest.
- Teach the importance of contacting her healthcare provider if discomfort becomes severe. Discomfort is expected, however, acute pain or discomfort that cannot be relieved may be an indication of complications.
- Suggest eating small meals, drinking ginger tea, taking calcium carbonate (Tums) after meals (do not use excessively), decreasing the use of spices or acid foods if bothersome, and increasing protein intake. These measures may reduce heartburn.
- Encourage exercises such as pelvic tilt or tailor sit. Will help flexibility and may help ease low back pain.

Nursing Diagnosis: INTERRUPTED FAMILY PROCESSES[1]

Related Factors: anticipated dramatic increase in family size; maternal activity intolerance and discomforts; concern about fetal status; and possibility of malformations.

Goals, Outcomes, and Evaluation Criteria

The woman and/or her partner will:
- provide mutual support.
- participate in decision making.
- explain how to access disciplines needed to support high-risk pregnancy.
- acknowledge change in family roles/responsibilities and competency building.
- identify family/community resources and how to access them.
- participate in parenting preparation for multiples.

NIC Interventions[2]

Emotional Support (5270)—Provision of reassurance, acceptance, and encouragement during times of stress.
Counseling (5240)—Use of an interactive helping process focusing on the needs, problems, or feelings of the patient and

significant others to enhance or support coping, problem solving, and interpersonal relationships.
Family Integrity Promotion: Childbearing Family (7104)—Facilitation of the growth of individuals or families who are adding an infant to the family unit.
Family Process Maintenance (7130)—Minimization of family process disruption effects.
Family Support (7140)—Promotion of family values, interests, and goals.
Support System Enhancement (5440)—Facilitation of support to patient by family, friends, and community.

Nursing Activities and Rationales

Assessments

- Assess the woman's/partner's reaction to multifetal pregnancy. Identifies negative or positive reactions to multifetal pregnancy and whether or not interventions are needed to assist the couple with forming positive expectations.
- Assess learning needs and provide information and resources to meet those needs. Parents of multiples and high-risk pregnant women need additional information and education to help them understand all this entails.
- Assess for potentially destructive interactions between family members and identify positive qualities. Multifetal pregnancy may create a crisis situation for the family resulting in dysfunctional family relationships. Identifying both positive interactions and abnormal interactions that may require intervention helps the nurse determine the need for referral and counseling.
- Assess degree of financial burden multiple births will have on family resources. Financial strain is a significant factor contributing to destructive interactions and breakdown of family cohesiveness. If noted, a referral may be needed to community resources and programs.
- Assess presence of family support system. Additional family support may be needed as the couple adjusts to the sudden increase in the size of their family. If family members are not available, identify other sources of assistance. The couple may need to build networks for later support.

Independent Nursing Actions

- Encourage self-care strategies. Adequate nutrition, rest, improvement of relationships, stress management skills, and opportunities for growth into the new role will help the woman and her partner transition into their new roles.
- Encourage childbirth preparation classes. Childbirth and parenting classes prepare the woman/partner for the event and help them understand what decisions need to be made.
- Provide list of community resources and services available. The couple may be unaware of community resources available to them.
- Encourage verbalization of specific concerns. Determines if teaching and counseling are needed.

- Help woman/partner develop health seeking behaviors and ways to access community resources. The couple may be unaware of resources such as parents of multiples groups and parents as teachers for early childhood development learning.
- Explore couple's specific concerns. Enables the development of a specific plan of action that fits their needs.
- Ensure that risk-management procedures are in place. These are necessary in case the birth of twins presents a crisis situation to the woman/couple to protect the safety of the mother and infants.

Patient/Family Teaching

- Teach skills necessary for caring for more than one infant. The woman/couple may need to learn time management or other skills that will allow them to cope with the increase in family size.
- Teach basic infant care skills. New parents may be unprepared to care for more than one infant. Increasing their knowledge of how to care for their infants will decrease their anxiety.
- Teach feeding techniques and encourage classes on bottle feeding and/or breastfeeding. Preparation prior to birth of the infants will better prepare the woman/parents to care for the infants when they are born. They will need information about breastfeeding and supplementation or bottle feeding.

Nursing Diagnosis: RISK FOR ACTIVITY INTOLERANCE[1]

Related Factors: physiologic demands of multifetal pregnancy. See the generic NDCP "Activity Intolerance,[1]" which begins on p. 9 in Chapter 2.

Goals, Outcomes, and Evaluation Criteria

- Woman describes daily rest regimen.

NIC Interventions[2]

Self-Care Assistance (1800)—Assisting another to perform activities of daily living.

Sleep Enhancement (1850)—Facilitation of regular sleep/wake cycles.

Nursing Activities and Rationales

Assessments

- Assess available support systems. Evaluates the amount and quality of caregiver support available to the woman. From this information, the nurse can determine any deficits in internal support systems (family, friends, older children) and provide referrals to external caregiving sources.

- Assess severity of activity intolerance. Establishes a baseline for later comparison when evaluating effectiveness of interventions. Activity intolerance is a normal part of pregnancy that may be increased by the additional physical demands of multifetal pregnancy.

Independent Nursing Actions

- Assure the woman that it is okay and even desirable to rest when feeling fatigued. Gives the woman permission to rest when she needs to. Some women may feel guilty about taking time out to rest. Assuring her that rest is needed to conserve her energy and for the well-being of her pregnancy may increase the likelihood of resting before she becomes overly fatigued.
- Develop a specific daily rest regimen with the woman (e.g., 10 hours a night in bed, scheduled naps). Adequate rest and pacing of activities promote maternal and fetal well-being. Specifying a plan of action with the woman's input increases likelihood of compliance behaviors.
- Arrange for assistance with self-care as needed. Family and/or friends may provide needed assistance if available. Outside agencies may be needed if a deficit in support is identified or to provide relief for primary caregivers.

Patient/Family Teaching

- Teach the need for balancing activities with rest. Excessive activity or inadequate rest will increase fatigue, which can contribute to the development of complications and threaten the well-being of the pregnancy.
- Teach the necessity for at least 8 hours of uninterrupted sleep when possible. Uninterrupted sleep allows for restoration of energy, which may decrease daytime fatigue.

HYPERTENSIVE DISORDERS OF PREGNANCY

Hypertensive disorders complicate 6–8% of pregnancies and can result in life-threatening events for mother and fetus. Preeclampsia, a pregnancy-specific syndrome, is seen in about 80% of cases and chronic hypertension composes the remaining 20% of cases (Leeman & Fontaine, 2008). Terms characterizing these disorders have changed over time. Standard criteria for common use of terms are defined by the National High Blood Pressure Education Program Working Group on High Blood Pressure in Pregnancy (2000). Elevated blood pressure states occurring during pregnancy are differentiated by whether they occurred during pregnancy, labor, or early postpartum to a previously normotensive, nonproteinuric woman or if they were superimposed on a preexisting condition.

Two terms, *gestational hypertension*, which replaced the term *pregnancy-induced hypertension*, and *preeclampsia/eclampsia*, both refer to a disorder occurring in a previously normal, healthy woman. Two other terms, *chronic hypertension* and *preeclampsia superimposed on hypertension*, are related to a hypertensive disorder that existed prior to the pregnancy. This care plan focuses on nursing care for preeclampsia.

Both gestational and chronic elevation of blood pressure are defined as (1) systolic blood pressure of 140 mmHg or greater, or (2) diastolic blood pressure of 90 mmHg or greater, or (3) mean arterial pressure of 105 mmHg or greater, and (4) new onset of hypertension based on two elevated measurements within 7 days. A woman should be closely observed if her measurements demonstrate an elevation of more than 30 mmHg systolic and more than 15 mmHg diastolic above baseline obtained in early pregnancy (National High Blood Pressure, 2000). Hypertensive states of pregnancy are classified as:

- *Gestational hypertension.* The development of mild hypertension during pregnancy by a previously normotensive patient; absence of proteinuria; normal laboratory testing; may be transient and diagnosed retrospectively.
- *Preeclampsia.* The development of gestational hypertension plus proteinuria after 20 weeks of gestation or in early postpartum period; in presence of trophoblastic disease, it can develop before 20 weeks of gestation.
- *Eclampsia.* Development of seizures or coma by the woman with preeclampsia that cannot be attributed to other causes.
- *Chronic hypertension.* Hypertension present before pregnancy or blood pressure 140/90 mmHg or higher before 20 weeks' gestation on two occasions 6 hours apart.
- *Preeclampsia superimposed on chronic hypertension.* Development of preeclampsia or eclampsia by a woman with chronic hypertension. New onset or increased proteinuria, thrombocytopenia, or increases in hepatic enzymes may complicate previous well-controlled hypertension.

HELLP syndrome (hemolysis, elevated liver enzymes, and low platelet count) is a laboratory diagnosis of a variant of severe preeclampsia with hematologic and hepatic involvement. A cascade of events results in lysis of red blood cells, activation of platelet adherence and fibrin deposits, and elevation of liver enzymes with impaired liver function. Rarely, a subcapsular hematoma develops in the liver. Proteinuria may or may not be present. For intrapartal care, refer to "Intrapartum Preeclampsia," beginning on p. 271 in Chapter 8.

Key Nursing Activities

- Monitor women at risk for developing preeclampsia and teach danger signs for early detection and reporting of same.
- Monitor BP with vital signs, weight, reflexes, clonus, edema, laboratory results, and evaluation of symptoms for danger signs during each prenatal visit.
- Monitor fetal well-being, heart rate, and activity and complete fetal surveillance as ordered.
- Teach self-care and support the woman during treatment to foster adherence to the medical regimen to minimize her risks.

- Maintain calm environment and routine monitoring for toxicity and side effects if the woman is hospitalized or being treated with magnesium sulfate ($MgSO_4$).

Etiologies and Risk Factors

Risk factors for preeclampsia include:

- Primigravidae (6–8 times greater risk)
- Multipara with new father for this pregnancy at same risk as primigravida
- Age younger than 18 years or older than 35 years
- African American race
- Diabetes mellitus
- Increased placental mass due to multifetal gestation (5 times greater risk)
- Hydatidiform molar pregnancy (10 times greater risk)
- History of hypertension, renal disease, or any condition in which circulation is impaired or vasoconstriction/vasospasm are present
- Preeclampsia in a previous pregnancy
- Family history of preeclampsia or eclampsia
- Immunologic factors, e.g., antiphospholipid syndrome
- Obesity

Risks for the pregnancy and fetus from eclampsia include:

- Risks to the fetus are 1–8% with mild preeclampsia, increasing to 12% with severe preeclampsia, and as high as 60% with eclampsia and HELLP syndrome.
- Placental insufficiency, which can cause intrauterine growth retardation, oligohydramnios, nonreassuring fetal status, and placental abruption. Morbidity and mortality for fetus are because of prematurity associated with preterm delivery or premature separation of the placenta or abruptio placentae.
- Maternal morbidity and mortality can occur with abruptio placentae, seizures, acute renal or hepatic failure, pulmonary edema or embolism, stroke, cardiac dysfunction with myocardial infarction, and cerebral hemorrhage.

Preeclampsia is a pregnancy-specific syndrome ranging from very mild to severe symptoms. Although the exact cause of preeclampsia is not fully understood, the underlying pathophysiology is based on responses to decreased perfusion, vasospasm, endothelial cell damage, and platelet aggregation. Elevation of blood pressure is accompanied by a systemic disorder involving multiple organs with both maternal and fetal manifestations. It begins with alterations in placental perfusion (stage 1) and then develops into a maternal syndrome (stage 2). Changes that take place include:

- *Uteroplacental insufficiency.* The placental arteries fail to create spiral arterioles that function so that cytotrophoblastic tissue can migrate and displace the musculoelastic structures to widen and increase blood flow. This failure of normal development decreases blood flow and impedes normal development and attachment of the placenta. This leads to decreased placental perfusion and subsequent placental hypoxia. Lack of oxygen to the placenta triggers a release of toxic substances that damage endothelial cells throughout the organs of the body. Endothelial cells line all blood vessels contributing to vessel wall integrity, preventing coagulation, modulating contractility, and providing immune and inflammatory response regulation. The onset of the maternal syndrome is from endothelial damage, loss of vasodilation, increasing blood pressure, and loss of multiorgan system regulation. Blood pressure elevation may be reflective of the extent of trophoblastic invasion by the placenta.

- *Renal compromise.* As the process continues, the kidneys sustain glomerular endothelial damage from fibrin deposits and reduction of blood flow. This results in decreased glomerular filtration rate. Increased capillary permeability in the kidneys allows albumin to escape into the urine, causing proteinuria and decreasing serum albumin levels. The reduced glomerular filtration rate results in decreased urine output and increased serum levels of creatinine, blood urea nitrogen, uric acid, and sodium. Vasospasms, worsening of preeclampsia, and sodium retention contribute to oliguria and edema.

- *Fluid and electrolyte imbalance.* During normal pregnancy, fluid tends to shift from the intracellular to the extracellular compartment because of normal hemodilution (pregnancy reduces colloid osmotic pressure in the intravascular compartment). In preeclampsia, there is further movement of fluid in that direction, causing edema from increased capillary permeability. This further decreases plasma colloid osmotic pressure and moves even more fluid to the extracellular spaces. It also increases sensitivity to the pressor effects of angiotensin II and endothelin, which causes decreased production of endothelium relaxing faction and subsequent damage to endothelial cells. Decreased intravascular volume causes increased blood viscosity and elevated hematocrit. In a normal pregnancy, the ratio of *thromboxane* (a vasoconstrictor) and *prostacyclin* (a vasodilator) is 1:1. Women with preeclampsia produce much more thromboxane than prostacyclin. This imbalance results in vasoconstriction and platelet aggregation. The coagulation cascade is activated, causing increased platelets and fibrin deposits at sites of the damage. As preeclampsia worsens, more systems are affected, which indicates that the condition is progressing. More changes are seen as more systems are involved.

- *Pulmonary involvement.* Pulmonary edema may develop, the most common reasons being volume overload due to left ventricular failure from high vascular resistance, IV fluids infused during treatment, and postpartum diuresis. Other causative factors include decreased colloid osmotic pressure or endothelial injury causing increasing pulmonary capillary permeability and fluid leak.

- *Central nervous involvement.* Endothelial damage to the cortical region of the brain results in fibrin deposition, edema, and cerebral hemorrhage. Physical signs and symptoms are hyperreflexia, clonus, severe headaches, visual disturbances, and changes in consciousness leading up to seizure and eclampsia.

- *Ophthalmic involvement.* Visual changes may occur, which may be related to arteriolar narrowing. They include scotoma, photophobia, blurring, and diplopia from retinal arteriolar spasms.

- *Hemodynamic changes.* Signs are related to systemic fluid shifts, including elevated blood pressure, pulmonary edema, volume overload, and oliguria (as previously discussed).

- *Coagulation involvement.* Endothelial damage activates the clotting cascade with decreased production of platelets. Thrombocytopenia and hemolysis can be initiated. This can lead to DIC in 10% of preeclamptic patients. Refer to the collaborative care plan, "Potential Complication: Disseminated Intravascular Coagulation," beginning on p. 26 in Chapter 3, or refer to a critical care textbook for further information about DIC.

- *Hepatic involvement.* Loss of perfusion to the liver and fibrin deposits can result in mild hepatocellular necrosis as evidenced by increased liver enzymes or severe dysfunction as seen in HELLP syndrome. Approximately 10% of patients may have periportal hemorrhagic necrosis, which can cause subcapsular hematoma. On rare occasions, this can rupture, resulting in maternal death. Hyperbilirubinemia may be present if increased lysis of red blood cells occurs. Right upper quadrant pain or epigastric pain may signal liver involvement and needs to be evaluated. Refer to HELLP syndrome discussed earlier in this chapter.

- *Eclampsia.* Severe persistent headache, visual changes (described earlier), epigastric pain, and restlessness can be precursors to seizures. In 20% of patients who have seizures, no elevation of blood pressure is present.

▋ Signs and Symptoms

Signs and symptoms correlate with the system affected. It is helpful to understand the link to the expression of the problem (type of hypertension) to the expression of the symptoms as the disorder progresses and becomes more serious. Accurate assessment can lead to early detection of worsening preeclampsia so that initiation of treatment can begin at the earliest possible time.

Chronic Hypertension

- Hypertension diagnosed either before pregnancy or diagnosed before 20 weeks' gestation

Gestational Hypertension

- Mild elevations in BP; systolic BP greater than or equal to 140 mmHg or diastolic greater than or equal to 90
- No other signs or symptoms of preeclampsia; no proteinuria or subjective symptoms
- No history of preexisting hypertension

Mild Preeclampsia

- BP greater than 140/90 mmHg, mean arterial pressure greater than 105 mmHg
- Proteinuria; normal serum creatinine

- Absent thrombocytopenia, normal or minimal elevation of aspartate aminotransferase
- Urine output matching intake, greater than or equal to 30 ml/hr or greater than 650 ml/24 hr
- Normal reflexes, no clonus
- Absent or transient headache, transient irritability, or change in affect
- No visual problems
- No nausea or epigastric pain
- Weight gain more than anticipated for gestation (expected gain in second and third trimesters is slightly less than 1 lb/wk)
- Fetal effects: reduced placental perfusion, no apparent premature placental aging

Severe Preeclampsia

Severe preeclampsia may develop suddenly.

- BP 160 mmHg systolic or 110 mmHg diastolic or greater; recorded on at least 2 occasions at least 6 hours apart, with patient on bed rest; mean arterial pressure greater than 105 mmHg
- Proteinuria greater that 2 g in 24 hours; 2+ or 3+ on dipstick
- Thrombocytopenia present, also marked alanine aminotransferase elevation
- Urine output 20 ml/hr or less than 400–500 ml in 24 hr (oliguria)
- Hyperreflexia greater than 3; possible ankle clonus
- Severe headache with altered state of consciousness, confusion, drowsiness, dizziness
- Visual disturbances present: blurred vision, diplopia, scotoma, blind spots on funduscopy
- Epigastric pain, right upper quadrant pain
- Pulmonary edema or cyanosis (dyspnea, auscultation of crackles or rhonchi)
- Increased weight gain and/or possible edema (especially of the face, fingers)
- Fetal effects: intrauterine growth restriction due to decreased placental perfusion; at birth, premature aging of placenta apparent with broken syncytia, ischemic necroses, and intervillous fibrin deposition present

Eclampsia

- Seizures, convulsions, or coma in a woman with preeclampsia, not attributable to other causes. One third of women develop eclampsia during pregnancy; one third during labor; and one third within 72 hours postpartum.

▌ Diagnostic Studies

- 24-hour urine collections for protein and/or creatinine clearance. Proteinuria is defined as equal to or greater than 30 mg/dl (equal to or greater than 1+ on dipstick) at least 2 random urine samples collected at least 6 hours apart; or equal to or greater than 0.3 g in a 24-hour specimen. Elevation of creatinine clearance in range of 130–180 ml/min. Reflective of glomerular damage or recovery and is part of criteria for diagnosis of preeclampsia.
- CBC or hemoglobin/hematocrit. Detects hemoconcentration. Increased with preeclampsia and decreased with hemolysis in HELLP; normal 12–16 g/dl, 37–47%.
- Platelets. Normal 150,000–400,000/mm^3. In preeclampsia, platelets may be unchanged or lowered; in HELLP, platelets will be lowered due to aggregation and fewer in circulation.
- Clotting studies, including prothrombin, partial prothrombin time. Normal 12–14 sec/60–70 sec; remain unchanged.
- Fibrinogen (normal 200–400 mg/dl)/fibrin split products (normal is absent). In preeclampsia, fibrinogen is 300–600 mg/dl; in HELLP, fibrinogen will be lower due to accumulation of fibrin in blood vessels; fibrinogen normally does not split, may or may not be present in preeclampsia, but will be present in HELLP because of cascading of events previously discussed.
- Liver function studies. Liver enzymes—lactate dehydrogenase (normal 45–90 units/L); aspartate aminotransferase (normal 4–20 units/L); alanine aminotransferase (normal 3–21 units/L). Determines if liver compromise has occurred; lactase dehydrogenase will elevate initially and may be seen in preeclampsia. Aspartate aminotransferase or alanine aminotransferase may be minimally elevated or normal. In HELLP, all will be elevated due to hepatic damage.
- Renal function tests. Blood urea nitrogen (normal 10–20 mg/dl); uric acid (normal 2–6.6 mg/dl); creatinine (normal 0.5–1.1 mg/dl). Blood urea nitrogen and uric acid are elevated because of reduced glomerular filtration rate, and creatinine clearance is decreased in both preeclampsia and HELLP.
- Burr cells or schistocytes. Normally absent, will not be seen in preeclampsia, but are present in HELLP because of blood cell changes.
- Bilirubin total (normal 0.1–1 mg/dl). Indicates lyses of RBCs and is by-product of cellular death. It is less than 1.2 mg/dl in preeclampsia; in HELLP it is increased to greater than 1.2 mg/dl.
- Electrolytes. Detects fluid and electrolyte imbalances (e.g., hypernatremia/hyponatremia).
- Ultrasound or serial sonography. Determines fetal size and position; evaluates and grades placenta, which is where changes initially occur. Should be done every 3 weeks to confirm and compare fetal growth.
- Amniocentesis. Assesses for fetal lung maturity and fetal readiness to be delivered because birth is the cure for preeclampsia.
- Nonstress tests (NST) and biophysical profile (BPP). Determines fetal well-being and is routinely done twice weekly for fetal surveillance.
- MgSO$_4$ levels. Monitors for maintenance of therapeutic range and to prevent toxicity.

■ *Medical Management*

Mild Preeclampsia (Home Care)

- Expectant management at home may be an option for monitoring women with mild gestational hypertension or mild preeclampsia with no subjective complaints and access to care and hospitals.
- Must have frequent evaluation at home or in office or clinic (2–3 times per week) for BP, fetal well-being, fetal activity, preterm labor, and signs of progression.
- If home care nursing is not available, woman must be taught to perform self-assessment daily to include weight, urine dipstick protein evaluation, BP measurement, and fetal movement counting.
- Laboratory tests may be done weekly.
- Bed rest in side-lying, lateral recumbent position, continuous or in 2–3 hour blocks of time at least twice daily as determined by severity of condition; diversion activities are important.
- Well-balanced diet with moderate-to-high protein content (60–70 g/day) and sufficient water intake and roughage. Avoid alcohol and limit caffeine intake. Replaces protein lost in the urine and maintains healthful diet to support pregnancy.
- Water therapy may be used. Water immersion in tub or swimming pool has shown to be helpful in reducing blood pressure.
- Ensure the woman/family know and are willing to report signs and symptoms of worsening condition, including BP changes, protein in urine, weight gain, decreased fetal movement, and signs of abruptio placentae, uterine irritability, and premature labor.
- Fetal surveillance, including fetal movement daily, ultrasound every three weeks, NST once or twice weekly, and BPP as needed.

Mild Preeclampsia (Hospital Care)

- Ideally, hospitalize for evaluation of maternal and fetal condition.
- If at or near term, induce labor with oxytocin; vaginal birth is delivery of choice; epidural analgesia is recommended if needed.
- Bed rest, primarily on left side. Increases venous return and improves renal and placental perfusion.
- Well-balanced diet with moderate-to-high protein content (60–70 g/day), sufficient water intake, roughage, avoidance of alcohol, and limited caffeine intake. Replaces protein lost in the urine and maintains healthful diet to support pregnancy.
- Monitor BP, lung sounds, reflexes, fetal status, laboratory data, and liver and renal function. Evaluates for progression of preeclampsia.

Severe Preeclampsia (Required Hospitalization)

- Administration of intravenous hydralazine and/or labetalol. Control BP, thereby maintaining uterine and placental blood flow.
- Administration of IV magnesium sulfate per protocol with adequate monitoring to avoid toxicity. Prevents and treats seizures in a woman with severe preeclampsia or eclampsia. This medication requires careful hourly monitoring to avoid side effects and complications. Refer to "Potential Complications of Use of Magnesium Sulfate Therapy to Control Seizures," beginning on p. 177 in this care plan.
- Ensure that calcium gluconate is available. Counters magnesium toxicity if it develops.
- Replace fluids and electrolytes as prescribed based on laboratory studies and maintain accurate intake and output. Accurate I and O is essential because of risk of fluid overload and resulting pulmonary edema.
- Auscultate lung sounds over anterior and posterior chest, including all five lobes. Detects signs of pulmonary edema. Crackles and rhonchi are abnormal lung sounds that indicate the presence of pulmonary edema or respiratory compromise.
- Perform fetal surveillance and monitoring. Fetal status must be evaluated because of risks to the fetus from the disorder and medications.
- Assess for early labor or abruptio. These can occur with preeclampsia. Uterine irritability or changes in softness of abdomen should be noted and reported immediately.
- Provide a calm, quiet, and darkened environment. Prevents stimulation, which may trigger seizures.
- Regulate visitors but do not completely restrict. Continues calm environment. Woman may find it more upsetting to not see visitors, but visits must be regulated to avoid overstimulation.

At 28–32 weeks' gestation:

- Administer corticosteroids (betamethasone or dexamethasone). Accelerates fetal lung maturity. About 24–36 hours is needed to complete required doses.
- Monitor for fetal distress. Expectant management includes frequent evaluation and delivery at 34 weeks' gestation or before if there is maternal or fetal distress. Aggressive management includes administration of steroids and delivery within 72 hours by induction if cervix favorable, by cesarean if not.

■ *Collaborative Problems*

Potential complications of hypertensive disorders and preeclampsia include the following:

- Ineffective tissue perfusion (pulmonary, renal, cerebral, cardiac, hepatic, peripheral) (a nursing diagnosis)
- Eclampsia (seizures) and/or coma
- HELLP syndrome

- Hemorrhage secondary to placental separation, HELLP syndrome, and/or DIC
- Fetal compromise

Potential complications of magnesium sulfate therapy include the following:

- CNS depression
- Fluid overload
- Magnesium toxicity

COLLABORATIVE (STANDARDIZED CARE) FOR ALL WOMEN WITH GESTATIONAL HYPERTENSION

Perform comprehensive assessment to identify individual needs for teaching, emotional support, and physical care.

Nursing Diagnosis: INEFFECTIVE TISSUE PERFUSION (PULMONARY, CARDIOVASCULAR, RENAL, CEREBRAL, AND HEPATIC)[1]

Related Factors: vasospasm, vasoconstriction, and increased systemic vascular resistance; decreased colloid osmotic pressure in the intravascular compartment due to normal physiologic edema; loss of fluid from the intravascular to the extracellular compartment, and systemic endothelial cellular damage.

Goals, Outcomes, and Evaluation Criteria

- Woman maintains blood pressure at or near baseline throughout pregnancy.
- Woman remains free of danger signs and symptoms of preeclampsia, elevating blood pressure, proteinuria, hyperreflexia, clonus, headaches, visual disturbances, edema, and free of signs of premature labor or abruptio placentae.
- Woman maintains weight within expected range for gestation and maintains appropriate fetal growth.
- Woman verbalizes understanding of preeclampsia and self-care measures required.
- Woman achieves positive pregnancy outcomes.

NIC Interventions[2]

Cerebral Perfusion Promotion (2550)—Promotion of adequate perfusion and limitation of complications for a patient experiencing or at risk for inadequate cerebral perfusion.

Circulatory Care: Arterial Insufficiency (4062)—Promotion of arterial circulation.

Fluid Management (4120)—Promotion of fluid balance and prevention of complications resulting from abnormal or undesired fluid levels.

Fluid Monitoring (4130)—Collection and analysis of patient data to regulate fluid balance.

Fluid/Electrolyte Management (2080)—Regulation and prevention of complications from altered fluid and/or electrolyte levels.

Neurologic Monitoring (2620)—Collection and analysis of patient data to prevent or minimize neurologic complications.

Respiratory Monitoring (3350)—Collection and analysis of patient data to ensure airway patency and adequate gas exchange.

Risk Identification (6610)—Analysis of potential risk factors, determination of health risks, and prioritization of risk-reduction strategies for an individual or group.

Surveillance (6650)—Purposeful and ongoing acquisition, interpretation, and synthesis of patient data for clinical decision making.

Vital Signs Monitoring (6680)—Collection and analysis of cardiovascular, respiratory, and body temperature data to determine and prevent complications.

Nursing Activities and Rationales

Assessments

- Assess for risk factors by obtaining a full history and completing exam on the first prenatal visit. Identifies those women who are at increased risk so that hypertension can be detected early in the disease process and carefully assessed on each subsequent visit.
- Establish baseline (BP, VSs, lung sounds, presence of edema, signs and symptoms of preeclampsia) on first prenatal visit. Provides a source for later comparison so that small changes will be detected early on future visits.
- Monitor weight and fundal height at each prenatal visit or daily weight if hospitalized or on home care. Indicates fluid retention and circulation status. Fundal height indicates adequate fetal growth. Oligohydramnios or IUGR can be indicative of poor placental perfusion.
- Assess laboratory data. Detects alterations that indicate renal, hematologic, cerebral, peripheral, or hepatic perfusion problems (see "Diagnostic Studies," on p. 173 and "Signs and Symptoms" on p. 172).
- Assess maternal heart rate pattern. Decreased perfusion, alterations in fluid volume and electrolyte levels, and renal damage affect circulation and cause corresponding changes in heart rate pattern, such as tachycardia.
- Assess peripheral circulation (e.g., edema, skin color, temperature of extremities, capillary refill time, peripheral pulses). The peripheral pulse should be equal to the apical heart rate; skin color should be normal; temperature warm to touch; and capillary refill time less than 3 sec. Dependent

edema is normal in pregnancy; however, edema in nondependent areas such as the face, hands, and sacrum is a sign of preeclampsia.

- Assess for pain. Headaches, especially frontal, are a sign of preeclampsia; epigastric pain is a sign of liver congestion; and edema and decreased perfusion may cause pain and discomfort at other sites.

- Assess for signs of CNS irritability. Changes in pupil reaction and eye movement, changes in deep tendon reflexes, and clonus are indications of central nervous system irritability resulting from edema and decreased perfusion. Hyperreactivity indicates progression from preeclampsia to severe preeclampsia.

- If hospitalized, measure every voiding if woman does not have an indwelling catheter. Output of less than 30 ml/hr (or less than 700 ml/24 hours) is a sign of renal compromise. Intake should approximately correlate with output.

- If hospitalized, measure hourly urine protein, or measure with each voiding (per healthcare provider order). A reading of 3+ or 4+ is a sign of glomerular compromise and severe preeclampsia.

- Measure hourly urine specific gravity as ordered. Readings greater than 1.040 correlate with oliguria and proteinuria.

- Assess for visual changes (dark spots or flashing lights in the field of vision). This is a sign of impending eclampsia.

- Assess for loss of vision (usually temporary). This is a sign of impending cerebral hemorrhage, the most urgent complication of eclampsia.

- Assess home environment, woman's ability to assume self-care responsibilities, support systems, language, age, culture, beliefs, and effects of illness. Determines if home care is an option for her care. It is important to know her access to care and her ability to care for self. If a support system is not present, she will need to be hospitalized when her condition worsens.

Independent Nursing Actions

- Establish rapport and trusting relationship during the first-trimester prenatal visits. Helps ensure compliance for return visits for future assessments.

- Encourage frequent rest periods and aid with position changes avoiding lying on back in lateral recumbent position. Relieves stress and fatigue, which can exacerbate symptoms. Changing positions increases uteroplacental blood flow and tissue perfusion, and avoiding back position increases uterine profusion, preventing compression of inferior vena cava and aorta.

Collaborative Activities (When Hospitalized)

- Administer IV fluids as prescribed or maintain IV access via heparin lock. Maintains fluid balance and provides access for blood if needed. In preeclampsia, the intravascular compartment loses fluid and hypovolemia can occur very quickly. It is difficult to establish venous access in hypovolemic individuals. An IV line also may be necessary for administration of medications.

- Administer medications as prescribed and monitor for therapeutic and side effects. Antihypertensive medications require BP monitoring before and after administration. $MgSO_4$ administration requires frequent assessment of the BP, respiratory rate, urinary output of at least 30 ml per hour, the presence of deep tendon reflexes, clonus check, level of consciousness, fetal status, and laboratory levels for therapeutic or toxic magnesium levels.

- Administer oxygen as prescribed. Promotes adequate oxygenation of maternal and fetal tissues. If perfusion is decreased, then it is important that the blood that does circulate to the tissues be as rich in oxygen as possible.

Patient/Family Teaching

- Teach the importance of rest and avoidance of back-lying position, use of preferred side-lying position, and how it improves renal perfusion. The kidneys are more efficient during sleep. The kidneys receive a greater blood supply when demands by other organs are reduced. Also, when the body is horizontal, blood does not pool as much in the lower extremities, thereby increasing the circulating volume available to the kidneys. Understanding may promote compliance with activity restrictions.

- Teach about hypertension and preeclampsia and the complications that can occur if not managed and controlled. May promote adherence to the treatment plan by increasing the woman's understanding of the threat to the fetus and her own health if the disease progresses.

- Teach about diet and self-care as mentioned previously. Increases the probability of a positive outcome for mother and fetus.

Potential Complications of Preeclampsia: ECLAMPSIA (SEIZURES), COMA

Refer to "Intrapartal Preeclampsia," which begins on p. 271 in Chapter 8.

Potential Complication of Preeclampsia: HELLP SYNDROME

Refer to "Intrapartal Preeclampsia," which begins on p. 271 in Chapter 8.

Potential Complication of Preeclampsia: FETAL COMPROMISE

Refer to the generic collaborative care plan, "Potential Complication: Fetal Compromise (Nonreassuring Fetal Heart Rate Tracing)," which begins on p. 27 in Chapter 3. Also refer to "Antepartum Fetal Monitoring and Other Diagnostic Tests," beginning on p. 60 in Chapter 4.

Focus Assessments

- Assess for symptoms of preeclampsia. Determines risk to fetal status.
- Perform continuous fetal monitoring as indicated if medications are continuous. When interpreting FHR pattern, note whether the woman is receiving magnesium sulfate or other medications. These medications may decrease FHR variability and cause CNS depression of the newborn.
- Assess fetal movement. Fetal activity is reassuring for both the nurse and the mother because it indicates fetal well-being.

Preventive Nursing Activities

- Encourage the woman to remain in lateral position or use wedge under buttock if supine. Increases venous return and promotes optimal blood flow to the placenta by preventing compression of the aorta and inferior vena cava by the gravid uterus.
- Ensure that emergency delivery pack, suction, oxygen, and emergency medications (such as calcium gluconate if on magnesium sulfate) are at bedside or nearby. For immediate use in case of seizure or emergency delivery.

Potential Complications of Use of Magnesium Sulfate Therapy to Control Seizures: CNS AND NEUROMUSCULAR DEPRESSION, RESPIRATORY DEPRESSION, AND DECREASED CARDIAC CONDUCTION

Focus Assessments

- Monitor BP, pulse, and respirations closely while administering loading dose; then every 15–30 minutes, depending on the woman's condition. Slow administration will relieve some of the flushing and potential nausea and vomiting that

can occur from $MgSO_4$. It is administered to prevent and control seizures. It can cause a lowering of the BP as a result of relaxation of smooth muscle. It interferes with the release of acetylcholine at nerve synapses, decreases neuromuscular and CNS irritability, and depresses cardiac conduction; therefore, heart rate and respirations may be slowed.

- Carefully monitor urine output. If therapeutic effects occur, arteriolar spasms will be relaxed, kidney perfusion will improve, fluid will move from interstitial spaces to the intravascular space, and diuresis will occur. Serum magnesium levels rise in the presence of oliguria because it is excreted in the urine; therefore, output must be closely monitored.
- Assess for signs of magnesium toxicity (e.g., hyporeflexia, respiratory rate less than 12 breaths/min, lethargy, hypotension, urine output less than 30 ml/hr, altered mental status). Loss of reflexes is often the first sign that toxicity is developing. If respirations, urinary output, or reflexes fall below specified levels, magnesium sulfate is discontinued and calcium gluconate may need to be administered for reversal of drug effects.
- Monitor serum magnesium levels. Determines if blood levels are therapeutic without producing toxicity. Therapeutic levels are in the range of 4–7 mg/dl. Some signs of toxicity (e.g., loss of reflexes) occur at levels of 8–12 mg/dl, but some women are more sensitive to medication so physical assessments are essential. Magnesium sulfate is excreted by the kidneys; when kidney function is affected by preeclampsia; toxic magnesium levels develop quickly.

Preventive Nursing Activities

- Administer as a secondary piggyback IV and by volumetric pump since dosages are small and critical. This allows for better control of infusion and the ability to discontinue the infusion if necessary while still retaining mainline fluids. An initial dose of 4–6 g of magnesium sulfate per protocol or provider's order is infused over 15–20 minutes and then maintained at 2 g/hr. Fans, cool cloths, or removal of heavy bedding may be helpful since magnesium causes flushing and nausea, and vomiting often develops. An emesis basin should be close by.
- Ensure that calcium gluconate is available at bedside. Antagonist of $MgSO_4$; administered IV push in case of severe toxicity with respiratory depression per order or protocol.
- Insert indwelling urinary catheter (for severe preeclampsia or if hourly I and O is needed). Facilitates monitoring of output. The woman will be on bed rest and may or may not have bathroom privileges. If urine output decreases, a catheter provides more accurate urine output measurement.
- Regulate fluid intake during magnesium therapy. Prevents fluid overload and pulmonary edema that can occur easily from this condition.

INDIVIDUALIZED (NURSING DIAGNOSIS) CARE PLANS

This section includes care plans that have been developed to meet unique patient needs.

Nursing Diagnosis: FLUID VOLUME EXCESS (EXTRACELLULAR)[1]

Related Factors: fluid shift from intravascular to extracellular tissues; normal physiologic hemodilution of pregnancy; sodium and water retention; and compromised renal function.

Goals, Outcomes, and Evaluation Criteria

- Serum electrolytes within normal limits.
- Serum blood urea nitrogen, creatinine, and uric acid within safe range.
- BP stable.
- Temperature within normal limits
- Urinary output greater than 30 ml/hr.
- Lungs clear to auscultation.
- Absence of generalized (face, fingers) edema.

NIC Interventions[2]

Fluid Management (4120)—Promotion of fluid balance and prevention of complications resulting from abnormal or undesired fluid levels.

Fluid Monitoring (4130)—Collection and analysis of patient data to regulate fluid balance.

Fluid/Electrolyte Management (2080)—Regulation and prevention of complications from altered fluid and/or electrolyte levels.

Nursing Activities and Rationales

Assessments

- Assess weight and pattern of weight gain on every prenatal visit, using the same scale. If hospitalized, weigh daily on the same scale at approximately the same time of day, and dressed in the same clothing. Weight measurement is a good indicator of fluid gains or losses. Normal weight gain during the second and third trimesters is slightly less than 1 pound a week. A sudden weight gain of 2 kg/week is usually associated with preeclampsia. A weight gain of 3 kg/month is a sign of preeclampsia. Weighing on the same scale, at approximately the same time of day, and with the same type of clothing provides a more accurate assessment of the weight gain or loss.
- Assess respiratory status. For respiratory assessments, see NDCP for "Ineffective Tissue Perfusion (Pulmonary,

Cardiovascular, Renal, Cerebral, and Hepatic),[1]" beginning on p. 175 in this chapter.
- Assess for presence of generalized and pitting edema. Pregnant women normally develop dependent edema in their feet and ankles because of elevated progesterone levels and hemodilution of pregnancy. Generalized edema is not normal. The presence of pitting edema in the pretibial area, face, hands, and sacrum is an indicator of fluid retention.
- Ask the woman if her face seems more puffy or swollen and if her rings fit tighter than usual. The woman may be the first to recognize signs of fluid retention, but family members often notice and comment even before the woman notices. Edema other than pedal can be an indicator of shifting fluids.
- Assess urine color and amount hourly and at 24-hour intervals, if the woman is hospitalized. Urine becomes more concentrated as fluid shifts from the intravascular to extracellular areas. When in the tissues, fluid is not delivered to, filtered by, or eliminated from the kidneys. As glomerular filtration decreases and renal damage occurs, urine output will decrease and become concentrated and blood-tinged. Cellular debris may be visible.

Independent Nursing Actions

- Assist the woman to a comfortable position and encourage her to elevate feet and legs and lie on her left side. Decreases peripheral and dependent edema and promotes optimal blood return to the heart.

Collaborative Activities

- Administer IV fluids as prescribed. Even though there is an excess of fluid in tissues, the intravascular system is experiencing a deficit. If the woman starts to bleed (e.g., HELLP syndrome, DIC), hypovolemia can occur very quickly because of the preexisting low intravascular fluid volume. Fluid volume replacement is based on urinary output and insensible fluid losses.

Patient/Family Teaching

- Teach the woman the importance of maintaining I and O records. Allows the woman some control of her situation by being an active participant in her care. The woman will not be hospitalized unless preeclampsia becomes severe. Maintaining accurate records will help the nurse determine fluid status and the need for intervention.
- Teach the woman how to collect needed urine specimens. Urine collections are often needed to determine quantity, creatinine clearance, and proteinuria. Accuracy of collection can be better insured if the woman understands how to collect her specimen and the importance of maintaining procedural protocols.
- Teach about the use of dietary sodium. Excessive sodium intake may increase water retention. Sodium is not restricted but should not be used excessively, either.

- Teach to maintain adequate oral fluid intake. Even though there is an excess of fluid in tissues, the intravascular system is experiencing a deficit.
- Teach to include adequate protein in her diet. Protein lost in the urine must be replaced to support tissue repair and maintain energy.

Nursing Diagnosis: ANXIETY[1]

Related Factors: threat to maternal and/or fetal well-being and concern about preeclampsia and risks to self and fetus. See the generic NDCPs, "Anxiety[1]" and "Fear,[1]" beginning on pp. 10 and 15, respectively, in Chapter 2.

Goals, Outcomes, and Evaluation Criteria

- Woman reports use of relaxation techniques and other coping strategies.
- Woman verbalizes her fears and concerns freely.
- Woman reports decreased feelings and symptoms of anxiety.

Nursing Activities and Rationales

Assessments

- Assess prior experiences with hypertension and/or pre-eclampsia. Determines if the woman has prior negative or positive experiences with hypertension that are currently influencing her reactions to her condition.
- Assess knowledge of hypertension and preeclampsia. The woman may have received home care before admission, heard reports from others, looked it up on the Internet, or received education through the healthcare provider's office. The nurse needs a baseline to individualize the teaching plan and eliminate misconceptions to reduce fear and anxiety.
- Assess for factors that create anxiety for the woman. Determines factors that need to be avoided or altered to prevent increased anxiety during this stressful period of time.
- Assess the woman's support systems. Determines if the woman has adequate support systems or needs to be referred for community assistance.

Independent Nursing Actions

- Actively listen to the woman's concerns about herself, her condition, and her fears. Validates the woman's feelings and conveys a sense of caring and concern. By identifying the woman's fears and concerns, appropriate interventions can be planned to reduce or eliminate those fears.

Patient/Family Teaching

- Provide a safe, calm, quiet environment to teach family and to provide emotional support. Facilitates coping.
- Encourage verbalization of anxiety, concerns, and fears. Decreases emotional response and allows venting of feelings.

- Involve woman and family in the management of her preeclamptic condition. Promotes greater sense of control of the situation.
- Aid woman in identifying and utilizing appropriate coping strategies and support systems. Reduces fear, anxiety, and lack of control in unknown situation.
- Teach and explore ways to relax, desensitize anxious feelings, and stop thoughts that are persistent by using relaxation, breathing, and other coping strategies. Helps prevent anxiety, gives the woman something to concentrate on, and diverts her attention away from fear, which may improve tissue perfusion.
- Teach about plan of care, treatments, and timeline of events. Facilitates woman's understanding of the possibilities for treatment in realistic terms, and answers her questions so she can better verbalize the aspect of care about which she is anxious.

Nursing Diagnosis: DEFICIENT KNOWLEDGE REGARDING TREATMENT PLAN FOR HYPERTENSIVE DISORDERS OF PREGNANCY: MANAGEMENT OF ACTIVITY, DIET, AND MEDICATIONS[1]

Teaching specific to hypertension has been integrated into the preceding care plans. Also see the generic NDCP, "Deficient Knowledge,[1]" which begins on p. 13 in Chapter 2.

LATE ANTEPARTUM BLEEDING

Vaginal bleeding may occur any time during pregnancy. Approximately 50% of bleeding in late pregnancy is due to abruptio placentae and placenta previa. Other causes are vaso previa, invasive placenta, cervical carcinoma, polyps, cervical or vaginal infection, velamentous insertion of the cord, and placenta succenturiate. This care plan will focus on the two most common. An *abruptio placenta* is the detachment of all or part of a normal placenta from its implantation site in the uterus. It occurs in approximately 1% of pregnancies with increased incidence in subsequent pregnancies. Abruption is classified as *grade 1* (mild, 10–20% separation), *grade 2* (moderate, 20–50% separation), or *grade 3* (severe, greater than 50% separation). Maternal bleeding is classified as *marginal* or *apparent* (separation near the edge with active bleeding), *central* or *concealed* (separation at center with entrapment of blood), and *missed* or *combined* (with separation at edge and center of placenta, with some active bleeding and some trapped). Abruptio placentae can occur prior to or during labor in about 1% of pregnancies and is a leading cause of vaginal bleeding in the last half of gestation.

Placenta previa is the implantation of the placenta in the lower uterine segment near or over the internal cervical os. The incidence is 1 in 200 births. Placenta previa is classified according to the degree to which the cervical os is covered by the placenta; that is, *complete* (total), *incomplete* (partial), *marginal*, or *low lying* (planted in the lower uterine segment, but not reaching the os). Either condition can precipitate a hemorrhagic disorder with extensive bleeding and both are medical emergencies.

▌ Key Nursing Activities

- Obtain history and assessment to help determine the cause of the bleeding.
- Monitor for hemorrhage and shock; institute measures for prevention or early treatment.
- Monitor for fetal well-being and assess for presence of fetal distress and bleeding.
- Monitor for and assist with preventing the onset of labor.
- Provide emotional support and information.

▌ Etiologies and Risk Factors

The etiologies of abruptio placentae and placenta previa are unknown. Risk factors for abruptio placentae include pregnancy-induced or chronic hypertension, previous abruption in a previous pregnancy, trauma to the abdomen, cigarette use, cocaine use, PROM, hydramnios, infection, advanced maternal age, clotting disorders, and hyperhomocystinuria. Complications include shock, disseminated intravascular coagulation, renal failure, and pituitary necrosis (Sheehan syndrome) with resulting disruption of lactation. Bleeding in the early part of pregnancy is associated with increased risk for abruption. Perinatal morality is approximately 14 in 1,000. Other problems are fetal hypoxia, prematurity, intrauterine growth restriction, and neurologic defects.

Factors that increase the risk of placenta previa are previous placenta previa, endometrial scarring from previous uterine surgeries (including cesarean section and induced abortion), decreased endometrial vascularization (hypertension, diabetes, uterine tumor, drug usage, cigarette smoking, advancing maternal age), and increased placental mass as in multiple pregnancy. Maternal complications include hemorrhage and hypovolemic shock, invasive placenta (accrete, increta, and percreta), septicemia, thrombosis, renal failure, Rh sensitization, and postpartum anemia. Fetal and neonatal effects include prematurity, malpresentation, intrauterine growth restriction, and fetal anemia (Gilbert, 2010).

▌ Signs and Symptoms

Suspect placenta previa or placental abruption whenever there is vaginal bleeding after 20 weeks' gestation.

Abruptio Placentae

Classic presentation is vaginal bleeding and abdominal pain; however, abruption can occur with neither of these. The extent of the abruption correlates with the risk of stillbirth. This condition can present as disseminated intravascular coagulopathy in severe concealed abruption. Symptoms vary with the degree of the condition, which can be mild, moderate, or severe, as explained next.

- Mild. Vital signs normal, total blood loss less than 500 ml, dark vaginal bleeding (mild to moderate), vague lower abdominal or back discomfort, no uterine tenderness or irritability, normal FHR pattern, normal fibrinogen of 450 mg/dl.
- Moderate. VSs include normal BP, mild shock with maternal tachycardia, narrowed pulse pressure, orthostatic hypotension, tachypnea; total blood loss of 1,000–1,500 ml, dark vaginal bleeding (mild to severe), gradual or abrupt onset of abdominal pain, uterine tenderness, increased uterine tone, early signs of disseminated intravascular coagulation (DIC) and fibrinogen 150–300 mg/dl; FHR shows nonreassuring signs of possible fetal distress.
- Severe. Moderate shock with decreased maternal BP, maternal tachycardia, narrowed pulse pressure, severe orthostatic hypotension, significant tachypnea; total blood loss more than 1,500 ml; dark vaginal bleeding, moderate to excessive; abrupt onset of uterine pain (tearing, knifelike, continuous); developing DIC; fibrinogen less than 150 mg/dl; FHR shows signs of fetal distress; and fetal death can occur. DIC is a secondary event activated by a lack of coagulation factors. The process of fibrinolysis activation in response to coagulation occurs, creating a cascade that results in rampant coagulation and simultaneous massive bleeding, both internal and external with resultant ischemia. Refer to a maternity care textbook, critical care textbook, or the collaborative care plan, "Disseminated Intravascular Coagulation," beginning on p. 26 in Chapter 3.

Placenta Previa

Two classical presentations of placenta previa are *antepartum hemorrhage* (painless, bright red) and *fetal malpresentation* in later pregnancy (fetus stays high because placenta is occupying lower uterine segment). Early diagnosis of placenta previa can change with progression of pregnancy, and normal migration of the placenta can result in normal placement in 90% of cases detected within the first half of the pregnancy.

▌ Diagnostic Studies

- Transabdominal and transvaginal ultrasound. Rules out or confirms placenta previa because it identifies placental location, determines degree of separation and presence of bleeding, position of fetus, fetal status, and gestational age.

- Amniocentesis. Performed with placenta previa to determine fetal lung maturity with lecithin/sphingomyelin ratio or presence of fetal glycerol.
- Speculum exam. Rules out local causes of bleeding (cervicitis, cervical polyps, heavy show, cervical carcinoma); performed if ultrasound reveals a normally implanted placenta; preferably done only after 34 weeks' gestation.
- CBC, platelets, fibrinogen, coagulation studies. Decreased Hgb and Hct, possible elevated WBC. Low platelets and decreased fibrinogen indicate progressing disseminated intravascular coagulopathy (DIC). Coagulation studies important for DIC treatment.
- Kleihauer-Betke test on maternal blood; or amniotic fluid index on amniotic fluid. Detects fetal blood in amniotic fluid and estimates fetal blood loss. Allows quantification of fetomaternal transfusion to guide dosing of Rh(O) immunoglobulin for Rh-negative women.

Medical Management

Medical management varies with the gestational age of the fetus, fetal well-being or compromise, and the severity of blood loss occurring from the placenta previa or abruptio placenta.

Abruptio Placentae

Delivery is the treatment of choice if the fetus is at term or if the fetus or mother is in jeopardy. If fetus is younger than 36 weeks' gestation and not in distress, and if bleeding is not severe, expectant management may be used.

Abruption Mild and Bleeding Minimal, Gestation Preterm

- Observation in hospital to facilitate rapid intervention with cesarean delivery.
- Close observation for signs of concealed or external bleeding.
- Fetal surveillance and monitoring until 72 hours have passed without bleeding, hypertension, or abnormal FHR pattern.
- Monitor for preterm labor; tocolysis is contraindicated.
- Corticosteroids given if indicated. Accelerates fetal lung maturity.

Moderate to Severe Bleeding, Any Gestation

- Monitor maternal volume status; pad count and weighing for blood loss calculation.
- IV hydration and volume expansion; accurate intake and output documentation.
- Blood administration, cryoprecipitate, platelets, fresh frozen plasma replacements.
- Oxygen therapy.
- Correct coagulation defect if present.

- Vaginal or cesarean delivery; use of oxytocin to induce labor contraindicated.

Placenta Previa

Expectant Management

- Observation and probable hospitalization (if fetus is younger than 36 weeks and bleeding is minimal or has stopped).
- Bed rest with bathroom privileges (if fetus is younger than 36 weeks and bleeding is minimal or has stopped).
- Close observation for bleeding. Hold maternal blood sample at all times for immediate type and cross-match.
- IV infusions; then heparin lock to maintain venous access.
- Continuous fetal monitoring initially, then every 4 hours once stabilized. If bleeding continues, fetus is older than 36 weeks, fetal lung maturity has been documented by amniocentesis, or labor begins, cesarean birth is performed. If previa is partial or low lying and bleeding is minimal, vaginal delivery may be attempted.
- Ultrasonography frequently until term; amniotic fluid index checked with NST, and modified biophysical profile performed twice weekly. Contraction stress tests contraindicated.
- Corticosteroids. Accelerate fetal lung maturation between 24 and 34 weeks' gestation.
- Monitor for signs of preterm uterine contraction; administration of tocolytics, preferably magnesium sulfate. Prevents preterm labor.
- Initiate iron supplementation. Builds iron stores.
- Amniocentesis. Determines lung maturity between 34 and 36 weeks because risk for bleeding increases with gestational age.

Collaborative Problems

Potential complications of placenta previa or placental abruption include the following:

- Hemorrhage, hypovolemic shock (antepartum and/or postpartum)
- DIC
- Preterm birth (greatest risk to fetus)
- PROM
- Fetal hypoxia
- Anemia (antepartal or postpartal)
- Infection (antepartal or postpartal)

COLLABORATIVE (STANDARDIZED) CARE FOR ALL WOMEN WITH ANTEPARTAL HEMORRHAGES

Perform comprehensive assessment to identify individual needs for teaching, emotional support, and physical care.

Potential Complications of Abruptio Placenta or Placenta Previa: HEMORRHAGE, HYPOVOLEMIC SHOCK, DIC

Refer to the generic collaborative care plans, "Potential Complication: Disseminated Intravascular Coagulation" and "Potential Complication: Hemorrhage," beginning on pp. 26 and 28, respectively, in Chapter 3.

Focus Assessments

- Assess vital signs and assess for vaginal bleeding, abdominal tenderness, pain, and rigidity. Helps differentiate abruptio placenta from placenta previa. Detects blood loss and progressing condition to alert provider of need to escalate care.
- Assess level of consciousness. Hypovolemia decreases the amount of circulating blood and therefore oxygen delivered to the maternal brain, causing decreased level of consciousness.
- Assess pulse oximetry. Evaluates level of oxygenation and effectiveness of treatments.
- Measure I and O, and insert indwelling urinary catheter. Urine output is a better indicator of blood loss than vital signs. Vital signs may be normal even with heavy blood loss because of the increased volume of blood during pregnancy. I and O indicates adequacy of renal perfusion and provides measure of fluid loss and adequacy of fluid replacement. Output of 30 ml/hr reflects adequate renal perfusion; this varies, though, depending on rate of fluid replacement. As a rule, I and O should be approximately equal. Maintain IV line or IV access as determined by maternal stability.
- Assess hemodynamic monitoring (e.g., central venous pressure) if ordered. For early determination of severity of blood loss.
- Review fibrin split products and coagulation studies, including fibrinogen levels, platelet count, activated partial thromboplastin, and partial thromboplastin time and prothrombin time. Provides information about the cause of the bleeding. Presence of fibrin split products, decreased platelet and fibrinogen levels, and prolonged partial thromboplastin time and prothrombin time are signs of DIC. Fibrinogen level should be at least 100 mg/dl for adequate clotting to occur. Clotting studies may be repeated frequently.
- Assess clot retraction. If blood clots in a plain glass (red-top) tube within 10 minutes, it contains at least 100 mg/dl fibrinogen. This is a good way to check blood-clotting ability while waiting for results of formal clotting studies.
- Monitor for hemolytic or allergic reaction to blood products, if administered. Allows for early intervention, which may prevent serious complication.
- Institute continuous fetal monitoring. Assesses fetal status and distress and assesses for uterine irritability. Follow plans for fetal surveillance.

- Assess for persistent and increased bleeding. Indicates the need to prepare the woman for cesarean birth. Do preoperative teaching and answer all questions.

Preventive Nursing Activities

- Institute bed rest, usually with bathroom privileges. Activity stimulates bleeding and increases oxygen demands.
- Avoid vaginal and rectal exams. May increase amount of bleeding, especially in placenta previa.
- Administer corticosteroids as prescribed. Enhances fetal lung maturity.
- Administer iron as prescribed. Builds iron stores.
- Administer blood as prescribed. Fresh frozen plasma or cryoprecipitate may be given to maintain a fibrinogen level of at least 100–150 mg/dl. In addition to decreasing BP and uteroplacental and maternal tissue perfusion, maternal hemorrhage results in a loss of formed elements of the blood (e.g., erythrocytes). Whole blood replaces formed elements, increases the oxygen-carrying capacity of the blood, and helps to prevent fetal hypoxia and/or fetal death.
- Obtain Rh antibody titer as ordered. Rarely, Rh sensitization occurs when fetal blood enters the maternal circulation. An Rh-negative woman may be given RhoD immune globulin if the fetus is Rh-positive.
- Prepare for immediate cesarean birth. If vaginal delivery is not possible (e.g., in most cases of placenta previa), and if bleeding is excessive, fetal distress occurs, or if labor cannot be stopped, surgery may be needed to save the life of the baby and/or the mother. Profound hemorrhage can occur at any time and without warning.
- For women being managed expectantly at home, teach the importance of bed rest, as well as symptoms of complications (e.g., bleeding, UCs) that must be reported. Helps to ensure that the woman will comply with the therapeutic regimen and will contact the care provider for timely intervention. Include daily fetal activity charts, pelvic rest, and need for weekly biophysical profile and doctor's visits in teaching.
- Provide continuous emotional support. Prolonged hospitalization with bed rest is difficult. The mother's concern for the outcome of the pregnancy is continually present.

Potential Complication of Abruptio Placentae or Placenta Previa: PRETERM BIRTH, PROM

Focus Assessments

- Assess uterine contractions. Indicates onset of labor. May require administration of tocolytics (e.g., before 36 weeks' gestation, if fetal lungs are mature). Uterine hyperstimulation may be noted in cases of abruptio placentae.

- If UCs occur, notify care provider, do not do vaginal exam. Exam may need to be done with speculum to avoid digital stimulation if low-lying placenta. If cervical dilation occurs along with UCs, it will probably not be possible to maintain the pregnancy.
- Assess for rupture of membranes. Indicates the likelihood that the pregnancy cannot be maintained; increases the risk for infection.
- Assist with amniocentesis. In placenta previa, determines lecithin/sphingomyelin ratio for fetal lung maturity.
- Fetal surveillance (e.g., monitoring, fetal activity, NST, BPP, amniocentesis). Determines fetal well-being, and information used in decisions about continuing the pregnancy.

Preventive Nursing Activities

- Advise against intercourse, nipple stimulation, and any activity that produces orgasm. Orgasm involves rhythmic contractions of the uterus. Nipple stimulation and prostaglandins in semen can stimulate UCs even if orgasm does not occur.
- Prepare for complications of hemorrhage and birth. Infant may need to be resuscitated. Further bleeding may occur.

Potential Complication of Abruptio Placentae or Placenta Previa: FETAL HYPOXIA

Focus Assessments

- Monitor FHR continuously. Assesses fetal well-being. Fetus responds to hypoxia first with tachycardia and later with bradycardia. Late decelerations and loss of FHR variability are also nonreassuring.
- Assess fetal movement. Fetus responds to hypoxia first with increased activity and later with decreased activity.
- Assess fetal BPP. Noninvasive way to evaluate fetal status and determine the need for birth. Fetal response to hypoxia is alteration in movement, muscle tone, breathing, and heart rate pattern. BPP is an accurate indicator of impending fetal death.
- Assess lecithin/sphingomyelin ratio. Determines fetal lung maturity and helps in decision making about medical interventions. May not be needed if corticosteroids are administered.
- Perform NST. Evaluates changes in FHR in response to fetal movements. A reactive test suggests an intact fetal central nervous system; a nonreactive test suggests fetal hypoxia and the need for further tests.

- Review Kleihauer-Betke test on maternal blood, or amniotic fluid index test on amniotic fluid. Detects fetal blood in amniotic fluid and estimates fetal blood loss.
- Assess maternal blood loss. Maternal blood loss reduces uteroplacental perfusion.

Preventive Nursing Activities

- Administer blood as ordered. In addition to decreasing BP and uteroplacental perfusion, maternal hemorrhage results in a loss of formed elements of the blood (e.g., erythrocytes). Whole blood replaces formed elements, increases the oxygen-carrying capacity of the blood, and helps to prevent fetal hypoxia and/or fetal death.
- Have the woman assume lateral position (alternating left and right) unless contraindicated. If supine position must be used, elevate hips. Promotes venous return by relieving pressure on the aorta and inferior vena cava. This increases uteroplacental circulation and fetal oxygenation. Elevating the hips in supine position prevents compression of the vena cava. Both positions help ensure adequate blood supply to the maternal brain.
- Avoid Trendelenburg position. May compromise maternal respirations and, therefore, oxygenation.
- Administer oxygen per order or protocol. Increases the oxygen available to the fetus. Because total maternal RBCs are reduced with bleeding, it is important that the remaining hemoglobin be fully saturated with oxygen.
- Stop oxytocin immediately if it is being used. Oxytocin stimulates UCs, which may be necessary to delay delivery, prevent vaginal birth until cesarean delivery is accomplished, or relieve stress on the fetus.
- Administer betamethasone per order or protocol. Accelerates fetal lung maturation when it is anticipated that gestation will not continue to term.
- Prepare for maternal and neonatal complications with birth; e.g., insert a large-bore (16-gauge) needle for IV line. A large-bore needle allows for rapid infusion of blood.
  - Abruptio Placentae. Vaginal birth is often feasible and is desirable when there is severe coagulopathy or fetal demise. Perinatal mortality is high because of fetal hypoxia, preterm birth, and small-for-gestational-age status that accompany antepartal hemorrhagic conditions.
  - Placenta Previa. Cesarean birth is usually necessary. Bleeding may continue even after birth of the infant because the living ligature (interlacing muscles) is absent in the lower part of the uterus where the placenta was implanted.
- For a woman being managed at home, teach to monitor fetal activity, fetal movement counting, and signs of labor. Establishes fetal viability and ensures that the woman will know when to contact healthcare provider or birthing center.

Potential Complication of Abruptio Placentae or Placenta Previa: ANEMIA

Refer to the generic collaborative care plan "Potential Complication: Anemia," which begins on p. 25 in Chapter 3.

Focus Assessments

- Assess Hgb and Hct. The Hct reflects the RBC volume, which is decreased in acute and chronic blood loss.
- Temperature and other signs of infection. Anemia increases the woman's risk for infection. Loss of RBCs affects the immune system's ability to fight infection.

Preventive Nursing Activities

- Administer iron supplement as prescribed. Builds iron stores.
- Be prepared for complications at birth. Anemia decreases the woman's ability to tolerate blood loss at birth.

Potential Complication of Abruptio Placentae or Placenta Previa: INTRAUTERINE INFECTION

Refer to the generic collaborative care plan, "Potential Complication: Infection," which begins on p. 29 in Chapter 3.

Focus Assessments

- Assess VSs and for indicators of infections. Chills, fever, and increased pulse, respirations, and BP are indicators of infection that can result from exposure of placental tissue and lowered resistance secondary to anemia.
- Monitor WBC count and differential. WBC count greater than 15,000 per mm³ and a differential shift to the left are associated with infection. In pregnancy, a normal WBC count may be slightly higher than the nonpregnant normal of 5,000 to 10,000 mm³.
- Monitor laboratory results for RBC count and erythrocyte sedimentation rate. Increased RBCs and erythrocyte sedimentation rate are signs of infection.
- Assess for uterine tenderness and malodorous vaginal discharge. These are early signs of reproductive tract infection.

INDIVIDUALIZED (NURSING DIAGNOSIS) CARE PLANS

The care plans in this section were designed to address unique patient needs.

Nursing Diagnosis: ANXIETY/ FEAR[1]

Related Factors: seriousness of maternal condition and threat of fetal harm or fetal demise. Refer to the generic NDCPs, "Anxiety[1]" and "Fear,[1]" which begin on p. 10 and 15, respectively, in Chapter 2.

Goals, Outcomes, and Evaluation Criteria

Woman and/or partner (family):

- Verbalize and demonstrate ability to concentrate.
- Report adequate sleep and rest.
- Report that anxious feelings are tolerable/manageable.
- Ask for help, as needed.

Nursing Activities and Rationales

Independent Nursing Actions

- Acknowledge and facilitate the woman's spiritual and cultural needs. Spiritual support helps relieve anxiety. In the event of fetal death, the mother may have specific wishes regarding baptism of the infant and disposal/burial of the products of conception.
- Use a calm, reassuring, supportive approach. Facilitates coping. Women take cues from their caregivers' behavior; a hurried, tense nurse provokes more anxiety.
- Involve the woman and her family in decision making as much as possible, but do not insist on participation during periods of high anxiety. When anxiety level is high, it interferes with cognitive functioning; efforts to make decisions at such a time create more anxiety.
- Maintain a presence at the bedside during periods of anxiety/fear; use silence, as appropriate. Do not necessarily expect verbal interaction from the woman. Promotes safety and reduces fear; if the woman is overwhelmed with stimuli, talking may add even more stress.
- Encourage an attitude of realistic hope. Although the situation may be grave, overall maternal morbidity is only about 5% and mortality is less than 1% with placenta previa. The greatest risk to the fetus is preterm birth. With abruptio placentae, the maternal mortality rate is about 1%; perinatal mortality ranges from 15% to 30%.
- Encourage talking or crying as a means to decrease the emotional response. Releases tension.
- Communicate empathy and understanding of the woman's experience, either verbally or with touch (e.g., hold hand, apply light touch on the shoulder or gentle pressure at wrist). Helps to reduce anxiety by promoting a feeling of safety and trust. Touch can be reassuring and communicate caring.
- Involve significant others in the woman's care; explain to them how they can help. The woman may receive her most

effective emotional support from those closest to her. Family members may wish to help but may need coaching as to the specific details. They may be hesitant because they see the nurse as the expert or because they are afraid of hurting the woman.

- Discuss the situation with the woman and partner/family, providing factual information about diagnosis, treatment, and prognosis. Helps ensure that emotional reaction is in response to the real, rather than an imagined, situation (some fears may be unrealistic and ungrounded). Knowledge helps to promote a sense of control over the situation.
- Answer questions about health status honestly. Builds trust and reduces anxiety.

Patient/Family Teaching

- Instruct on use of relaxation techniques such as slow, purposeful deep breathing, guided imagery, and progressive muscle relaxation. Enables the woman to retain control of emotions and physical symptoms created by fear.
- Explain all tests and procedures, including sensations likely to be experienced. Knowing what to expect helps woman/family to better cope.
- Repeat information as needed. Facilitates assimilation and recall of information, which are decreased during severe anxiety.

Nursing Diagnosis: INTERRUPTED FAMILY PROCESSES[1]

Related Factors: hospitalization or prescribed bed rest/inactivity at home.

▌ Goals, Outcomes, and Evaluation Criteria

Woman and/or partner (or family):

- Comply with activity restrictions.
- Provide mutual support for each family member.
- Demonstrate role flexibility (e.g., reallocate tasks and functions usually performed by the woman).
- Seek help and use available social supports (e.g., extended family).
- Report that family life is essentially normal and that usual routines are being maintained.
- Adapt family schedule to accommodate the woman's bed rest restrictions.
- Provide diversional activities for the woman on bed rest.

▌ NIC Interventions[2]

Family Integrity Promotion (7100)—Promotion of family cohesion and unity.

Family Process Maintenance (7130)—Minimization of family process disruption effects.
Family Support (7140)—Promotion of family values, interests, and goals.
Financial Resource Assistance (7380)—Assisting an individual/family to secure and manage finances to meet healthcare needs.
Role Enhancement (5370)—Assisting a patient, significant other, and/or family to improve relationships by clarifying and supplementing specific role behaviors.
Support System Enhancement (5440)—Facilitation of support to patient by family, friends, and community.

▌ Nursing Activities and Rationales

Assessments

- Determine typical family processes, roles, and relationships. Assists care providers in suggesting ways to achieve family tasks and support member's usual roles.
- Explore with the family the need for additional help (e.g., with housework) and their ability to pay for it. Identifies the need for referrals.

Independent Nursing Actions

- Encourage the woman to participate in family decisions (e.g., schedules, allocation of tasks) and activities (e.g., plan menus, make grocery lists, reorganize files, work on household budget, mend, update address book) as much as possible. Supports maintenance of her usual role and enhances self-esteem; helps to ensure usual family functioning.
- Suggest diversional activities the woman enjoys and can do while on bed rest (e.g., read information about childbirth or high-risk pregnancy, do passive exercises, keep a journal, shop by phone or Internet, do crafts, work on photo albums, call or email friends, have a facial or manicure). The woman may find it difficult to comply with bed rest for a variety of reasons, including boredom. Diversional activities may decrease boredom and improve adherence to the treatment plan.

Collaborative Activities

- Inform woman/family about available resources (e.g., Medicaid or other public assistance) if needed; make referrals as needed. Woman/family may not be aware that assistance is available.
- Assist with contacting support agencies and filling out applications. Relieves stress on the woman and family, who may be overwhelmed by stressors (e.g., illness, effect on the woman's job).

Nursing Diagnosis: ACUTE PAIN[1]

Related Factors: UCs, cervical dilation, and retroplacental hemorrhage (with abruptio placentae). Refer to the generic NDCP, "Pain,[1]" beginning on p. 18 in Chapter 2.

Goals, Outcomes, and Evaluation Criteria

- Woman expresses satisfaction with pain control (e.g., less than 3 on a 1–10 scale).
- Woman demonstrates ability to concentrate and participate in decisions about own care.
- Woman reports receiving an adequate amount of sleep/rest.
- Absence of physical signs of pain (e.g., facial expression, restlessness, changes in VSs, moaning).

NIC Interventions[2]

Analgesic Administration (2210)—Use of pharmacologic agents to reduce or eliminate pain.

Environmental Management: Comfort (6482)—Manipulation of the patient's surroundings for promotion of optimal comfort.

Pain Management (1400)—Alleviation of pain or a reduction in pain to a level of comfort that is acceptable to the patient.

Simple Guided Imagery (6000)—Purposeful use of imagination to achieve relaxation and/or direct attention away from undesirable sensations.

Nursing Activities and Rationales

Assessments

- Palpate UCs and assess for abdominal tenderness and rigidity. Pain may be caused by UCs; strength of contractions is best evaluated by palpation unless an internal monitor is used. With abruptio placentae, pain and rigidity may be caused by retroplacental hemorrhage.

Independent Nursing Actions

- Institute measures to decrease anxiety. See the generic NDCP, "Anxiety,[1]" which begins on p. 10 in Chapter 2. Anxiety increases the perception of pain.
- Remove sources of discomfort in the environment (e.g., damp vaginal pad or underpad, wrinkled bed linens). Removes additional sources of discomfort.
- Use noninvasive pain control measures for mild to moderate pain (e.g., cutaneous stimulation, guided imagery, therapeutic touch). Noninvasive pain control measures may be adequate to control pain and eliminate the need for narcotics. Narcotics cross the placenta and, therefore, can depress the fetus/newborn if given close to the time of birth. Predicting time of birth in these conditions is difficult because emergency delivery may be required at any time if severe hemorrhage or fetal distress occurs.
- Consider the woman's cultural background when assessing and evaluating pain. Expressions of pain vary among cultures, causing the nurse to over- or underestimate the severity of the woman's pain.

Collaborative Activities

- Administer sedatives or narcotics, per order or protocol. Sedatives promote rest, which increases the energy needed

to cope with pain. Fatigue increases the perception of pain. Narcotics alter the transmission and perception of pain impulses in the CNS.

TOXOPLASMOSIS, OTHER INFECTIONS, RUBELLA, CYTOMEGALOVIRUS, HERPES SIMPLEX VIRUS, AND SEXUALLY TRANSMITTED INFECTIONS

STIs, bacterial and viral, can complicate pregnancies and fetal outcomes. Treatment and management differ depending on the infection; therefore, screening during the initial prenatal visit and later in pregnancy is indicated. Toxoplasmosis, other infections (e.g., hepatitis, syphilis, gonorrhea, rubella, varicella, HIV, parvovirus) cytomegalovirus, and herpes simplex virus (TORCH) are a group of infections affecting pregnancy. There is a TORCH laboratory screening panel, but the diseases in this panel may be grouped differently depending on the laboratory doing the testing. While the acronym has fallen out of favor in medical literature in recent years, it still appears in many nursing textbooks. When investigating a certain disease, one should search for it by name.

In this care plan, TORCH will be used to introduce disease processes that, if acquired in pregnancy, can cause significant morbidity and mortality to both mother and fetus. Some infections can be transmitted to the fetus in utero, while others are transmitted during passage through the birth canal.

Because most TORCH infections can cross the placenta, exposure of the mother during the first 12 weeks of pregnancy can cause fetal developmental anomalies. TORCH infections are usually minor for the mother, but they can cause serious complications in the fetus/neonate, including miscarriage, congenital heart defects, deafness, IUGR, mental retardation, encephalitis, and fetal death.

Bacterial STIs covered in this care plan include *Chlamydia*, gonorrhea, syphilis, and group B β-hemolytic *Streptococcus* (GBS). Viral STIs covered include human immunodeficiency virus (see "HIV in Pregnancy," which begins on p. 125 in Chapter 5), herpes simplex virus (HSV) 1 and 2, hepatitis, and human papillomavirus (HPV). Prevention is the most effective means to avoid adverse consequences and reduce transmission of these infections to others and to the fetus.

Key Nursing Activities

- Teach about disease prevention during prenatal care.
- Screen for and identify the specific prenatal infection.
- Prevent new infections, reinfection, or transmission of the infection to others.
- Facilitate and encourage compliance with treatment and follow-up.

- Anticipate and prepare the woman for complications that may occur in the fetus/neonate.

Etiologies and Risk Factors

Risks for STIs should be assessed through careful history and physical assessment. Factors that should be noted include history of STI or pelvic inflammatory disease, number of past or current sexual partners, and types of sexual activity. Lifestyle behaviors that place the woman at greater risk are IV drug use or partner with IV drug use, smoking, alcohol use, inadequate or poor nutrition, and high levels of stress or fatigue.

Etiologies and risk factors vary according to the particular pathogen and potential for exposure. Pathogens include the following:

- *Toxoplasmosis.* Protozoan infection or oocytes transmission occurs from eating raw or undercooked meat (cyst is destroyed with heat), drinking unpasteurized goat's milk, from handling infected cat feces from litter box or dirt in which cats have defecated (garden dirt could be on vegetables—the woman should use gloves and properly wash the vegetables), and transplacental transmission to fetus. About 38% of American women already have antibodies to this disease but could suffer an initial infection during pregnancy, especially in the first trimester.
- *Hepatitis A.* Transmission occurs through fecal–oral route by ingestion of contaminated food or polluted water or from person-to-person contact.
- *Hepatitis B.* Transmission of DNA virus through direct contact; household items; sexual contact; perinatal transmission; and body fluids—blood (including that found on used needles), saliva, sweat, tears, vaginal secretions, and semen. Fetus is at risk for contact with disease due to vertical transmission. Hepatitis B risk factors in individuals are (1) being of Central African, Haitian, Southeast Asian, Middle Eastern, Pacific Island, or Alaskan descent; (2) being an IV drug user; (3) having multiple sexual partners; (4) working in a healthcare field with blood or needlestick exposure; and (5) receiving multiple blood transfusions.
- *Hepatitis C.* Blood-borne transmission. Those with hepatitis C risk factors are (1) IV drug users or women who ever injected an illegal drug; (2) women who received clotting factor products before 1987; (3) recipients of blood transfusions or organ transplants before 1992; (4) healthcare workers with blood or needlestick exposure.
- *Rubella.* This is also known as German measles and as 3-day measles. It is a viral infection transmitted by droplets. The mother experiences mild disease, with the greatest risk during the first trimester.
- *CMV.* Viral infection transmitted by close contact, semen, cervical and vaginal secretions, human milk, placental tissue, urine, feces, and banked blood. Women at risk are daycare workers, institutional workers, and healthcare workers.
- *HSV.* Sexually transmitted virus.
- *GBS.* Normal flora of vagina in some women. GBS risk factors for a pregnant woman: positive in previous pregnancy, preterm birth, premature rupture of membranes for 18 hours' duration

or more, intrapartum maternal fever of higher than 38°C, and positive history for early-onset neonatal GBS.
- *Chlamydia.* Sexually transmitted bacterial infection.
- *Gonorrhea.* Sexually transmitted bacterial infection.
- *HPV.* Sexually transmitted viral infection. Insignificant effect on pregnancy.
- *Syphilis.* Sexually transmitted bacterial infection.

Signs and Symptoms

TORCH infections generally produce influenza-like symptoms in the mother (e.g., nausea, vomiting, anorexia, weight loss, malaise, and activity intolerance); fetal and neonatal effects tend to be more serious. Symptoms of STIs vary according to the particular disease but may include fever; positive cultures; elevated titers; dysuria; urinary frequency; itchy, burning, painful genital lesions; and vaginal discharge. Some TORCH infections and STIs may be asymptomatic. Conditions based on the various diseases follow.

- *Toxoplasmosis.* Possibly asymptomatic; acute infection similar to influenza: malaise, myalgia, rash, splenomegaly, lymphadenopathy.
- *Rubella.* Rash, low-grade fever, prodromal headache, coryza, lymphadenopathy, photophobia.
- *CMV.* Asymptomatic, or possible mononucleosis-like syndrome; possible cervical discharge. Most common cause of viral uterine infection; may cause chronic infection.
- *HSV.* Prodrome for 2–10 days followed by neuralgia, paresthesia, hypoesthesias. Painful vesicles rupture after approximately 6 days, forming dry crusts that last about 8 days on the genitalia and cervix; dysuria; fever; malaise; inguinal lymphadenopathy. Recurrent infections are milder and shorter.
- *HPV.* Visible warty growths that may be single or multiple (condylomata acuminate), flesh colored, pale pink or red, raised or flat, small or large, or cauliflower-like clusters.
- *Hepatitis A.* Fever, malaise, nausea, abdominal discomfort, usually self-limiting.
- *Hepatitis B.* Chronic low-grade fever, rash, arthralgia, anorexia, nausea and vomiting, fatigue, skin rashes, abdominal pain, jaundice, tender and enlarged liver.
- *Hepatitis C.* Mostly asymptomatic.
- *HIV.* Refer to "HIV in Pregnancy," which begins on p. 125 in Chapter 5.
- *GBS. Streptococcus agalactiae,* asymptomatic, or symptoms of urinary tract infection in pregnant women. Normal vaginal flora in nonpregnant women (with 10–30% being asymptomatic carriers). It is an important factor in perinatal and neonatal morbidity and mortality. GBS can cause infection transmitted during the infant's passage through the birth canal. Intrapartum treatment with ampicillin, cefazolin, or clindamycin is recommended.
- *Chlamydia trachomatis.* Often asymptomatic or nonspecific. May present with cervicitis, urinary frequency and dysuria, pelvic pain, dyspareunia, or postcoital bleeding. Can progress to pelvic inflammatory disease due to late detection.

- *Gonorrhea. Neisseria gonorrhoeae* may coexist with *Chlamydia* in 20–40% of cases.
  - ▶ *Early.* Frequently asymptomatic, but may have purulent cervical discharge; menstrual irregularities. Infrequently vague abdominal pain; low backache; or urinary frequency and dysuria; cervical motion tenderness.
  - ▶ *Late.* Lower abdominal pain, distention, and pelvic pain; rectal itching or pain, profuse anal discharge, joint and tendon pain, dysuria, dyspareunia, vulva swelling or itching; inguinal or cervical adenopathy; Bartholin, urethral, and Skene glands tender to palpation.
- *Syphilis. Treponema pallidum.*
  - ▶ *Primary.* Highly infectious, painless chancre(s) at entry point, which erodes to form a shallow, indurated ulcer; painless, enlarged single lymph node; low-grade fever; malaise, may last 3–6 weeks.
  - ▶ *Secondary.* Occurs 6 weeks to 6 months later than primary infection. Symmetrical maculopapular rash on face, palms, and soles characterized by brown sores about penny size; generalized lymphadenopathy; fever, sore throat, headache, malaise, and fatigue; genital condylomata lata, patchy hair loss.
  - ▶ *Latent.* Can be from 5–20 years after infection. Asymptomatic but seroreactive and is infectious during first year of this stage.
  - ▶ *Tertiary.* If untreated, about one third of women develop tertiary syphilis, with neurologic, cardiovascular, musculoskeletal, or multiorgan system complications including liver, bones, and skin.
- *Human papilloma virus (HPV).* Visible genital lesions (warts), usually painless; chronic vaginal discharge or pruritus can occur.

▌ *Diagnostic Studies*

- Urinalysis, culture, and sensitivity. Asymptomatic bacteriuria may be present; urinary tract infection (UTI) may be caused by GBS, gonorrhea, or other STIs.
- Toxoplasmosis. Serum for antibody titers, with history of exposure; microscopic identification of protozoa. IgM and IgG antibodies can be detected; indirect fluorescent antibody test and indirect hemoagglutination test and Sabin-Feldman dye tests are used to establish diagnosis. Also, polymerase chain reaction in amniotic fluid determines presence of protozoa.
- Rubella titer. Hemagglutination inhibition; serum for antibody titers; if titer is 1:18 or greater, it is evidence of immunity. Does not discriminate between present or past illness.
- CMV titer. Serology positive; presence of CMV in the urine or endocervical secretions; rise in IgM levels and identification of CMV antibodies within the serum IgM fraction. Only 80% of CMV can be detected.
- Herpes simplex. Careful history for past symptoms or lesions; physical examination for lymphadenopathy and lesions. Diagnosis is confirmed by viral culture of active lesions.
- Hepatitis A serology. Detects the immunoglobulin (IgM) antibody; confirms infection.

- Hepatitis B serology. All women should be screened at the first prenatal visit and screening should be repeated later in pregnancy for those who have high-risk behaviors or are from high-risk groups (e.g., Asians, Central Americans, native Caribbean Islanders). Testing is complex since three values, HBcAg, HbeAg, and anti HBc, are screened for since the disease changes according to stage. Combined with liver studies if positive to determine extent of disease.
- Hepatitis C serology. Screening for those at risk, but not routine. Enzyme immunoassay test for anti-hepatitis C virus is the preferred test. If positive, recombinant immunoblot assay is done.
- HIV screening. Serologic test for antibodies to HIV. (Refer to "HIV in Pregnancy," which begins on p. 125 in Chapter 5.)
- Group B beta-hemolytic streptococcus screening. Cultures from anorectal and vaginal areas should be obtained from all women at 36–37 weeks' gestation.
- Chlamydia. Cervical cultures at the first prenatal visit and in the last trimester at about 35 weeks' gestation.
- Gonorrhea. Rectal, cervical, and pharyngeal cultures at first prenatal visit; repeat in third trimester (35 weeks with *chlamydia*).
- Syphilis. Screen at first prenatal visit, again in late third trimester (28 weeks), and at delivery if high risk. VDRL and rapid plasma regain (RPR) are used as screening tests but may give false-positive results. To confirm positive results, positive dark field microscopy for *Treponema pallidum* from chancre exudate or secondary lesion. Positive fluorescent treponemal antibody absorbed (FTA-ABS) and microhemagglutination assays for antibody to *T. pallidum* (MHA-TP).
- Human papillomavirus. Physical inspection of the vulva, perineum, anus, vagina, and cervix whenever HPV lesions are suspected or seen in one area; women with vulvar HPV or partners with HPV should have a Pap smear.
- Complete blood count. White blood cells elevated over 12,000 indicate infection.
- Ultrasound and fetal surveillance. Evaluates for presence of fetal abnormalities, growth patterns, and placenta development.

▌ *Medical Management*

Treatment of STIs includes notification and treatment of all sex partners and follow-up screening to be certain that treatment was effective. Because of the teratogenic effects of some medications, treatment of some infections is different for pregnant than for nonpregnant women. The treatments for the various conditions follow.

- Toxoplasmosis. Pyrimethamine and sulfadiazine combination, leucovorin calcium (to counteract the bond marrow suppression of pyrimethamine), folinic acid, and spiramycin. These are potentially harmful to the fetus, but in acute maternal infection, treatment is essential and will be started after 16 weeks' gestation because of teratogenic effect of pyrimethamine. Spiramycin does not cross the placenta but may be less effective. Sulfadiazine and erythromycin may be used during the first half of pregnancy.

- Rubella. No treatment available. Up to 15% of women of child-bearing age are not immune to rubella. Vaccination of pregnant women is not recommended because of the risk of developing a rubella infection. All women without antibody protection should be vaccinated postpartum but only when leaving the unit because the live virus is used in the vaccination and could infect others due to shedding. Contraception for 3 months is essential.
- CMV. No treatment available in pregnancy or for the infected newborn. Symptomatic care.
- HSV. Oral acyclovir 400 mg three times a day for 7 days for treatment of first clinical episode or severe recurrent infection; in severe maternal HSV infection, IV acyclovir is administered. Avoidance of artificial rupture of membranes, fetal scalp electrode, and pH; instrumental delivery. Cesarean delivery if active lesions at time of delivery to prevent transmission.
- Hepatitis A. Treatment is supportive; immune globulin (hepatitis A immunoglobulin); condition is self-limiting and does not result in chronic infection.
- Hepatitis B. No specific treatment; bed rest, high-protein, low-fat diet; increased fluids; avoid drugs and alcohol that affect liver; if exposed to hepatitis B virus, hepatitis B immune globulin and begin hepatitis B vaccine series within 14 days of contact. Needs self-management teaching due to chronicity of disease and carrier state. May breastfeed if infant is immunized at birth.
- Hepatitis C. Liver studies and routine prenatal care. If high viral load, avoid artificial rupture of membranes and fetal scalp electrode. Interferon is not recommended during pregnancy but is used in postpartum period after liver biopsy. Risk of vertical transmission very low. Baby should be screened at 1 year of age.
- HIV. Antiretrovirals (to reduce the likelihood of transmission of HIV to the fetus). Refer to "HIV of Pregnancy" beginning on p. 125 in Chapter 5.
- GBS. Penicillin or ampicillin during labor; also cefazolin (clindamycin for those allergic to penicillin); if given earlier, recolonization can occur with subsequent infection of the infant.
- Chlamydia. Oral azithromycin 1 g once or amoxicillin, 500 mg orally three times a day for 7 days. Erythromycin is an alternative drug. Treatment of sexual partners.
- Gonorrhea. Cefixime, 400 mg, or ceftriaxone, 125 mg IM plus azithromycin, 1 g, or amoxicillin. Spectinomycin IM is an alternative drug if allergic to cephalosporin. Treatment of sexual partners.
- Syphilis. Benzathine penicillin G; no proven alternatives to penicillin in pregnancy. Those treated may have Jarisch-Herxheimer reaction (fever, myalgia, headache, mild hypotension, tachycardia, decreased fetal activity, and uterine contractions). Monthly quantitative nontreponemal serologic tests are required for remainder of pregnancy. If fourfold rise,

then retreatment is necessary. Management of sexual partners.
- Human papillomavirus. External warts treated with cryotherapy with liquid nitrogen or cryoprobe or TCA or BCA 80–90% weekly; podophyllum, imiquimod, and podofilox should not be used during pregnancy (CDC, 2006).

Collaborative Problems

Potential complications are associated with specific infectious diseases as follows:

- Potential complication of toxoplasmosis. Neonatal disorders such as convulsion, coma, microcephaly, hydrocephalus, blindness, deafness, and mental retardation (severity depends on gestational age). Retinochoroiditis may be the only recognizable damage in mild cases.
- Potential complication of hepatitis A, B, or C. Infection of the neonate, infant at birth (or acquisition of carrier state).
- Potential complication of rubella. Measles can cause miscarriage, IUGR, congenital anomalies (heart, eyes, ears, brain, and congenital rubella syndrome), systemic infection, and death.
- Potential complication of CMV. No maternal risks; neonatal eye, ear, and dental defects; learning disabilities; neurologic complications (cerebral palsy, microcephaly, hydrocephaly); small for gestational age; anemia; and hyperbilirubinemia.
- Potential complication of HSV. Miscarriage, birth anomalies, intrauterine growth restriction, PTL, neonatal infection with jaundice, seizures, neurologic damage, and death.
- Potential complication of GBS. Urinary tract infection, preterm labor (PTL), preterm rupture of membranes (PROM), chorioamnionitis, postpartum sepsis, preterm birth, early-onset sepsis.
- Potential complication of *Chlamydia*. Pelvic inflammatory disease, PROM, PTL, neonatal eye infections, and pneumonia.
- Potential complication of gonorrhea. Pelvic inflammatory disease, miscarriage, PROM, PTL, intraamniotic infection, preterm birth, sepsis, postpartum endometritis, pelvic inflammatory disease, and neonatal eye infections.
- Potential complication of HPV. If lesions are large, they can cause dystocia, impede vaginal delivery, and cause bleeding from lacerations. There is a small chance of laryngeal papillomas in infants exposed to the virus during birth.
- Potential complication of syphilis. Miscarriage, prematurity, stillbirth, congenital multisystem failure (heart, lungs, spleen, liver, pancreas, bone, nervous system), and mental retardation.

COLLABORATIVE (STANDARDIZED) CARE FOR ALL WOMEN WITH TORCH OR SEXUALLY TRANSMITTED INFECTIONS

Perform a comprehensive assessment to identify individual needs for teaching, emotional support, and physical care. Care plans for several complications have been combined because many of the interventions are identical. For example, all the complications can be prevented if the maternal infection can be treated before it is transmitted to the fetus.

Potential Complications of Maternal TORCH or Sexually Transmitted Infections: IUGR, SPONTANEOUS ABORTION, PROM, PRETERM LABOR, AND FETAL DEATH

Also refer to the generic collaborative care plans, "Potential Complication: Fetal Compromise (Nonreassuring Fetal Heart Rate)," "Potential Complication: Premature Rupture of Membranes," and "Potential Complication: Preterm Labor," beginning on pp. 27, 30, and 31, respectively, in Chapter 3.

Focus Assessments

- Screen for and identify the specific prenatal infection. See "Diagnostic Studies" on p. 188. The type of infectious organism determines the mode of treatment. Also, several infections are asymptomatic, even though they may have serious effects on the fetus (e.g., up to 30% of women who have positive cultures for GBS are asymptomatic).
- Monitor and teach the woman to monitor for fetal activity. A decrease in fetal movement has been shown to be a precursor to severe fetal compromise. If the woman feels fewer than 10 movements in a 12-hour period, she should contact her care provider immediately.
- Assess status of maternal membranes. Intact membranes provide a barrier to some infectious organisms that can be transmitted via the ascending route.
- Monitor fundal height (measurement and ultrasonography). Establishes IUGR. Fundal height should correlate with fetal gestational age. Infections such as rubella and toxoplasmosis can result in IUGR.
- If the woman is infected with HSV or CMV, determine whether infection is primary or recurrent. Neither virus is cured; both recur, especially in times of stress. However, recurrent CMV is not problematic for the fetus. The newborn can be infected with both primary and recurrent HSV-II; however, viral shedding time is reduced in recurrent infection.

Preventive Nursing Activities

- Counsel to seek care at earliest stage of symptoms. Helps prevent neonatal complications. Even though maternal symptoms may be minor, fetal complications may be serious. Prompt intervention may promote a positive outcome.

- Urge to comply with treatment and follow-up care. Essential for preventing reinfection.
- Provide information about the complications that may occur in the fetus/neonate. Knowledge that harm can come to the neonate may motivate the mother to comply with treatment.
- Provide information about symptoms of PROM and premature labor. Enables the woman to seek early treatment and perhaps prevent fetal loss.
- Prepare for transfer to tertiary care center if indicated (e.g., to treat PROM or premature labor). Optimal treatment of high-risk woman and fetus/newborn is more likely in a setting with special equipment and specially trained staff.

Potential Complications of Maternal TORCH or Sexually Transmitted Infections: MATERNAL CHORIOAMNIONITIS AND/OR POSTPARTUM INFECTION

Use generic NDCP, "Risk for Infection,[1]" beginning on p. 21 in Chapter 2; NDCP, "Risk for Reinfection; Risk for Transmission of Infection to Others," beginning on this page in this section; "Premature Rupture of Membranes," which begins on p. 206 in this chapter; the NDCP, "Chorioamnionitis and/or Postpartum Infection," which begins on p. 190 in this topic; and "Postpartum Infection," which begins on p. 347 in Chapter 10.

Potential Complications of Maternal TORCH or Sexually Transmitted Infections: FETAL OR NEONATAL INFECTION (TRANSPLACENTAL OR DURING BIRTH), FETAL MALFORMATIONS, AND ANOMALIES

Focus Assessments

- Determine specific infectious organism and determine gestation. The gestation at which the woman contracts the infection partially determines the effects on the fetus. For example, if rubella is contracted in the first trimester, the fetus will definitely have teratogenic effects; however, if contracted in the second trimester, the fetus has only a 50% chance of being affected. As another example, women who contract hepatitis B in the third trimester have about a 60% chance of transmitting it to the infant at delivery; however, when contracted in first and second trimesters, hepatitis rarely affects the fetus.

Preventive Activities

- Provide information about medications that have teratogenic effects on the fetus. For example, the fetus can be damaged both by toxoplasmosis and by the pyrimethamine and sulfadiazine medications used to treat it.
- Prepare to treat the newborn, as indicated. For some infections, the newborn can be effectively treated at birth. For example, administering hepatitis B immune globulin and hepatitis B vaccine immediately after delivery prevents the newborn from becoming infected with the virus (two follow-up immunizations are necessary); administration of penicillin effectively treats syphilis in the newborn.
- Review available options and support woman/family as they decide to terminate pregnancy, induce labor, or proceed to cesarean birth, as indicated. Some conditions have such profound effects on the fetus that the woman may be advised to terminate the pregnancy (e.g., toxoplasmosis prior to 20 weeks' gestation and rubella in the first trimester). In cases of fetal distress, it may be necessary to induce labor. In other situations, cesarean birth may be indicated (e.g., in the presence of active HSV-II lesions at onset of labor).
- Bathe the newborn immediately after delivery prior to any injections. This helps prevent infection with organisms acquired during birth (e.g., hepatitis B).

INDIVIDUALIZED (NURSING DIAGNOSIS) CARE PLANS

The care plans in this section were developed to address unique patient needs.

Nursing Diagnosis: RISK FOR REINFECTION; RISK FOR TRANSMISSION OF INFECTION TO OTHERS

Related Factors: deficient knowledge of modes of transmission, misinformation, deficient knowledge of safer sex methods, high-risk lifestyle, failure to receive follow-up care, and embarrassment about contacting sex partners.

Goals, Outcomes, and Evaluation Criteria

Woman and partner(s) will:

- Be free of infection (other than viral).
- Experience remission or stabilization of the infection, if viral.

- Identify risky behaviors and find ways to avoid and change behaviors.
- Comply with prescribed treatment and follow-up care.

NIC Interventions[2]

Communicable Disease Management (8820)—Working with a community to decrease and manage the incidence and prevalence of contagious diseases in a specific population.

High-Risk Pregnancy Care (6800)—Identification and management of a high-risk pregnancy to promote healthy outcomes for mother and baby.

Immunization/Vaccination Management (6530)—Monitoring immunization status, facilitating access to immunizations, and provision of immunizations to prevent communicable disease.

Infection Control (6540)—Minimizing the acquisition and transmission of infectious agents.

Infection Protection (6550)—Prevention and early detection of infection in a patient at risk.

Nursing Activities and Rationales

Assessments

- Inquire about the woman's sexual history, practices, and partners. Provides database for identifying effective interventions to prevent transmission of the infection.
- Determine elements of woman's lifestyle that create risk for infection transmission and reinfection. For example, having multiple sex partners increases the risk of being reinfected and transmitting the infection to others; IV drug users are at high risk for HSV-II, hepatitis B virus, and HIV/AIDS.

Independent Nursing Actions

- Discuss the use and importance of safer sexual practices. Increases awareness and motivation to avoid behaviors that lead to infection transmission.
- Provide confidential, nonjudgmental communication. Provides emotional support; increases self-esteem; promotes trust, and, therefore, increases likelihood of following the therapeutic regimen.
- Provide emotional support for the woman who must ask her partner(s) to seek treatment. The woman may be embarrassed and/or concerned about confidentiality. She may fear admitting that she has not been monogamous, or she may be upset to know that her partner was not monogamous.
- When sexual partners should be treated, provide specific ways of talking with or notifying them; offer literature or role play the situation. The woman may wish to notify partner(s), but not know how to do so. Counseling improves compliance and case finding.
- Observe appropriate infection control measures. Standard precautions are used in care of all persons; additional precautions (e.g., barrier precautions) are required for invasive procedures such as labor and birth.

Patient/Family Teaching

- Provide information about safe sex practices. For STIs, both partners must be treated for the infection; condoms must be used; and orogenital sex must be avoided until follow-up tests indicate eradication of the organism.
- Provide information about the specific disease, including cause, mode of transmission, symptoms, and treatment for both partners. Enhances knowledge base and corrects misinformation; increases likelihood of compliance with therapeutic regimen. Treatment is necessary even if the woman does not have symptoms.
- Explain the importance of completing the medication regimen, notification and treatment of all sex partners (for STIs), and follow-up care. To completely eradicate the infectious organism. Disappearance of symptoms does not mean that further treatment is unnecessary.
- Stress importance of taking all of the medication, even if symptoms disappear in a few days; discuss risks, benefits, and side effects. Provides knowledge necessary for successful completion of treatment regimen and helps ensure that organism is completely eradicated. Also helps ensure compliance.
- Stress teaching, support networks if indicated for disease, and follow-up care. Essential for self-management and proper care.

Nursing Diagnosis: PAIN AND IMPAIRED TISSUE INTEGRITY (PERINEAL)[1]

Related Factors: effects of infectious process; excoriation from scratching pruritic areas; and hygiene practices. Also refer to the generic NDCP, "Pain,[1]" beginning on p. 18 in Chapter 2.

▋ Goals, Outcomes, and Evaluation Criteria

- Woman verbalizes relief or control of discomfort.
- Woman demonstrates or reports correct use of appropriate comfort measures.
- Healing of lesions will not be delayed by scratches and excoriation.

▋ NIC Interventions[2]

Pain Management (1400)—Alleviation of pain or a reduction in pain to a level of comfort that is acceptable to the patient.
Perineal Care (1750)—Maintenance of perineal skin integrity and relief of perineal discomfort.

▋ Nursing Interventions and Rationales

Assessments

- Inspect the condition of the perineum, amount and characteristics of drainage, and extent of discomfort. Determines the status of any lesions, whether additional excoriation or secondary infection is occurring, and individualizes interventions.

Independent Nursing Actions

- For a hospitalized, acutely ill woman, provide perineal care. Provides supportive physical care and relieves discomfort.

Patient/Family Teaching

- If the woman has pain on urination, suggest voiding in warm sitz bath. Relaxes perineum to facilitate voiding; provides sensation of warmth to compete with pain stimulus.
- Suggest that the woman wear loose-fitting underwear and jeans/pants (or wear skirts). Reduces mechanical irritation of lesions.
- Suggest that the woman wear cotton underwear. Cotton is more absorbent than man-made fibers; it also allows for better circulation of air.
- Teach the woman to avoid using feminine hygiene sprays, perfumed soaps, bubble bath, and bath oils; douching; and perfumed or colored toilet paper. May cause perineal irritation and skin breakdown, making invasion by bacteria or virus easier.
- Urge the woman to bathe perineum frequently with mild, nonperfumed, nondeodorant soap; and to rinse well and dry thoroughly. Keeps urine and vaginal secretions from coming in contact with lesions; keeping dry helps prevent secondary infections.
- Teach the woman to perform self-vulvar examination. Encourages participation in self-care and early detection in the future if reoccurrence.

Collaborative Activities

- Teach to administer prescribed lidocaine hydrochloride ointment to lesions. Provides local anesthesia; used for herpetic lesions.
- Teach about prescribed oral analgesics such as acetaminophen and codeine. Aspirin can inhibit platelet aggregation and, therefore, increase risk of maternal and fetal hemorrhage. Acetaminophen acts as an antipyretic and peripherally to reduce pain. Codeine acts in the central nervous system to reduce pain. Note that antipyretics can mask fever that accompanies infection.

▋ Other Nursing Diagnoses

Also assess for the following nursing diagnoses, which are frequently present with this condition.

- Complicated grieving[1] related to anticipated fetal anomalies or fetal death.
- Deficient knowledge[1] related to treatment of infection, transmission and reinfection, high-risk behaviors, and self-care/proper care for prevention of diseases/self-management if chronic disease.

- Impaired health maintenance[1] related to practicing prevention of STIs as evidenced by positive diagnosis of STI.

VAGINAL INFECTIONS

Vaginal secretions are increased during pregnancy and must be differentiated from vaginal discharge resulting from infection. Vaginitis is caused by microorganisms. Sometimes changes in vaginal pH can predispose to overgrowth of normal flora, resulting in an infectious process. Vaginal infections can be symptomatic or asymptomatic; some are transmitted sexually; some are not. The most common vaginal infections are bacterial vaginosis, candidiasis, and trichomoniasis.

▮ *Key Nursing Activities*

- Teach about the infection, its cause, problems it causes for the mother, and that the fetus is not affected, to promote understanding of disease process.
- Assist with tests to identify specific organism involved.
- Teach the side effects of her medications.
- Teach self-care activities to prevent reoccurrence of infection.

▮ *Etiologies and Risk Factors*

- *Bacterial vaginosis (BV).* The organisms causing BV are anaerobic bacteria, such as *Gardnerella vaginalis*; *Mobiluncus*, *Mycoplasma hominis*, and *Prevotella*. A disturbance in the normal vaginal flora initiated by sexual intercourse, hormonal shifts, state of pregnancy, antibiotics treatment, and use of nonoxynol-9 spermicides can have a bactericidal effect on lactobacilli, which help maintain normal flora balance in the vaginal environment. Douching and feminine hygiene products can also affect vaginal pH.
- *Candidiasis.* About 90% of cases are caused by *Candida albicans,* a fungus. Predisposing factors include antibiotic therapy, diabetes, pregnancy, obesity, diets high in sugars, use of corticosteroids, exogenous hormones, immunosuppressed states, tight-fitting clothing, and underwear made of nonabsorbent materials. May be sexually transmitted.
- *Trichomoniasis.* An STI caused by a flagellated protozoan, *Trichomonas vaginalis.* It may also be contracted by swimming in contaminated water, sitting in hot tubs, or using contaminated towels.

▮ *Signs and Symptoms*

In general, symptoms include vulvovaginitis and changes in vaginal secretions. They are not systemic.

BV

- May be asymptomatic.
- Profuse vaginal discharge (thin; white, gray, or milky); but discharge may not be present.
- Characteristic fishy odor if vaginal discharge is present; increased odor after intercourse.

- Alkaline pH greater than 4.5.
- Does not cause vaginal itching or dysuria; no cervical or vaginal inflammation.

Candidiasis

- Vulvar and vaginal inflammation; pruritus (mild or intense).
- Thick, white, cottage-cheese-like vaginal discharge.
- Yeasty odor.
- Dyspareunia.
- Pain when urine flows over the vulva.

Trichomoniasis

- May be asymptomatic.
- Copious, yellowish to greenish, frothy, or malodorous vaginal discharge.
- Inflammation of the vagina; pH alkaline (greater than 4.5).
- Cervical findings include strawberry spots (erythema) on cervix; punctuate hemorrhages; friability or bleeding when touched.
- Spotting after intercourse.
- Irritation and constant perineal pruritus.

▮ *Diagnostic Studies*

- Speculum examination of the vagina and cervix.
- Microscopic examination of vaginal secretions (both normal saline and 10% K+ smears)
  - ▸ Bacterial vaginosis. Presence of clue cells (vaginal epithelial cells coated with bacteria).
  - ▸ Candidiasis. Presence of hyphae and pseudohyphae on 10% K+ wet prep; positive Gram stain smear.
  - ▸ Trichomoniasis. Presence of one-celled flagellate trichomonads on normal saline wet prep; positive culture revealed on Papanicolaou smear (should also test for gonorrhea, because it is commonly present with trichomoniasis).
- Whiff test. Release of fishy odor when vaginal secretions mixed with a solution of potassium hydroxide is indicative of bacterial vaginosis.
- pH tesing. Alkaline environment (greater than 4.5) with BV and trichomoniasis, lower than 4.7 with candidiasis.

▮ *Medical Management*

The following therapies are recommended for pregnant women. Only symptomatic women should be treated for bacterial vaginosis and candidiasis.

- *Bacterial vaginosis.* Oral metronidazole (Flagyl) for 1 week, or oral clindamycin for 1 week. Clindamycin cream is not recommended during second half of pregnancy because of increased risk for low birth weight and neonatal infections. No alcohol while on medication to avoid nausea and vomiting, cramping and headache.
- *Candidiasis.* Intravaginal azole agents: butoconazole, clotrimazole, miconazole (available over the counter), and terconazole

(prescription). Also applied to perineum and perianal area to reduce itching and inflammation. Sitz baths twice daily, abstaining from intercourse, avoiding bubble baths, and wearing cotton undergarments may also be helpful in reducing discomfort. Eating yogurt or probiotic foods helps adjust vaginal pH and restore lactobacillus.

- *Trichomoniasis.* Oral metronidazole (Flagyl) in a single dose of 2 g with male sexual partner(s) treated to avoid further transmission even if asymptomatic. Precautions with alcohol and vinegar products for 48 hours because of side effects noted under BV.

▌ *Collaborative Problems*

Potential complications of vaginitis in pregnancy include the following:

Bacterial Vaginosis

- Spontaneous abortion, PROM, and preterm labor
- Postpartum endometritis
- Neonatal septicemia

Candidiasis

- Thrush (a mouth infection in the newborn if candidiasis is present at the time of birth)
- Trichomoniasis
- Preterm labor and birth
- PROM

COLLABORATIVE (STANDARDIZED) CARE FOR ALL WOMEN WITH VAGINAL INFECTIONS

Perform comprehensive assessment to identify individual needs for teaching, emotional support, and physical care.

▌ Potential Complications of Vaginal Infections: PRETERM LABOR AND BIRTH/PROM

Refer to the generic collaborative care plans, "Potential Complication: Premature Rupture of Membranes" and "Potential Complication: Preterm Labor," which begin on pp. 30 and 31 in Chapter 3; and "Recurrent Pregnancy Loss (Cervical Insufficiency)," which begins on p. 155 in this chapter, and the collaborative care plan, "Potential Complication of Maternal TORCH or Sexually Transmitted Infections: IUGR, Spontaneous Abortion, PROM, Preterm Labor, and Fetal Death," which begins on p. 190 in this chapter.

INDIVIDUALIZED (NURSING DIAGNOSIS) CARE PLANS

The care plans in this section were developed to address unique patient needs.

▌ Nursing Diagnosis: DEFICIENT KNOWLEDGE OF MEDICATIONS, PREVENTING REINFECTION, AND COMFORT MEASURES[1]

Also refer to the generic NDCP, "Deficient Knowledge,[1]" beginning on p. 13, in Chapter 2; the generic NDCP, "Pain,[1]" which begins on p. 18 in Chapter 2; and the generic NDCP, "Risk for Infection,[1]" which begins on p. 21, also in Chapter 2.

▌ *Goals, Outcomes, and Evaluation Criteria*

- Woman states that she is using measures to prevent reinfection.
- Woman verbalizes measures to relieve perineal discomfort.
- Woman takes medication in prescribed manner.
- Woman verbalizes understanding of her disease process and its possible implications for her pregnancy.

▌ *NIC Interventions[2]*

Teaching: Disease Process (5602)—Assisting the patient to understand information related to a specific disease process.

Teaching: Prescribed Medication (5616)—Preparing a patient to safely take prescribed medications and monitor for their effects.

Teaching: Safe Sex (5622)—Providing instruction concerning sexual protection during sexual activity.

▌ *Nursing Activities and Rationales*

Assessments

- Inquire whether this is the first or a recurrent infection. Establishes learning needs; helps determine appropriate therapies.
- Monitor perineal erythema, pruritus, excoriation, discharge, and discomfort. Facilitates diagnosis, appropriate management, and effectiveness of treatment.

Patient/Family Teaching

- Teach comfort measures for pruritus and pain. Pain and itching are common symptoms of vaginitis.
- For women with trichomoniasis, stress the importance of treating the male partner and abstaining from sexual intercourse during treatment. Prevents reinfection.

- Teach women with BV and candidiasis the importance of abstaining from sexual intercourse. The trauma may contribute to further inflammation and introduction of more organisms.
- Teach women to avoid douching. Douching increases the risk for BV, chlamydia, pelvic inflammatory disease, HIV transmission, and cervical cancer and has no benefits.
- Teach the woman taking metronidazole to avoid alcoholic beverages and vinegar products. Alcohol creates adverse reactions (abdominal pain, nausea and vomiting, flushing, headache) when taking metronidazole. Metronidazole is contraindicated while breastfeeding, although it can be taken throughout the pregnancy. Previously, it was not given during the first trimester, but studies have confirmed its safety; therefore, the guidelines have been updated.

▌ *Other Nursing Diagnoses*

Also assess for Impaired Skin Integrity[1] related to excoriation and scratching secondary to pruritus, which is frequently present with this condition.

URINARY TRACT INFECTION

Normal physiologic changes predispose the pregnant woman to urinary tract infections (UTIs). Under the influence of progesterone, muscle tone and activity of the ureters decrease, resulting in increased risk of urinary stasis. Urinary pH and glycogen levels are elevated, bladder tone decreases, capacity increases, and emptying tends to be incomplete.

These changes, combined with a short urethra and decreased perineal hygiene because the pregnant uterus gets in the way, increase the chance of UTI. Because UTIs ascend, it is important to diagnose and treat lower UTIs (cystitis and urethritis) early to prevent the development of an upper UTI (pyelonephritis). Lower tract cystitis progresses to pyelonephritis in 15–50% of cases, which causes significant morbidity for mother and baby. Asymptomatic bacteriuria progresses to pyelonephritis in 20–40% of cases. The increased risk for pyelonephritis is likely related to the anatomic and physiologic changes in pregnancy and is seen most commonly in the third trimester when stasis and hydronephrosis are most apparent.

Pregnant women can have asymptomatic bacteriuria (2–7%), which, if untreated, can progress to UTI. Prenatal screening is part of routine care to prevent infections from progressing and complicating the pregnancy. Women who are immunosuppressed, have diabetes mellitus, sickle cell anemia, neurogenic bladder, or recurrent or persistent UTIs prior to pregnancy are at increased risk for complicated UTIs during pregnancy.

▌ *Key Nursing Activities*

- Assess urine at each prenatal visit.
- Administer and teach the woman about medications.
- Teach self-care measures and prevention strategies.
- Monitor for complications (e.g., effects of pyelonephritis on the pregnancy).

▌ *Etiologies and Risk Factors*

- Most common causative pathogen is *Escherichia coli* (70% of cases) normally present in the bowel; coliform organisms are part of normal perineal flora and may be introduced into urethra during intercourse or improper wiping.
- Other causative pathogens are *Staphylococcus saprophyticus* (pyelonephritis); group B *Streptococcus* (10%); *Klebsiella* or *Enterobacter* (3%); and *Proteus* (2%). *Chlamydia trachomatis* and *Neisseria gonorrhoeae* have also been implicated in urinary tract symptoms and have sexual transmission.
- Short urethra.
- Perineal flora that continually contaminate perineum.
- Female predisposition toward incomplete emptying of the urinary bladder.
- Suppressing the desire to urinate.
- Transfer of microorganisms during sexual intercourse.
- Use of a diaphragm and a spermicide.
- Delayed postcoital micturition and not voiding prior to intercourse.
- General poor health and lowered resistance (pregnancy depresses immune system to maintain pregnancy).

▌ *Signs and Symptoms*

- *Asymptomatic bacteriuria.* Bacteria present in urine on culture, but with no accompanying symptoms.
- *Cystitis, urethritis (lower UTI).* Dysuria, urgency, frequency, hematuria, low-grade fever (101°F or 38.3°C), hesitancy or dribbling, suprapubic tenderness.
- *Acute pyelonephritis.* Sudden onset of chills, high fever, and flank pain; back pain and positive costovertebral angle tenderness. May be accompanied by nausea, vomiting, malaise, flulike symptoms.

▌ *Diagnostic Studies*

- Asymptomatic bacteriuria. At first prenatal visit, screen with clean catch, midstream urinalysis. Culture may also be done as baseline. At each routine visit, urine will be dipped and tested for presence of nitrates and leukocyte esterase. If positive, urinalysis and culture will be done.
- Lower UTI. Clean catch, midstream urinalysis shows abnormally high number of leukocytes and bacteria. Urine culture shows increased leukocytes and more than 100,000 colonies of bacteria per milliliter of urine.

- Acute pyelonephritis. Fluorescent antibody titer (FA-test) positive; creatinine clearance (low); marked bacteremia in urine culture; pyuria, WBC casts in the urine.
- CBC, electrolytes, blood urea nitrogen, serum creatinine. Assesses for anemia and kidney function if pyelonephritis is present.

▌ Medical Management

Treatment depends on the causative organism. Culture and sensitivity indicate which antibiotic is most effective. Penicillins, cephalosporins, and nitrofurantoin have been used for years without problems to the fetus. The causative organisms and treatments follow:

- Asymptomatic bacteriuria. Oral sulfonamides in early pregnancy (no trimethoprim, e.g., Bactrim), cephalexin and nitrofurantoin in late pregnancy (no sulfonamides or nitrofurantoin due to hemolysis in fetus). Amoxicillin is no longer used for asymptomatic bacteriuria unless it is shown to be effective in sensitivity study because of 20–40% resistance of *Escherichia coli* to penicillin, which renders it ineffective. Cephalexin is a good choice because it is also effective in treating pyelonephritis; it is not, however, effective against *Enterococcus*.
- Cystitis and urethritis. Oral sulfonamides in early pregnancy; cephalexin or nitrofurantoin in third trimester to late pregnancy (no sulfonamides).
- Acute pyelonephritis. Hospitalization; hydration; IV antibiotics (e.g., gentamicin, cephalosporins); IM ceftriaxone; supportive therapy for comfort; follow-up urine cultures and possible blood cultures; evaluation of CBC, serum creatinine, and electrolyte levels; I and O; frequent monitoring of mother and fetus; use of antipyretics; suppressive therapy possible with oral nitrofurantoin.
- Medications contraindicated in pregnancy are tetracyclines, fluoroquinolones, erythromycin, and chloramphenicol. Some drugs are contraindicated depending on the trimester, e.g., trimethoprim in the first trimester, sulfonamides in the first and last trimesters, and nitrofurantoin in the third trimester.

▌ Collaborative Problems

Potential Complication of Asymptomatic Bacteriuria and/or Cystitis

- Ascending UTI (cystitis, acute pyelonephritis)

Potential Complications of Acute Pyelonephritis

- Premature labor and birth leading to increased infant morbidity and mortality
- IUGR
- Hypertension
- Preeclampsia
- Maternal anemia
- Amnionitis

- Perinephric cellulitis and abscess
- Septic shock
- Renal dysfunction
- Hematologic dysfunction
- Pulmonary injury due to endotoxins and pulmonary edema

COLLABORATIVE (STANDARDIZED) CARE FOR ALL WOMEN WITH URINARY TRACT INFECTIONS

Perform a comprehensive assessment to identify individual needs for teaching, emotional support, and physical care.

▌ Potential Complications of Asymptomatic Bacteriuria and/or Cystitis: ASCENDING UTI

Ascending UTI includes cystitis and pyelonephritis.

Focus Assessments

- Monitor signs and symptoms of cystitis and monitor urine culture and sensitivity results. Ensures that the woman's infection (or bacteriuria) is eradicated.
- Monitor and teach the woman to monitor for symptoms of pyelonephritis. If pyelonephritis develops, hospitalization and intravenous antibiotic therapy are indicated to prevent serious maternal and fetal complications. Note that labor, appendicitis, and abruptio placenta may be mistakenly diagnosed; careful assessment facilitates correct diagnosis.

Preventive Nursing Activities

- Stress the importance of taking the entire course of antibiotics and returning for follow-up urinary cultures. Ensures that the infection is entirely eradicated.
- Teach signs, symptoms, therapy, and possible complications of cystitis. Promotes early identification and treatment; prevents ascending infection.
- Teach self-care measures to help prevent cystitis, including:
  - Hydrate with water; avoiding sodas, caffeine, and alcohol. Soda, caffeine, and alcohol have a high acid content and irritate the urinary bladder.
  - Do not suppress the urge to void, and void frequently. Prevents bladder distention and urinary stasis.
  - Urinate before going to bed at night and before and after intercourse. The longer urine stays in the bladder, the more opportunity there is for bacteria to multiply. Bacteria can be introduced into the urethra during intercourse; voiding flushes them downward.
  - Maintain a good fluid intake; explain that if the urine looks dark, fluid should be increased. Increases urine

volume and promotes flushing of bacteria downward in the renal system.

- Take cranberry pills and/or 500 mg vitamin C daily. Helps acidify the urine, possibly preventing recurrence of infection. Avoid juice because too much sugar can exacerbate symptoms.
- Eat yogurt and drink acidophilus milk. May help prevent UTI and vaginal infections by enhancing growth of normal flora.
- Wear cotton underwear and maintain good perineal care (front to back wiping, cleaning urethra first when bathing, and using a clean washcloth each time.) Prevents buildup of moisture in the genital area. Moisture fosters bacterial growth. Most bacteria enter the urethra by being spread from the anal area.
- Using liquid soap instead of bar soap and wash hands often. Prevents bacterial colonization on soap. Clean hands help prevent the spread of most infections.

Potential Complication of Acute Pyelonephritis: INCREASED RISK OF PREMATURE BIRTH

Refer to the generic collaborative care plan, "Preterm Labor and Spontaneous Abortion," next, and "Premature Rupture of Membranes," which begins on p. 206, in this chapter.

PRETERM LABOR AND SPONTANEOUS ABORTION

A term pregnancy is approximately 40 weeks in length, but a natural termination of pregnancy can occur before that time. Prior to 20 weeks' gestation, the fetus is considered nonviable, and the expulsion of the fetus is called a *spontaneous abortion*. A threatened abortion is when continuation of the pregnancy is in doubt but still possible. *Miscarriage* is a term often used instead of abortion because the term abortion can have social stigma. Spontaneous abortions complicate 10–30% of all clinically apparent pregnancies and are classified as follows:

- *Inevitable abortion/imminent abortion.* The cervix has dilated and continuation of the pregnancy is impossible; symptoms are present including mild, moderate, or severe cramping, and tissue in cervix.
- *Incomplete abortion.* The products of conception are only partially expelled from the uterus; the placenta may be retained; associated with heavy, profuse bleeding, mild cramping, and passage of tissue.
- *Complete abortion.* Total evacuation of the products of conception from the uterus; signs may only include slight bleeding

with brownish color on assessment since passage of tissue and bleeding are past.

- *Missed abortion.* The embryo or fetus dies, but the products of conception are retained in the uterus; may be associated with spotting and malodorous discharge.
- *Recurrent pregnancy loss (formerly called habitual abortion).* Spontaneous loss of fetus prior to 20 weeks on three or more occurrences. Refer to topic "Recurrent Pregnancy Loss (Cervical Insufficiency)," beginning on p. 155 in this chapter.
- *Septic abortion.* The products of conception are infected; may occur from prolonged unrecognized rupture of membranes; pregnancy with intrauterine device; or after unsuccessful attempts to terminate early pregnancy; may be associated with malodorous variable bleeding and passage of tissue.

After 20 weeks' gestation and up to the end of 36 weeks' completed gestation, delivery of a live fetus is considered a *preterm birth*. If contractions and cervical changes are identified early, it is sometimes possible to arrest preterm labor, preventing the birth of a premature infant. Preterm labor complicates approximately 12% of all pregnancies. Diagnosis is made when there are four contractions in a 20-minute period and the cervix is dilated more than 2 cm and 80% or greater effaced.

Key Nursing Activities

Spontaneous Early Pregnancy Bleeding

- Collect and organize key assessments.
- Teach regarding treatment and plan of care.
- Prepare woman for diagnostic procedures.
- Provide physical care during bleeding.
- Assess coping mechanisms, support system, and offer emotional support.
- Prepare the woman and partner for the possibility of fetal loss.
- Provide discharge teaching and follow-up call for continuity of care.

Preterm Labor

- Assess woman who presents in preterm labor.
- Teach differentiation between false labor and true labor.
- Monitor maternal and fetal response to medications when hospitalized.
- Assess coping mechanisms, support system, and offer support emotionally and physically.
- Provide discharge planning if labor is stopped and woman is able to return home.

Etiologies and Risk Factors

The precipitating factors associated with spontaneous abortion and preterm birth are similar.

Spontaneous Abortion

Most spontaneous abortions occur within the first 12 weeks of pregnancy as a result of chromosomal abnormalities in the embryo or fetus, developmental defects, placental anomalies, hormonal disruptions, luteal phase defects, chronic maternal diseases, and infections. Maternal substance abuse of tobacco, alcohol, caffeine, and illicit drugs can affect pregnancy outcome. Other causes include exposure to teratogens, poor maternal nutrition and obesity, maternal age older than 36, physical abnormalities (uterine anomalies, insufficient cervix), immunologic response by the mother against the embryo (antiphospholipid syndrome), and clotting disorders (inherited thrombophilic defect). Cause cannot be found in 50% of women after thorough assessment and evaluations.

Preterm Labor

Modifiable risk factors include the following:

- Tobacco, alcohol, and illegal substances use (esp. cocaine and methamphetamine [Methedrine])
- Low prepregnancy weight or low weight gain with poor maternal nutrition
- Vaginal infections
- Asymptomatic group B streptococcal bacteriuria
- Domestic violence
- Periodontal disease
- Maternal stress
- Long working hours or strenuous work

Nonmodifiable risk factors that may contribute to risk include the following:

- Socially disadvantaged status; lack of support
- Less than high school education
- Extremes of maternal age
- Multiple gestation
- African American descent (is also increased in Asian or nonwhite races)
- Unmarried or not in stable relationship

Pregnancy, reproductive, and medical factors that increase risk include the following:

- Pregnancy complications such as preeclampsia, hyperthyroidism, anemia, hepatitis, cholestasis, heart disease, diabetes, premature rupture of membranes (significant in one third of PTL pts.), lack of prenatal care, polyhydramnios, placenta previa or abruptio placenta, trauma.
- Reproductive risk factors, such as multiple gestation, no or inadequate prenatal care, cervical abnormality, in vitro fertilization, polyhydramnios, uterine anomalies, abruptio placenta or placenta previa.
- Medical conditions such as autoimmune disorders, thromboembolic disorders, diabetes, renal or cardiovascular diseases, hypertension, anemia, or presence of vaginal infections.
- The greatest risk factor is previous history of preterm labor (Gilbert, 2010).

Preterm labor can lead to delivery of preterm infant whose immaturity can lead to many problems, increase in possibility of birth trauma, and increased transition to extrauterine life. Refer to "Preterm Newborn," beginning on p. 412 in Chapter 12.

▌ Signs and Symptoms

Clinical manifestations vary depending upon the specific situation. Most common findings, however, are:

Subjective. Increased pelvic pressure, backache, uterine cramping with early pregnancy loss; abdominal pain, back pain, pelvic pain, and menstrual-like cramping with preterm labor.

Objective. Increased vaginal discharge, change in character of vaginal discharge (clear to bloody), passage of blood clots or tissues may occur with spontaneous abortion (see previous section for specificity due to type of loss); possible leakage of fluid seen with both. Preterm labor is characterized by shortening, effacement, and/or dilation of cervix and more than five regular uterine contractions an hour, lasting more than 1 hour. Uterine activity can cause diarrhea and urinary frequency. Increased cramping will be experienced if urinary tract infection coexists.

▌ Diagnostic Studies

- Pregnancy test. Verifies the presence of early pregnancy; not evaluated in later pregnancy because other signs of pregnancy are present.
- Hormonal assays (hCG, estrogen, progesterone). Establishes presence of pregnancy and adequacy of hormones for pregnancy retention. Hormone levels increase rapidly during early pregnancy; decreasing levels indicate that the pregnancy is not functioning normally. Serial hCGs must be done for comparison over several-day period during possible early pregnancy loss. Low progesterone can be indicative of lowered ability to maintain rich uterine lining for fetal growth. Salivary estradiol levels increase before preterm birth.
- Ultrasonography. Determines gestation, fetal age, and viability; detects placenta attachment and cord perfusion; determines blighted ovum, fetus growing less than expected, and absence of fetal heart rate in evaluation of viable pregnancy; detects hidden bleeding behind placenta and placental grading.
- Transvaginal ultrasound (PTL). Determines cervical length and internal os dilation; dilatation of internal os and shortening of cervix are associated with progression in labor.
- Sterile vaginal exam. Determines cervical dilation and effacement, observation of bleeding or fluid leakage, anatomic view to assess if presence of polyps, cervicitis, or erosion. Recent intercourse can cause spotting and sperm can be visualized on vaginal smear when screening for vaginal infections; presence of yeast, *Trichomonas*, or clue cells indicate bacterial vaginosis.
- Vaginal culture. Rules out infection (which can cause preterm labor). Presence of infection can be cause for cervical or vaginal

bleeding rather than spontaneous abortion and needs to be ruled out. Cultures for gonorrhea, *Chlamydia*, and beta-*Streptococcus* should all be obtained and treated if present prior to birth.

- Fetal fibronectin (PTL). Present in vaginal secretions within 2 weeks of onset of delivery; detects preterm labor between 24 and 32 weeks' gestation. The detection of fetal fibronectin in vaginal secretions with intact membranes suggests impending preterm labor. Results may be inaccurate if bleeding, recent intercourse, or amniotic fluid is present. A negative result is indicative of no pending labor in the next 7 days.
- CBC, platelets. Detects hemoglobin and hematocrit to determine if anemia is present from blood loss. Infections can be noted, which can precipitate spontaneous abortion or preterm labor. Low platelets can be associated with clotting disorders, which can cause pregnancy loss.
- Type and screen with cross-match. Safety measure in the event blood replacement is needed due to blood loss and to determine Rh status if Rho(D) immune globulin treatment is indicated after loss of pregnancy if Rh negative.
- C-reactive protein. Detects the presence of active inflammatory conditions that may precipitate preterm labor.
- Human placental lactogen (hPL). Evaluates placental function in a high-risk pregnancy.
- Urinalysis and culture. Rules out infection that can irritate uterus causing premature cramping and contractions due to inflammation.
- Electronic fetal monitoring. Establishes baseline and the presence of abnormalities (e.g., decelerations or decreased FHR variability) that can indicate fetal stress. Also documents the frequency of contractions. Palpation of the actual contraction can aid in determining the strength of contraction since external monitoring does not assess for strength.

▮ *Medical Management*

Threatened Spontaneous Abortion

- Activity restrictions, including pelvic rest, no intercourse or orgasm, no douching or anything in vagina including tampons. Sedation at times because of accompanying pain and need for reduced activity.
- Fluid hydration. Dehydration can occur with blood loss and can aggravate the uterus.
- Pain control is needed especially since anxiety increases pain. This is an upsetting situation for most women.

Other Types of Spontaneous Abortion

- Fluid hydration
- Transfusion, if needed
- Dilation and curettage or suction curettage
- Expectant management
- Antibiotic therapy
- Rho(D) immune globulin treatment administration indicated if Rh negative

Preterm Labor

- Bed rest, including pelvic rest, no intercourse or orgasm, and at times sedation. Needs to avoid resting on back to increase perfusion to uterus and fetus.
- Fluid hydration.
- Tocolytic therapy with terbutaline, ritodrine, magnesium sulfate, calcium channel blockers, prostaglandin synthetase inhibitors.
- Antibiotic therapy if infection is present.
- Steroid therapy to enhance lung maturation.
- Amniocentesis to obtain lecithin/sphingomyelin ratio if steroid therapy will be helpful.
- Assessment to determine if membranes are still intact so pregnancy can continue if labor is stopped.

Tocolytic Therapy for PTL

Beta Sympathomimetics

- Action. Augments or duplicates the norepinephrine and epinephrine effects on the tissues innervated by adrenergic nerve fibers, alpha and beta.
- Contraindications. Cardiovascular problems, hypertension, uncontrolled maternal hyperthyroidism, and migraines.
- Examples. IV or subcutaneous terbutaline.
- Goal. Stop uterine contractions.
- Dosing. 0.01 mg/min intravenous, increasing dose by 0.01 mg/min every 10–30 min until contractions stop or side effects are intolerable; subcutaneous injections of 0.25 mg every 30–60 min up to three doses.
- Maternal side effects. Hypotension, light-headedness, tremors, flushed feeling, anxiety, tachycardia, heart palpitations and skipping of heartbeat, hyperglycemia, decreased serum potassium, decreased hematocrit, nausea, and bronchial relaxation.
- Fetal effects. Tachycardia most common.
- Precautions. Do not administer if maternal heart rate over 120. Assess for pulmonary edema and cardiac dysrhythmias and cerebral vasospasm.

Magnesium Sulfate

- Action. Relaxes the smooth muscle of the uterus by substituting itself for calcium.
- Contraindications. Myasthenia gravis.
- Dosing. As ordered or 4–6 g intravenously over 20–30 min (see discussion in care plan); oral dosing for maintenance: magnesium gluconate.
- Sign of toxicity. Depressed respirations less than 12, absence of deep tendon reflexes, severe hypotension, or extreme muscle relaxation.
- Antidote. Calcium gluconate 1 g IV (10 ml of a 10% solution) over 3 minutes.

Calcium Channel Blockers

- Action. Blocks movement of calcium into the smooth muscle of the uterus, blocking uterine contractions.

- Example. Nifedipine.
- Dosing. 10 mg by mouth every 20 min up to three doses, then maintenance.
- Maternal side effects. Flushing, headache, fatigue, mild hypotension, dizziness, peripheral edema, tachycardia.
- Fetal side effects. Secondary to decreased uteroplacental perfusion from maternal hypotension.
- Precautions. Hold if maternal heart rate exceeds 120 bpm or blood pressure drops below 90/50 mmHg.

Prostaglandin Inhibitors

- Action. Inhibits prostaglandin synthesis.
- Examples. Indomethacin, ibuprofen.
- Dosing. Indomethacin, 50–100 mg orally or rectally with maintenance of 25–50 mg oral every 4 hours for 24–48 hours.
- Maternal side effects. Uncommon but may have heartburn or nausea; can mask a fever.
- Fetal side effects. Closure of ductus arteriosus. Do not use past 32 weeks' gestation because it interferes with this.

Collaborative Problems

Potential complications of spontaneous abortion or preterm labor include the following:

- Maternal hemorrhage
- Maternal infection
- Fetal loss

Potential complications of tocolytic therapy include the following:

- Fluid volume excess
- Pulmonary edema
- Cardiac dysrhythmias; myocardial ischemia
- Central nervous system depression
- Metabolic and electrolyte alterations
- Magnesium toxicity

COLLABORATIVE (STANDARDIZED) CARE FOR ALL WOMEN WITH SPONTANEOUS ABORTION OR PRETERM LABOR

Perform a comprehensive assessment to identify individual needs for teaching, emotional support, and physical care.

Potential Complication of Spontaneous Abortion and Preterm Labor: HEMORRHAGE

Refer to the generic collaborative care plan, "Potential Complication: Hemorrhage," on p. 28 in Chapter 3.

Potential Complication of Spontaneous Abortion and Preterm Labor: INFECTION

Refer to the generic collaborative care plan, "Potential Complication: Infection," which begins on p. 29 in Chapter 3.

Potential Complication of Spontaneous Abortion or Preterm Labor: FETAL LOSS

Refer to the generic collaborative care plan, "Potential Complication: Fetal Compromise (Nonreassuring Fetal Heart Rate)," which begins on p. 27 in Chapter 3.

Focus Assessments (Abortion/Miscarriage)

- Assess bleeding in early pregnancy (amount, duration, type, timing, color, pain, how many pads), proper dating with last menstrual period, and VSs. Evaluates for hypotension, hypovolemia, fever, and Rh status. If Rh status is negative and pregnancy is lost, Rho(D) immune globulin treatment will be needed. Also ensures that labs are ordered and sonogram is scheduled.
- Discuss treatment options, if offered, and help with decision making as needed. The woman/couple may have to decide between medical intervention with dilatation and curettage or expectant management. They may need assistance or support with making their decision.
- Discuss the possibility of loss and impact on family, emotional support and discharge planning with available community services and spiritual support. Provides additional support or resources to the woman/couple.
- Provide an empathetic, caring environment to help the mother/couple/family adjust to the reality of perinatal death. Supportive and emotional care when loss occurs includes a discussion of grief, differences between men's and women's grief processes, and the need to concretize the experience. Facilitates grief and coping and demonstrates compassion and understanding.
- Reassure woman/couple/family that follow-up counseling needs are common and they may recur at odd times or at the anniversary of the loss. They may need to work on their relationship since loss can cause marital disharmony, and grief is different for each person. Each parent needs to have time to process the loss. Supports potential need for counseling if woman/couple is grieving or woman is experiencing postpartum depression.

Focus Assessments (Preterm Labor)

- Assess fetal heart tones and movement. Determines fetal well-being. Normally the fetus moves 10 times an hour. If fetal movement decreases by half during 1 hour it may indicate lack of fetal well-being.

- Palpate contractions and document activity. Over four contractions in 20 minutes is one of the indicators for PTL.
- Assess VSs and for presence of vaginal leakage of fluid or bleeding. Vaginal exams are avoided because digital exams can stimulate contractions. If vaginal leak is present, check pH to evaluate for rupture of membranes.

Preventive Nursing Activities (PTL)

- Maintain bed rest, positioned off vena cava to avoid hypotension, preferably on sides. Relieves pressure of the fetus on the cervix and major arteries to promote perfusion. Encourage the woman to change positions frequently for comfort.
- Ensure adequate hydration. Prevents premature labor. When dehydration occurs, the pituitary gland is activated to secrete antidiuretic hormone, which stimulates the release of oxytocin. Oxytocin stimulates UCs.
- Frequent urination is encouraged. A full bladder causes uterine irritability.
- Administer tocolytics as prescribed. May stop labor.
- Explain actions of medication and side effects. May be effective in stopping premature labor. Magnesium sulfate is a CNS depressant that halts labor by decreasing acetylcholine and blocking neuromuscular transmission. Beta-adrenergic drugs such as ritodrine hydrochloride and terbutaline are beta-adrenergic agonists. They reduce intracellular concentrations of calcium by preventing the conversion of adenosine triphosphate into cyclic adenosine monophosphate, making myometrial muscle contractions ineffective and halting labor. Nifedipine is a calcium-channel-blocking agent that prevents muscular uptake of calcium, which also stops myometrial contractions (see "Medical Management").
- Assess response to tocolytics. Determines effectiveness of drugs in stopping premature labor and birth. Monitor for toxicity and respond quickly if interventions are needed.
- Administer antenatal glucocorticoids if ordered. Accelerate fetal lung maturity.
- Provide supportive emotional care and explain all procedures. Expectation of a preterm baby is an area of concern with many unknowns, creating stress for the mother, the father, and the entire family. A listening ear and caring attitude can reduce stress, which also decreases pain and contractions.

Potential Complications of Tocolytic Therapy:
FLUID VOLUME EXCESS, PULMONARY EDEMA, CARDIAC DYSRHYTHMIAS,

CENTRAL NERVOUS SYSTEM DEPRESSION, AND MAGNESIUM TOXICITY

Focus Assessments

- Assess vital signs. Detects complications occurring from tocolytic therapy (e.g., fluid volume excess, pulmonary edema, or cardiac dysrhythmias due to $\beta2$ stimulation from ritodrine or terbutaline or as a side effect of $MgSO_4$). Notify care provider if pulse exceeds 120 beats/min (though some increase is an expected side effect of β-adrenergic tocolytics) or if there are signs of magnesium toxicity.
- Assess lung sounds (crackles and rhonchi) and respiratory status (shortness of breath). Detects complications occurring from tocolytic therapy (see preceding rationale).
- Assess neurologic status. Detects changes that may indicate neurologic depression from $MgSO_4$ (e.g., restlessness, tremors, headaches, light-headedness, drowsiness, depression, or absence of deep tendon reflexes, blurred vision) from drug therapy.
- Assess cardiopulmonary status and for chest pain. Detects changes that may indicate cardiac compromise, such as palpitations, vascular collapse, pulmonary edema, peripheral edema, or deep vein thrombosis.
- Assess reflexes and clonus. Hypotonia is sign of magnesium toxicity.
- Monitor for nausea, vomiting, and headache. These are side effects of tocolytic drugs; they are expected side effects and not necessarily a reason to discontinue therapy.
- Assess magnesium level (when the woman is receiving $MgSO_4$). Detects elevated magnesium levels, which can precipitate cardiac dysrhythmias or neurologic complications. The therapeutic range of magnesium is 4–8 mg/dl. If over 10 mg/dl, toxicity is approaching.
- Monitor for magnesium toxicity, flushing, lethargy, vomiting (common responses to drug) but progressing to hypotonia, pulmonary edema, respiratory depression, and subsequent cardiac arrest. Enables rapid response to toxicity. Hourly monitoring is required at a minimum, and more frequent monitoring might be necessary. Magnesium toxicity is reversed with calcium gluconate, which should be kept immediately available at the woman's bedside.
- Keep strict measure of I and O. Helps assess for side effects of tocolytics. Urine output less than 30 ml/hr suggests fluid volume deficit or inadequate renal perfusion.
- Assess daily weight. Determines water retention.
- Assess urine and check for ketones. Altered glucose metabolism is a side effect of terbutaline (Brethine).
- Assess electrolytes and blood glucose levels. Identifies hyperglycemia and hypokalemia, which are side effects of tocolytics, so they can be managed. Women with diabetes may need to increase their insulin dosage as advised by their practitioner.

- Assess hourly while on medication. Enables rapid identification of and intervention for drug side effects or toxicities should they occur.

Preventive Nursing Activities

- Place calcium gluconate at the bedside. In the event of magnesium toxicity, calcium gluconate is the antidote.
- Limit total oral and IV fluid intake to 2,400–3,000 ml/day. Helps prevent fluid overload and pulmonary edema.
- Teach and prepare for discharge if labor is stopped. Teach couple signs of preterm labor and reasons to seek additional care.
- Advise about the need for diversional activity planning. The woman may be at home on bed rest, which may require diversional activities for compliance. Also, assess supportive network since she may need extra household help.

INDIVIDUALIZED (NURSING DIAGNOSIS) CARE PLANS

The care plans in this section were developed to address unique patient needs.

▌ Nursing Diagnosis: PAIN[1]

Related Factors: uterine cramping, vaginal dilation, and effacement in PTL. Refer to the generic NDCP "Pain,[1]" beginning on p. 18 in Chapter 2.

▌ *Goals, Outcomes, and Evaluation Criteria*

- Woman recognizes and reports pain.
- Contractions are arrested.

▌ *NIC Interventions[2]*

Medication Aministration (2300)—Preparing, giving, and evaluating the effectiveness of prescription and nonprescription drugs.

▌ *Nursing Activities and Rationales*

Assessments

- Monitor for therapeutic and adverse effects of medications. Determines the effectiveness of therapy and identifies complications that may require discontinuing therapy or treatment. Response to pain medications and comfort measures are important to document.

Patient/Family Teaching

- Inform the woman that backache, abdominal cramping, contractions, and pelvic pressure may indicate preterm labor. Some women only refer to pain and do not describe discomfort in other terms unless taught about distinction of

symptoms. The woman is the one who will most likely identify the initiation of labor and needs to be acutely aware of the physical changes and terms to accurately describe to her provider. Understanding may allow for early intervention and prevention of a preterm birth.

- Instruct to report sensations of pain as soon as they are identified. Early intervention may arrest contractions or alleviate pain before it becomes too severe or labor has progressed too far to be stopped.
- Describe nonpharmacologic methods to manage pain. Relaxation techniques, distraction, warm/cold applications, guided imagery, etc., are techniques that serve as adjuncts to pharmacologic methods and provide the woman some control over her pain.

Collaborative Activities

- Administer tocolytics and analgesics as prescribed. Tocolytics alleviate pain by decreasing the UCs; analgesics work centrally or peripherally, depending on the medication used, to decrease perception of pain.

▌ Nursing Diagnosis: ANXIETY/ FEAR[1]

Related Factors: unknown outcome of pregnancy; feared loss of fetus, loss of control. Refer to the generic NDCPs, "Anxiety[1]" and "Fear,[1]" which begin on pp. 10 and 15, respectively, in Chapter 2.

▌ *Nursing Activities and Rationales*

Assessments

- Identify personal strengths, coping mechanisms, and social supports. Establishes a basis for further care planning. Coping strategies that have been successful in the past are likely to be successful during current stressful situation. The presence of a strong social support system increases the woman's ability to cope with the stress of her current situation.
- Determine what the loss of the pregnancy or an early delivery means to the woman. Involve family as willing to participate in process. Facilitates decision making and coping. Fears related to premature birth or loss of a wanted pregnancy can be very distressful to the woman and her partner. Identifying the degree of stress helps direct the plan of care.
- Reinforce previous teaching and realistic expectations. Ensures the woman has factual information and understands her risks and the situation. Some people who experience fear will have unrealistic fears and exaggerate the situation. If realistic teaching is done, it may help decrease fears about the unknown.
- Assess stressors and discuss management. Reduces anxiety.

- Explain and teach about all procedures and medications; answer all questions. Anxiety will decrease if information is freely shared and questions are welcomed.

Independent Nursing Actions

- Encourage self-care activities (rest, adequate nutrition). Maintains a woman's health and stamina and allows for a sense of control over her situation.
- Listen with empathy and acceptance. Demonstrates compassion and understanding and facilitates trust.
- Aid in problem solving and decision making with stress management techniques. Planning to reduce other stressors, household responsibilities, and workload can reduce stress and anxiety so increased self-care and relaxation can occur. If physical stressors are reduced, mental anxiety can also be reduced.

Collaborative Activities

- Refer to pastoral care or counseling services for present need or for future needs. Provides additional support or resources to the woman.
- Refer to support agencies, such as Compassionate Friends, SHARE, and so forth. Provides system for long-term social support.
- Assess for potential for depression or mood disorders postpartum. Allows for referrals and early intervention as needed and appropriate.
- Refer for birth control after miscarriage. Prevents pregnancy before woman/couple has adjusted to loss or before couple is ready for another pregnancy.
- Refer to support agency and/or counseling if preterm labor results in premature infant. Prematurity is also a stressor and is a loss of the perfect child and pregnancy. Parents of premature infants need teaching and time to adjust to a high-needs infant. Refer to "Preterm Newborn," which begins on p. 412 in Chapter 12.

▌ Nursing Diagnosis: SPIRITUAL DISTRESS[1]

Related Factors: guilt regarding fetal loss/preterm labor.

▌ *Goals, Outcomes, and Evaluation Criteria*

- Woman identifies and verbalizes feelings about loss.
- Woman participates in usual spiritual practices (e.g., prayer, meditation).
- Woman discusses spiritual practices and concerns, as well as cultural needs.
- Woman maintains personal needs for sleep, nutrition, hygiene.
- Woman expresses inner peace, meaning, and purpose in life.
- Woman works through normal grief process and discussion of possible guilt.

▌ *NIC Interventions[2]*

Grief Work Facilitation: Perinatal Death (5294)—Assistance with the resolution of a perinatal loss.
Guilt Work Facilitation (5300)—Helping another to cope with painful feelings of responsibility, actual or perceived.
Spiritual Growth Facilitation (5426)—Facilitation of growth in patient's capacity to identify, connect with, and call upon the source of meaning, purpose, comfort, strength, and hope in his/her life.

▌ *Nursing Activities and Rationales*

Assessments

- Determine previous experience with spontaneous abortion or premature labor. Establishes a basis for intervention. Depending on the outcome of the previous experience, it may positively or negatively affect the woman's ability to cope with her current situation.
- Assess feelings, beliefs, or concerns about activities that may have initiated the spontaneous abortion/preterm labor, including cultural preferences and values. Enables the verbalization of any irrational belief and discussion of the factual findings or understanding about the early loss. The woman may blame herself or her partner for her current situation. Identifying her feelings and beliefs helps with planning appropriate interventions. She may feel like she has not fulfilled her responsibility to her family because of the loss, that she's lost face, or that she has specific religious needs for resolution over the loss. Expressions of grief can be from wailing to no response depending on the culture. Support in some cultures comes from the partner only and in others only female relatives or friends are called upon for support. Nurses need to be open to a patient's grief response. Acceptance helps facilitate the grief process.
- Identify strengths, coping mechanisms, support systems, and spiritual rituals. Determines possible resources for ongoing care and support.
- Discuss ways to concretize experience. Stillbirth, early fetal death, and prematurity have rituals and burials associated with each experience. Miscarriage is not as recognized; however, personal rituals and memories are just as important to integrate into the mother's/father's life experience and honor the loss of the potential child that was hoped for and has no replacement.
- Reassure the mother/father that grieving is a process and takes time. Facilitates the grief process. Encourage the woman/partner/family to be patient with grieving in different ways and seek counseling if the process becomes difficult for the relationships.

Independent Nursing Actions

- Encourage and arrange time for uninterrupted expression of spiritual or personal rituals. Demonstrates support for spiritual activities that are comforting to the woman/ partner/family.

- Assist to problem solve and identify ways to express anger. Facilitates resolution of guilt and grief and allows for spiritual growth.
- Be available to listen, hand hold, etc. Portrays compassion and concern and helps establish trust.

Collaborative Activities

- Provide information about support groups (e.g. SHARE, Compassionate Friends). The woman may be unaware of community resources that are available to her or how to access them.
- Provide referrals as needed to pastoral care, social services, counseling services, genetic counselor. Provides additional sources of emotional and spiritual support.
- Provide information about postpartum depression and refer to physician as appropriate. Sometimes a situational depression can be helped with short-term antidepressants or sleeping aids if insomnia is present.

Patient/Family Teaching

- Discuss the stages of loss and grief. Facilitates the woman's understanding of her reactions to the situation.
- Teach normal responses to grief and normal timeline. Teach the woman that her partner may not necessarily grieve in the same way and that counseling may be helpful. Understanding the range of normal responses and time needed to heal forms a reference to further understand grieving and loss.
- Offer suggestions on activities to help heal the loss and feelings of guilt or loss of self-esteem. Journaling, writing, personal rituals, prayer, and support groups with others who have similar experiences are all possibilities that people find helpful.
- Discuss postpartum depression or mood disorders and teach the family the signs and symptoms and importance of seeking care. The potential for occurrence can be after an early loss as well as full-term pregnancy. The family can recognize these before the woman does.

▌Nursing Diagnosis: INEFFECTIVE THERAPEUTIC REGIMEN MANAGEMENT[1]

Related Factors: Deficient Knowledge,[1] lack of understanding, lack of support systems, and so forth.

▌ *Goals, Outcomes, and Evaluation Criteria*

- Woman describes rationale for treatment regimen.

- Woman avoids behaviors, activities, and increased stress associated with increased risk for preterm labor.
- Woman follows prescribed plan of care.

▌ *NIC Interventions[2]*

Health System Guidance (7400)—Facilitating a patient's location and use of appropriate health services.

High-Risk Pregnancy Care (6800)—Identification and management of a high-risk pregnancy to promote healthy outcomes for mother and baby.

Labor Suppression (6860)—Controlling uterine contractions prior to 37 weeks of gestation to prevent preterm birth.

Teaching: Disease Process (5602)—Assisting the patient to understand information related to a specific disease process.

▌ *Nursing Activities and Rationales*

Assessments

- Determine understanding of fetal development, the signs of spontaneous abortion/preterm labor, and treatment plan. Provides a basis for teaching regarding therapeutic regimen.
- Assess baseline understanding of condition and fill in gaps in knowledge. Increases the woman's understanding and corrects misinformation. Include a family member who the woman wants involved in her care because she may not be able to take information in while she is cramping, contracting, or in physical pain. She may only be able to take in small amounts of information at a time.

Independent Nursing Actions

- Keep the woman and her family informed about the status of the pregnancy. Keeps lines of communication open and the family involved to increase compliance with necessary interventions and decrease fear and anxiety.
- Arrange for prenatal classes. Provides childbirth education opportunities while she is on bed rest.

Patient/Family Teaching

- Teach the woman signs and symptoms of preterm labor and how to differentiate between false and true labor. Aids in her ability to self-assess and obtain intervention as needed.
- Provide information about fetal development, signs of spontaneous abortion/preterm labor, procedures, and treatment as needed. Enhances the woman's understanding of her condition and care. The woman is most likely the person who will identify the onset of labor. Early recognition on her part will ensure early treatment and possible control of labor.
- Provide a tour of the neonatal intensive care unit for PTL. Decreases the woman's anxiety in the event that admission to the unit is necessary.
- Inform woman about home care needs—medication administration and side effects, restrictions in physical

and sexual activity, diet and hydration needs. Increases the woman's understanding of her condition to promote self-management of care.
- Teach the woman how to palpate UCs and assess fetal movement and fetal movement and fetal kick counting. Increases her self-awareness in regard to uterine and fetal activity. She will need to identify and monitor her own contractions while at home and be able to report indications of preterm labor.
- Inform the woman about when and how to contact her healthcare provider. Facilitates early intervention if preterm labor begins.

Nursing Diagnosis: DEFICIENT DIVERSIONAL ACTIVITY[1]

Related Factors: bed rest and/or other prescribed activity limitations.

▮ *Goals, Outcomes, and Evaluation Criteria*

- Woman identifies and uses diversional activities.
- Woman interacts with family, friends, and others.
- Woman verbalizes diminished feelings of boredom.

▮ *NIC Interventions[2]*

Recreation Therapy (5360)—Purposeful use of recreation to promote relaxation and enhancement of social skills.
Visitation Facilitation (7560)—Promoting beneficial visits by family and friends.

▮ *Nursing Activities and Rationales*

Assessments

- Assess feelings and concerns about bed rest. Determines if and what type of intervention is needed. Women vary in their need for diversional activities.
- Determine hobbies and recreational interests. Establishes a basis for care planning. Women with more sedentary lifestyle habits may adapt to bed rest more readily than those who are active.
- Monitor response to recreational activities. Determines level of enjoyment and possible harmful effects.

Independent Nursing Actions

- Assist the woman to creatively explore personally meaningful activities. Allows the woman to diversify and take time to explore interests at this quiet time in her pregnancy.
- Discuss maintaining connection to friends and family through phone calls, letter writing, emails, and the Internet. Allows the woman to feel connected even though she is homebound.

- Explore ways for the woman to remain an active participant in home management and decision making. Promotes a sense of control.
- Encourage visits and calls from family and friends. Provides opportunities for social interaction and reassurance of family support.
- Vary the physical environment and daily routine. Reduces monotony, which contributes to boredom and may interfere with compliance.

Collaborative Activities

- Collaborate with recreational, occupational, and music therapists. Provides diversional activities, such as crafts, games, puzzles, cards, reading materials, movies, etc., in order to reduce boredom and provides opportunities for interaction with others.

Patient/Family Teaching

- Teach about stress management and relaxation techniques. Helps manage tension resulting from confinement.

Nursing Diagnosis: INTERRUPTED FAMILY PROCESSES[1]

Related Factors: the impact of spontaneous abortion/preterm labor; loss of fetus; hospitalization of the woman; and disruption of family routines.

▮ *Goals, Outcomes, and Evaluation Criteria*

- Family identifies feelings and beliefs about loss.
- Family adapts to situation by adjusting roles and responsibilities.
- Family supports all family members.
- Family seeks assistance and support as needed.

▮ *NIC Interventions[2]*

Family Integrity Promotion (7100)—Promotion of family cohesion and unity.
Family Process Maintenance (7130)—Minimization of family process disruption effects.

▮ *Nursing Activities and Rationales*

Assessments

- Encourage verbalization of feelings, beliefs, and concerns. Identifies irrational feelings so that misconceptions can be corrected.
- Identify effects of situation on family roles, responsibilities, and functioning. Determines need for intervention.

Enforced bed rest on the mother may be difficult for all family members.

- Determine the family's strengths, coping mechanisms, and support systems. Establishes the basis for care planning. Building on strengths will help the plan be more effective. Coping mechanisms that have worked in the past are likely to be successful during the present situation.

Independent Nursing Actions

- Listen with empathy. Establishes a trusting relationship and demonstrates a nonjudgmental, caring attitude.
- Keep family informed about the woman's and fetus's condition. Maintains open communication and decreases anxiety. Lack of knowledge or understanding increases fear and anxiety.
- Provide for opportunities for family communication and visitation. Promotes family solidarity and opportunities for support.

Collaborative Activities

- Refer to social services, pastoral care, counseling services, and genetic therapy as needed. The family may be unaware of community resources and how to access those resources. Additional resources may facilitate family functioning, understanding, and cohesiveness.
- Provide information about support groups. Allows family additional sources of support.

Patient/Family Teaching

- Instruct family regarding the normal process of loss and grief. Facilitates understanding of the family's reaction to the situation.
- Counsel family regarding effective coping mechanisms. Equips family to deal constructively with the situation. Family members may or may not be aware of their use of ineffective coping mechanisms.

▌ *Other Nursing Diagnoses*

Also assess for the following nursing diagnoses, which are frequently present with this condition:

- Risk for Infection[1] related to retained products of conception.
- Situational Low Self-Esteem[1] related to inability to successfully carry a pregnancy to term.

PREMATURE RUPTURE OF MEMBRANES

Preterm birth complicates approximately 12% of all births in the United States, one third of which involve premature rupture of membranes. Premature rupture of membranes (PROM) refers to the spontaneous rupture of the amniotic sac prior to the onset of labor. PROM may occur at any gestation time in a pregnancy. The timing of the rupture and fetal status determine treatment interventions and outcomes of the pregnancy. *Preterm PROM (PPROM)* is rupture before 37 weeks' gestation. *Prolonged PROM* is rupture more than 24 hours before birth, referring to the latency period prior to birth. The longer membranes are ruptured, the greater the risk for infection.

PROM occurs when there is a localized weakening of the membrane from changes in collagen or from increased intraamniotic pressure. Bacteria ascending from the vagina create enzymes and inflammatory processes that thin the membrane and finally break through the sac. PROM increases the risk for intrauterine infection (chorioamnionitis) that can lead to life-threatening septicemia if not recognized and treated.

▌ *Key Nursing Activities*

- Monitor for infection (vital signs, assessments, cultures) and be prepared to treat infection and decrease risk for cord prolapse and preterm birth.
- Assist with medical therapies to maintain the pregnancy and/or mature fetal lungs.
- Assess gestational age, document time and date of rupture of membranes, assess fetal heart rate, and help with fetal surveillance.
- Provide information about condition and treatments, and offer emotional support during time of uncertainty.
- Assess for signs of labor.

▌ *Etiologies and Risk Factors*

The exact cause of PROM is unknown; but current scientific evidence supports 30–40% of cases occurring from ascending bacterial infections from the vagina entering the amniotic fluid through breaks in the sac (Behrman & Butler, 2007). Other predisposing conditions for PROM include:

- increased uterine pressure with multiple gestation and polyhydramnios
- inflammation from cervicitis or amnionitis
- placenta previa, abruptio placentae
- abnormalities of internal cervical os
- multiple amniocenteses
- urinary tract infection
- bacterial vaginosis or group B streptococci, gonorrhea
- therapeutic abortion

There is an increased risk in women who

- have a history of previous PROM in another pregnancy
- are socioeconomically disadvantaged
- are/were sexually promiscuous teenagers
- have nutritional deficiencies (especially regarding zinc, vitamins D and E, and copper)
- smoke

▌ Signs and Symptoms

Subjective. Continuous small leak or gush of fluid from the vagina prior to onset of labor. Some women describe the feeling as leaking of urine. Some will describe a pop or gush. Backache may be present. Abdominal cramping may or may not be present.

Objective. Clear or slightly pink or green-tinged fluid from the vagina prior to the onset of labor; gross pooling of amniotic fluid in the vaginal vault visible on sterile speculum exam. Fever may be present if infection has started.

▌ Diagnostic Studies

These are tests for diagnosing PROM. Tests for identifying complications from PROM are found under the associated collaborative care plans.

- Sterile speculum exam. Visualizes cervix and pooling of fluid. Enables fluid sample to be obtained. Vaginal digital exam should be avoided because it increases risk for infection. Dilatation is determined visually on speculum exam.
- Nitrazine test. Nitrazine paper turns blue due to alkaline nature of ammonic fluid, which is pH 7.1–7.3.
- Fern test of vaginal secretions. Visualization of microscopic exam of dried fluid will show a fernlike pattern.
- Amniocentesis. Determines fetal lung maturity and presence of infection.
- Intrauterine dye. When diagnosis is uncertain, a dye may be inserted via amniocentesis to see if it will color the vaginal secretions. Vaginal secretions turn color if fluid is leaking.
- Ultrasound and fetal surveillance with BPP is common. Determines gestational age, fetal status, level of amniotic fluid, and placenta grading.
- External uterine and fetal monitoring. Evaluates fetal well-being and presence, frequency, and duration of contractions.
- Blood Rh factor and antibody screen. Determines need for Rh-immune globulin in the event the woman is Rh negative.
- Cultures. Determines pathogen if infection of fluid is suspected.

▌ Medical Management

Medical management depends upon the gestational age of the fetus as well as the presence of infection.

General

- Documentation of gestational age through review of records and ultrasound.
- Confirm or rule out PROM.
- Fetal monitoring to evaluate fetal well-being; assessment of stressors through fetal heart rate and movement monitoring, nonstress tests, BPP, and amniotic fluid index.
- Assessment of amniotic fluid for presence of infection may occur in addition to vital signs assessment, uterine tenderness, and maternal white blood cell count.

- Hospitalization is usually necessary.
- Home care may be appropriate if fetus is below viable age (23 weeks to 34 weeks of gestation), no fetal compromise, absence of infection, and fetus is not in immediate danger. Criteria for home care includes cervical dilation of 3 cm or less, documented PROM of longer than 72 hours, no signs or symptoms of chorioamnionitis or pyelonephritis, no signs or symptoms of preterm labor, woman is willing to comply with strict pelvic rest, and no fetal malpresentation creating risk of prolapsed cord. The presence of a responsible adult 24 hours each day and immediate availability of transportation to the hospital may also be required.
- Corticosteroids (betamethasone or dexamethasone) are indicated if less than 34 weeks and no chorioamnionitis.
- Prophylactic antibiotic therapy, especially in presence of group B streptococcus.
- Tocolysis is controversial.
- Before 23 weeks of gestation, care must be individualized due to extreme prematurity. (Extreme prematurity is beyond the scope of this book. For further information, refer to a maternity or obstetrics textbook.)

Term (37 Weeks' Gestation or More)

- Monitoring and preparation for birth.
- Induction if spontaneous labor does not begin within 12–16 hours.
- Antibiotic prophylaxis for group B streptococcus.

Near Term (34–36 Weeks' Gestation Completed)

- The preferred treatment of term PROM is birth.
- If in active labor, allow to progress.
- If not in labor, induction is indicated if signs and symptoms of infection are present. When the risk to the fetus of the continued pregnancy is greater than the risks associated with preterm delivery, labor is induced. The exact number of weeks' gestation at which labor is induced differs among practitioners and is based on their patient population and morbidity/mortality statistics. Some, for example, have found that babies born at or after 34 weeks' gestation generally do well.
- Labor may be induced/augmented with oxytocin to shorten the interval between membrane rupture and delivery. Misoprostol has been shown to be comparable to oxytocin in some studies.
- Prostaglandin suppositories may be used to prepare an unripe cervix for induction but are controversial because of problems with infection.
- Prophylactic antibiotics may also be used (e.g., ampicillin, betamicin). Group B streptococcus (GBS) prophylaxis is indicated if unknown status and rupture of membranes exceeds 18 hours.

Preterm (32–33 Weeks' Gestation Completed)

- Provide expectant management in the hospital, including bed rest and possible tocolysis if UCs begin.
- Vaginal cultures for GBS, chlamydia, and gonorrhea. Prophylaxis for group B streptococcus and treatment if present.
- Monitor FHR and UCs to evaluate.
- If labor begins and infection or fetal distress occurs, delivery is warranted.
- Corticosteroids (to promote fetal lung maturity) and broad-spectrum parenteral antibiotics (to prevent infection) may be given.

Previable Fetus (e.g., Fewer Than 24 Weeks' Gestation Completed)

- Patient counseling.
- If labor or infection is present, deliver.
- For all other situations, perform either immediate termination of the pregnancy (if the woman chooses) or expectant management at home. This includes bed rest, avoidance of intercourse, self-monitoring of temperature, awaiting UCs, and (if gestational age of 25–35 weeks is attained) hospitalization for daily fetal evaluation and prompt intervention when labor occurs.
- Corticosteroids and GBS prophylaxis are not recommended.

▮ *Collaborative Problems*

Potential complications of PROM include the following:

- Risk for infection (chorioamnionitis)
- Umbilical cord prolapse
- Placental abruption
- Fetal compromise (deformities, decreased respiratory movement, fetal structural development because of amniotic bands caused by decreased amniotic fluid, fetal asphyxia resulting from cord compression because of decreased amniotic fluid, respiratory distress syndrome, infection, fetal hypoxia)
- Fetal risks (premature birth, prolapsed cord, oligohydramnios, meconium presence and risk of aspiration pneumonia, intestinal obstruction, diaphragmatic hernia, clubfoot, scoliosis, and hip dislocation)

Potential complications of chorioamnionitis include the following:

- Congenital pneumonia
- Sepsis (maternal and fetal)
- Meningitis
- Pulmonary hypoplasia

COLLABORATIVE (STANDARDIZED) CARE FOR ALL WOMEN WITH PREMATURE RUPTURE OF MEMBRANES

Perform comprehensive assessment to identify individual needs for teaching, emotional support, and physical care.

▮ Nursing Diagnosis: RISK FOR INFECTION (CHORIOAMNIONITIS AND ENDOMETRITIS)[1]

Related Factors: rupture of membranes more than 13 hours before labor. Refer to the generic NDCP, "Risk for Infection,"[1] which begins on p. 21 in Chapter 2, and the collaborative care plan, "Potential Complication: Infection," beginning on p. 29 in Chapter 3.

▮ *Goals, Outcomes, and Evaluation Criteria*

Also see the generic NDCP, "Risk for Infection,"[1] which begins on p. 21 in Chapter 2.

- Woman will remain free of chorioamnionitis, as evidenced by VSs within normal limits for woman (e.g., temperature less than 100.4°F), WBCs less than 15,000, C-reactive protein within normal limits, amniotic fluid clear and free of foul odor.
- Pregnancy will be maintained until fetal lungs mature.

▮ *Nursing Activities and Rationales*

Focus Assessments

- Assess and verify membrane rupture by sterile speculum examination (see "Diagnostic Studies").
- Determine the duration of the rupture of membranes. There is a high incidence (10%) of intrauterine infection associated with PROM. The risk for infection may be directly related to the time involved. Also, onset of labor occurs within 24 hours in 60–80% of women with PROM.
- Assess for elevation of temperature every 4 hours and maternal pulse and blood pressure. Note if there is a change in vaginal discharge, especially for odor and purulence. It is necessary to be vigilant for detecting presence of infection with PROM because chorioamnionitis compromises both mother and baby. Early signs of infection are elevation of temperature and tachycardia.
- Assess for uterine contractions. Preterm labor, a leading cause of perinatal morbidity and mortality, occurs in most cases where intrauterine infection is present. Also, when

intrauterine infection is present, both the mother and the fetus are at risk for sepsis; the neonate is also at risk for congenital pneumonia and meningitis.

- Observe for abdominal pain or tenderness. These are signs of intrauterine infection.
- Assess laboratory results for signs of infection—elevated WBCs and C-reactive protein; cloudy, foul-smelling amniotic fluid. Elevation of WBCs indicates infection. Normal C-reactive protein is a reassuring sign of absence of infection. The presence of WBCs or Gram-negative bacteria in amniotic fluid is an indicator of infection.
- Review urinalysis report. Urinalysis may indicate urinary tract infection that needs treatment because it can cause uterine irritability and early labor and is a source for potential ascending infection.
- Obtain vaginal cultures as ordered or per protocol. Determines presence of pathogenic organisms such as *Chlamydia*, group B streptococci (GBS), *Trichomonas*, or gonorrhea.

Independent Nursing Actions

- Maintain aseptic technique, e.g., for perineal care, catheterization. Prevents introduction of pathogens into the vagina.
- Avoid digital vaginal examinations. Vaginal examinations introduce pathogens into the vagina and may stimulate UCs.

Patient/Family Teaching

- Instruct on good perineal hygiene. Cleansing and wiping from front to back help prevent transfer of organisms from the anus and perineal area to the vagina where they can ascend to the uterus.
- Instruct the woman to monitor her temperature four times a day if going home. Detects infection, which facilitates early treatment.
- Advise to call the primary care provider if her temperature is greater than 100.4°F (38°C) or if she develops uterine tenderness, foul-smelling vaginal discharge (for woman at home), or early labor signs. If signs of infection are reported early, early treatment may prevent maternal sepsis and chorioamnionitis, as well as neonatal infections. She will return to the laboratory for white blood cell counts as often as twice weekly.
- Instruct the couple to put nothing in the vagina and emphasize the need for pelvic rest, no douching, and no tub baths. Prevents the introduction of pathogens into the vagina.
- Teach the importance of activity restriction. The woman will likely be advised to stay on bed rest with bathroom privileges unless the provider states otherwise. She needs to be in lateral position.

- Explain the implications of PROM and all treatment methods. Helps to prepare the couple for possible outcomes, such as preterm birth, cesarean birth, and the possibility of fetal or neonatal demise. Also provides the woman with information needed for self-care.

Potential Complications of PROM: PLACENTAL ABRUPTION

Focus Assessments

- Assess for vaginal bleeding, abdominal pain, and strong uterine contractions that do not let up. These are signs of placental abruption. (See "Late Antepartum Bleeding," beginning on p. 179 in this chapter.)

Preventive Nursing Activities

- Explain the importance of bed rest. Facilitates compliance with plan to prevent stimulating uterine contractions.
- Teach the woman (being followed at home) to notify her provider immediately if signs of placental abruption develop. Placental abruption is a medical emergency. Treatment must begin immediately in order to prevent maternal hemorrhage and fetal demise.

Potential Complications (Fetal) of PROM (Prior to 37 Weeks' Gestation): PREMATURITY AND RESPIRATORY DISTRESS SYNDROME

Focus Assessments

- Monitor fetal heart rate, activity, and NSTs. Helps determine the fetus's ability to withstand the stresses of labor.
- Assess fetal lung maturity studies (if fetus is nearing 34 weeks' gestation). Assists with decision making about whether to try to prolong the pregnancy. This is seldom done when corticosteroids are routinely given as a standard of care.
- Administer corticosteroids as prescribed or per protocol. Administered over a 24-hour period to enhance fetal lung maturity.
- Assess uterine and fetal activity. These are signs that labor is occurring. For 60–80% of women, labor occurs within 24 hours of PROM.

- Assess for symptoms of maternal infection. Preterm labor occurs in most cases in which intrauterine infection is present.

Preventive Nursing Activities

- Prepare for complications with the newborn. The most common neonatal complication with PROM prior to 37 weeks' gestation is respiratory distress syndrome. Other complications include anoxia due to cord prolapse or compression, sepsis, and neonatal pneumonia and meningitis.
- Encourage modified bed rest. Maternal activity can stimulate uterine contractions.
- Administer tocolytics if ordered as prescribed. Although tocolytics are not usually indicated for PROM, they may be ordered for short-term use to allow for administration of corticosteroids (to mature the fetal lungs) before the birth.
- Instruct the woman on signs of preterm labor. This is especially important for women being managed at home so that intervention can begin as soon as possible.

Potential Complication (Fetal) of PROM: UMBILICAL CORD PROLAPSE

Focus Assessments

- Monitor fetal heart rate and activity. Variable decelerations and other rate changes may indicate umbilical cord compression.
- Assess ultrasound. Determines amniotic fluid volume; oligohydramnios increases the likelihood of cord prolapse.
- Assess for cord prolapsed by performing frequent visualization of the vagina to detect presence of umbilical cord, palpating umbilical cord via sterile vaginal exam, or through maternal statements such as, "It feels like something came out." These are signs of cord prolapse, which necessitates immediate action to prevent fetal anoxia.

Preventive Nursing Activities

- Keep patient on modified bed rest. Before 37 weeks' gestation, the fetus is small and the head is not engaged in the pelvis. When the membranes rupture, the cord may pass the fetal head and emerge through the cervix into the vagina. Because of the effects of gravity, this is more likely to occur when the woman is in an upright position.
- In the event of cord prolapse, institute emergency interventions, such as:
  - Place the woman in slight Trendelenburg position. Prevents more cord from coming into the vagina; prevents the weight of the fetus from compressing the cord against the maternal pelvis.
  - Insert a sterile-gloved hand into the mother's vagina and apply gentle pressure to the fetal presenting part. Prevents the weight of the fetus from compressing the cord against the maternal pelvis.
  - Have someone else immediately call the provider. Summons help for the nurse. The nurse cannot leave the patient and cannot remove the pressure on the fetal presenting part; however, emergency birth is essential, so the provider must be notified immediately.

Potential Complications (Maternal) of Glucocorticoid Therapy: INFECTION, PULMONARY EDEMA, AND HYPERGLYCEMIA

Focus Assessments

- Assess for signs of infection (e.g., temperature, WBCs, foul-smelling vaginal fluid, malaise). Steroid therapy may mask signs of infection; therefore, it increases the risk of sepsis in women with PROM. There is also concern regarding immunosuppression related to steroid administration.
- Monitor blood glucose levels. Corticosteroids may increase serum glucose levels, especially in a woman with diabetes.
- Assess lung sounds. Detects pulmonary edema, a possible side effect of glucocorticoid therapy.

Preventive Nursing Activities

- Use and teach good hand-washing and hygiene practices. Prevents infection, which may be masked by the corticosteroids.

INDIVIDUALIZED (NURSING DIAGNOSIS) CARE PLANS

The care plans in this section were developed to address unique patient needs.

Nursing Diagnosis: ANXIETY/ FEAR[1]

Related Factors: outcome of pregnancy (e.g., the possibility of preterm birth and/or fetal death); concern about threats to self (e.g., infection and sepsis). Refer to the generic NDCPs, "Anxiety[1]" and "Fear,"[1] which begin on pp. 10 and 15, respectively, in Chapter 2.

Goals, Outcomes, and Evaluation Criteria; NIC Interventions

See the NDCPs, "Anxiety[1]" and "Fear,[1]" which begin on pp. 10 and 15, respectively, in Chapter 2.

Nursing Activities and Rationales

Independent Nursing Actions

• Encourage an attitude of realistic hope. If labor can be delayed until fetal lungs are mature, and if infection can be prevented, a good outcome can be anticipated, which may reduce anxiety and fear.

Patient/Family Teaching

• Provide factual information about diagnosis, treatment, and prognosis (e.g., the need for bed rest, the possibility of premature birth, cesarean birth, and/or fetal or neonatal loss). Provides information the woman needs to participate in her own care. Provides anticipatory guidance to support coping in the event of a poor outcome.

Nursing Diagnosis: DEFICIENT DIVERSIONAL ACTIVITY[1]

Related Factors: prescribed bed rest.

Goals, Outcomes, and Evaluation Criteria; NIC Interventions

See the NDCP, "Deficient Diversional Activity,[1]" beginning on p. 12 of Chapter 2.

Nursing Activities and Rationales

Assessments

• Inquire about interests and activities before PROM (e.g., reading, sports). A related activity may be an acceptable substitute.

• Assess level of anxiety and ability to concentrate. If the woman is having difficulty concentrating, activities requiring extended attention span may create frustration and feelings of failure.

Independent Nursing Actions

• Provide frequent contact. Set up a schedule so that the woman will know when to expect contact or activities. Prolonged confinement may cause the woman to become depressed or to disengage by sleeping excessively or refusing visitors.

• Spend time with the woman without providing physical care. Engaging the woman in conversation without focusing on her condition will divert her attention and help pass the time.

• Suggest new interests (e.g., crafts, Internet). Renting or borrowing a computer that can be connected to social networks or other sources may provide intellectual stimulation and access to chat groups.

• Facilitate visiting by family and friends. Provides distraction and emotional support.

Collaborative Activities

• Consult with dietary services to provide dietary changes, if possible. Meals and menu selection become very important to the confined woman.

• Collaborate with volunteers and physical and/or occupational therapy to plan an acceptable activity program. Take care to not overload the woman with books, projects, etc. for which she has no interest.

Other Nursing Diagnoses

Also assess for the following nursing diagnoses, which are frequently present with this condition:

• Ineffective Coping[1] related to situational crisis, uncertain outcome, threat to mother and fetus, perceived lack of control over the situation, or inadequate support.

• Impaired Home Maintenance[1] related to imposed bed rest or hospitalization.

CLINICAL INTERRUPTION OF PREGNANCY: SURGICAL AND MEDICATION ABORTION

Induced abortion, also referred to as *elective abortion* and *therapeutic abortion*, refers to the planned termination of pregnancy before 20 weeks' gestation at the woman's request (elective) or for reasons of maternal or fetal health (therapeutic). Ninety percent of abortions are performed during the first trimester, when the maternal mortality rate is less than the mortality rate after normal term delivery. Greater than one in five pregnancies ends in abortion. Women might choose to terminate a pregnancy when genetic abnormalities are such that they are incompatible with life, compromise life, or shorten life expectancy.

Abortion was legalized in 1973 to protect the mother from abortion complications. In the first trimester, abortion is allowed with collaboration between the woman and her medical provider without state intervention. In the second trimester, individual states can regulate procedures as long as the reason is associated with preserving the woman's health. Third-trimester terminations are limited or even prohibited by state regulation. With increasing multiple fetuses from fertility intervention, there may be the option to perform a fetal reduction. A discussion of this option is beyond the scope of this care plan. Refer to a maternal or obstetrics textbook for further information.

Nearly half of pregnancies in the United States are unintentional, thus the nurse's role must include option counseling. A woman may need time to process a positive pregnancy test. She has three options for her pregnancy such as completing it to term, relinquishment if untimely, and termination. Knowledge of choice and review of all options are important.

When unexpected results come back from a prenatal screening test, alpha fetoprotein test, or triple screen, chromosomal abnormalities that are not compatible with life may be present. Just as in the previous paragraph, a woman in this situation has to make decisions about whether she wishes to continue her pregnancy. The option that will be discussed in this care plan is abortion, the clinical interruption of pregnancy and planned termination of a pregnancy.

Key Nursing Activities

- Assess the woman's health, conduct history, physical exam, establish gestational age, and review laboratory findings, noting Rh factor and need for Rho(D) immune globulin treatment.
- Offer emotional support, information, alternatives, and risks to the procedure.
- Teach regarding preparation and procedures and confirm signed consent.
- Monitor for complications and assist with recovery process.
- Teach regarding self- and home care and the importance of follow-up appointment.
- Support the grieving process because a pregnancy loss has occurred.
- Discuss emotional impact of pregnancy loss and screen for postpartum depression from shifting hormones after termination of pregnancy.
- Treat patient with respect and maintain confidentiality.

Indications for Induced Abortion

- Preservation of life or health of the mother
- Fetal genetic disorders (e.g., chromosomal abnormalities, microcephaly)
- Rape or incest
- Pregnant woman's request

Signs and Symptoms

- Verbalization of desire to terminate pregnancy
- Documentation of fetal abnormality that may be incompatible with life
- Life situational crisis and decision made to choose abortion

Diagnostic Studies

- Sonogram. Determines size of fetus prior to second-trimester abortion.

- HCG serum or urine test. Validates existence of pregnancy.
- Blood type and Rh factor determination. Establishes the presence of isoimmunization or sensitization prior to administering Rho(D) immune globulin treatment and determines blood type in case transfusion is needed postabortion.
- Complete blood count, WBC count, and differential. Rules out the presence of infection, anemia, or other factors that can affect the outcome of the abortion.
- Screening for *Chlamydia*, gonorrhea, and other STIs. Prevents introduction of pathogens into pelvic organs by instruments.
- Coagulation studies, liver function tests, and other studies. May be ordered if patient has medical conditions that require further testing.

Medical Management

- Counseling prior to any procedure. Ensures time for obtaining information, verbalizing understanding of procedures and recovery, and careful decision making. A choice needs to be made about which procedure is to be done, consent given, and postprocedural birth control options must be determined.
- Counseling regarding congenital fetal anomaly if diagnosed. Ensures family understands the anomaly, the impact on the fetus, and implications for the family; treatment options available to manage the anomaly; and availability of experts and counselors if needed. A genetic counselor may be needed and used.
- Type of procedure is determined by gestational age, expertise of provider, patient preference, clinical importance of obtaining a specimen for further testing, and presence of other clinical conditions.
- Cultures must be obtained and infections, if present, treated prior to procedure.
- Pain management following procedure if surgical procedure is elected, or pain support when passing products of conception at home if medical option is elected.
- Need for follow-up appointment to evaluate for missed abortion, bleeding, reduction of pregnancy symptoms, and infection or other problems such as grief or depression, and the need for appropriate referrals.

First-Trimester Abortions (Up to 14 Weeks; 8–12 Weeks Ideal Timing)

- Vacuum aspiration (vacuum or suction curettage). Minor procedure completed after lidocaine paracervical block. Oral medication for anxiety or conscious sedation is also sometimes used. Contents of uterus are evacuated by suction within about 5 minutes or less. Recovery takes from 1 hour to 3 hours and includes monitoring VSs, pain status, uterine involution, and bleeding.
- Mifepristone (RU 486)/misoprostol. Combination drug therapy approved by FDA to medically terminate pregnancy up to the 49th day of the pregnancy, or 63 days after the

start of the last menstrual period. Mifepristone terminates pregnancy by interfering with the action of progesterone, a hormone that maintains pregnancy. Misoprostol stimulates uterine contractions. Dosing is a two-step process. An oral dose of mifepristone is followed by an oral or vaginal dose of misoprostol in 48 hours if abortion has not occurred. Follow-up is required 2 weeks after dosing to verify abortion. If abortion is not complete, a surgical procedure is necessary. The woman is sent home to abort after the first dose of medication, which usually occurs within 24 hours. Pain medication is given because cramping and bleeding will occur. Warm packs may be used for comfort.

- Methotrexate/misoprostol. Cytotoxic drug that causes early abortion by blocking folic acid in fetal cells to block division; process is similar to mifepristone/misoprostol. Contraindications to medical abortion include ectopic pregnancy, in place intrauterine device, adrenal failure, current long-term corticosteroid use, bleeding disorder or current anticoagulant drug use, seizure disorder that is uncontrolled, inherited porphyrias, or inflammatory bowel disease. If the woman is breastfeeding, milk must be discarded.

Second-Trimester Abortions

Second-trimester abortions are performed up to 20 weeks' gestation; few states allow abortions past this gestational age.

- Dilatation and evacuation. Cervical priming and mechanical dilation are necessary to adequately evacuate the contents of the uterus with suction and curettage. Cervical preparation is accomplished with osmotic dilators/prostaglandins the evening before the abortion. Recovery is similar to first-trimester abortions. Complications associated with surgical abortion include retained placenta with associated hemorrhage or infection, failed abortion, live birth (in late 2nd-trimester terminations), uterine rupture, cervical injury, and uterine perforation.
  - Prophylactic antibiotic therapy. Tetracycline, clindamycin, and metronidazole are used to prevent infection.
  - Oral ergonovine postoperatively. Prevents retention of products of conception.
  - Rho(D) immune globulin treatment. Administered if candidate to prevent isoimmunization.
  - Provision of contraception method prior to going home is essential.

▌ Collaborative Problems

Potential complications of abortion include the following:

- Infection
- Hemorrhage
- Retained products of conception

COLLABORATIVE (STANDARDIZED) CARE FOR ALL WOMEN UNDERGOING ELECTIVE ABORTION

See the generic collaborative care plans "Potential Complication: Infection" and "Potential Complication: Hemorrhage," which begin on pp. 29 and 28, respectively, in Chapter 3. Perform comprehensive assessment to identify individual needs for teaching, emotional support, and physical care.

Focus Assessments (Second-Trimester Abortion)

- Assess uterine tone frequently following second-trimester abortion procedure. It is most important to make sure the uterus is clamping down after a second-trimester abortion procedure because there is greater possibility of atony after later abortions than with those prior to 10 weeks.

▌ Preventive Nursing Actions

Medical Abortion

- Teach the woman to monitor for side effects of medications. Nausea, vomiting, diarrhea, headache, dizziness, fever, and chills are side effects of mifepristone (RU 486)/misoprostol. These usually subside in a few hours after administration. Allergic reaction is a more serious adverse reaction.
- Review the parameters for postabortion bleeding and expectation of recovery. Bleeding can last up to 13 days. Enables the woman to anticipate changes in her physical status when she returns home.
- Teach the woman to report excessive vaginal bleeding and the need to comply with follow-up appointment in 2 weeks after 2nd dose of medication. Ensures early recognition of complications and facilitates early intervention such as surgical aspiration of uterine contents due to bleeding or treatment failure or blood transfusion.

Surgical Abortion

- Review discharge instructions. Helps ensure compliance. Discharge instructions include nothing in her vagina for 3 weeks, may shower daily, avoid douches, and watch for signs of potential complications. Call healthcare provider if fever over 100.4°F (38°C), chills (signs of infection); bleeding is greater than two saturated pads in 2 hours or heavy bleeding lasts a few days (retained products or uterine atony or infection); purulent or odorous discharge; severe abdominal pain, cramping, or backache; abdominal tenderness with pressure (signs of infection); or no menstrual cycle for 6 weeks after procedure (possible retention).

Nursing Diagnosis: RISK FOR DECISIONAL CONFLICT[1]

Related Factors: options and decisions regarding elective abortion and plan for this pregnancy; perceived threat to personal value system; unclear personal values/beliefs; lack of social system support; lack of experience or interference with decision making; multiple or divergent sources of information; lack of relevant information; situational distress; fetus with severe abnormality; and difficulty with decision-making process.

Goals, Outcomes, and Evaluation Criteria

- Absence of physical signs of distress.
- Woman participates in decision making.
- Woman verbalizes understanding of procedures.
- Woman uses coping strategies effectively.
- Woman verbalizes fears/concerns.
- Woman accepts assistance and support from family/partner.

NIC Interventions[2]

Coping Enhancement (5230)—Assisting a patient to adapt to perceived stressors, changes, or threats that interfere with meeting life demands and roles.

Counseling (5240)—Use of an interactive helping process focusing on the needs, problems, or feelings of the patient and significant others to enhance or support coping, problem solving, and interpersonal relationships.

Decision-Making Support (5250)—Providing information and support for a patient who is making a decision regarding health care.

Emotional Support (5270)—Provision of reassurance, acceptance, and encouragement during times of stress.

Mutual Goal Setting (4410)—Collaborating with patient to identify and prioritize care goals, then developing a plan for achieving those goals.

Nursing Activities and Rationales

Assessments

- Assess the woman's values and beliefs about the pregnancy and options available to her; listen to her and support her decision-making process; explore her thoughts/feelings about her pregnancy and discuss the pros/cons and risks/benefits of each of her available options. Establishes a baseline understanding of the woman's belief system so that the nurse can support those beliefs while the woman/couple make decisions about terminating the pregnancy or other decisions.
- Assess the woman for feelings of conflict regarding the alternatives that conflict with values, ethics, and/or spiritual beliefs. Verbalization of feelings assists the patient to discuss options and alternatives and provides the nurse with information that will be used in supporting the decisions made by the patient.

- Assess for possibility of domestic violence and what her home life is like. If partner is supportive include that person so she is not so alone. The nurse needs to be aware of risks and if she has special needs. Women who are pregnant are at higher risk for domestic violence and should always be assessed for it.
- Help the woman identify support persons and systems and assess risks for her. The woman needs to know who will help her. If support system is not in place, she will need assistance locating appropriate community resources.

Independent Nursing Actions

- If fetal anomaly is known to be present, make sure all information is reviewed with the woman/partner by her provider or genetic counselor so she can make the best decision for her and her partner about the outcome for her pregnancy. Helps the woman make an informed decision. All information should be explained in plain language and in a way that is clearly understood, leaving no gray areas or areas of doubt about the potential outcome of the pregnancy, fetal anomaly being incompatible with life, or causing severe impairment of the child, etc.
- Support decisional process and reserve any judgment, but help her decide on timetable because the type of pregnancy termination is dependent on gestational age. Conveys supportive, nonjudgmental attitude, but helps the woman maintain a realistic focus.
- If the woman makes her decision to terminate her pregnancy, support her decision and refer her to the proper facility and provider. Demonstrates acceptance, relieves anxiety, and facilitates the woman's access to the appropriate healthcare facility.
- Offer support by giving the woman permission to grieve, encouraging her to forgive herself and give up guilt, identify her support systems, and include her partner and family in the process. Demonstrates support and facilitates healing. The woman's feelings of guilt and being alone need to be discussed. She needs to be encouraged to include her partner and family in the process so they can heal as a couple and family unit and provide needed support for each other.

Collaborative Activities

- Refer for counseling as appropriate. Identify those at increased risk for distress, grieving, or depression and provide resources for care. Elective abortion is a difficult choice for some women. Counseling may be needed to help the woman adjust to her decision to terminate her pregnancy. Grieving is common and it takes time to find resolution.

Patient/Family Teaching

- Teach the woman all options and safe methods of abortion. Helps the woman make an informed decision and select the method of abortion that is most acceptable to her.

- Teach the woman about her chosen procedure, preparations, and postabortion care. Increased knowledge may positively impact the woman's ability to cope with her decision.
- Teach birth control options for her after the procedure and need for follow-up care. Facilitates the identification of physical and mental complications that can follow abortion. Mental complications such as depression are just as important to identify and address as physical problems.

Nursing Diagnosis: PAIN[1]

Related Factors: the effects of a procedure and/or postoperative events. See the generic NDCP, "Pain,[1]" on p. 18 in Chapter 2.

Goals, Outcomes, and Evaluation Criteria

- Woman expresses satisfaction with pain control (e.g., less than 3 on a 1–10 scale).
- Woman demonstrates ability to concentrate and participate in decisions about her own care.
- Woman exhibits no physical signs of pain (e.g., facial expression, restlessness, changes in VSs, moaning).

NIC Interventions[2]

Environmental Management: Comfort (6482)—Manipulation of the patient's surroundings for promotion of optimal comfort.

Therapeutic Touch (5465)—Attuning to the universal healing field, seeking to act as an instrument for healing influence, and using the natural sensitivity of the hands to gently focus and direct the intervention process.

Nursing Activities and Rationales

Assessments

- Determine nature, severity, and location of pain using a 1–10 scale. Facilitates planning appropriate interventions, e.g., nonpharmacologic measures versus analgesics.
- Assess for emotional distress. Emotional pain may contribute to sensation of physical pain.
- Assess uterus and for bleeding to determine if it is within normal recovery parameters. Retained contents can increase bleeding, cramping, and pain.

Independent Nursing Actions

- Institute measures to decrease anxiety. Anxiety increases the perception of pain. (See the NDCP, "Anxiety,[1]" on p. 10 in Chapter 2.)
- Allow support person to be nearby. Support can reduce anxiety, which may reduce pain.
- Implement comfort measures. Position changes, warm packs, and massage can be calming, which may reduce pain.

- Offer hydration and light food when recovery has progressed and it is allowable. Hydration and food are comforting and may reduce the perception of pain.

Collaborative Activities

- For severe pain, administer analgesics per order or protocol. Analgesics (aspirin, NSAIDs) alter the perception of pain and may have anti-inflammatory properties that reduce localized swelling and tenderness.

Patient/Family Teaching

- Explain all procedures and answer questions about diagnosis and prognosis. Information often decreases anxiety, which may reduce pain.
- Provide discharge teaching about self-care and pain control. Facilitates the woman's self-care at home and her use of pharmacologic and nonpharmacologic measures to control her pain.

Nursing Diagnosis: SPIRITUAL DISTRESS[1]

Related Factors: conflicting moral, ethical, and religious beliefs regarding elective termination of pregnancy as evidenced by patient verbalizations.

Goals, Outcomes, and Evaluation Criteria

- Woman expresses meaning and purpose in life following pregnancy termination.
- Woman uses prayer to assist in decision making regarding terminating the pregnancy.
- Woman verbalizes a sense of inner peace and self-control.

NIC Interventions[2]

Anticipatory Guidance (5210)—Preparation of patient for an anticipated developmental and/or situational crisis.

Coping Enhancement (5230)—Assisting a patient to adapt to perceived stressors, changes, or threats that interfere with meeting life demands and roles.

Counseling (5240)—Use of an interactive process focusing on the needs, problems, or feelings of the patient and significant others to enhance coping, problem solving, and interpersonal relationships.

Guilt Work Facilitation (5300)—Helping another to cope with painful feelings of responsibility—actual or perceived.

Spiritual Growth Facilitation (5426)—Facilitation of growth in patient's capacity to identify, connect with, and call upon the source of meaning, purpose, comfort, strength, and hope in his/her life.

Support Group (5430)—Use of a group environment to provide emotional support and health-related information for members.

■ *Nursing Activities and Rationales*

Assessments

- Assess the woman's values and beliefs that may conflict with or support decisions regarding termination of her pregnancy. Establishes a baseline understanding of the woman's belief system so that the nurse can support those beliefs while the woman/couple make decisions regarding abortion.
- Assess the woman's feelings of conflict regarding alternatives (abortion, adoption, etc.) and how they fit with her values, ethics, and/or spiritual beliefs. Verbalization of feelings assists her with sorting out options and alternatives and provides the nurse with information that can be used in supporting decisions made by the patient.
- Assess whether the patient has an objective, realistic understanding of her situation. It is important that the woman be well grounded in reality so that she understands the long-term ramifications of her decisions.
- Evaluate need for counseling if the woman demonstrates signs of grief, depression, or continued conflict after her abortion. Some women continue to grieve an abortion and pregnancy loss, which can reoccur with another pregnancy. Counseling can help the woman resolve conflicts and possibly prevent postpregnancy depression or mood disorders that can occur with termination.
- Determine the patient's usual way of problem solving when decisions do not align with her values, ethics, or spiritual beliefs. Discussing the woman's usual decision-making framework will assist the nurse in providing guidance to continued use of that process.

Independent Nursing Actions

- Offer support and acceptance of her as a person in her struggle. A person who is struggling with decisions needs to feel that she can voice her feelings without judgment and that her issues are heard by the nurse.
- Acknowledge the patient's spiritual and cultural background. The fact that a woman has decided to terminate a pregnancy does not mean that she does not have deep spiritual convictions. Acknowledging her beliefs demonstrates acceptance and willingness to assist her with problem solving while considering her belief system.

Collaborative Activities

- Refer the patient to pastoral care provider of choice or spiritual advisor as appropriate. The woman who terminates a pregnancy may feel that she has committed a mortal sin. A pastoral care provider may be able to provide additional guidance and support in decision making regarding elective termination of pregnancy.
- Refer for birth control counseling. The woman may not have the knowledge or financial resources to obtain and consistently use reliable birth control methods.

Patient/Family Teaching

- Maintain a sense of hope when teaching the family about options for terminating a pregnancy. Once the decision to terminate a pregnancy has been made, the situation needs to be presented realistically, but with hope and positive adaptation emphasized.
- Inform the patient of alternative courses of action based upon her beliefs and values. Careful consideration of other options may help the woman come to a decision that is acceptable and compatible with her belief system. She may be unaware of other options available to her.
- Provide information that the patient requests regarding diagnosis, treatment, and prognosis. Providing the patient with accurate information assists the patient in making informed decisions. The woman demonstrates her readiness to learn when she seeks out information.

■ *Other Nursing Diagnoses*

- Knowledge Deficiency.[1] See the NDCP, "Deficient Knowledge,[1]" beginning on p. 13 in Chapter 2.
- Anxiety.[1] See the NDCP, "Anxiety,[1]" beginning on p. 10 in Chapter 2.
- Fear.[1] See the NDCP, "Fear,[1]" beginning on p. 15 in Chapter 2.

ENDNOTES

1. Nursing Diagnoses—Definitions and Classification 2009–2011. Copyright © 2009, 2007, 2005, 2003, 2001, 1998, 1996, 1994 by NANDA International. Used by arrangement with Blackwell Publishing Limited, a company of John Wiley & Sons, Inc. In order to make safe and effective judgments using NANDA-I nursing diagnoses it is essential that nurses refer to the definitions and defining characteristics of the diagnoses listed in this work.
2. Bulechek, G. M., Butcher, H. K., Dochterman, J. M. (2008). *Nursing Interventions Classification* (5th ed). St. Louis, MO: Elsevier, by permission.

REFERENCES

Behrman, R. E., & Butler, A. S. (Eds.). (2007). *Preterm birth: Causes, consequences, and prevention.* Committee on Understanding Premature Birth and Assuring Healthy Outcomes. National Academy of Sciences. Washington, DC: National Academies Press. Retrieved from http://www.ncbi.nlm.nih.gov/bookshelf/br.fcgi?book=nap11622&part=a20012272ddd00135

Bulechek, G. M., Butcher, H. K., & McCloskey, J. (2009). *Nursing Interventions Classification.* St. Louis, MO: Mosby/Elsevier.

Centers for Disease Control and Prevention. (2006). Sexually transmitted diseases treatment guidelines 2006. *Morbidity and Mortality Weekly Report, 55*(RR–11), 1–94.

Gilbert, E. S. (2010). *Manual of high risk pregnancy and delivery* (5th ed.). St. Louis, MO: Mosby.

Kaiser, L., & Allen, L. H. (2008). ADA report: Position of the American Dietetic Association: Nutrition and lifestyle for a healthy pregnancy outcome. *Journal of the American Dietetic Association.* Retrieved from http://www.eatright.org/search.aspx?search=pregnancy

Koren, G., Boskovic, R., Hard, M., Maltepe, C., Navioz, Y., & Einarson, A. (2002). Motherisk-PUQE (pregnancy-unique quantification of emesis and nausea) scoring system for nausea and vomiting of pregnancy. *American Journal of Obstetrics and Gynecology, 186*(5 Suppl Understanding), S228–S231.

Leeman, L., & Fontaine, P. (2008, July). Hypertensive disorders of pregnancy. *American Family Physician, 78*(1), 93–100.

Luke, B. (2005). Nutrition and multiple gestation. *Seminars in Perinatology, 29*(5), 349–354.

Mattson, S., & Smith, J. E. (2010). *Core curriculum for maternal-newborn nursing* (2nd ed.). St. Louis, MO: Mosby.

Meighan, M., & Wood, A. F. (2005). The impact of hyperemesis gravidarum on maternal role assumption. *Journal of Obstetrical Gynecological Neonatal Nursing, 34*(2), 172–179.

National High Blood Pressure Education Program. Working Group on High Blood Pressure in Pregnancy. (2000). Report of the National High Blood Pressure Education Program Working Group on High Blood Pressure in Pregnancy. *American Journal of Obstetricians and Gynecologists, 183*(1), S1–S22. Retrieved from http://www.ncbi.nlm.nih.gov/pubmed/10920346

Rasmussen, K. M., & Yaktine, A. L. (Eds.). (2009). *Weight gain during pregnancy: Reexamining the guidelines.* Committee to Reexamine IOM Pregnancy Weight Guidelines. Institute of Medicine and National Research Council of the National Academies. Washington, DC: National Academies Press. Retrieved from http://books.nap.edu/openbook.php?record_id=12584

RESOURCES

Acharya, G., Eschler, B., Grønberg, M., Hentemann, M., Ottersen, T., & Maltau, J. M. (2006). Noninvasive cerclage for the management of cervical incompetence: A prospective study. *Obstetrical & Gynecological Survey, 61*(4), 221–222. doi: 10.1097/01.ogx.0000206343.06995.36

American College of Obstetricians and Gynecologists (ACOG). (2002). ACOG practice bulletin (No. 33): Diagnosis and management of preeclampsia and eclampsia. *Obstetrics and Gynecology, 99*(1), 159–167.

American College of Obstetricians and Gynecologists (ACOG). (2003). ACOG practice bulletin: Management of preterm labor. *International Journal of Gynecology and Obstetrics, 82*(1), 127–135.

American College of Obstetricians and Gynecologists (ACOG). (2004). ACOG practice bulletin. Clinical management guideline for obstetrician-gynecologists: Nausea and vomiting of pregnancy. *Obstetrics and Gynecology, 103*(4), 803–811.

American College of Obstetricians and Gynecologists (ACOG). (2005). ACOG practice bulletin (No. 67): Clinical management guidelines for obstetrician-gynecologist: Medical management of abortion. *Obstetrics & Gynecology, 106*(4), 871–882.

American College of Obstetricians and Gynecologists (ACOG). (2007). ACOG practice bulletin (No. 80): Premature rupture of membranes: Clinical management guidelines for obstetrician-gynecologists. *Obstetrics and Gynecology, 109*(4), 1007–1019.

American College of Obstetricians and Gynecologists (ACOG). (2008). ACOG practice bulletin: Medical management of ectopic pregnancy. *Obstetrics and Gynecology, 111*(6), 1479–1485.

Aruda, M. M., Waddicor, K., Frese, L., Cole, J. C. M., & Burke, P. (2010). Early pregnancy in adolescents: Diagnosis, assessment, options, counseling, and referral. *Journal of Pediatric Health Care, 24*(1), 4–13.

Bazaco, M. C., Albrecht, S. A., & Malek, A. M. (2008). Preventing foodborne infection in pregnant women and infants. *Nursing for Women's Health, 12*(1), 48–55.

Bess, K. A., & Wood, T. L. (2006). Understanding gestational trophoblastic disease: How nurses can help those dealing with a diagnosis. *American Women's Health and Obstetrical Neonatal Nursing Lifelines, 10*(4), 320–326.

Biggs, W. D., & Williams, R. M. (2008). Common gynecologic infections. *Primary Care Clinical Office Practices, 36*(1), 33–51.

Brier, N. (2008). Grief following miscarriage: A comprehensive review of the literature. *Journal of Women's Health, 17*(3), 451–464.

Britistan, S., & Gilliam, M. (2009). First trimester surgical abortion. *Clinical Obstetrics and Gynecology, 52*(2), 151–159.

Cunningham, F. G., Leveno, K. J., Gilstrap, L. C., Hauth, J. C., Wenstrom, K. D., & Bloom, S. L. (Eds.). (2010). *William's obstetrics* (23rd ed.). Boston, MA: McGraw-Hill.

Curran, C. A. (2003). Intrapartum emergencies. *Journal of Obstetric, Gynecological Neonatal Nursing, 32*(6), 802–813.

Damato, E. G., Anthony, M. K., & Maloni, J. A. (2009). Correlates of negative and positive mood state in mothers of twins. *Journal of Pediatric Nursing, 24*(5), 369–377.

Daskalakis, G. J. (2009). Prematurity prevention: The role of cerclage. *Current Opinion in Obstetrics and Gynecology, 21*(2), 148–152.

Davidson M. R., London M. L., & Ladewig, P. A. (2007). *Olds' maternal-newborn nursing and women's health across the lifespan* (8th ed.). Upper Saddle River, NJ: Prentice Hall Health.

Davis, M. (2004). Nausea and vomiting of pregnancy: An evidence-based review. *Journal of Perinatal Neonatal Nursing, 18*(4), 312–328.

Drummond, S., & Fritz, E. (2008). Management of a partial molar pregnancy: A case study report. *Journal of Perinatal Neonatal Nursing, 23*(2), 115–123.

Easterwood, B. (2004). Silent lullabies: Helping parents cope with early pregnancy loss. *AWONN Lifelines, 8*(4), 356–360.

Fejzo, M. S., Poursharif, B., Korst, L. M., Munch, S., MacGibbon, K. W., Romero, R. & Goodwin, T. M. (2009). Symptoms and pregnancy outcomes associated with extreme weight loss among women with hyperemesis gravidarum. *Journal of Women's Health, 18*(12), 1981–1987.

Goodnight, W., & Newman, R. (2009). Optimal nutrition for improved twin pregnancy outcome. *Obstetrics and Gynecology, 114*(5), 1121–1134.

Harris, A. A. (2004). Supportive counseling before and after elective pregnancy termination. *Journal of Midwifery and Women's Health, 49*(2), 105–112.

Hays, J., & Fox, M. (2009). Cervical dilation in second-trimester abortion. *Clinical Obstetrics and Gynecology, 52*(2), 171–178.

Hoover, K. W., Tao, G., & Kent, C. K. (2010). Trends in the diagnosis and treatment of ectopic pregnancy in the United States. *Obstetrics and Gynecology, 115*(3), 495–502.

Howard, E. D. (2006). Family-centered care in the context of fetal abnormality. *Journal of Perinatal Neonatal Nursing, 20*(3), 237–242.

Hoyt, G. (2006). Bleeding in pregnancy: What's the diagnosis? *Nursing 36*(5 Suppl E D), 16–18.

Jackson, K. M., & Mele, N. L. (2009). Twin-to-twin transfusion syndrome: What nurses need to know. *Nursing for Women's Health, 13*(3), 226–233.

Jenning-Sanders, A. (2009). A case study approach to hyperemesis gravidarum: Home care implications. *Home Healthcare Nurse, 27*(6), 347–351.

Kata, A. (2001). Waiting for something to happen: Hospitalization with placenta previa. *Birth, 28*(3), 186–191.

Kriebs, J. M. (2008). Breaking the cycle of infection: TORCH and other infections in woman's health. *Journal of Midwifery and Women's Health, 53*(3), 173–174.

Kriebs, J. M. (2008). Understanding herpes simplex virus: Transmission, diagnosis, and considerations in pregnancy management. *Journal of Midwifery and Women's Health, 53*(3), 202–208.

Kriebs, J. M., & Fahey, J. O. (2006, November–December). Ectopic pregnancy. *Journal of Midwifery & Women's Health, 51*(6), 431–419.

Lamondy, A. M. (2006). Hyperemesis gravidarum and the role of the infusion nurse. *Journal of Infusion Nursing, 29*(2), 89–100.

Leonard, L. G., & Denton, J. (2006, June). Preparation for parent multiple birth children. *Early Human Development, 82*(6), 371–378.

Lipp, A. (2008). Supporting the significant other in women undergoing abortion. *British Journal of Nursing, 17*(19), 1232–1236.

Lowdermilk, D. L., & Perry, S. E. (2007). *Maternity & Women's Health Care* (7th ed.). St. Louis, MO: Mosby.

Macejko, A. M., & Schaeffer, A. J. (2007). Asymptomatic bacteriuria and symptomatic urinary tract infections during pregnancy. *Urologic Clinics of North America, 34*(1), 35–42.

MacMullen, N. J., Dulski, L. A., & Meagher, B. (2005). Red alert: Perinatal hemorrhage. *Maternal and Child Nursing, 30*(1), 46–51.

Maloni, J. A., Margevicius, S. P., & Damato, E. G. (2006). Multiple gestation: Side effects of antepartum bed rest. *Biological Research for Nursing, 8*(2), 115–128.

Marowitz, A. (2007). Midwifery management of prelabor rupture of membranes at term. *Journal of Midwifery and Women's Health, 52*(3), 199–206.

Montoya, J. G., & Remington, J. S. (2008, August 15). Management of *Toxoplasma gondii* infection during pregnancy. *Clinical Infectious Diseases, 47*(4), 554–566.

Morgan, K. L. (2004). Management of UTIs during pregnancy. *Maternal and Child Nursing, 29*(4), 254–258.

North American Nursing Diagnosis Association International (NANDA). (2009). *Nursing diagnoses, 2009–2011: Definitions and classification.* Ames, IA: John Wiley & Sons.

O'Reilly, M. (2009). Careful counsel: Management of unintended pregnancy. *Journal of the American Academy of Nurse Practitioners, 21*(11), 596–602.

Oyelese, Y., & Ananth, C. V. (2006). Placental abruption. *Obstetrics and Gynecology, 108*(4), 1005–1016.

Perry, S. E., Hockenberry, M. J., Lowdermilk, D. L., & Wilson, D. (2009). *Wong's maternal child nursing care* (4th ed.). St. Louis, MO: Mosby.

Peters, R., & Flack, J. M. (2004). Hypertensive disorders of pregnancy. *Journal of Obstetrical Gynecological and Neonatal Nursing, 33*(2), 209–220.

Quinlan, J. D., & Hill, D. A. (2003). Nausea and vomiting of pregnancy. *American Family Physician, 68*(1), 121–128.

Schnarr, J., & Smaill, F. (2008). Asymptomatic bacteriuria and symptomatic urinary tract infections in pregnancy. *European Journal of Clinical Investigation, 38*(Suppl 2), 50–57.

Simmonds, K. E., & Likis, F. E. (2005). Providing options counseling for women with unintended pregnancies. *Journal of Obstetrical Gynecological and Neonatal Nursing, 34*(3), 373–379.

Soper, J. T. (2006, July). Gestational trophoblastic disease. *Obstetrics and Gynecology, 108*(1), 176–187.

Stringer, M., Gennaro, S., Deatrick, J. A., & Founds, S. (2008). Symptoms described by African American women evaluated for preterm labor. *Journal of Obstetrical Gynecological and Neonatal Nursing, 37*(2), 196–202.

Stringer, M., & Miesnik, S. R. (2004). Nursing care of the patient with preterm premature rupture of membranes. *Maternal and Child Nursing, 29*(3), 144–150.

Strong, T. H., Jr. (2001, December). Alternative therapies of morning sickness. *Clinical Obstetrics and Gynecology, 44*(4), 653–660.

Tan, P. C., Jacob, R. M., Quek, K. F., & Omar, S. Z. (2007). Pregnancy outcome in hyperemesis gravidarum and the effect of laboratory clinical indicators of hyperemesis severity. *Journal of Obstetrics and Gynecology, 33*(4), 457–464.

Taylor, D., Hwang, A., & Stewart, F. (2004). Care for women choosing medication abortion. *Nurse Practitioner, 29*(10), 65–70.

Thorstensen, K. A. (2000). Midwifery management of first trimester bleeding and early pregnancy loss. *Journal of Midwifery and Women's Health, 45*(6), 481–97.

Tran, S. H., Cheng, Y. W., Kaimal, A. J., & Caughey, A. B. (2008). Length of rupture of membranes in the setting of premature rupture of membranes at term and infectious maternal morbidity. *American Journal of Obstetrics and Gynecology, 198*(6), 700e3, 700.e1–700.e5.

Waters, T. P., & Mercer, B. (2009, September). The management of preterm premature rupture of the membranes near the limit of fetal viability. *American Journal of Obstetrics and Gynecology, 201*(3), 230–240. doi: 10.1016/l.ajog.2009.06.049

Whitney, K. (2009). Placental site trophoblastic tumor. *American Journal of Nursing, 109*(12), 32–37.

Williams, G. B. (2001). Short term grief after an elective abortion. *Journal of Obstetrical Gynecological and Neonatal Nursing, 30*(2), 174–184.

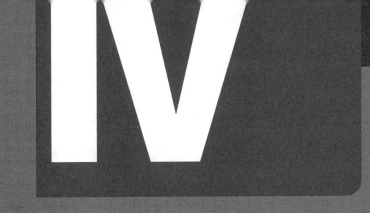

IV

INTRAPARTUM CARE

NORMAL INTRAPARTUM

Cynthia Waits

NORMAL LABOR: FIRST STAGE

Labor is a natural process in which, after approximately 282 days of pregnancy, the fetus, placenta, and membranes are moved through the birth canal and expelled. In at least 95% of all labors, birth is in the occiput (vertex) presentation. Labor is normal when it occurs near term, is completed in 24 hours, there is a single fetus in vertex presentation, and there are no complications. The course of normal labor consists of progressive uterine contractions, effacement and dilation of the cervix, and descent of the fetus. Birth is a complex set of events that occur representing a reversal of the uterine role from a relaxed to an active myometrium. Prior to labor, it functioned to prevent birth, but in labor, it functions as an active participant to activate birth. First-stage labor is characterized by dilation and effacement of the cervix; it is divided into the following three phases: latent, active, and transition.

Key Nursing Activities

- Complete a thorough assessment focusing on prior obstetrical history, current pregnancy, and labor signs.
- Maintain optimal maternal and fetal well-being.
- Identify and treat anxiety; facilitate coping of woman and partner.
- Provide nonpharmacologic pain relief measures.
- Observe, assess for, and prevent or minimize complications.
- Promote parent–infant attachment.
- Establish obstetric baseline on admission to labor unit. Key baseline assessments are:
  ‣ Assess UCs for location, regularity, intensity, and duration.
  ‣ Perform Leopold's maneuvers for fetal lie.
  ‣ If no bleeding, perform sterile vaginal examination to assess status of membranes, cervical dilation and effacement, presenting part, and station.
  ‣ Review patient profile (e.g., for last menstrual period, estimated date of confinement, age).
  ‣ Take vital signs (temperature, pulse, respirations, BP; compare with prepregnant and prenatal levels).

‣ Assess for peripheral edema and reflexes/clonus.
‣ Biochemical assessments. Standard lab screening to include blood for Hgb and Hct, serology, type and cross-match or type and screen; Pap test, blood group, Rh and antibody screening; rubella titer, glucose screening, group B Streptococcus, hepatitis B, urine dipstick or urinalysis, clean-catch urine sample for protein, glucose, and bacteria; STI screening; or additional screening as indicated such as genetic screening (chorionic villi sampling, amniocentesis, maternal serum alpha-fetoprotein, etc.).
‣ Use universal precautions when there is possibility of exposure to blood and body fluids, as during labor and birth (e.g., when changing underpads, when testing amniotic fluid, when assisting with artificial rupture of membranes, and with intravenous [IV] access).
- Establish fetal assessment on admission to labor unit, including:
  ‣ FHR with external Doppler or fetal monitor (baseline heart rate, variability, accelerations, decelerations, or unusual characteristics).
  ‣ Ultrasonography.
  ‣ Fetal movement counting.
  ‣ Nonstress test (NST) reports.
  ‣ Biophysical profiles.
  ‣ Contraction stress test.
  ‣ Doppler flow studies.
  ‣ Growth abnormalities (e.g., intrauterine growth restriction, large for gestational age or small for gestational age).

Etiologies and Risk Factors

Labor is thought to be triggered by one or more of the following factors, which seem to be associated with myometrial irritability:
- Oxytocin release by the posterior pituitary.
- Estrogen stimulation resulting from progesterone withdrawal.
- Increased maternal prostaglandin and fetal cortisol levels.
- Uterine distention.
- Increasing intrauterine pressure.
- Aging of the placenta.
- Pressure of the presenting part on the cervix and lower uterine segment.

Signs and Symptoms

Signs of impending labor include lightening, false labor, and bloody show. Signs of true labor include:
- UCs showing a consistent pattern of increasing frequency, intensity, and duration; the force of labor is from the UC acting on resistance of the cervix.
- Walking increases the UCs because it increases myometrial activity.
- Discomfort beginning in lower back, sweeps around to lower abdomen and groin, feeling like menstrual cramps.
- Progressive dilation and effacement of the cervix (varies widely among women). No consensus on the appropriate length of

labor, although averages were defined by the Friedman curve in the 1950s. This curve is less accurate when anesthesia is used, labor is augmented, or maternal weight is greater than those of women used to originally define the scale.

- UCs continue even when sleeping.
- Sedation does not stop UCs.
- Physical and behavioral findings in the latent phase include:
- Irregular, brief, and mild UCs in which the mucous plug may be expelled.
- Cervical dilation of 0–3 cm.
- Cervical effacement in primiparas usually complete before dilation; in multiparas, it occurs along with dilation.
- UCs mild, irregular, cramps with dull backache 3–30 min apart, 30–40 sec duration.
- Scant pink or brown vaginal discharge or mucous plug.
- Station for primiparas usually 0; for multiparas, 0–2.
- FHTs clearest at or below umbilicus, depending on fetal position.
- Latent phase may last from 8–24 hours for primiparas; usually lasts 5–10 hours for multiparas; however, there are no absolute values for the expected length of the first stage. First stage is much longer than the second and third stages combined; and the latent phase of the first stage is typically longer than the active and transition phases. The duration of each phase is affected by parity, maternal position, fetal position/presentation, and level of activity.
- Pain controlled fairly well, the woman is able to ambulate and talk through UCs.
- Excited, alert, follows directions; may be talkative or silent, calm or tense; confident or anxious.
- Physical and behavioral findings in active phase include:
- Cervical dilation: 4–7 cm.
- UCs moderate to strong by palpation, more regular, 2–3 min apart, 40–70 sec duration.
- Scant to moderate pink or bloody vaginal mucus.
- Station of 0 to + 1.
- FHT clearest slightly below umbilicus or lower abdomen.
- Active phase lasts about 3–6 hours.
- Serious demeanor; doubts ability to control pain; apprehensive; inner focus; evidence of fatigue; some difficulty following instructions; does not wish to be left alone, quiet, accepts coaching efforts by nurse and significant other.
- Increasing discomfort, trembling of thighs and legs, pressure on bladder and rectum, persistent backache with occiput posterior fetal position.
- Physical and behavioral findings in transition phase include:
- Cervical dilation: 8–10 cm.
- UCs strong to very strong by palpation, regular, 2–3 min apart, 45–90 sec duration, urge to push.
- Copious amount of bloody vaginal mucus.
- Station: + 2 to + 3.
- FHT clearest directly above symphysis pubis.
- Transition phase lasts about 0.5–2 hours (primigravida 3–4 hours and multigravida varies).

- Severe pain; fears loss of control; irritability; does not volunteer communication; nausea and vomiting; circumoral pallor; perspiration; shaking of thighs; feeling of pressure on anus and need to defecate, membranes may rupture if they have not already; ambulation difficult; irritable, self-absorbed, need for support increases.

Diagnostic Studies

A diagnosis of labor is based on physical findings. Testing is done only to monitor maternal and fetal well-being or if a complication is suspected.

- Fern test of fluid from vagina. Tests for rupture of membranes; crystalline frondlike, fern pattern indicates amniotic fluid.
- Nitrazine test of vaginal fluid. Determines whether membranes have ruptured; if test tape remains yellow to olive green, membranes are probably intact; if tape turns blue-green to deep blue, the fluid pH is high and it is probably amniotic fluid.
- AmniSure fetal membranes rupture test. Determines the presence of amniotic fluid in vaginal secretions of pregnant women. Swab of vaginal fluid is obtained and then dipped into a vial of solvent for one minute. Test strip is then dipped into the vial with solvent for 5–10 minutes. Strip is read as no rupture, ruptured, or invalid depending on the line colors on the test strip.
- Ultrasound examination of amniotic fluid volume. Supportive lab testing for PROM.
- Fetal heart monitoring. During labor this is not, strictly speaking, a diagnostic test; it is used to monitor for fetal distress during labor.

Medical Management

- Fetal heart rate monitoring. Assesses fetal well-being.
- Assessment of vital signs (VSs) and clinical findings. Ensures maternal well-being.
- Monitoring the progress of labor.
- Monitoring for complications of labor.
- Medications to manage pain, as needed. These may include:
  ▸ Sedatives. Relieve anxiety and induce sleep in early latent labor and in absence of pain.
  ▸ Systemic narcotic analgesics (e.g., fentanyl [Sublimaze]). Act in the central nervous system to alter the transmission and perception of pain.
  ▸ Mixed narcotic agonist-antagonists: butorphanol (Stadol), nalbuphine (Nubain). Action similar to narcotic analgesics, but interfere with the actions of narcotics if there are any in the woman's system.
  ▸ Antiemetics and analgesic potentiators: hydroxyzine (Vistaril), promethazine (Phenergan), promazine (Sparine). Act at the chemoreceptor trigger zone to relieve nausea.
  ▸ Local and regional anesthesia (e.g., pudendal block, epidural block, paracervical block); commonly used agents are 0.25–1% solutions of lidocaine (Xylocaine), bupivacaine (Marcaine), chloroprocaine (Nesacaine), tetracaine (Pontocaine), and mepivacaine (Carbocaine). Act locally

or regionally to block transmission of pain along specific nerves.

▸ Epidural and intrathecal narcotics. Act in the central nervous system (CNS) to relieve pain.

▸ Intravenous solutions. For hydration and to serve as a route for administration of emergency medications.

Collaborative Problems

Potential Complications of Labor

- Fetal distress/anoxia (reduced placental perfusion, head/cord compression, hyperventilation, etc.)
- Cord prolapse
- Dystocia (e.g., failure to progress, malpresentation)
- Precipitous labor/delivery
- Uterine rupture
- Placental abruption
- Uterine hyperstimulation

Potential Complications of Epidural Anesthesia

- Maternal hypotension
- Fetal hypoxia
- Urinary retention
- Decreased awareness of lower body sensations

Potential Complications of Narcotic Analgesia

- Maternal respiratory depression
- Maternal hypotension
- Maternal falls
- Newborn respiratory depression

COLLABORATIVE (STANDARDIZED) CARE FOR ALL WOMEN IN NORMAL FIRST-STAGE LABOR

Perform comprehensive assessment to identify individual needs for teaching, emotional support, and physical care.

Potential Complications of Labor: FETAL DISTRESS/ANOXIA, CORD PROLAPSED, DYSTOCIA, PRECIPITOUS LABOR, UTERINE RUPTURE, AND PLACENTAL ABRUPTION

Refer to "Intrapartum Fetal Monitoring," beginning on p. 244 in this chapter. Also refer to "Dystocia/Dysfunctional Labor," which begins on p. 265; "External Version," beginning on p. 297; "Uterine Rupture," beginning on p. 295; and "Forceps- or Vacuum-Assisted Birth," which begins on p. 301, all in Chapter 8.

▌ Nursing Activities and Rationales

Focus Assessments

- Review prenatal and admission records for maternal conditions that can decrease uteroplacental circulation (e.g., diabetes, gestational hypertension); review results of antepartum nonstress test or contraction stress tests. Identifies high-risk situations that are likely to compromise fetal oxygenation.

- Review prenatal and admission records for indications of IUGR, multiple gestation, more than five previous births. Identifies conditions that increase the incidence of cord prolapse and other labor complications.

- Monitor maternal blood pressure, pulse, and respirations every 4 hours in the latent phase, hourly in active phase, and every 15–30 minutes during transition (as long as VSs are within normal range). Maternal condition affects fetal status. Maternal hypotension reduces placental perfusion and, thus, fetal oxygenation; normal maternal respirations are vital for maintaining the O_2–CO_2 balance in the blood.

- Perform Leopold's maneuver or otherwise determine fetal position, lie, and presentation. The incidence of prolapsed cord is greater with abnormal lie, especially footling breech and shoulder presentations, because the presenting part does not totally engage and block the cervical os. Malposition and malpresentation can cause difficult labor or dystocia (e.g., in breech presentation, the fetal part is not as effective in applying pressure to the cervix as in vertex position).

- If there is no vaginal bleeding on admission, perform a vaginal exam to assess cervical dilation; monitor dilation periodically as necessary. Determines labor status. Failure of cervix to dilate is one cause of dystocia.

- Inspect perineum on admission and when membranes rupture for visible cord in the vagina. Feel for cord in the vagina when performing vaginal exams. Cord prolapse is an obstetric emergency that requires immediate cesarean birth. When the umbilical cord precedes the presenting part, it becomes trapped between the presenting part and the maternal pelvis; the vessels in the cord are compressed, leading to fetal hypoxia/acidosis.

- Monitor UCs. An external monitor cannot determine intensity of UCs; the nurse must palpate or use an internal uterine pressure catheter [IUPC]. Notify healthcare provider if frequency is less than 2 per min, duration greater than 90 sec, or if uterus does not relax completely between UCs (rising baseline on the monitor). Identifies hypo- or hypertonicity of the uterus and monitors progress of labor. UCs are quantified by the number of contractions present in a 10-minute window averaged over 30 minutes. Normal is five UC or fewer in 10 min; tachysystole is greater than five UC in 10 min averaged over 30 min. Contractions should be 90 sec or less in duration; the uterus should return to baseline on the monitor (i.e., relax completely) between contractions. IUPC pressure should be less than 30 mmHg resting and less than 50 mmHg during a contraction. Hypertonicity of the uterus decreases oxygenation in the intervillous spaces, causing fetal distress. Hypotonicity prolongs labor, leading to maternal fatigue and fetal distress.

- Obtain baseline FHR on admission and frequently per unit procedures. Record baseline rate and variability; correlate accelerations/decelerations with UCs and fetal activity. If continuous electronic monitoring is not done, the FHR should be assessed hourly in latent phase and every 30 minutes in the active and transition phases. See "Intrapartum Fetal Monitoring," beginning on p. 244 in this chapter. FHR reflects fetal oxygenation. Any of the potential complications of labor can lead to fetal hypoxia. For example, bradycardia (FHR less than 120 bpm) and persistent variable decelerations may indicate cord prolapse. Note: continuous electronic FHR monitoring for all laboring women is not supported by research. Notify healthcare provider if absent or marked variability, no acceleration, or acceleration greater than 2 minutes, prolonged late decelerations, or sinusoidal pattern. The 2008 NIHD definitions include three categories (normal, indeterminate, and abnormal) for defining and identifying meaningful and evidence-based management of intrapartum fetal compromise (Robinson & Nelson, 2008).

- If FHR is not in the 110–160 range and/or decelerations or decreased variability occur, or if maternal risk factors occur, apply external monitor. Continuous external monitoring is routine in many, but not all, settings. Monitoring is recommended if any fetal or maternal abnormalities or complications are suspected because the FHR provides information about how well the fetus is tolerating labor.

- For a breech presentation, assess FHR more frequently. Breech presentation is a high-risk rather than a normal condition. It occurs in about 3% of term births and often requires surgical delivery.

- Monitor progress of labor. Correlate UC pattern, cervical dilation and effacement, and fetal descent, and note the length of time in each phase. Prolonged labor creates maternal exhaustion and increases the risk for fetal hypoxia. Fetal descent of less than 1 cm/hr (primipara) or less than 2 cm/hr (multipara) suggests cephalopelvic disproportion or malposition. The risk of fetal death increases when the active phase lasts for more than 15 hours. Monitoring labor also detects precipitous labor.

- Monitor fetal descent (station) by vaginal examinations. Descent should be 1 cm/hr for primiparas and 1.5 cm/hr for multiparas. Slower descent may signal dystocia. Prolonged head compression can stimulate a vagal response, resulting in fetal bradycardia.

- Note color, amount, and odor of amniotic fluid when membranes rupture. Record with time of rupture. Green amniotic fluid may indicate fetal hypoxia. Hypoxia causes the fetal anal sphincter to relax and release meconium. Foul-smelling fluid signals infection, while scanty fluid may indicate poorly controlled maternal diabetes. All of these stress the fetus.

- Assess energy level and review admission record for activity and rest prior to onset of UCs. Maternal fatigue contributes to dystocia.

- Determine time of last bowel movement. Presence of feces in the bowel may interfere with fetal descent and possibly inhibit UCs.

- When membranes rupture, either spontaneously or artificially, note the time; note the amount, color, and odor of the fluid; take the FHR. Oligohydramnios contributes to dystocia and fetal distress; foul-smelling fluid is a sign of infection; greenish-tinged fluid may indicate fetal hypoxia, which causes vagal stimulation, relaxation of the fetal sphincter, and passage of meconium.

- Observe for acute, severe abdominal pain with minimal to diffuse external bleeding; observe for increase in pulse and decrease in BP; monitor FHR; observe for abrupt cessation of UCs; and review prenatal record for risk factors for uterine rupture or abruption (e.g., prior uterine surgery or cesarean birth; fetal malpresentation, grand multiparity, illicit drug use). These are symptoms of uterine rupture (which is rare in the United States). Concealed hemorrhage may occur and be undetected until the woman shows symptoms of hypovolemic shock. The first sign of uterine rupture may be nonreassuring FHR or abrupt cessation of UCs.

Preventive Nursing Activities

- Teach or reinforce measures that help the woman to relax between UCs. Uteroplacental blood flow is interrupted during a contraction; it is reestablished between UCs. Stress can cause a dysfunctional labor pattern by causing an imbalance of epinephrine and norepinephrine. It helps prevent fatigue that can develop with a prolonged labor. Rest and relaxation conserve energy by reducing glucose utilization. Tense muscles increase resistance to fetal descent.

- During the antepartum period, advise the woman to call the healthcare provider or go to the clinic/office when her membranes rupture. Cord prolapse can occur with rupture of membranes (ROM); there are few outward signs of prolapse, so a vaginal exam is necessary; immediate intervention is needed if prolapse occurs. ROM may be the beginning of labor. Prolonged ROM (more than 24 hours) increases the risk of maternal and fetal infection, especially if positive for group B Streptococcus, which indicates prompt antibiotic treatment.

- Ensure maternal hydration with IV or oral fluids. Maintains circulating blood volume, which maintains BP and thus placental perfusion and fetal oxygenation.

- Have the woman void every 1–2 hours and palpate for bladder distention. A full bladder can interfere with fetal descent and possibly inhibit UCs.
- Encourage left lateral or semi-Fowler's position but avoid supine position. In supine position, the gravid uterus compresses the ascending vena cava, resulting in decreased cardiac output and, thus, in decreased placental perfusion and decreased oxygen to the fetus. Changing position can prevent or correct fetal hypoxia.
- During latent phase, the woman may be up and walking about unless her membranes have ruptured and the fetal head is unengaged. Walking makes use of gravity and may stimulate UCs to help decrease the length of the labor. However, if the membranes rupture, the effects of gravity may cause the umbilical cord to wash out with the fluid, past the unengaged fetal parts and into the vagina.
- During active phase, the woman may prefer an upright position. Upright position may shorten labor, does not increase discomfort or cause fetal distress, and can decrease operative births by 50%.
- Intervene to prevent and reduce anxiety. Anxiety can decrease uterine contractility. (See the NDCP "Anxiety,[1]" beginning on p. 227 in this topic.)

Potential Complications of Epidural Anesthesia: URINARY RETENTION, MATERNAL HYPOTENSION, AND POSSIBLE FETAL HYPOXIA

Refer to "Epidural Anesthesia/Analgesia," beginning on p. 248 in this chapter.

Potential Complications of Narcotic (and Narcotic Agonist-Antagonist) Analgesia: MATERNAL RESPIRATORY DEPRESSION, MATERNAL HYPOTENSION, AND NEWBORN RESPIRATORY DEPRESSION

Focus Assessments

- Assess for contraindications to use of narcotics and agonist-antagonists (e.g., butorphanol tartrate and nalbuphine hydrochloride). Narcotics are contraindicated if there is the possibility of current narcotic drug dependence, history of asthma, or sensitivity to sulfites. If the woman has been using narcotics, administration of an agonist-antagonist will precipitate withdrawal by reversing the effect of the other opioids.
- Check level of consciousness before and after administering. The primary action sites for narcotics are in the brain; sedation is a side effect.
- Assess vital signs (especially respirations and BP) before and after administering. Narcotics depress respirations and BP through their effects on the CNS. Maternal respiratory depression decreases the amount of oxygen in blood delivered to the fetus; hypotension decreases placental perfusion.
- Assess FHR before and after administering. Determines direct and indirect side effects of the medication.
- Assess for nausea. Nausea is a side effect caused by stimulation of the chemoreceptor trigger zone.

Preventive Nursing Activities

- Provide bedpan for urination and place side rails in up position. Prevents falls. Side effects of pain medications may include dizziness, sedation, and urinary urgency.
- Consider placing an indwelling urinary catheter if the woman has an epidural anesthesia. Placement of a urinary catheter should not be routine because similar to the woman with a walking epidural medication, there still may be some sensation to void.
- Time administration of the medication, considering route of administration (intramuscular or IV), so that it will be metabolized before the birth of the infant. Prevents respiratory depression in the newborn. Timing depends on the rapidity with which labor is progressing, and the peak of action and the duration of the medication. As a general rule, do not give narcotics within 1 hour of anticipated birth.
- Have naloxone (Narcan) available in the birthing unit. Reverses mild maternal respiratory depression, sedation, and hypotension caused by butorphanol, nalbuphine, or other narcotics. Reverses respiratory depression in the newborn.

Nursing Diagnosis: RISK FOR INFECTION[1]

Related Factors: invasive procedures (e.g., vaginal exams, placement of an internal monitoring device), and ruptured membranes. Refer to the generic NDCP, "Risk for Infection,[1]" which begins on p. 21 in Chapter 2.

NIC Interventions[2]

Intrapartal Care (6830)—Monitoring and management of stages one and two of the birth process.

■ *Goals, Outcomes, and Evaluation Criteria*
- Woman's temperature remains within normal limits.
- Amniotic fluid is clear and odor free.
- Woman remains free of puerperal infection.

■ *Nursing Activities and Rationales*

Assessments

- Monitor maternal temperature every 4 hours if membranes intact; hourly if ruptured. Elevated temperature may indicate infection; fever occurs as a result of endotoxins in the cell walls of bacteria and viruses. Fever is a body defense mechanism that kills or inhibits the growth of many microorganisms. However, an elevated temperature does not necessarily indicate infection. The increased metabolic rate during labor may also cause a slight temperature elevation. Because bacterial growth does not occur immediately, more frequent monitoring is unnecessary unless temperature is elevated or infection existed before labor. If birth does not occur within 4 hours after ROM, mother and fetus are at risk for infections. The more time that elapses between ROM and birth of the infant, the higher the incidence of ascending infection, especially if the mother or infant is group B Streptococcus positive.
- Perform Nitrazine paper test, fern test, and/or AmniSure test on vaginal secretions. Be aware that blood in the secretions increases the alkalinity and may give a false reading on the Nitrazine paper. Determines whether membranes have ruptured; if test tape remains yellow to olive green, membranes are probably intact; if tape turns blue-green to deep blue, the fluid Ph is high (alkaline) and it is probably amniotic fluid; AmniSure strip reads as positive or negative for rupture.
- When membranes rupture, either spontaneously or artificially, note the time; note the amount, color, and odor of the fluid; and take the FHR. Foul-smelling fluid is a sign of infection; greenish-tinged fluid indicates passage of meconium caused by fetal hypoxia, which may indicate preexisting intrauterine infection. FHR is indicator of fetal well-being or stress.
- Assess WBC count results. An increase of greater than 30% in a 6-hour period is indicative of pathology. Normal WBC count in labor may be as high as $25,000/mm^3$, so this must be differentiated from the elevated WBC count typically caused by infection.

Independent Nursing Actions

- During labor, provide perineal care after defecation or urination, and as needed, using medical asepsis. Change linens and underpad as needed for cleanliness. Removes pathogens and medium for their growth. The woman may not be able to provide self-care because of analgesics or epidural anesthesia.
- Use sterile gloves for vaginal examinations. Perform only as many vaginal exams as absolutely necessary to evaluate labor progress. Prevents introduction of pathogens into the vagina.

■ Nursing Diagnosis: RISK FOR DEFICIENT FLUID VOLUME[1]

Related Factors: decreased oral fluid intake, diaphoresis associated with the work of labor, and mouth breathing.

■ *Goals, Outcomes, and Evaluation Criteria*
- Woman is free of abnormal thirst.
- Mucous membranes are moist.
- Woman has elastic skin turgor.
- Intake is approximately equal to output.
- Urine output is 30–50 ml/hr.
- BP is within normal limits (WNL).
- Woman is afebrile.
- Peripheral pulses are strong; the rate is WNL.
- Urine-specific gravity is 1.005–1.030.

■ *NIC Interventions[2]*

Fluid Management (4120)—Promotion of fluid balance and prevention of complications resulting from abnormal or undesired fluid levels.

Fluid Monitoring (4130)—Collection and analysis of patient data to regulate fluid balance.

Intrapartal Care (6830)—Monitoring and management of stages one and two of the birth process.

Intravenous (IV) Therapy (4200)—Administration and monitoring of intravenous fluids and medications.

■ *Nursing Activities and Rationales*

Assessments

- Monitor hydration status—skin turgor, mucous membranes, eyes, subjective feelings of thirst. Smooth, supple skin, moist mucous membranes, absence of thirst, and firm eyeballs are evidence of good hydration.
- Monitor intake and output and note amount of diaphoresis. Determines fluid balance; intake should approximately equal output.
- Measure urine-specific gravity, as needed. Normal range is 1.005–1.030. Urine-specific gravity in excess of 1.030 is an indication of dehydration. When blood volume is decreased, aldosterone is released, increasing the reabsorption of sodium (and, with it, water) from the kidney tubules. This reduces urine output and increases specific gravity.

- Assess temperature every 4 hr (or every hr after ROM). Elevated temperature is a symptom of dehydration. Decreased fluid volume affects the ability to perspire; loss of the cooling effect produced by perspiring results in elevated temperature.
- Monitor for increased pulse and decreased BP and monitor peripheral pulse volume. These are late signs of dehydration and/or hypovolemia. Fluid deficit may cause decreased intravascular and/or extracellular volume, which causes the BP to fall; the body attempts to compensate by increasing the heart rate.

Independent Nursing Actions

- Administer and monitor IV infusion as prescribed. Prevents dehydration/hypovolemia and subsequent acidosis in the woman who cannot have anything by mouth.
- Provide ice chips unless medical order contraindicates them. Women may be kept on nothing by mouth status because gastric emptying time is prolonged in labor. Therefore, if the woman vomits, it may result in aspiration, a source of obstetric morbidity. However, this practice is being questioned. Even with fasting, gastric contents remain in the stomach, and they may even be more acidic when the woman is on nothing by mouth status. In addition, an adequate intake of fluids and calories is needed to meet the energy demands and fluid losses associated with labor. It is fairly common practice to allow clear liquids during early labor. IV solutions vary from lactated Ringer's solution to dextrose in lactated Ringer's solution.
- If diaphoresis occurs, provide measures to keep the woman cool (e.g., cool washcloth to face and body, remove bedspread and any excess clothing, decrease room temperature). Provides comfort and minimizes fluid loss. The work of labor tends to elevate the body temperature, diaphoresis occurs as the body attempts to cool.

INDIVIDUALIZED (NURSING DIAGNOSIS) CARE PLANS

The care plans in this section were developed to address unique patient needs.

▌ Nursing Diagnosis: ANXIETY[1]

Related Factors: misinformation or lack of information, late or no prenatal care, no previous experience, lack of recall, unfamiliar surroundings and procedures, fatigue, excitement, and triggered memories of childhood sexual abuse. Refer to the generic NDCPs "Anxiety,[1]" which begins on p. 10 and "Deficient Knowledge,[1]" which begins on p. 13 in Chapter 2.

▌ Goals, Outcomes, and Evaluation Criteria

- Woman uses breathing and relaxation techniques.
- Woman states that anxiety is manageable.
- Woman's anxiety level is appropriate to the situation.

▌ Nursing Activities and Rationales

Assessments

- Assess level of childbirth preparation. Determines whether lack of information may be contributing to anxiety.
- Assess age, ethnicity, primary language, degree of acculturation, use of personal space, communication patterns. Provides data for meeting psychosocial needs.
- During admission process, assess for a history of sexual abuse. Labor and birth can trigger memories of childhood sexual abuse. The effects of childhood sexual abuse can be manifested in a woman's reluctance to address her healthcare needs, poor relationships with caregivers, anxieties and fears about her upcoming delivery, disappointment with the birth experience and further trauma from giving birth, emotional problems in the postpartum period that extend to bonding difficulties and parenting. Some estimates are that one in three women has experienced sexual abuse, so it is important to assess.
- Observe for increased anxiety or unexpected/unusual pain during vaginal exams or other procedures involving body exposure. It may be too personal and difficult for the woman to discuss abuse with the nurse. However, exposure, examinations, and procedures can trigger a memory at any time. Women with higher anxiety have less confidence in their abilities to perform relaxation techniques and higher degrees of pain during labor and birth. Evidence supports that early labor assessment with an individualized plan of care may improve outcomes in an uncomplicated pregnancy.
- Evaluate FHR, UCs, and maternal VSs. Anxiety can cause excess release of epinephrine and norepinephrine, elevating the pulse and BP. Anxiety can also depress UCs by depleting glucose reserves and, therefore, the synthesis of adenosine triphosphate, which is needed to provide energy for UCs.

Independent Nursing Actions

- Provide privacy during examinations and procedures; drape, pull curtains, shut door to minimize exposure. Demonstrates respect for the woman. Promotes trusting relationship.
- Support cultural or religious practices/rituals as much as possible. These are a source of comfort and strength; enhances coping, reduces anxiety.
- Support woman's spirituality or faith as appropriate. These may serve as a source of inner strength to the

woman. The incorporation of prayer, meditation, chanting, reading, or reciting scriptures can help the woman cope with labor.

- Assist with breathing and relaxation techniques. Assists the woman to cope with anxious feelings. The woman may have difficulty focusing, either because of anxiety or because of the discomforts of labor. Also to relax tense muscles, which interfere with fetal descent and contribute to fatigue; fatigue, in turn, increases pain perception and contributes to inability to cope with pain. Breathing awareness and use of different breathing levels can increase the woman's confidence and ability to cope with UCs.

- Talk with the couple/woman about their expectations for labor and birth, their plans for the baby, whether they have chosen a name, and so forth. Helps woman to focus on the positive aspects of the situation; provides diversion.

- Verbalize confidence in the woman's/couple's ability to cope with labor (e.g., "You're doing a good job," or "You can do this."). Give positive feedback for correct breathing, relaxation techniques, and pushing, for example. Provides reassurance and a sense of control; encourages continuation of positive behaviors.

- Provide presence and remain with the woman as much as possible. Relieves fear of abandonment and conveys caring.

- Provide diversion as needed (e.g., walking about the unit, if condition permits; television, massage, music, showering, birthing ball). Prevents focusing on anxious feelings and fears; helps time pass more quickly.

- Review, reinforce, or teach regarding the labor process and associated procedures. Information gives the woman a sense of control and reduces anxiety. Anxiety evokes stress, which stimulates an adrenal-corticoid response that sets off a chain of physiologic events that can reduce myometrial activity and decrease glucose stores needed by the contracting uterus, increase BP, and cause vasoconstriction. These decrease blood flow to the placenta and fetus and decrease circulation to the uterus.

- Explain that childhood sexual abuse is common in our society and that childbirth may trigger memories; ask permission before all procedures and explain why they are needed; assure the woman that she can say "stop" at any time; and reassure her that the sensations she feels are good because they will bring her baby. Anticipatory guidance may relieve some of the anxiety should memories be triggered. These interventions give control to the woman and affirm her body's capabilities. Note: This intervention may be unfamiliar to some nurses. It is recommended because unreported sexual abuse is common in today's society and memories of it may have been repressed.

Nursing Diagnosis: INEFFECTIVE BREATHING PATTERN (HYPERVENTILATION)[1]

Related Factors: breathing too rapidly and deeply over a prolonged period of time when trying to cope with contractions, in response to pain, and misuse of breathing techniques.

Goals, Outcomes, and Evaluation Criteria

- Woman states relief from symptoms of hyperventilation.
- Woman's respiratory rate returns to prenatal and admission baseline.

NIC Interventions[2]

Anxiety Reduction (5820)—Minimizing apprehension, dread, foreboding, or uneasiness related to an unidentified source of anticipated danger.

Intrapartal Care (6830)—Monitoring and management of stages one and two of the birth process.

Respiratory Monitoring (3350)—Collection and analysis of patient data to ensure airway patency and adequate gas exchange.

Nursing Activities and Rationales

Assessments

- Assess for symptoms of hyperventilation. Hyperventilation is a result of an imbalance of oxygen and carbon dioxide. Prolonged rapid, deep breathing causes too much carbon dioxide to be exhaled, and too much oxygen remains in the body.

- Monitor rate and depth of respiration. Ensures intervention if breathing is too fast, before hyperventilation occurs; evaluates effectiveness of interventions for hyperventilation.

Independent Nursing Actions

- Coach the woman to slow her breathing rate and take shallow breaths. Restores O_2–CO_2 balance by preventing excessive loss of carbonic acid. With instruction, she may be able to correct the problem. Cleansing breaths at the start and completion of a UC may serve as a signal to begin and end the UC focused and in control.

- If necessary, count out loud for the woman. Helps her pace her breathing during the UCs.

- Encourage the woman to relax and use relaxation techniques as needed. See the NDCP "Anxiety,[1]" which begins on p. 227 in this topic. Anxiety may increase the respiratory rate.

- Remain with the woman. Provides reassurance and decreases anxiety.

- If symptoms continue or become more severe, have the woman breathe into a paper bag, a surgical mask, or into her cupped hands. Causes rebreathing of CO_2 to restore O_2–CO_2 balance.

Nursing Diagnosis: INEFFECTIVE COPING[1]

Related Factors: stress of labor, worry about potential complications of labor, history of ineffective coping skills, inadequate emotional support, fatigue, situational or maturational crisis, unrealistic expectations, lack of knowledge, and lack of confidence.

Goals, Outcomes, and Evaluation Criteria

- Woman relaxes with and between UCs.
- Woman responds appropriately to verbal stimuli.
- Woman follows simple directions; e.g., "Breathe with me, 1-2-3."
- Woman makes eye contact.
- Woman verbalizes a sense of control; e.g., "I can do it a little longer."
- Woman asks for help, as needed; e.g., "John, please don't go to lunch now; I need you."

NIC Interventions[2]

Anxiety Reduction (5820)—Minimizing apprehension, dread, foreboding, or uneasiness related to an unidentified source of anticipated danger.
Calming Technique (5880)—Reducing anxiety in a patient experiencing acute distress.
Intrapartal Care (6830)—Monitoring and management of stages one and two of the birth process.
Presence (5340)—Being with another, both physically and psychologically, during times of need.

Nursing Activities and Rationales

Assessments

- Assess maternal and family stressors, use of coping skills, ability to accept help with coping, and existing support systems. Effective coping requires the ability to identify and solve problems and adapt to change. Labor and birth are a situational crisis that calls for increased coping and adaptation.
- Assess cultural background and observe the mother's verbal and nonverbal responses to pain. What appears to be ineffective coping may merely be a culturally accepted mode of dealing with pain (e.g., what appears to be withdrawal may be a cultural expectation that one must be stoic with pain).

- Assess for factors (e.g., age, lack of partner) that may increase vulnerability to stress. For example, women without a support person and adolescent women may be more vulnerable to stress and less able to remain in control with UCs.
- Assess for factors that may contribute to ineffective coping (e.g., misinformation, unrealistic expectations). Knowing the causes of the problem enables the nurse to individualize interventions to meet the specific needs of the woman/couple.
- Evaluate the efforts of the partner to provide support, and teach or role model as needed. Especially in transition, the woman is likely to be calmer when her coach and/or the nurse is calm. Because she may feel dependent and out of control, it is especially important for her to feel that those around her are in control.
- Assess for negative coping—inability to perform breathing techniques, thrashing about, screaming, requests for medication very early in labor (e.g., at 1–2 cm of cervical dilation, when UCs are still mild to palpation). Each woman responds uniquely to labor and to the discomfort of UCs. Ineffective coping strategies may increase anxiety and decrease confidence in her ability to perform relaxation techniques, which increases the perception of pain and the number of requests for medication.
- Assess UC pattern and intensity, cervical dilation, and fetal position, presentation, and lie. Identifies factors that may be increasing the amount of discomfort and determines whether maternal behaviors represent ineffective coping or an unusual labor situation.

Independent Nursing Actions

- Assist the woman to identify new behaviors or techniques to help her cope. As she uses her coping skills effectively, her feelings of autonomy, control, and self-esteem will increase.
- Support the woman's helpful coping behaviors and support systems. Supports her continued success in using coping behaviors and in receiving support.
- Stay with the woman as much as possible; provide support for the partner; provide a doula, if possible, if the woman is alone. Women are dependent during labor, and fears of abandonment may surface, interfering with the ability to cope. Having a supportive other meets dependency needs and provides support. Positive outcomes have been achieved from the use of doulas to provide information and support during labor and birth.
- Relieve anxiety. See the generic NDCP, "Anxiety,[1]" beginning on p. 10 in Chapter 2, and the NCDP, "Anxiety,[1]" which begins on p. 227 in this topic.
- If the partner/doula is providing adequate coaching, do not verbalize further instructions during a contraction.

This may be confusing to the woman, cause her to lose focus, and result in loss of control. It is easier to focus and follow the direction of one voice.

- Provide pharmacologic and nonpharmacologic pain-relief measures. Pain is a stressor, and minimizing stressors improves ability to cope. Conversely, an inability to cope increases anxiety and, thus, increases perception of pain. See the NDCP, "Pain,[1]" next.

Nursing Diagnosis: PAIN[1]

Related Factors: cervical dilation, muscle hypoxia, uncomfortable position, lack of a position change, diaphoresis, full bladder, dry mouth, and leaking of amniotic fluid. During the first stage, pain arises primarily from dilation of the cervix—but also from hypoxia of the uterine muscle cells during contraction, stretching of the lower uterine segment, and pressure on adjacent structures.

Use this section with the generic NDCP, "Pain,[1]" beginning on p. 18 in Chapter 2. Also use the collaborative care plan, "Potential Complications of Narcotic (and Narcotic Agonist-Antagonist) Analgesia: Maternal Respiratory Depression, Maternal Hypotension, and Newborn Respiratory Depression," beginning on p. 225 in this topic.

Goals, Outcomes, and Evaluation Criteria

- Woman expresses satisfaction with pain relief measures.
- Woman copes satisfactorily with UCs, using breathing and other relaxation techniques.
- Woman follows coach's/nurse's directions during UCs.
- There is an absence of physiologic signs of pain.

NIC Interventions[2]

Analgesic Administration (2210)—Use of pharmacologic agents to reduce or eliminate pain.

Analgesic Administration: Intraspinal (2214)—Administration of pharmacologic agents into the epidural or intrathecal space to reduce or eliminate pain.

Anxiety Reduction (5820)—Minimizing apprehension, dread, foreboding, or uneasiness related to an unidentified source of anticipated danger.

Cutaneous Stimulation (1340)—Stimulation of the skin and underlying tissues for the purpose of decreasing undesirable signs and symptoms such as pain, muscle spasm, or inflammation.

Distraction (5900)—Purposeful focusing of attention away from undesirable sensations.

Environmental Management: Comfort (6482)—Manipulation of the patient's surroundings for promotion of optimal comfort.

Intrapartal Care (6830)—Monitoring and management of stages one and two of the birth process.

Pain Management (1400)—Alleviation of pain or a reduction in pain to a level of comfort that is acceptable to the patient.

Touch (5460)—Providing comfort and communication through purposeful tactile contact.

Nursing Activities and Rationales

Assessments

- Assess the amount and type of preparation for childbirth the couple has had (e.g., classes). Preparation for childbirth reduces the need for analgesia during labor.
- Monitor for signs of anxiety. A moderate amount of anxiety about the pain enhances the ability to cope with it; however, too much anxiety interferes with coping.
- Monitor VSs and observe for signs of pain. Frequent physiologic manifestations of pain are increased heart rate, respirations, and BP; dilated pupils; and muscle tension. Muscle tension can impede the progress of labor.
- Observe for side effects of analgesics/epidural anesthesia. Refer to "Epidural Anesthesia/Analgesia," beginning on p. 250 in this chapter. Also refer to the collaborative care plan, "Potential Complications of Narcotic (and Narcotic Agonist-Antagonist) Analgesia: Maternal Respiratory Depression, Maternal Hypotension, and Newborn Respiratory Depression," beginning on p. 227 of this topic.

Independent Nursing Actions

- Perform interventions to decrease anxiety. Anxiety exacerbates pain-fear-pain cycle. Increases catecholamines, increases physical distress, and may result in myometrial dysfunction and ineffectual labor. See the NDCP, "Anxiety,[1]" beginning on p. 227 in this topic.
- Encourage voiding every 1–2 hrs and palpate for bladder distention. Catheterize if necessary. Epidural analgesia/anesthesia may take away the sensation of the need to void. A full bladder can increase discomfort. Opioid analgesics may cause urinary retention.
- Encourage distractions such as talking, watching TV, reading, playing cards, using a focal point, and guided imagery. These interventions work best early in labor; they are less effective in transition or when UCs are very painful. Distracts the woman's attention from the UCs.
- Encourage and assist to reposition frequently. Prevents tissue ischemia and muscle stiffness.
- Encourage ambulation if the following criteria are met: in latent or active first stage, has not had an analgesic, membranes are intact, no vaginal bleeding, no fetal distress. Ambulation provides diversion because the woman focuses on stimuli other than the UCs. Criteria provide for the safety of the mother and the fetus.
- Encourage the woman to use pelvic rocking or use effleurage; encourage the partner to provide back rubs; use cold or warm compresses to the back; or use birthing ball. Reduces abdominal and back discomfort.
- Use touch (e.g., hold the woman's hand, rub her back), as appropriate. A sensory experience (e.g., back rub) can

provide distraction; the woman focuses on the stimulus rather than the pain. Some women want physical contact; others do not. It is common for a woman to want touch during early labor, but to pull away from touch during transition. Nurses must consider the patient's personal space and cultural background when determining appropriate touch during labor.

- Assist with use of breathing and relaxation techniques, as necessary. Provides distraction, contributes to a sense of control, and decreases the perception of pain in the cerebral cortex.

- Provide information about, and demonstrate as necessary, various techniques the partner can use to encourage relaxation and pain control. By giving the woman/couple a choice, the intervention is likely to be more effective. This enhances self-esteem and coping, as well.

- Offer partner care. Physical labor support can be exhausting for the partner/significant other. To maintain energy, the nurse can offer respite time and encourage frequent meals. Also offer pillows and blankets so that short naps or rest periods can be obtained.

- Take the woman's culture into account when evaluating pain expression and pain relief. For accurate evaluation. In some cultures, one is expected to communicate even mild pain; in others one is expected to tolerate pain stoically. Absence of crying and moaning does not necessarily mean there is no pain; just as loud crying and moaning may not mean that the woman wants pain medication at that time.

- Encourage the woman to rest between UCs. Teach and/or demonstrate muscle relaxation techniques, as needed. Relieves muscle tension, which can lead to fatigue. Fatigue increases the perception of pain and makes it difficult for the woman to cope with the UCs.

- Cluster nursing activities so the woman can have periods of rest. Keep the room quiet. Reduces fatigue, which interferes with the woman's ability to cope with UCs.

- Assist to take a warm shower, directing warm water over the woman's lower back and abdomen. Enhances relaxation and reduces pain.

- If a whirlpool bath is used, use only after active labor is established. Water temperature should be 37°C or less. Have the woman drink fluids while in the bath. Warm water baths/whirlpools increase relaxation and promote labor progress. Fluids are needed to maintain fluid balance and the beneficial effects of the hydrotherapy. After about 2 hours, and as UCs become more intense, the effectiveness of hydrotherapy tends to decrease.

- Administer analgesics if the woman wishes and if nonpharmacologic measures are not effective. Frequently this is an intravenous narcotic or narcotic agonist-antagonist. Alternatively, assist with administration of epidural analgesia/anesthesia. When UCs become too intense for the woman to cope, analgesics control the pain and allow her to rest between contractions, promote relaxation, and shorten labor. If given too early, however, they may slow the labor process; if narcotics are given within 1 hour of the birth, the newborn may have respiratory depression.

- Support the mother's choice of analgesia or her decision to use nonpharmacologic measures. Reduces feelings of failure and guilt if she had wished to have an unmedicated birth.

- Support and assist with alternative therapies (e.g., acupressure, acupuncture, reflexology). As long as the practices are not harmful to the woman, they may be of assistance in relieving pain.

- Provide other comfort measures (e.g., keep the bed clean and dry and room temperature comfortable, and provide a cold cloth for the face and petroleum jelly for the lips; provide lip care). Removes sources of irritation that may increase the woman's perception of pain.

Nursing Diagnosis: NAUSEA[1]

Related Factors: transition phase of the first stage, delayed gastric emptying time, hyperventilation, and narcotic analgesics.

Goals, Outcomes, and Evaluation Criteria

- Woman expresses that nausea is relieved.
- There is an absence of symptoms of nausea.
- There is an absence of anxiety regarding the nausea.

NIC Interventions[2]

Aspiration Precautions (3200)—Prevention or minimization of risk factors in the patient at risk for aspiration.
Nausea Management (1450)—Prevention and alleviation of nausea.
Vomiting Management (1570)—Prevention and alleviation of vomiting.

Nursing Activities and Rationales

Assessments

- Measure intake and output and measure or estimate emesis volume. Determines fluid balance. Refer to the NDCP, "Risk for Deficient Fluid Volume,[1]" on p. 228 in this topic.
- Identify factors that may cause or contribute to vomiting. (See "Related Factors," preceding.) When possible, interventions should address the cause rather than just the symptoms of a problem.

Independent Nursing Actions

- Control environmental factors such as aversive smells, sounds, and visual stimulation. These may cause nausea.
- Intervene to control anxiety, fear, and fatigue. These contribute to nausea. Refer to the NDCPs, "Anxiety,[1]" and "Fatigue,[1]" which begin on pp. 10 and 14, respectively.

- Wait 30 minutes after the woman vomits before offering fluids; begin with ice chips and then clear liquids. Maintains hydration and prevents further vomiting. Whether or not to provide fluids depends on the stage and progress of labor and the medical order.
- Elevate head of bed to at least 45 degrees, or position on left side with head turned to side. Helps prevent aspiration of vomitus.
- Apply cool cloths to forehead, sponge the face, keep gown clean. Provides comfort.
- Support the woman's head during vomiting. Provides comfort.
- If vomiting occurs, provide oral hygiene; clean nose and mouth. Removes unpleasant taste and odors that may cause further nausea. Keep in mind, though, that oral hygiene sometimes stimulates nausea and vomiting.
- Administer antiemetic medications such as promethazine (Phenergan), if ordered. Acts in the CNS on the chemoreceptor trigger zone to decrease nausea.

Patient/Family Teaching

- Explain that nausea and vomiting are normal in active and transition labor, that it is a sign that labor is progressing, and that the symptoms are temporary. Provides reassurance and minimizes anxiety.

▌ Other Nursing Diagnoses

Also assess for the following nursing diagnoses, which are frequently present with this condition:

- Fatigue[1] related to long or difficult labor or to sleep deprivation before labor.
- Deficient Knowledge[1] of labor processes and procedures related to no previous experience, late or no prenatal care.
- Urinary Retention[1] related to effects of epidural anesthesia or opioid analgesia.

NORMAL LABOR: SECOND STAGE

Labor is normal when it occurs near term, is completed in 24 hours, there is a single fetus in vertex presentation, and there are no complications. The course of normal labor consists of progressive uterine contractions, effacement and dilation of the cervix, and descent of the fetus. Second-stage labor begins with complete cervical dilation and ends with the expulsion of the fetus. During the second stage, the presenting part presses on the stretch receptors of the pelvic floor. This stimulates the pushing reflex and causes the release of oxytocin from the posterior pituitary, which provokes stronger uterine contractions (UCs).

▌ Key Nursing Activities

- Monitor FHR and maternal BP between contractions.
- Palpate contractions until the birth.

- Assist with positioning and encourage with pushing (open glottis technique).
- Provide comfort measures (e.g., warm perineal compresses, visualization techniques).
- Scrub perineal area prior to delivery.
- Assist the provider with preparing for the birth (e.g., assist with sterile gowning and gloving).
- Note and record the time of birth, time of placenta, type of birth, operative birth, fetal position, type of laceration or episiotomy, type of incision, umbilical cord gases (as requested by provider).
- Promote parent–infant attachment.

CAUTION: Use universal precautions when there is possibility of exposure to blood and body fluids. Goggles or glasses and a splash apron or a protective plastic apron are recommended during the birth process because of the likelihood of splashes from amniotic fluid or blood.

▌ Signs and Symptoms

- Complete cervical dilation of 10 cm.
- Complete cervical effacement (100%).
- Uterine contractions (UCs) strong, 2–3 min apart, and with a duration 60–90 seconds.
- Urge to push begins.
- Membranes may rupture.
- An episode of vomiting may occur.
- Copious bloody mucus.
- Woman may become more verbal, scream, and act out of control; she becomes more focused on the bearing-down efforts.
- Fetal station: descent continues at 1 cm/hr in primiparas and 2 cm/hr in multiparas until presenting part reaches perineal floor.
- Perineum bulges, then flattens, then crowning occurs.
- Infant is born.
- Duration of second stage can be from about 15 minutes to 2 hours, depending on parity and whether the woman has had regional analgesia/anesthesia.

▌ Diagnostic Studies

- Vaginal examination. Detects progressive cervical dilation and effacement, as well as fetal station and position.
- Blood gas analysis on cord blood. Determines fetal response to labor; however, this practice varies by practitioner.

▌ Medical Management

- FHR monitoring. Assesses fetal well-being.
- Assessment of VSs and clinical findings. Ensures maternal well-being.
- Monitoring for complications of birth.
- Episiotomy, if indicated.
- Hand maneuvers to prevent trauma when the fetal head has distended the perineum.
- Manual or vacuum rotation of fetal head (e.g., from occiput posterior to occiput anterior).

- Clamp and cut umbilical cord.
- Suction the newborn's nose and mouth. Removes mucus.

▌ *Collaborative Problems*

Potential complications of labor include the following:
- Fetal distress/anoxia (reduced placental perfusion, head/cord compression, hyperventilation, etc.)
- Dystocia (dysfunctional UCs, malpresentation)
- Uterine rupture
- Placental abruption

Potential complications of epidural anesthesia include the following:
- Maternal hypotension
- Fetal hypoxia
- Bladder distention
- Ineffective bearing down with UCs

COLLABORATIVE (STANDARDIZED) CARE FOR ALL WOMEN IN NORMAL SECOND-STAGE LABOR

Perform a comprehensive assessment to identify individual needs for teaching, emotional support, and physical care.

▌ Potential Complications of Labor: FETAL DISTRESS/ANOXIA, DYSTOCIA, AND UTERINE RUPTURE

Refer to "Intrapartum Fetal Monitoring," beginning on p. 242 in this chapter. Also refer to "Dystocia/Dysfunctional Labor," which begins on p. 263; "Uterine Rupture," which begins on p. 293; and "Forceps- or Vacuum-Assisted Birth," which begins on p. 299, all in Chapter 8.

Focus Assessments

- Monitor maternal BP, heart rate, and respirations after each UC (some recommendations are every 5–15 min). Maternal condition affects fetal status. Maternal hypotension reduces placental perfusion and, thus, fetal oxygenation; normal maternal respirations are vital for maintaining the oxygen–carbon dioxide balance in the blood.
- Monitor UCs continually (with electronic monitor and manual palpation). Detects dysfunctional contractions or hypertonic contractions.
- Monitor FHR continually or after every UC. Observe rate (which should be 110–160 beats/min); observe for severe or prolonged variable or late decelerations; and observe variability. Detects fetal hypoxia or bradycardia that may

occur as a result of vagal stimulation during head compression. Placental perfusion may be decreased by anesthesia, by Valsalva maneuver during pushing contractions, or by incorrect positioning. Early or variable FHR decelerations may occur during UCs because of head compression or a nuchal or short umbilical cord, but they should return to baseline between UCs. Late decelerations are less likely in a normal labor; they are usually associated with gestational hypertension, diabetes, or other complications; or with maternal anesthesia. Variability suggests an intact fetal nervous system; it should range from 6 to 10 bpm.

- Continue to assess fetal station, presentation, and position. Detects malpresentation (if not detected before second stage) and ensures intervention, as needed, by changing maternal position. For example, posterior position tends to prolong second stage; but placing the woman in lateral recumbent position or in hands-and-knees position may rotate the fetal occiput from posterior to anterior position. Rapid descent, as in precipitous labor, may cause fetal head trauma because the bones do not have time to adjust to the size of the birth canal.
- Frequently assess the effect of maternal positions (lying, sitting, squatting, etc.) on fetal status and descent. There is no single, correct position for childbirth. Angles between the fetus and the woman's pelvis change as the infant descends through the birth canal. A different position may facilitate descent or rotation of the presenting part.
- Assess length of first stage and level of woman's fatigue. Labor consumes a great deal of energy because of the UCs in stage 1 and the muscular effort of bearing down in stage 2. A woman who has had a long first stage or who was not rested at the beginning of labor may be too exhausted to push effectively during stage 2.
- When membranes rupture, note the time and the amount, color, and odor of the fluid. Green-colored amniotic fluid may indicate fetal hypoxia. Hypoxia causes the fetal anal sphincter to relax and release meconium. Foul-smelling fluid signals infection; scanty fluid may indicate poorly controlled maternal diabetes. All of these stress the fetus.

Preventive Nursing Activities

- Be sure an emergency delivery kit is available in the labor room (in institutions where birth occurs in a delivery room instead of the labor room). Ensures that the necessary equipment and supplies are available in the event of precipitous birth or other emergency that prevents transfer to the delivery room.
- Encourage laboring down while the fetus descends passively. This allows the urge to push for women with regional analgesia since it may take as long as 2 hours for the urge to occur. A lateral position facilitates passive fetal descent until the head is low enough to stimulate the Ferguson

reflex, which is caused by the fetus pressing the Ferguson plexus of nerves.

- Assist with episiotomy, if necessary. Although routine use of an episiotomy remains controversial, it shortens the second stage and may prevent fetal trauma when labor is long or forceful or when the fetus is large.
- Assist with use of forceps if the woman's efforts do not rotate the fetal head and promote adequate fetal descent. When maternal efforts are unsuccessful, low forceps birth may be necessary.
- Be prepared to assist with procedures such as vacuum rotation from occiput posterior to occiput anterior or to prepare for cesarean birth. A midforceps rotation from occiput posterior to occiput anterior position may be necessary. There is increased risk of fetal injury with this procedure; nevertheless, it is preferred to birth in occiput posterior position, which presents a risk of fetal neck trauma. Cesarean birth may be necessary when cephalopelvic disproportion occurs, when there is persistent occiput posterior position, when there is fetal distress, or in prolonged second stage labor.
- Provide comfort measures, such as a cool cloth to the forehead, and coach the woman to relax between UCs. Uteroplacental blood flow is interrupted during a contraction; it is reestablished between UCs. Stress can cause a dysfunctional labor pattern by causing an imbalance of epinephrine and norepinephrine. Also helps prevent fatigue that can develop with a prolonged labor. Rest and relaxation reduce glucose utilization and conserve energy needed for pushing. Tense muscles increase resistance to fetal descent.
- Encourage a lateral recumbent, Fowler's, standing, hands-and-knees, or squatting position for the labor and birth if not contraindicated. The choice of position is influenced by provider preference. If the lithotomy position must be used, elevate the woman's back 30–40 degrees. Prevents occlusion of the inferior vena cava by the gravid uterus, promotes venous return, and prevents hypotension and decreased placental perfusion. May also promote comfort. These positions make use of gravity to enhance fetal descent. There are a number of disadvantages to the lithotomy position (refer to an obstetrics text for more details), but it is often used to enhance the maintenance of asepsis, monitoring of the FHR, and performing the episiotomy. The nurse should explain the benefit of upright positions for second stage of labor even though no single position is appropriate for all labors.
- Coach the woman to take several deep breaths when the contraction begins, then through pursed lips, exhale slowly every 5–6 sec while pushing; take another breath and continue the exhale breathing and pushing as long as the UC lasts, but with no more than 3 pushing efforts per contraction. Also coach to inhale every 10–20 seconds while pushing. Promotes maternal oxygenation. The Valsalva maneuver, which occurs when the woman holds her breath while pushing, increases intrathoracic pressure due to her closed glottis. This causes a decrease in cardiac output and blood pressure that decreases the maternal heart rate, reduces the PO_2, and increases PCO_2; this can result in fetal hypoxia and acidosis.

- Intervene to prevent and reduce anxiety. Anxiety can decrease placental perfusion and uterine contractility.
- Encourage maternal movement and position changes if descent is not occurring. The upright position makes use of gravity to bring about descent. Squatting aligns the fetus with the birth canal and facilitates pelvic and perineal relaxation. Even though no single position is appropriate for all labors, suggested positions include squatting, standing, semirecumbent, and upright kneeling.
- Encourage the woman to take panting breaths or to exhale slowly through pursed lips as the baby's head crowns. Helps prevent fetal trauma by allowing for gradual accommodation of the fetal head to the birth canal and ensuring slow birth of the fetal head.

Potential Complications of Epidural Anesthesia: MATERNAL HYPOTENSION, FETAL HYPOXIA, BLADDER DISTENTION, AND INEFFECTIVE BEARING DOWN WITH UCS

Refer to "Epidural Anesthesia/Analgesia," beginning on p. 248 in this chapter.

Nursing Diagnosis: RISK FOR INFECTION[1]

Related Factors: invasive procedures (e.g., vaginal exams, placement of internal monitoring device, forceps or vacuum extraction), ruptured membranes, or prolonged labor. Refer to the generic NDCP, "Risk for Infection,[1]" which begins on p. 21 in Chapter 2.

NIC Interventions[2]

Intrapartal Care (6830)—Monitoring and management of stages one and two of the birth process.

Nursing Activities and Rationales

Assessments

- Assess maternal temperature and heart rate. Elevated temperature may indicate infection; fever occurs as a result of endotoxins in the cell walls of bacteria and viruses. Fever is an immune system defense mechanism that kills or inhibits the growth of many microorganisms. Elevated temperature does not necessarily indicate infection. The increased metabolic rate during labor may also cause a slight temperature elevation.

- When membranes rupture, either spontaneously or artificially, note time and amount, color, and odor of the fluid; assess the FHR. Foul-smelling fluid is a sign of infection; greenish-tinged fluid indicates passage of meconium caused by fetal hypoxia, which may indicate preexisting intrauterine infection. FHR is indicator of fetal well-being or stress.

Independent Nursing Actions

- Use medical asepsis to perform perineal care; sterile asepsis for perineal prep for birth; remove feces expelled during pushing; change linens and underpad as needed for cleanliness. Removes pathogens and medium for their growth.
- Use sterile gloves for vaginal examinations. Perform only as many vaginal exams as absolutely necessary to evaluate labor progress. Prevents introduction of pathogens into the vagina and subsequent endometrial infection.

Nursing Diagnosis: RISK FOR MATERNAL INJURY (PERINEAL OR CERVICAL LACERATIONS/ BRUISING, MUSCLE/LIGAMENT STRAIN, AND FALLS)[1]

Related Factors: forceps-assisted birth, large fetus, hypertonic uterine contractions, perineal tension while pushing; falls; and muscle strain due to inappropriate positioning of the mother's legs in stirrups.

Goals, Outcomes, and Evaluation Criteria

- Woman remains free of perineal and cervical lacerations.
- Woman remains free of muscle strain.
- Woman remains free of falls and injury.

NIC Interventions[2]

Fall Prevention (6490)—Instituting precautions with patient at risk for injury from falling.
Intrapartal Care (6830)—Monitoring and management of stages one and two of the birth process.
Positioning: Intraoperative (0842)—Moving the patient or body part to promote surgical exposure while reducing the risk of discomfort and complications.

Nursing Activities and Rationales

Assessments

- Palpate for bladder fullness and catheterize as needed. Helps prevent bladder trauma from the presenting part and makes room for the descent of the presenting part into the pelvis.

Independent Nursing Actions

- Encourage the woman to take panting breaths or to exhale slowly through pursed lips as the baby's head crowns. Ensures slow birth of the fetal head and avoids perineal trauma.
- Repeat instructions with each UC. Amnesia between UCs often occurs during the second stage.
- Assist with positioning. Encourage the woman to relax her perineal muscles and use abdominal muscles in pushing. Place in an upright position for pushing and in left Sims position for the birth, if possible. Promotes gradual stretching of perineal and vaginal tissue and, therefore, helps prevent trauma and lacerations of the cervix, vagina, urethra, and perineum. Upright positions for pushing reduce the need for episiotomy. For example, squatting aligns the fetus with the birth canal and facilitates pelvic and perineal relaxation. Sims position reduces perineal tension during the birth and reduces need for episiotomy.
- When placing the woman in lithotomy position (the most commonly used birthing position in the United States), pad the stirrups and place both legs simultaneously into the stirrups. Be sure the calves are supported and there is no pressure on the popliteal space. Prevents muscle and ligament strain and avoids interfering with popliteal circulation, which contributes to postpartal thrombophlebitis and nerve damage.
- Be sure that stirrups are the same height, if lithotomy position is used. Prevents strain on back ligaments as the woman bears down.
- Never apply fundal pressure when shoulder dystocia is suspected. The practice of applying fundal pressure for shoulder dystocia is controversial because it compromises fetal and maternal safety and should not be attempted by the nurse. The use of McRoberts maneuver, which involves flexing the woman's thighs against her abdomen, is the first maneuver to assist in delivering the impacted shoulder.

Collaborative Activities

- Assist with episiotomy, if necessary. Episiotomy is thought to prevent perineal tears in rapid labor, when the infant is large, or when there is perineal tension. However, routine use of episiotomy is controversial. Midline episiotomies tend to heal better and with less pain but they are associated with increased perineal trauma and extensive tearing. If tearing occurs, it may extend into the rectum. Mediolateral episiotomies reduce the incidence of perineal lacerations but are more difficult to repair and to heal.

Nursing Diagnosis: RISK FOR FLUID VOLUME DEFICIT[1]

See the NDCP, "Risk for Deficient Fluid Volume,[1]" beginning on p. 228 in the topic "Normal Labor: First Stage," which begins on p. 223 in this chapter.

Nursing Diagnosis: RISK FOR IMPAIRED PARENT–INFANT/ CHILD ATTACHMENT[1]

Related Factors: anxiety, physical/environmental/situational barriers, and lack of privacy. Use this NDCP with the generic NDCP, "Risk for Impaired Parent–Infant/Child Attachment,[1]" which begins on p. 19 in Chapter 2.

▌ NIC Interventions[2]

Environmental Management: Attachment Process (6481)— Manipulation of the patient's surroundings to facilitate the development of the parent–infant relationships.

▌ Nursing Activities and Rationales

Assessments

- Assess level of childbirth preparation and past deliveries if relevant (prior to active labor). Determines whether lack of information may be contributing to the anxiety. Anxiety can interfere with attachment process.
- Assess age, ethnicity, degree of acculturation, use of personal space, communication patterns. Provides data for meeting psychosocial needs. The amount of early physical contact desired is different among cultures.
- Assess anxiety level. Anxiety can interfere with attachment.

Independent Nursing Actions

- When starting maternal IV, use tubing long enough to allow for freedom of movement. Also consider local anesthesia when starting the IV. Decreases anxiety and pain associated with needle puncture, and long tubing enables the woman to hold and examine the infant.
- Limit number of people in delivery room, considering the parents' preferences. Enables parents to focus on the newborn and on each other.
- Place the infant on the mother's body immediately after birth. Provide opportunity for parents to see and hold the baby immediately after birth. Perform as many assessments or interventions as possible with the infant on the

mother's body or being held. Early physical contact promotes maternal and paternal attachment. Newborns have highly developed senses that allow them to actively participate in interactions from birth.

- Keep parents informed of the care that is being given to the newborn at birth. If possible, position infant warmer so that the parents can see the newborn while care is given. Birth is an emotionally charged time for all members of the family. As they verbally express amazement and pride, their feelings of accomplishment and joy strengthen family bonds.
- Encourage early breastfeeding. Promotes attachment. Stimulates maternal release of prolactin, which initiates the onset of lactation.
- Encourage parents to do whatever they feel comfortable doing in the way of holding and caring for the newborn. Some want immediate time; others may prefer to wait until after third stage birth and episiotomy repair are completed and the infant is clean and dry. The parents' wishes should be supported.

INDIVIDUALIZED (NURSING DIAGNOSIS) CARE PLANS

The care plans in this section were developed to address unique patient needs.

Nursing Diagnosis: PAIN[1]

Related Factors: muscle hypoxia, uncomfortable position, lack of a position change, diaphoresis, full bladder, dry mouth, pressure of presenting part, stretching of the vagina and perineum, intense uterine contractions, and episiotomy. Use with the generic NDCP, "Pain,[1]" which begins on p. 18 in Chapter 2. Also refer to the NDCP, "Pain,[1]" which begins on p. 230 in the topic, "Normal Labor: First Stage," beginning on p. 221 in this chapter. Also refer to "Epidural Anesthesia/Analgesia," beginning on p. 248 in this chapter.

▌ Goals, Outcomes, and Evaluation Criteria

- Woman rests between UCs.

▌ NIC Interventions

Some interventions are the same as in the first stage. However, some, such as cutaneous stimulation and distraction, are not as effective in managing second-stage pain.

▌ Nursing Activities and Rationales

Assessments

- Assess level of pain and its location and causes. Enables choice of best intervention. Pain may not be coming from the obvious sources (UCs and pressure of the descending fetus); it may be that the woman has a cramp in her leg, for example.

- Assess for bladder distention. Catheterize if necessary because a full bladder may increase pain.

Independent Nursing Actions

- Provide comfort measures, such as a cool cloth to the face and neck; clean underpads; perineal care; mouth care. Helps relieve pain by promoting psychologic comfort, demonstrating caring, and promoting physical comfort.
- Assist the woman to assume the position she finds most comfortable for pushing, keeping in mind that squatting, lateral recumbent, or semi-Fowler's position enhance the effectiveness of bearing-down efforts. Support the legs as needed during pushing. Proper positioning reduces discomfort.
- Encourage the woman to relax her perineum as she pushes with her abdomen. Allows the tissues to stretch and reduces the amount of pressure created by the fetal presenting part.
- Assist the woman to bear down as she feels the need to do so during UCs. Let her know when to push if she has had epidural anesthesia. Epidural anesthetics may interfere with the woman's ability to feel the UCs.
- Catheterize (between UCs) if the bladder is distended. A full bladder can increase discomfort. Opioid analgesics may cause urine retention.

Collaborative Activities

- Assist with administration of local anesthetic before episiotomy. Anesthetizes the perineum and prevents pain from incision and suturing.

■ Nursing Diagnosis: ANXIETY[1]

Related Factors: inability to control defecation when bearing down and lack of knowledge about and inexperience with perineal sensations associated with the urge to push. Refer to the generic NDCPs, "Anxiety,[1]" which begins on p. 10, and "Deficient Knowledge,[1]" which begins on p. 13, in Chapter 2. Also refer to the NDCP, "Anxiety,[1]" beginning on p. 227 in the topic "Normal Labor: First Stage," which begins on p. 221 in this chapter.

■ *Nursing Activities and Rationales*

Assessments

- Observe for a decrease in the woman's voluntary bearing-down efforts. Sometimes when a woman reaches second stage, she experiences a lack of readiness to complete the process (e.g., reluctance to care for another baby, desire to wait until her support person arrives, fear about the new and painful sensations of second stage). When this happens, the nurse must address the woman's concerns and coach her to push effectively.

Independent Nursing Actions

- Continue to provide explanations and information without waiting for the woman/partner to ask; prepare her for sensations she will experience. Anticipatory guidance relieves anxiety and helps the woman/couple to achieve a satisfying birth experience.
- Continue to provide feedback to the woman and partner. Reduces anxiety by providing reassurance that they are performing well.
- Use music as the woman desires. Enhances relaxation, thereby reducing stress and anxiety.
- Encourage the partner and other family members as desired to participate during the second stage. Family members may hesitate to continue helping as the situation seems more intense for fear of interfering or being in the way.
- Adhere to the parents' birth plan if the labor and delivery are normal and without complications. Promotes a satisfying birth experience.

■ Nursing Diagnosis: INEFFECTIVE BREATHING PATTERN (HYPERVENTILATION)[1]

See the NDCP, "Hyperventilation," which begins on p. 230 in the topic "Normal Labor: First Stage," which begins on p. 223 in this chapter.

■ Nursing Diagnosis: FATIGUE[1]

Related Factors: long or difficult labor, sleep deprivation before labor, prolonged first- and/or second-stage labor, overwhelming physical and emotional demands of labor, unrelieved pain, and prolonged nothing-by-mouth status. See the generic NDCP, "Fatigue,[1]" which begins on p. 14 in Chapter 2.

■ *Goals, Outcomes, and Evaluation Criteria*

- Woman pushes effectively with UCs.
- Woman follows coach's instructions.

■ *NIC Interventions[2]*

Intrapartal Care (6830)—Monitoring and management of stages one and two of the birth process.

■ *Nursing Activities and Rationales*

Assessments

- Note length of first stage. A woman who has experienced a long or difficult first stage may be too exhausted to push effectively in the second stage. Refer to the Freedman curve in an obstetrics textbook for more information.

- Monitor fetal presentation, position, and station; monitor length of second stage. Fetal malposition or malpresentation may prolong second stage, causing energy depletion. Recognition of the problem allows for interventions such as changing the woman's position.

Independent Nursing Actions

- Encourage the woman to relax completely between UCs. Conserves energy needed for pushing and expulsion of the fetus. A great deal of muscular effort is used during the second stage.
- Support or show the partner how to support the woman's back and shoulders during bearing-down efforts (or support her body in other positions, as needed). She may be too tired to raise her back and shoulders from the bed without help. Enables her to assume position most effective for pushing.

Collaborative Activities

- Provide oral glucose or IV with glucose, as permitted. A great deal of muscular effort is used during the second stage. Because the woman may be on nothing-by-mouth status and without the intake of calories for many hours, energy deficit occurs.

Patient/Family Teaching

- Teach and/or reinforce correct use of relaxation techniques. Muscle tension increases fatigue; it may also impede fetal descent and prolong the second stage. Because of the intensity of the second stage, the couple may not remember what they have learned about relaxation techniques, or they may not be able to concentrate well enough to perform them.

▌ *Other Nursing Diagnoses*

Also assess for the following nursing diagnosis, which is frequently present with this condition.

- Deficient Knowledge[1] of labor processes and procedures related to no previous experience, late or no prenatal care.

NORMAL LABOR: THIRD STAGE

The third stage begins when the baby is born and ends with expulsion of the placenta. The placenta is attached to the decidual layer of the endometrium by fibrous anchor villi. After the birth, strong uterine contractions cause the placental site to shrink. This causes the anchor villi to break and the placenta to separate from the decidua. If the uterus does not contract, the placental site does not shrink, so the placenta will not detach. The third stage is the shortest labor stage. It can last from 1 to 30 minutes; the average length is 3–5 minutes.

▌ *Key Nursing Activities*

- Assess for placental separation and note and record time of expulsion.
- Prepare the woman for the sensations she will experience.
- Observe for complications (e.g., hemorrhage).
- Administer oxytocics per medical order.
- Promote parent–infant attachment.
- Use standard precautions when there is possibility of exposure to blood and body fluids. Goggles or glasses and a splash apron or a protective plastic apron are recommended during the birth process because of the likelihood of splashes from amniotic fluid or blood.

▌ *Signs and Symptoms*

The woman may show signs of fatigue. Also, after the birth, cardiac output increases, causing a decreased pulse rate and temporary increase in BP. Signs of placental separation include the following:

- A firm, contracted uterus.
- The uterus changes from a discoid to a globular shape as the placenta descends into the lower uterine segment.
- A sudden gush of dark red blood and/or clots from the vagina.
- An additional length of the umbilical cord slips out of the vagina as the placenta gets closer to the introitus (lengthening of the umbilical cord).
- Vaginal or rectal exam reveal vaginal fullness, or fetal membranes appear at the introitus.

▌ *Diagnostic Studies*

No diagnostic tests are applicable.

▌ *Medical Management*

- Prompt separation and expulsion of the placenta in the easiest and safest manner. Avoid excessive traction on the umbilical cord. Can cause uterine inversion, breaking of the cord, retention of placental fragments and increased blood loss.
- Examination of the placenta. Make sure that no fragments have remained in the uterine cavity.
- Manual inspection of uterus and birth canal. For tears and lacerations.
- Episiotomy repair.
- Oxytocin. Prevents hemorrhage after the placenta is removed.

▌ *Collaborative Problems*

Potential Complications of Third-Stage Labor

- Hemorrhage
- Rupture of a preexisting cerebral aneurysm
- Pulmonary emboli; amniotic fluid embolism

- Uterine inversion
- Delayed placental separation

COLLABORATIVE (STANDARDIZED) CARE FOR ALL WOMEN IN NORMAL THIRD-STAGE LABOR

Perform a comprehensive assessment to identify individual needs for teaching, emotional support, and physical care.

Potential Complications of Labor: HEMORRHAGE, RUPTURE OF A PREEXISTING CEREBRAL ANEURYSM, PULMONARY EMBOLI, AMNIOTIC FLUID EMBOLISM, UTERINE INVERSION, AND UTERINE RUPTURE

Refer to the generic collaborative care plan, "Potential Complication: Hemorrhage," which begins on p. 28 in Chapter 3. Also refer to "Postpartum Hemorrhage," beginning on p. 343 in Chapter 10.

Focus Assessments

- Observe for excessive blood loss. Maternal blood loss should be less than 500 ml or less than 1% of body weight. After the expulsion of the placenta, the uterine muscles should contract and compress intramyometrial blood vessels. Hemostasis is achieved in this manner rather than by platelet aggregation and clot formation.
- Palpate the uterus before and after placental expulsion. Before, to be sure it is contracting enough to achieve expulsion; after, to identify the potential for hemorrhage.
- Note mechanism of placental expulsion. Duncan's mechanism occurs when the rough, maternal surface of the placenta presents first; Schultze's mechanism occurs when the fetal (shiny) surface of the placenta presents first. Duncan's mechanism carries a higher risk of retained placental fragments.
- Note and record information about any retained placental fragments and manual or instrumental removal. Retained placental fragments contribute to postpartum hemorrhage by preventing complete contraction of the uterus and by contributing to postpartum infection.
- Note abnormal placental invasion when the placenta does not deliver. This is usually seen in women who have had four or more cesarean births or in births accompanied

by placenta previa. The etiology is unknown; it has been attributed to a defect in or damage to the deciduas basalis.

- Observe for pallor and cyanosis, decreased urinary output, lightheadedness, restlessness, irritability, altered level of consciousness, and disorientation. These are symptoms of inadequate blood circulation to the skin and organs (e.g., kidneys and brain).
- Observe for increased pulse and respirations and decreased BP. These are signs of hemorrhage. Loss of blood volume causes a fall in BP; pulse and respirations increase in attempt to compensate.
- Observe for restlessness, dyspnea, cyanosis, hypotension, tachycardia, shock, coagulation failure (e.g., petechiae, bleeding from venipuncture sites), uterine atony, pulmonary edema, respiratory arrest. These are signs of amniotic fluid embolism (AFE). AFE occurs when amniotic fluid, carrying debris such as vernix and meconium, enters maternal circulation and obstructs pulmonary vessels. Amniotic fluid can enter maternal circulation whenever there is an opening in the maternal uterine veins and enough intrauterine pressure to force the fluid into them (e.g., at placental separation). Maternal and fetal mortality are high when AFE occurs; early detection of the problem allows for immediate emergency measures to be carried out.
- Observe for severe headache with nausea and vomiting, stroke symptoms, slurred speech, deviation of the eyes, and other central nervous system manifestations. Signs of ruptured cerebral aneurysm. An aneurysm is most likely to rupture during periods of activity (e.g., the increased intracranial pressure during bearing down in second- and third-stage labor). Symptoms depend on the location, extent, and duration of the bleeding. Hemorrhage usually occurs with no warning; symptoms are usually rapid and severe; there is poor prognosis for recovery.
- Observe for uterine inversion (uterus visible at introitus; or with partial inversion, pain and severe bleeding). Although rare, inversion is life threatening. The first signs are usually hemorrhage and shock. It presents with sudden and agonizing pelvic pain. The fundus cannot be palpated. It can occur spontaneously or may be forced by pulling on the umbilical cord. There is increased intra-abdominal pressure (with cough or bearing down). It requires emergency intervention. The possibility of uterine inversion is a good reason for avoiding fundal pressure!
- Uterine rupture can occur from midforceps rotation of the fetus to achieve a vaginal delivery or from multiple gestation, vaginal birth after cesarean, grand multiparity, or hyperstimulation. Observe for abdominal pain and tenderness, vomiting, syncope, tachycardia, pallor, change in fetal heart rate, or increased bleeding at time of birth, all of which can be signs of uterine rupture.

Preventive Nursing Activities

- For mothers who plan to breastfeed, put the baby to breast immediately after birth. Stimulates the release of oxytocin, which causes the uterine muscles to contract and remain firm; preventing hemorrhage.
- Administer IV or intramuscular oxytocin immediately after expulsion of the placenta, as ordered. Intramuscular methylergonovine maleate (Methergine) or prostaglandins, such as misoprostol, may be given. Stimulates the uterus to contract, compress intramyometrial blood vessels, and prevent hemorrhage. Methylergonovine maleate is contraindicated if maternal BP is elevated.
- If the uterus is not firm after placental expulsion, massage gently using both hands (one at the top of the fundus and one at the symphysis pubis) until it contracts. Prevents hemorrhage by compressing intramyometrial blood vessels.
- Assist with repair of episiotomy and/or birth canal lacerations. Lacerations contribute to hemorrhage.
- Maintain IV fluids as ordered. Fluid replacement helps maintain circulating volume in the event of excessive blood loss.
- If fundal pressure is required to help expel the placenta, encourage the woman to maintain abdominal relaxation. Relaxation is difficult because this procedure is painful. Fundal pressure may damage uterine supports and may cause uterine inversion, so it must be used with utmost care.
- Apply ice packs to perineum for the first 24 hours, leaving on no longer than 30 minutes at a time. Constricts blood vessels and reduces bleeding and bruising.

Potential Complication of Third-Stage Labor: DELAYED PLACENTAL SEPARATION

Focus Assessments

- Palpate fundus and observe for signs of placental separation, which are (1) a firm, contracted uterus, (2) uterus changing from discoid to a globular shape as placenta descends into the lower uterine segment, (3) a sudden gush of dark red blood from the vagina, (4) an additional length of umbilical cord slipping out of the vagina as the placenta moves closer to the introitus (lengthening of the umbilical cord), and (5) vaginal or rectal exam reveal svaginal fullness or fetal membranes appear at the introitus. Separation and expulsion should occur within 5 minutes, although it may take up to 30 minutes. Occasionally manual or instrument removal of the placenta, under anesthesia, may be necessary.

Preventive Nursing Activities

- Encourage the woman to continue to push with UCs. After the birth of the baby, her attention may be diverted from her pushing efforts. Additionally, she may be fatigued. Good bearing-down efforts will aid in separation and expulsion of the placenta.
- If fundal pressure is required to help expel the placenta, encourage the woman to maintain abdominal relaxation. Relaxation is difficult because this procedure is painful. Fundal pressure may also damage uterine supports and may cause uterine inversion.

Nursing Diagnosis: RISK FOR MATERNAL INJURY[1]

Related Factors: (maternal injury such as muscle/ligament strain; and falls) incorrect moving of woman's legs from stirrups or supports; drowsiness from analgesia; lack of feeling in legs, and inability to bear weight secondary to regional anesthesia. Use the NDCP, "Risk for Maternal Injury,[1]" beginning on p. 235 in the topic "Normal Labor: Second Stage," which begins on p. 232 in this chapter. The following risk factors and nursing activities should be added for the third stage.

Nursing Activities and Rationales

Assessments

- Assess level of consciousness and sensation in feet and legs. Determines the amount of protection/assistance needed to ensure safety in moving and transferring.

Independent Nursing Actions

- Remove both legs from the stirrups (if they were used) at the same time. To avoid muscle strain.
- When removing legs from the stirrups, hold them together, gently and slowly push them toward the woman's abdomen, back to the neutral position, and then gently lower them to her right side and then her left side. To promote circulation.
- If birth has occurred in a delivery room instead of the labor room, assist in transferring the woman from the delivery bed/table to a cart and to her recovery bed. Woman may be unable to move her legs due to effects of regional anesthesia. She may also have an altered level of conscious secondary to narcotic analgesics.

Nursing Diagnosis: RISK FOR INFECTION[1]

Refer to the generic NDCP, "Risk for Infection,[1]" which begins on p. 21 in Chapter 2. Also refer to the NDCP, "Risk for Infection,[1]" on p. 234 in "Normal Labor: Second Stage," in this chapter.

Nursing Activities and Rationales

Assessments

- Note urinalysis on admission. Determines presence of a urinary tract infection.
- Assess leukocytosis on admission. WBC count greater than 15,000/mm³ during intrapartum period indicates infection.
- Note foul-smelling lochia. May indicate presence of an anaerobic organism, in which case, blood cultures or endometrial culture may be indicated.

Independent Nursing Actions

- After placental expulsion and episiotomy repair, cleanse vulva and perineum with sterile water and antiseptic solution; apply sterile vaginal pad; and place clean absorbent pads on the bed beneath the woman. Removes pathogens, prevents ascending infection.
- Encourage fluid intake after delivery. Restores fluid balance and prevents dehydration.
- Observe vital signs. Increased pulse rate from baseline and fever are signs of infection.
- Patient teaching on importance of frequent hand washing especially after voiding and perineal care. Prevents contamination and possible infection.

Nursing Diagnosis: RISK FOR IMPAIRED PARENT–INFANT/ CHILD ATTACHMENT[1]

Use with the generic NDCP, "Risk for Impaired Parent–Infant/ Child Attachment,[1]" which begins on p. 19 in Chapter 2. Also refer to the NDCP, "Risk for Impaired Parent–Infant/Child Attachment,[1]" which begins on p. 236 in the topic "Normal Labor: Second Stage," in this chapter.

INDIVIDUALIZED (NURSING DIAGNOSIS) CARE PLANS

The care plans in this section were developed to address the woman's unique needs.

Nursing Diagnosis: PAIN[1]

Related Factors: perineal bruising and edema, episiotomy, and postbirth chills. Use with the generic NDCP, "Pain,[1]" which begins on p. 18 in Chapter 2. Also refer to NDCP, "Pain,[1]" which begins on p. 232 in the topic "Normal Labor: First Stage," in this chapter. Also refer to "Epidural Anesthesia/Analgesia," beginning

on p. 250 in this chapter. The related factors are different in the third stage; also some nursing interventions and activities appropriate to the second stage do not apply to the third stage.

Goals, Outcomes, and Evaluation Criteria

- Woman verbalizes adequate pain relief.
- Woman is free of discomfort that interferes with maternal–infant attachment.

Nursing Activities and Rationales

Collaborative Activities

- Assist with administration of local anesthetic before episiotomy or laceration repair, if needed. Anesthetizes the perineum; prevents pain from incision and suturing. Episiotomy may have been done without local anesthesia, and by the end of the third stage the regional anesthesia may have worn off.
- Provide distraction (e.g., breathing techniques, focus on the newborn) during episiotomy repair, as needed. Draws attention away from any pain associated with suturing.

Independent Nursing Actions

- Apply ice bags to the perineum after the placenta is expelled and perineal repair is done. Helps prevent edema by constricting local blood vessels. Produces local anesthesia and decreases pain.
- Apply dry underpads; change linens, if needed; change damp clothing. Providing warmth and cleanliness are psychologically comforting and reduce anxiety. Anxiety increases pain.
- Provide a warmed blanket. The sudden release of pressure on pelvic nerves, or perhaps a fetal-to-maternal transfusion that occurs with placental separation may cause chills. A warm blanket increases tissue perfusion and muscle relaxation.

Nursing Diagnosis: ANXIETY[1]

Related Factors: lack of knowledge of postbirth procedures and routines and lack of knowledge of postbirth sensations. Refer to the generic NDCPs "Anxiety,[1]" which begins on p. 10, and "Deficient Knowledge,[1]" which begins on p. 13, both in Chapter 2. Also refer to the NDCP, "Anxiety,[1]" beginning on p. 227 in the topic "Normal Labor: First Stage," in this chapter.

Assessments

- Ask whether the couple has any requests for disposal of the placenta. Many cultures have beliefs differing from those of the provider's/nurse's culture. Some may wish to take the placenta home with them, to be buried at a specific time or in a certain place. Some couples may be hesitant to ask for special consideration.

Independent Nursing Actions

- Explain that chills and leg tremors are normal. Provide explanations. Anticipatory guidance relieves anxiety and helps the woman/couple to achieve a satisfying birth experience.
- Introduce the woman/partner to the staff who will be caring for her during the postpartum period. Describe the unit routines and the care she can expect to receive during the next few hours. Continuity of care provides a feeling of security and decreases anxiety.
- Allow the parents time alone with their newborn. Promotes psychologic adaption by allowing early contact between the mother and infant while facilitating development of a positive relationship. Research shows that women who are single, unemployed, and depressed are at a high risk of having disturbed initial bonding with the infant.

INTRAPARTUM FETAL MONITORING

Because labor is stressful for the fetus, the nurse must monitor fetal well-being frequently during labor. The fetal heart rate (FHR) provides information about fetal hemodynamic and oxygen status. Nonreassuring patterns are an indication of fetal *hypoxemia* (a deficiency of oxygen in the blood), which can lead to *hypoxia* (inadequate supply of oxygen at the cellular level). The fetal oxygen supply can be compromised in the following ways:

- Maternal hypertension. Constriction of maternal vessels reduces the blood flow through the placenta and to the fetus.
- Maternal hypotension (e.g., as a result of supine hypotension, side effects of epidural anesthesia). Decreased intra-arterial pressure creates slower circulation through the placenta to the fetus.
- Maternal hemorrhage. Decreased blood volume lowers intra-arterial pressure, resulting in decreased fetoplacental circulation.
- Reduced oxygen content of maternal blood. For example, as a result of hemorrhage or anemia.
- Uterine hypertonicity (e.g., as caused by excessive doses of oxytocin). During a uterine contraction (UC), blood flow to the intervillous space in the placenta is reduced, so less oxygenated blood reaches the fetus.
- Placental vascular disorders (e.g., associated with hypertension or diabetes) or deterioration of the placenta (e.g., postdates). These impair fetoplacental blood flow.
- Problems with fetal circulation. Problems include compression of the umbilical cord, placental separation or abruption, head compression, vagal nerve stimulation, medication side effects, and dysrhythmias.
- Medical problems with the fetus. These may include hypothermia, hypothyroidism, or hypoglycemia.

Also refer to the topic, "Antepartum Fetal Monitoring and Other Diagnostic Tests," beginning on p. 60 in Chapter 4.

▌ Key Nursing Activities

- Constantly conduct fetal surveillance and documentation of fetal movement, maternal vital signs, and medications administered to the mother.
- Differentiate between reassuring and nonreassuring FHR patterns (standardized interpretation by staff and healthcare provider).
- For nonreassuring patterns, differentiate between those that indicate mild hypoxemia and those that indicate severe hypoxia.
- Report nonreassuring patterns to primary care provider, actions taken, and results.
- Provide specific, appropriate interventions for nonreassuring patterns.
- Document patient data and nursing interventions on the monitor strip as well as in the woman's electronic or written record.

▌ Indications for Electronic Fetal Monitoring

Some healthcare providers believe the procedure should be mandatory for all women in labor; but caution that there are more limitations than benefits.

- History of medical or obstetric problems that create a risk to mother or fetus, including:
  - ▸ Fetal factors (e.g., decreased fetal movement, multiple gestation, postdates)
  - ▸ Maternal factors (e.g., infection, gestational hypertension, previous cesarean birth)
  - ▸ Uterine factors (e.g., dysfunctional labor, oxytocin induction/augmentation)
  - ▸ Complications of pregnancy (e.g., PROM, preterm labor, partial placenta previa)
- Regional anesthesia

▌ Etiologies and Risk Factors

Etiologies and risk factors are not applicable. In the United States, intrapartum fetal monitoring is almost routinely used in hospitals and birthing centers. FHR monitoring can be done by *intermittent auscultation* with a fetoscope (which transmits sound via bone conduction through the examiner's head) or by using *ultrasound devices intermittently*. If intermittent auscultation is the primary method of fetal assessment, a one-to-one nurse-to-patient ratio is recommended. If this cannot be arranged, then *continuous electronic fetal monitoring* should be used, even though American College of Obstetricians and Gynecologists and the Association of Women's Health, Obstetric, and Neonatal Nurses recognize that intermittent monitoring for low-risk women is safe and comparable with continuous fetal monitoring in detection of fetal well-being.

▌ Electronic Fetal Monitoring Modes

- Doppler principle. This is done using an ultrasound device that is hand held. It transmits and receives reflected high-frequency ultrasound waves to obtain the fetal heart rate.

- External monitor. Transducers are placed on the maternal abdomen to assess FHR and UCs. This method does not provide information about the strength of UCs, and it provides minimal data about FHR variability. Telemetry can also be used so that the woman can be out of the bed and away from the monitor.
- Internal monitor. A spiral electrode is applied to the fetal presenting part to monitor the fetal electrocardiogram; a direct ECG assessment, which provides accurate information about the FHR variability and neurologic status. An intrauterine pressure catheter (IUPC) is inserted through the cervix into the uterine cavity to assess the UCs strength (it measures changes in the pressure inside the uterus). However, it requires that membranes be ruptured and that the cervix be sufficiently dilated. Also, the nurse must have special training to insert the equipment.

Signs and Symptoms

FHR is evaluated in relationship to UCs. Reassuring FHR patterns are, in general, characterized by:

- Baseline FHR of 110–160 bpm with no periodic changes
- Moderate baseline variability (amplitude range 6–25 beats per minute)
- Accelerations with fetal movement (abrupt increase in the FHR with a peak of 15 beats per minute with a duration of 15 seconds or more but less than 2 minutes from onset to return).

Nonreassuring FHR patterns, which indicate fetal hypoxemia, include the following:

- FHR ≥ 160 bpm.
- Severe bradycardia (< 70 bpm).
- Progressive increase or decrease in baseline rate.
- Severe variable decelerations (FHR < 60 bpm, lasting > 30–60 sec, with rising baseline, decreasing variability, or slow return to baseline; timing is variable in relation to UCs).
- Late decelerations, especially if they recur and cannot be corrected and are accompanied by decreasing variability or rising baseline FHR. Late decelerations are seen as a gradual decrease in FHR below the baseline and associated with a UC. They begin after the peak of the UC and do not return to baseline until well after the end of the contraction. Rate usually does not drop below 100 bpm, but depth of deceleration is proportional to the strength of the UC.
- Absent or minimal variability.
- Prolonged deceleration (2 min or more, but less than 10 minutes in duration).

Collaborative Problems

Potential complication of fetal monitoring includes maternal or fetal injury secondary to:

- Infection introduced by placement of internal transducer/electrode.
- Injury to fetal presenting part caused by electrode placement/removal.

- Inaccurate information obtained from the monitor.
- Inaccurate interpretation of or intervention for FHR patterns.

COLLABORATIVE (STANDARDIZED) CARE FOR ALL WOMEN WITH INTRAPARTUM FETAL MONITORING

Perform a comprehensive assessment to identify individual needs for teaching, emotional support, and physical care.

▍ Potential Complication of Fetal Monitoring: MATERNAL OR FETAL INJURY

Maternal or fetal injury may be secondary to infection introduced by placement of internal transducer/electrode, injury to fetal presenting part caused by electrode placement/removal, inaccurate information obtained from the monitor, and inaccurate interpretation of or intervention for FHR patterns.

Also refer to the generic collaborative care plan, "Potential Complication: Infection," beginning on p. 29 in Chapter 3.

Focus Assessments

- Monitor and record data in woman's record (e.g., FHR, variability, decelerations, accelerations, UCs, uterine resting tone); include method of monitoring and notification of primary care provider. Provides timely information for evaluation of maternal and fetal status and progress of labor.
- Document on the monitor strip (if it is the legal document according to facility policy) all assessments (e.g., cervical dilation and effacement, fetal station), interventions, procedures, and medications, along with the woman's responses; significant occurrences such as ROM, voiding, sterile vaginal exams; repositioning of monitor equipment or calibration of the monitor; notification of the primary care provider. Aids in accurate interpretation of monitor tracing. For example, procedures such as vaginal exams may stimulate fetal movement and increase FHR; certain medications may temporarily decrease FHR variability and require no intervention.
- Auscultate or assess monitor strip every 30 min in first stage of labor; every 15 min in second stage; more frequently (every 5 min) if condition warrants (e.g., for high-risk women); and every 5 minutes once pushing is initiated. For prompt identification of problems. As labor progresses, UCs become stronger and, therefore, more stressful to the fetus; so more frequent monitoring is required.
- Auscultate FHR with fetoscope (or use a handheld Doppler) if there is doubt as to the quality of the tracing,

while also assessing the maternal heart rate. Ensures accurate data are obtained.

- Palpate fundus at least every hr to assess strength of UCs. The tocotransducer (external monitoring) can assess only frequency and duration of UCs. When an IUPC is being used, palpation is a cross-check to ensure proper calibration and functioning of the equipment.

Preventive Nursing Activities

- Assist the woman when ambulating (e.g, to chair, to bathroom). External monitoring straps and devices need to be removed and reapplied. The wires/tubing from the internal monitor must be held carefully to prevent the woman from becoming entangled with them, causing dislodging of wires/tubing or causing the woman to fall. Also, the equipment is delicate and expensive; it can be damaged if dropped. Telemetry can be used if available to increase ambulation and be away from the monitor.
- Provide perineal care after voiding and prn during labor. Prevents infection by removing secretions that provide a dark, warm, moist medium for pathogen growth.
- Promptly report to care provider nonreassuring FHR rates and patterns, worsening of any pattern, or difficulty in obtaining an adequate FHR tracing or sound. Facilitates prompt intervention and helps prevent injury to fetus.
- For fetal tachycardia (FHR greater than 160 bpm for greater than 10 min), treat the cause, if possible (e.g., drugs, cigarettes, cocaine or amphetamine use by mother; disease states; medical reasons such as hyperthyroid, elevated maternal temperature, or infection); use cool sponge or prescribed antipyretics to reduce maternal fever; administer oxygen at 8–10 L/min per face mask; increase parenteral fluids; reduce maternal anxiety; determine fetal acid-base status. Prevents increased fetal distress. Tachycardia can occur as a result of maternal infection, medications, street drugs, and early fetal hypoxemia. If hypoxemia is the cause, oxygen will help increase the oxygen saturation of the blood circulated to the fetus.
- For fetal bradycardia (FHR less than 110 bpm for greater than 10 min). Bradycardia may result from fetal hypoxia, medications, prolonged cord compression, and maternal hypotension, hypoglycemia, or hypothermia; and fetal arrhythmia, cord entanglement, hypothermia, hypothyroidism, or hypoglycemia. If FHR accelerates in response to scalp stimulation, then the fetus probably has the ability to compensate physiologically for stress.
- If decreased FHR variability occurs, intervention depends on cause. No intervention is needed if variability is decreased temporarily (e.g., because of CNS depressants administered to the mother or because of fetal sleep, which usually lasts 20–30 min). Otherwise:
  - Digitally stimulate the fetal scalp. An FHR acceleration or a return to average variability is a reassuring response.

- Consider application of an internal electrode. Ability of external transducer to record variability is limited. Better evaluation can be made with an internal electrode.
  - Assist with fetal scalp blood sampling for pH. Evaluates fetal acid-base balance and aids in interpreting seriousness of decreased variability.
  - Prepare for birth (vaginal or cesarean) as indicated by primary care provider. Decreased variability, if accompanied by late decelerations, can indicate fetal hypoxia severe enough to warrant immediate birth.
- Be alert for absent variability. Absent variability can be caused by neural, humoral, or pharmacologic mechanisms. It can also be absent when the fetus has complete heart block. Chronic hypoxia may proceed absent variability and immediate delivery should be considered.
- If late decelerations occur:
  - Turn the woman to her side. Corrects deceleration caused by maternal positioning and moves gravid uterus off the vena cava, improving blood return to the heart, which in turn increases cardiac output and BP, and therefore placental–fetal blood flow.
  - Increase IV rate. Increases circulating volume and, therefore, cardiac output, BP, and fetoplacental blood flow.
  - Discontinue oxytocin if it is being used. Late decelerations are caused by uteroplacental insufficiency and lack of fetal reserve to cope with decreased blood flow that occurs during UCs. This is especially true if the uterus is being hyperstimulated by oxytocics.
  - Administer oxygen at 8–10 L/min per face mask. Increases the amount of circulating oxygen available to the fetus.
  - Wash out prostaglandin gel or suppository with a sodium biphosphate-sodium phosphate (Fleet enema) or by using the open end of the IV tubing attached to a bag of normal saline or lactated Ringer's solution. Decreases absorption of prostaglandin.
  - Prepare for birth if decelerations cannot be corrected. Persistent, repetitive late decelerations usually indicate fetal hypoxemia, which, if uncorrected, progresses to hypoxia, acidemia, and acidosis. It is an ominous sign if they cannot be corrected, especially when associated with fetal tachycardia and decreased variability.
- If variable decelerations occur, change maternal position, side to side. Variable decelerations may be related to brief cord compression; changing position may take weight of fetus off the cord.
- If severe variable decelerations occur and cannot be relieved by maternal position change:
  - Discontinue oxytocin, if infusing. Decreases the strength of the UCs and improves blood flow through intervillous spaces during contractions.
  - Administer oxygen at 8–10 L/min per face mask. Increases the oxygen content of the blood circulating to the fetus.

■ Inspect perineum and/or assist with vaginal or speculum examination. Detects cord prolapse or detects imminent delivery. Sometimes variable decelerations occur in stage 2 labor, and occasionally they are the first sign that a woman is completely dilated and that the fetal head is on the perineum.

■ Assist with amnioinfusion, if needed. Increases the amount of fluid in the uterus, floating the fetus off the compressed cord.

■ If variable decelerations occur during the second (pushing) stage of labor, urge the woman to push with every other (instead of every) contraction. In the second stage, the umbilical cord can easily become compressed during fetal descent. Alternating pushing gives the fetus time to recover after a contraction. Fetal depression occurs only if cord compression is severe or prolonged.

■ Assist with birth if pattern cannot be corrected. Prevents fetal anoxia.

• If a prolonged deceleration occurs (decrease in FHR of 15 beats/min or more below baseline and lasting more than 2 but less than 10 minutes), notify the physician immediately and initiate appropriate treatment. A prolonged deceleration may have a benign cause (e.g., epidural analgesia); however, if seen after severe variable decelerations or a series of late decelerations, it may signal impending fetal death.

For external monitoring:

■ Palpate fetal parts (Leopold's maneuvers) and position transducer to ensure clear, interpretable FHR data; reposition as needed. Ensures accurate information from the monitor. The high-frequency sound waves best transmit and reflect the mechanical action of the fetal heart when transducer is over the fetal back; this is usually in one of the lower quadrants of the abdomen if in vertex position.

■ Position the woman to obtain the best transducer readings, while maintaining optimum fetoplacental circulation. Lateral or semi-Fowler's position will usually facilitate monitoring and will keep the weight of the gravid uterus from compressing the abdominal aorta and vena cava. Supine position should not be used.

■ Position tocotransducer over uterine fundus above the umbilicus (reposition as needed). Tocotransducer is a pressure-sensitive device. It should be placed so that the UCs will depress the pressure-sensitive side next to the abdomen. Usually this is over the fundus.

■ Keep monitor straps snug, but comfortable. Facilitates accurate readings from the transducers while promoting maternal comfort and skin integrity.

■ Reposition monitor as needed after changing the woman's position, when the fetus is very active, or when reading becomes unclear. Ensures accurate data from the monitor. Position changes may change the location of the fetal parts.

■ Correlate FHR tracing with labor progress, analgesia, anesthesia, and other obstetrical or medical complications. Provides more accurate interpretation of monitor data; because so many factors affect the FHR, it cannot be evaluated in isolation.

For internal monitoring:

■ Use sterile technique when inserting electrode or transducer. Prevents introduction of pathogens into the vagina; when membranes are ruptured, there is no barrier to ascending infection.

■ Ensure that electrode wires are firmly attached to leg plate; reapply electrode gel to leg plate as necessary. Helps ensure that accurate data are obtained from the monitor.

■ When removing the electrode, turn it counterclockwise; never pull straight out from the presenting part. Prevents fetal injury from the spiral electrode.

■ Follow guidelines for catheter and electrode insertion (e.g., setting baseline rate, testing). Ensures that accurate information is obtained from the equipment.

■ Check for functioning by tapping catheter or applying fundal pressure or having the mother cough. This should cause the stylus to move higher up on the strip.

■ Keep IUPC taped to the woman's leg. Prevents dislodgment and ensures adequate data.

INDIVIDUALIZED (NURSING DIAGNOSIS) CARE PLANS

The care plans in this section were developed to address unique patient needs.

▌ Nursing Diagnosis: ANXIETY[1]/ FEAR[1]

Related Factors: use of unfamiliar equipment in an unfamiliar environment; the belief that electronic fetal monitoring may mean that something is wrong with the mother or the baby; and embarrassment regarding the nature of the procedures. Refer to the generic NDCPs, "Anxiety,[1]" and "Fear,[1]" beginning on pp. 10 and 15, respectively, in Chapter 2.

▌ *Nursing Activities and Rationales*
Independent Nursing Actions

• If there is difficulty in locating the FHR initially, explain that you are looking for the spot where the sounds are heard best. The woman may become anxious if you cannot readily locate the fetal heartbeat. She may be concerned about her baby or about your skill.

• Make eye contact frequently. It is important to nurse the woman, not the machine, in order to convey caring and relieve anxiety.

Patient/Family Teaching

- Explain and demonstrate how the monitor works; point out the FHR and the UCs on the monitor tracing; when adjustments must be made, explain why. Information increases understanding, gives the woman a sense of control, and removes fear of the unknown, thereby helping relieve anxiety that occurs in an unfamiliar environment with unfamiliar sights, sounds, and odors.
- Explain that the monitor need not interfere with breathing and relaxation techniques learned in childbirth preparation classes and that observing the UCs on the monitor may actually help them use their breathing techniques effectively. Restores control when the labor does not proceed as the woman/partner has anticipated/fantasized.
- Explain that the use of an external fetal monitor does not imply maternal or fetal jeopardy. Provides realistic reassurance.

Nursing Diagnosis: DISCOMFORT[1]

Related Factors: maternal position, limited mobility because of external monitoring straps and devices, application of internal electrode and transducer, and tightness of belts holding external transducers in place.

Goals, Outcomes, and Evaluation Criteria

- Woman expresses satisfaction with labor and birth experience.
- Woman expresses satisfactory level of comfort during labor.

NIC Interventions[2]

Bed Rest Care (0740)—Promotion of comfort and safety and prevention of complications for a patient unable to get out of bed.
Electronic Fetal Monitoring: Intrapartum (6772)—Electronic evaluation of fetal heart rate response to uterine contractions during intrapartal care.
Perineal Care (1750)—Maintenance of perineal skin integrity and relief of perineal discomfort.
Simple Massage (1480)—Stimulation of the skin and underlying tissues with varying degrees of hand pressure to decrease pain, produce relaxation, and/or improve circulation.

Nursing Activities and Rationales

Assessments

- Monitor for signs/symptoms of discomfort. Allows for interventions to relieve discomfort. Nurse should focus on the woman's response to the monitoring, not just on the monitor strip.

Independent Nursing Actions

- Remove external belts/equipment at least every 2 hrs; wash sites and apply new gel; change placement of belts, if possible. Removes perspiration under transducers, promotes circulation to the skin.
- Provide back massage. Promotes circulation, relaxes muscles, and promotes psychologic comfort. External monitoring essentially confines the woman to bed.
- Change underpads and keep perineum clean and dry. This is especially important when using internal monitor because the membrane must be ruptured and continual leaking of amniotic fluid and other vaginal secretions will occur, increasing as labor progresses.
- Be aware that with both internal and external monitors, the height of the UCs on the monitor strip does not determine the need for analgesia. The amount of pain experienced with UCs varies greatly among women, and many factors other than contraction intensity contribute to the pain.

Patient/Family Teaching

- Assure the woman that it is safe to move about in bed; encourage position changes at least every 2 hours, except for supine position. External monitoring essentially confines the woman to bed. Position changes decrease the hazards of immobility and relieve discomfort caused by muscle and joint stiffness that occurs with immobility.

AMNIOTOMY

Amniotomy is the artificial rupture of the amniotic membranes (AROM), using an instrument (AmniHook [amniotic membrane perforator] or latex finger cot [AmniCot]) inserted through the partially dilated cervix. A common obstetrical procedure, AROM may be performed to induce labor or to accelerate labor during the first stage. It is also performed to allow access to the fetus in order to apply an FHR monitor to the fetal scalp, to insert an intrauterine pressure catheter, or to obtain a fetal scalp blood sample. Amniotomy is a medical procedure performed by a physician or certified nurse midwife.

Key Nursing Activities

- Explain the procedure to the woman/partner and family.
- Monitor fetal well-being.
- Prevent infection.

Etiologies and Risk Factors

Etiologies and risk factors are not applicable.

Signs and Symptoms

Signs and symptoms are not applicable.

Diagnostic Studies

Diagnostic study includes FHR monitoring before and after the procedure.

▌ *Medical Management*

- Amniotomy is usually delayed until engagement has occurred. Decreases the risk for a prolapsed cord.
- The cervix must be dilated at least 2 cm: AROM requires that an instrument be inserted through the cervix.
- Once amniotomy is performed, birth must occur. Microorganisms can invade the intrauterine cavity after ROM.
- Molding and compression of the fetal head are increased with AROM. The cushioning effect of the amniotic fluid for the fetal head is lost.
- Amniotomy is not used alone as a method of induction. Evidence supports amniotomy alone as an ineffective method for inducing labor.

▌ *Collaborative Problems*

Potential Complications of Amniotomy

- Abruptio placentae. Due to rapid decompression of the uterus when the amniotic fluid is lost rapidly.
- Infection. Due to introduction of pathogens into the cervix and uterine cavity when the membranes no longer serve as a barrier.
- Amniotic fluid embolus. Due to rapid decompression of the uterus; small amounts of fluid can enter the maternal blood vessels under the edge of the placenta.
- Cord prolapse.
- Moderate to severe variable decelerations. May lead to a cesarean birth for nonreassuring fetal status.

COLLABORATIVE (STANDARDIZED) CARE FOR ALL WOMEN HAVING AN AMNIOTOMY

Perform a comprehensive assessment to identify individual needs for teaching, emotional support, and physical care.

▌ Potential Complications of Amniotomy: ABRUPTIO PLACENTAE, INFECTION, AMNIOTIC FLUID EMBOLUS, AND CORD PROLAPSE

Refer to the generic NDCP, "Risk for Infection,[1]" which begins on p. 21 in Chapter 2. Refer to the generic collaborative care plans, "Potential Complication: Hemorrhage," and "Potential Complication: Fetal Compromise," which begin on pp. 28 and 27, respectively, in Chapter 3. Also refer to the collaborative care plan for "Potential Complications of Labor: Fetal Distress/

Anoxia, Cord Prolapsed," beginning on p. 225 in "Normal Labor: First Stage" and the collaborative care plan for "Potential Complications of Labor: Hemorrhage, Rupture of a Preexisting Cerebral Aneurysm, Pulmonary Emboli, Amniotic Fluid Embolism, etc." beginning on p. 241 of "Normal Labor: Third Stage," in this chapter.

Focus Assessments

- Before AROM, assess fetal presentation, position, and station. Because of the danger of cord prolapse, some physicians do not perform amniotomy unless the fetal head is well engaged.
- Monitor FHR before and after AROM; if there are marked changes, check for cord prolapse. To compare the two results and evaluate fetal status. The fetus may already have been stressed, or the procedure may have created stress for the fetus. ROM increases the danger of cord prolapse, especially if the fetal presenting part is not well engaged, pressing down against the cervix.
- Observe the amniotic fluid for amount, color, odor, and presence of meconium or blood. Foul odor is a sign of infection. A greenish color indicates intrauterine passage of meconium, a sign of fetal distress.
- Monitor the woman's temperature every 2 hours. Detects developing infection.

Preventive Nursing Activities

- Be certain that sterile technique is observed. Prevents introduction of pathogenic microorganisms into the cervix/vagina.
- Arrange the woman in a side-lying position or supine with a left uterine tilt. Prevents maternal hypotension by keeping weight of gravid uterus off the vena cava (which would decrease cardiac output and, subsequently, fetal oxygenation).
- After the procedure, clean and dry the perineum and change the disposable underpad. Removes warm, moist medium in which infectious organisms can reproduce.
- Observe strict sterile technique during vaginal examinations; keep vaginal exams to a minimum. Reduces the chance of introducing an infection. ROM creates an open pathway for microorganisms to ascend into the uterus and cause infection.
- Maintain bed rest in a semi-Fowler's position unless the presenting part is engaged and firmly against the cervix. Decreases the chance of prolapsed cord.

INDIVIDUALIZED (NURSING DIAGNOSIS) CARE PLANS

The care plans in this section were developed to address unique patient needs.

Nursing Diagnosis: ANXIETY[1]/ FEAR[1]

Related Factors: lack of experience with or knowledge about amniotomy, fear of pain, or fear that the fetus may be harmed. See the generic NDCPs, "Anxiety[1]" and "Fear,[1]" which begin on pp. 10 and 15, respectively, in Chapter 2.

▋ Goals, Outcomes, and Evaluation Criteria

- Woman and/or partner (family) remain relaxed prior to, during, and after the amniotomy.

▋ Nursing Activities and Rationales

Patient Teaching

- Explain the procedure to the woman/couple, including sensations she will feel. Anticipatory guidance allows them to feel more in control of the situation and relieves anxiety.
- Correct any misinformation. For example, explain that amniotic fluid is constantly produced, even though the membranes are ruptured, and that the woman will not experience a dry birth. Knowledge removes the fear of the unknown or unrealistic fears.

EPIDURAL ANESTHESIA/ANALGESIA

Lumbar epidural anesthesia and analgesia are commonly used to provide pain relief during labor and birth. *Epidural anesthesia* involves injection of an anesthetic (e.g., lidocaine [Xylocaine]) into the epidural space to block pain impulses from the uterus to the central nervous system (CNS). The mother remains alert and relaxed, airway reflexes are intact, and gastric emptying is not delayed. However, this method has the disadvantage of causing hypotension and loss of motor function in the legs. *Epidural analgesia* involves injection of a narcotic analgesic (e.g., fentanyl, morphine) into the epidural space. These agents have the advantage of blocking pain impulses from the uterus without totally inhibiting perineal sensation or motor function, and they do not cause maternal hypotension. However, they do not usually provide adequate relief for second-stage labor pain, so they are combined with anesthetics. Epidural medication can be administered via a single injection or by continuous infusion (via pump) through a small, indwelling catheter. The degree of epidural anesthesia depends on the dose of anesthetic agent and level at which the catheter tip is placed. Evidence shows that withholding an epidural until the cervix is dilated to 4 cm does not increase the rate of cesarean delivery and may result in a shorter duration of labor. Therefore, there is little justification for withholding this form of pain relief in early labor.

Block and Anesthetic Types:

- Saddle block. Blocks perineum and inner thigh.
- Pudendal block. Blocks pudendal nerves from S2 to S4.
- Paracervical block. Blocks sensation of uterus, cervix, and upper vagina (used less often than the others because it can cause fetal bradycardia).
- Local anesthetics. Injected into the tissue of the perineum and vagina to provide anesthesia for episiotomy or repair of vaginal and perineal lacerations.

Combined intrathecal (spinal) epidural analgesia/anesthesia is a technique used for labor analgesia, for cesarean birth, and for limited procedures such as postpartum tubal ligation, postcesarean pain control, or repair of obstetric lacerations following a vaginal delivery. An epidural catheter is placed and an intraspinal opioid analgesic is administered through the epidural catheter. When active labor begins, or at the request of the woman, epidural anesthetic or a combination of anesthetic and analgesia is given. Combined, the spinal and epidural anesthetics offer the advantages of rapid onset of spinal analgesia along with the ability to use the indwelling epidural catheter to titrate medication as needed during the labor. It may also be used and dosed to provide anesthesia for an urgent cesarean delivery.

Intrathecal (spinal) analgesia alone may also be used. This is the administration of an opioid into the intraspinal space.

These care plans are specific to the care of women receiving epidural anesthesia/analgesia. They do not cover all the care that is needed during labor. For that information, refer to "Normal Labor: First Stage," "Normal Labor: Second Stage," and "Normal Labor: Third Stage," which begin on pp. 221, 232, and 238, respectively, in this chapter.

▋ Key Nursing Activities

- Explain procedure and sensations (or lack of sensations) felt by the woman.
- Monitor fetal well-being.
- Assess for complications and side effects of anesthesia agents.
- Assess for complications and side effects of narcotic analgesics.
- Have all equipment available and in working order prior to the procedure.

▋ Etiologies and Risk Factors

Epidural anesthesia is used for labor and for cesarean birth. Epidural analgesia is used both for labor and for pain relief during the first 24 hours after a cesarean birth.

▋ Diagnostic Studies

- FHR monitoring. Before and during the procedure and continuously while the epidural is in place or until birth.
- Hb and Hct (or CBC). Before administration. Determines presence of anemia.
- Prothrombin time and platelet count. Determines presence of coagulopathy or bleeding disorder.
- WBC count. Determines presence of infection.

Medical Management

- Protect airway in case general anesthesia is needed.
- Administer anesthetic agents and monitor for side effects.
- Administer epinephrine for hypotension.
- Administer epinephrine and parenteral antihistamines for anaphylaxis.
- Modify dose, volume, and type of anesthetic to allow the woman to push during second stage.
- Contraindications to epidural blocks include marked obesity, severe anemia, severe preeclampsia, previous history of anesthetic complications, antepartum hemorrhage, anticoagulant therapy or bleeding disorder, local or systemic infection, lack of trained staff, maternal refusal, and allergy to the anesthetic medication or medications in the same class.

Collaborative Problems

Potential Complications of Epidural Anesthesia and Analgesia

- Anaphylaxis
- Urinary retention

Potential Complications of Epidural Anesthesia

- Maternal hypotension
- High spinal anesthesia
- Medication toxicity
- Local infection at the site of injection
- Maternal inability to cooperate due to pain, anxiety, language barrier, or mental barrier

Potential Complications of Epidural Analgesia

- Itching
- Nausea and vomiting
- Respiratory depression

COLLABORATIVE (STANDARDIZED) CARE FOR ALL WOMEN RECEIVING EPIDURAL ANESTHESIA/ANALGESIA IN LABOR

Perform a comprehensive assessment to identify individual needs for teaching, emotional support, and physical care.

Potential Complication of Epidural Anesthesia and Analgesia: ANAPHYLAXIS

Focus Assessments

- Assess for allergies prior to the procedure. Screens for systemic allergic reactions related to drugs used for regional anesthesia/analgesia.
- Before administration, review history. Helps ensure that there are no contraindications to regional anesthesia/analgesia.
- Monitor for rash, rhinitis, fever, asthma, or pruritus. These are minor allergic reactions that do not constitute an emergency.
- Observe frequently for irritability, weakness, nausea and vomiting, and hives. Early signs of severe anaphylaxis; these progress to dyspnea, cyanosis, convulsions, and cardiac arrest.
- Observe frequently for sudden, severe bronchospasm, vasospasm, and severe hypotension. These are signs of the most dramatic form of severe anaphylaxis. Anaphylaxis can, of course, be caused by any medication. Anaphylactic symptoms, in general, occur as a result of contractions of smooth muscles.
- Monitor for excessive drowsiness. Side effect of narcotic analgesia that may require administration of a narcotic antagonist.

Preventive Nursing Activities

- Report symptoms of allergic reaction to anesthesiologist or physician. Anaphylaxis must be treated immediately to prevent death. Cardiopulmonary resuscitation may be necessary.
- Report FHR decelerations and decreased variability to the primary care provider. Maternal anaphylaxis may result in fetal hypoxia necessitating immediate delivery.

Potential Complication of Epidural Anesthesia and Analgesia: URINARY RETENTION

Focus Assessments

- Ask the woman if she feels the need to void. The woman will have decreased ability to feel her bladder filling; depending on whether it was a high-dose or low-dose epidural, she may be able to void on a bedpan and avoid catheterization and the risk for postpartum UTI. If she cannot void, catheterization will be necessary to prevent bladder injury and to make room for the descending fetus during labor.
- Palpate for bladder distention. The woman will probably be unable to feel the sensation of the need to void. The bladder will probably fill rapidly because of the rapid infusion of intravenous fluids prior to the procedure.

Preventive Nursing Activities

- Have the woman void just before the epidural is administered. Prevents or delays urinary retention.
- Encourage early ambulation after vaginal or cesarean birth. Facilitates bladder emptying.

Potential Complications of Epidural Anesthesia: HYPOTENSION, HIGH SPINAL ANESTHESIA, AND TOXICITY

Maternal hypotension is the most common complication of epidural block.

Focus Assessments

- Obtain baseline maternal VSs and FHR. Ensures that they are normal before procedure begins, and to provide a baseline for later evaluation.
- Assess woman's legs for flushing and warmth. Determines if anesthetic is entering the epidural space and whether peripheral vasodilation is occurring.
- Monitor BP, pulse, and respirations at least every 2 min for 20 min after initial injection of an anesthetic and following each additional dose; monitor every 5–15 min thereafter until dose wears off; evaluate against baseline readings. Changes in VS patterns, especially BP, signal the possibility of an adverse reaction. Blocking of sympathetic nerve fibers in the epidural space causes decreased peripheral resistance and subsequent hypotension. A rapid rise in maternal heart rate may indicate an injection into a vein. When maternal systolic BP drops below 100 mmHg, fetal hypoxia may occur. This is especially dramatic in pregnant women because vasoconstriction is the primary compensatory mechanism for raising the BP during pregnancy. Epidural anesthesia may cause a temporary elevation in temperature.
- Observe for signs of local anesthetic/analgesic toxicity (tinnitus, tingling, shivering, paresthesia, unexplained confusion or drowsiness, slurred speech, a metallic taste, and visual disturbances, as well as sudden and severe problems including seizures, cardiac arrhythmias, and cardiovascular collapse). If toxicity occurs, discontinue the medication and implement appropriate emergency intervention.
- Monitor O_2 saturation levels and respiratory rate frequently. Detects hypoxia related to suppressed respirations secondary to high anesthesia. Also, catheters can migrate. When this happens, the woman will start to exhibit signs of a rising level of motor and sensory blockade.
- Assess level of anesthesia. The higher the level of anesthesia, the greater the risk for respiratory depression due to paralysis of the diaphragm.

- Monitor UCs. Absence of contractions may indicate that the anesthetic is rising too high within the spinal column (spinal anesthesia). This can occur because of accidental perforation of the dural membrane during the administration of lumbar epidural anesthesia.
- Closely monitor FHR and progress of labor. The woman may not be aware of changes in the strength of the UCs, nor feel the pressure of fetal descent. Fetal distress from an epidural is rare but can occur if the medication is absorbed rapidly or if severe maternal hypotension occurs.
- If legs are in stirrups during birth, assess BP immediately upon taking the legs out of the stirrups. Elevation increases the circulating blood volume in the trunk; restoring circulation to the legs decreases the blood volume overall and can cause hypotension.

Preventive Nursing Activities

- Provide a safe physical environment. Essential resuscitation equipment, including self-inflating resuscitation bag and mask oxygen flow meter and mask, must be readily available; the suction must be functioning and the equipment tested daily. Also all IV lines must be correctly identified and labeled to avoid medication errors in the event of an emergency.
- Stay with the woman throughout the anesthesia process. For monitoring and early detection of hypovolemia or signs of toxicity. Association of Women's Health, Obstetric, Gynecologic, and Neonatal Nursing recommends a 1:1 nurse-to-patient ratio during the initiation of the epidural.
- Give a clear antacid before placement of the epidural. This may reduce the risk of aspiration if an epidural emergency occurs.
- Place the woman on her side if she must be supine for procedures (e.g., sterile vaginal examination); place a wedge/pad under her right hip. Prevents the uterus from compressing the ascending vena cava and descending aorta, which can decrease placental perfusion due to compromised venous return. Note that some anesthesiologists prefer that the woman be in a sitting position for catheter placement.
- Place the woman's head on a pillow during and after procedure. Prevents anesthetic from rising too high and stopping UCs or respiratory function.
- After the block is administered, help the woman assume a semireclining position (elevate head 25 degrees) and pad to effect a lateral uterine tilt. Provides even distribution of the block; after this is achieved, she may resume a lateral position.
- Maintain fluid hydration via intravenous route; administer a preload of 500–1000 ml of balanced saline solution over a 15–30 min period, then infuse continuously, according to agency protocol. Prevents hypotension by maintaining

intravascular pressure and volume; the increased volume compensates the peripheral vasodilation that occurs when epidural anesthesia is administered. Dextrose solutions can cause fetal hyperglycemia and rebound hypoglycemia in the first few hours after birth.

- Administer oxygen by face mask if needed. Counters hypotension by ensuring that the blood is well saturated with oxygen. Hypotension can occur in spite of adequate hydration and uterine displacement. Excessive hypotension may be life threatening to the fetus because it decreases placental perfusion. Oxygen also helps decrease the nausea that occurs with hypotension.

- If hypotension is severe or prolonged, elevate the woman's legs for 2–3 minutes. Increases blood return from the extremities, thereby increasing cardiac output.

- Notify provider or anesthesiologist immediately if FHR decelerations or decreased variability occur. These may occur if maternal hypotension develops; they reflect decreased placental perfusion.

- Educate the woman about treatment interventions that will be implemented if she experiences untoward reactions. Oxygen administration, repositioning, elevating extremities, and increasing fluids will be needed. Advanced preparation will reduce her anxiety and increase the likelihood of her cooperation if drug toxicity is experienced.

- If there is a 20–30% drop in systolic BP or a drop to less than 100 mmHg, maintain left lateral displacement of the uterus (e.g., with a folded blanket), increase the IV rate, and place the woman in a 10–20 degree Trendelenburg position. Ensures venous return to the heart and circulation to the brain. If BP is not restored in 1–2 min, a vasopressor (e.g., ephedrine) may be administered intravenously.

Potential Complication of Epidural (Narcotic) Analgesia: RESPIRATORY DEPRESSION

Focus Assessments

- Monitor respiratory rate and depth every 15 to 30 minutes for the first hour, and then every hour for 24 hrs (or per agency protocol). Respiratory depression is not a rare side effect of epidural narcotics and is a serious concern.

- Monitor oxygen saturation levels. Detects hypoxia related to suppressed respirations secondary to narcotic analgesic.

- Instruct the woman about the therapeutic actions of the regional anesthesia and to report any signs of toxicity. Ensures rapid implementation of emergency measures should toxicity develop.

Preventive Nursing Activities

- Administer naloxone hydrochloride if respiratory rate less than 10 breaths/min or if O_2 saturation less than 89% (or according to agency protocol). Naloxone hydrochloride is a narcotic antagonist that competes for receptor sites in the brain and reverses the effects of opioids.

- Administer O_2 by face mask and notify anesthesiologist if respiratory rate less than 10 breaths/min or of O_2 saturation less than 89%. Increases the percentage of oxygen in the air the woman is breathing and, therefore, increases the oxygen level in the blood. Anesthesiologist may be needed for emergency measures.

Potential Side Effects of Epidural Analgesics: ITCHING, NAUSEA, AND VOMITING

Collaborative Activities

- Administer antipruritics, as needed. Relieve itching. For example, antihistamines such as diphenhydramine HCl (Benadryl) compete with histamine for H1 receptor sites on effector cells.

- Administer antiemetics, as needed. For systemic relief of nausea and vomiting, usually by elevation of the chemoreceptor trigger zone threshold and/or promoting gastric emptying.

- If symptoms are not relieved, administer narcotic antagonists (e.g., naloxone HCl). Itching is a common side effect of epidural narcotic analgesia. Narcotic antagonists compete with narcotics for opioid receptor sites in the brain, thereby neutralizing their effects.

- Apply a cold washcloth or compress to site. May reduce itching and increases comfort.

INDIVIDUALIZED (NURSING DIAGNOSIS) CARE PLANS

The care plans in this section were developed to address unique patient needs.

Nursing Diagnosis: RISK FOR MATERNAL INJURY (E.G., FALLS)[1]

Related Factors: falls from partial motor paralysis secondary to injection of anesthetic drugs and drowsiness secondary to narcotic analgesics.

Goals, Outcomes, and Evaluation Criteria

- Woman accomplishes labor, birth, and recovery safely (e.g., without falls).
- Woman's skin and tissues remain free from injury (e.g., no bruises, strains).

NIC Interventions[2]

Environmental Management: Safety (6486)—Monitoring and manipulation of the physical environment to promote safety

Fall Prevention (6490)—Instituting special precautions with patient at risk for injury from falling.

Positioning (0840)—Deliberate placement of the patient or a body part to promote physiologic and/or psychologic well-being.

Surveillance: Safety (6654)—Purposeful and ongoing collection and analysis of information about the patient and the environment for use in promoting and maintaining patient safety.

Nursing Activities and Rationales

Assessments

- Assess for motor ability and sensation in legs. Determines how much activity the woman is capable of performing. The amount of immobility depends on the type and dose of medication used. Narcotic analgesia, used alone, should not interfere with being out of bed with assistance.

Independent Nursing Actions

- Offer bedpan or assist to bathroom if still able to ambulate; catheterize if necessary. Epidural anesthesia interferes with the motor function in the legs, so the woman may not be able to get out of bed. Although epidural analgesia does not affect motor function, it is sometimes given in combination with an anesthetic; also, the narcotic analgesic may produce some drowsiness. In addition, most women are unable to void while the block is still working.
- Raise side rails and place call bell within easy reach when nurse not at bedside. Prevents injury from falls; if the woman cannot obtain help when she needs it, she may attempt to get out of bed without help.
- Ensure that there is no prolonged pressure on the hips or legs; change positions hourly; do not allow one leg to rest, unpadded, on the other; keep bed linens loose across the feet; place both legs in stirrups to the same level and angle, moving them at the same time, and taking care to not put pressure on the popliteal angle. Ensures adequate peripheral circulation and prevents tissue injury.
- Prior to leaving the delivery suite, use a postanesthesia fall risk assessment scoring system. Assists the nurse in determining the woman's risk for post anesthesia falls.

Patient/Family Teaching

- Teach the need for staying in bed and calling for assistance as needed. The woman is at increased risk for injury

because, although motor control of the legs may not be totally absent, it is weak. Complete sensation and ability to control the legs should be present before ambulation is attempted.

Nursing Diagnosis: DEFICIENT KNOWLEDGE (OF EPIDURAL ANESTHESIA/ANALGESIA)[1]

Refer to the generic NDCP, "Deficient Knowledge,[1]" which begins on p. 13 in Chapter 2.

Assessments

- Verify that the woman has signed the consent form; clarify and describe procedures; and ask the primary care provider to further explain the procedure and its advantages and disadvantages, if necessary. The nurse may witness the signature of the patient giving consent for the procedure, but only a licensed anesthesia care provider can obtain informed consent prior to analgesia/anesthesia administration. The nurse may witness the signature of the patient stating the patient has been given all information about the procedure and the risks involved. Even if the woman has received information about anesthesia/analgesia earlier in pregnancy, she should be interviewed again early in labor so that she has time to consider alternative methods of pain relief.

Patient/Family Teaching

- Explain how the procedure will be done, what will be expected of her (e.g., to hold still during insertion of the epidural needle), and what she can expect to feel, how long it will take to administer the medication, and how long before it takes effect. Removes fear of the unknown and promotes cooperation during the procedure.
- Explain the numeric rating scale for rating pain. Used after the procedure to assess the adequacy of analgesia.
- If an indwelling epidural catheter is to be used, explain that she may feel a momentary shock in her leg, hip, or back; and that this is not a sign of injury and is temporary. Reduces fear in the event this occurs.

Nursing Diagnosis: RISK FOR MATERNAL HYPOTHERMIA[1]

Related Factors: normal vasodilation that occurs with pregnancy, effects of epidural anesthesia (which produces further vasodilation), cool environmental temperature, and as an effect of opiates (increased dilation and radiant heat loss).

▌ NIC Interventions[2]

Environmental Management (6480)—Manipulation of the patient's surroundings for therapeutic benefit.

Hypothermia Treatment (3800)—Rewarming and surveillance of a patient whose core body temperature is below 35°C (95°F).

Temperature Regulation (3900)—Attaining and/or maintaining body temperature within a normal range.

Vital Signs Monitoring (6680)—Collection and analysis of cardiovascular, respiratory, and body temperature data to determine and prevent complications.

▌ Nursing Activities and Rationales

Assessments

- Monitor temperature; if temperature is low, assess rectal temperature. Rectal temperature is a more accurate reflection of core body temperature. Hypothermia may result in cardiovascular, pulmonary, circulatory, renal, and other complications; therefore, it is important to detect and treat it immediately.

Independent Nursing Actions

- During labor and delivery, remove wet drapes, towels, underpads, and clothing. Prevents heat loss by evaporation.
- Ensure that birthing area is warm. Prevents heat loss by convection, conduction, and radiation.
- Cover the woman with a warm blanket after the birth. Prevents heat loss. Shivering may occur because of heat loss from the increased peripheral blood flow or by alteration of thermal input to the CNS when warm, but not cold, sensations have been suppressed.

▌ Nursing Diagnosis: RISK FOR INJURY[1]

Related Factors: maternal inability to cooperate because of cognitive deficit, inability to understand and follow directions, language barrier, fear, lack of previous experience, anxiety, lack of childbirth preparation, and so forth.

▌ Goals, Outcomes, and Evaluation Criteria

- Woman accepts support through the nurse–patient relationship.
- Woman follows directions from nurse and/or provider.

▌ NIC Interventions[2]

Environmental Management: Safety (6486)—Monitoring and manipulation of the physical environment to provide safety.

Presence (4340)—Being with another, both physically and psychologically, during times of need.

Risk Identification (6610)—Analysis of potential risk factors, determination of health risks, and prioritization of risk reduction strategies for an individual or group.

Surveillance: Safety (6654)—Purposeful and ongoing collection and analysis of information about the patient and the environment to use in promoting and maintaining patient safety.

▌ Nursing Activities and Rationales

Assessments

- Assess on admission to determine if the woman understands instructions or has a developmental delay. This may indicate a need for a guardian or mental health nurse to be present to give instructions and assist the nurse in caring for this patient.
- Assess woman's primary language on admission. An interpreter may be needed when explaining procedures or obtaining consent to elicit cooperation and ensure adequate communication.
- Assess education level on admission. Ensures patient understanding of procedures.
- Assess level of anxiety and mental state. Enables the use of anticipatory guidance and use of information about past coping mechanisms to provide safe care for the patient who is exhibiting fear or unusual behavior.

Preventive Nursing Activities

- Report to healthcare provider if patient becomes anxious or refuses procedures. Enables interventions to be implemented early to reduce anxiety and perform procedures safely.
- Use a slow, deliberate approach to patient. A rushed or hurried approach may elicit increased stress and anxiety from the patient. A calm approach may calm the patient.
- Ensure that an interpreter is with patient to translate medical terminology. Knowledge and understanding reduce anxiety.
- Explain all procedures to the woman. Knowledge and understanding reduce anxiety.
- Keep healthcare provider informed of patient progress and special needs. Enables a change in plan of care if deemed necessary.

▌ Other Nursing Diagnoses

Also assess for the following nursing diagnoses, which are frequently present with this condition:

- Anxiety/Fear[1] related to deficient knowledge regarding the procedure and its risks and fear of pain during the procedure.
- Pain[1] related to inadequate block, one-sided block, or block failure, and tenderness at the needle puncture site.
- Risk for Infection[1] related to insertion of the epidural catheter.

INDUCTION/AUGMENTATION OF LABOR

An *oxytocic* is any medication that stimulates uterine contractions; *oxytocin* is a polypeptide hormone produced by the hypothalamus and secreted from the posterior pituitary that acts as an oxytocic. *Prostaglandins* are a large group of unsaturated fatty acids that have many physiologic actions, one of which is to act as an oxytocic. *Induction* and *augmentation* refer to processes by which birth is achieved through the use of artificial methods to stimulate uterine contractions (UCs). The most common techniques are amniotomy and intravenous oxytocin (Pitocin) administration. Other techniques include mechanical and chemical procedures to ripen the cervix (e.g., laminaria tents, prostaglandin E intravaginal gel),and administration of prostaglandin to stimulate UCs. Usually, labor is induced by first ripening the cervix (if necessary), performing an amniotomy if the cervix is ripe, and then administering oxytocin or misoprostol to initiate UCs. Various protocols using low-dose, high-dose, and pulsatile regimens show no difference in the percentages of successful inductions. The low-dose regimen minimizes risks and side effects. Nursing care is the same for both induction and augmentation.

▌ Key Nursing Activities

- Review of indications, expected results, and side effects of each mechanical and pharmacologic agent used.
- Carefully follow protocols for oxytocin administration.
- Assess and document cervical status.
- Monitor UCs and labor progression.
- Monitor and support fetal well-being.
- Provide information and emotional support.

▌ Etiologies and Risk Factors

The following are not, strictly speaking, etiologies or risk factors. They are indications for labor induction/augmentation.

Medically Indicated Indicators (ACOG, 2009)

- Severe preeclampsia at or near term
- Gestational hypertension
- Medical problems (e.g., diabetes, Rh isoimmunization, renal disease)
- Prolonged PROM
- Chorioamnionitis
- Incomplete or inevitable abortion
- Abruptio placenta (risk factor)
- Mild abruptio placenta with no fetal stress or distress

Fetal Conditions

- IUGR, poorly functioning placenta
- Gestational age greater than 42 weeks
- Fetal death
- Anomalies

- Isoimmunization
- Category III FHR pattern per American Congress of Obstetrics and Gynecologists fetal heart rate monitoring practice guideline

Motives for Induction/Augmentation

- Patient or healthcare provider request
- Logistical reasons (e.g., rapid labor, distance from hospital)
- Psychosocial indications (partner availability due to job or service)

Criteria for Induction

In addition to the aforementioned reasons, fetal lung maturity or 39 weeks' gestation must have been achieved or be determined by:

- FHT from 20 weeks onward by nonelectronic fetoscope or for at least 30 weeks by Doppler.
- At least 36 weeks since positive serum or urine human chorionic gonadotropin test.
- Ultrasound measured at 6–12 weeks that supports gestational age.
- Ultrasound between 13 and 20 weeks confirming 39 weeks' gestation as determined by clinical history and physical exam.

▌ Signs and Symptoms

Physical findings vary according to the condition warranting the labor induction/augmentation (see "Etiologies and Risk Factors," preceding). Examples include:

- Maternal exhaustion during labor
- Maternal BP elevation, possibly with brisk deep tendon reflexes
- Greenish amniotic fluid
- UCs infrequent and of mild intensity and short duration
- Dysfunctional labor as indicated by prolonged first stage, lack of progress in cervical dilation and effacement, and/or lack of descent of fetal presenting part

▌ Diagnostic Studies

Tests vary, depending on the condition that is being diagnosed or ruled out.

- Serial ultrasounds. Evaluate fetal size, position, and gestational age; to locate the placenta.
- Pelvimetry. Ensures there is no cephalopelvic disproportion to contraindicate induction.
- Nonstress or contraction stress test. Evaluates fetal well-being or extent of fetal distress.
- Lecithin/sphingomyelin ratio (requires amniocentesis). Indicates fetal lung maturity; lecithin/sphingomyelin ratio of 2:1 correlates with a 35-week gestation.
- Phosphatidylglycerol. Evaluates fetal lung maturity.
- Fetal scalp pH. Evaluates acid-base status of fetus when FHR patterns are nonreassuring or confusing; a fetal scalp pH of 7.25 or more is considered normal.

- Nitrazine paper and/fern test/AmniSure. Confirms rupture of membranes.
- CBC with differential. Confirms presence of infection.
- Urinalysis. Identifies UTI or spilling of glucose or protein.
- Type and Rh. Evaluates for risk for isoimmunization.
- Digital examination of the cervix (for Bishop score). Prelabor numerical scoring system to evaluate inducibility of cervix. Assigns scores for cervical dilation, effacement, consistency, and position, as well as a score for fetal station; a score of 9 for nulliparas and 5 for multiparas is favorable for induction (ACOG, 2009).

▌ Medical Management

- Stripping of membranes may be first procedure performed. This is achieved by separating the lower uterine segment without rupturing the membranes; however, there is no research to support the effectiveness of this procedure.
- Rule out contraindications to induction of labor: patient refusal, placenta previa, transverse fetal lie, prolapsed umbilical cord, prior vertical (classic) uterine incision, active genital herpes infection.
- Evaluate readiness for labor including fetal maturity and cervical readiness.
- Perform amniotomy in conjunction with oxytocin.
- Insert an indwelling catheter tip into the cervix and inflate the balloon. Dilates the cervix.
- IV oxytocin (Pitocin)—10 U per 1 L of intravenous fluid (e.g., D5 lactated Ringer's solution or lactated Ringer's solution). This produces a concentration of 10 mU oxytocin per 1 ml of IV fluid. Dosage protocols vary among agencies but should not exceed ACOG recommended dosage of 40 mU/min (ACOG, 2009). A common protocol is to start at 0.5–1 mU/min and increase by 1–2 mU/min every 40–60 minutes until a good contraction pattern is achieved. An alternative protocol is to start at 1–2 mU/min and increase by 1 mU/min every 15 min until a good UC pattern is achieved. Once the cervix has dilated to 5–6 cm, decrease oxytocin dosage by similar increments. A third regimen is to start at 2 mU/min and increase by 2 mU/min every 30 min until the woman has at least 5 contractions lasting 45–90 seconds within a 10-minute period averaged over 30 minutes. The maximum dose of oxytocin for this method is 20 mU/min, administered via infusion pump, unless another dose is specifically ordered by the healthcare provider.
- Misoprostol (Cytotec), a synthetic prostaglandin E_1 analogue. Misoprostol is FDA approved for the prevention of stomach ulcers in patients taking oral NSAIDs. It is used off-label to ripen the cervix and induce labor when there is a Bishop score of 5 or less. Misoprostol is not approved by FDA for cervical ripening and not recommended for women with a history of prior cesarean section or uterine scarring.
- Prostaglandin E_2 (Cervadil). A cervical ripening agent that increases myometrial contractility. Approved by FDA in 1995, it is a controlled-release vaginal insert with a removable cord. It is not recommended for women who have a history of prior cesarean birth or uterine scar.

- Prostaglandin gel or pessary. Ripens the cervix, if necessary. There is no easy way to remove the gel if hyperstimulation occurs. Recommended for women who have a medical indication for inducing labor.
- Laminaria tent. A seaweed preparation inserted into the cervix that mechanically softens and dilates the cervix because it absorbs water.
- Assess for AROM. Delivery must occur within 24 hours after AROM.
- Cesarean birth in the event of failed induction/augmentation.
- Terbutaline or magnesium sulfate. Reduces uterine hyperactivity if hyperstimulation occurs.

▌ Collaborative Problems

Potential complications of amniotomy include the following:

- Infection
- Cord prolapse

Potential complications of hydroscopic cervical dilators (e.g., laminaria tents) include the following:

- Maternal postpartum and newborn infection
- Urinary retention

Potential complications of prostaglandin cervical ripening agents include the following:

- Hyperstimulation of the uterus
- Fetal distress

Potential complications of oxytocin or misoprostol (Cytotec) administration:

- Uterine hyperstimulation (that may result in placental abruption, uterine rupture, and fetal hypoxia)
- Water intoxication (oxytocin)
- Rapid labor (which may result in birth canal lacerations and trauma to the fetus)
- Intrapartum and postpartum hemorrhage

COLLABORATIVE (STANDARDIZED) CARE FOR ALL WOMEN HAVING INDUCTION OR AUGMENTATION OF LABOR

Perform comprehensive assessment to identify individual needs for teaching, emotional support, and physical care.

▌ Potential Complications of Amniotomy: INFECTION AND CORD PROLAPSE

See "Amniotomy," beginning on p. 246 in this chapter.

Potential Complications of Hydroscopic Cervical Dilators (e.g., Laminaria Tents): MATERNAL POSTPARTUM AND NEWBORN INFECTION AND URINARY RETENTION

Refer to the generic collaborative care plan, "Infection," beginning on p. 29 in Chapter 3.

Focus Assessments

- Assess cervical dilation after leaving dilator in place for 6–12 hours. If further cervical dilation is desired, fresh dilators must be inserted.
- Assess for ROM and observe and document amount, color, and odor of amniotic fluid. Birth must occur within 24 hours after ROM in order to reduce the risk for infection. Normal amniotic fluid should be clear and odorless; a greenish tint occurs when the fetus passes meconium in utero, which can result from fetal stress.
- Assess UCs, vaginal bleeding, uterine tenderness, pain, and urinary retention. Evaluates maternal well-being and the possibility that labor has begun. It is likely that the mother has some medical indication for labor induction, so it is important to identify any symptoms that might indicate a developing complication, whether from the cervical dilator or other etiology.
- Assess FHR regularly. Fetal distress is a contraindication for labor induction, so it is necessary to establish satisfactory condition of the fetus. See the generic collaborative care plan, "Potential Complication: Fetal Compromise," which begins on p. 27 in Chapter 3; and "Intrapartum Fetal Monitoring," which begins on p. 242 in this chapter.

Preventive Nursing Activities

- When inserting the dilator, lubricate cervix with bacteriostatic cream or jelly; saturate the sponges used to hold the dilators in place with povidone-iodine. Helps decrease the risk for postpartum and neonatal infection.
- Document the number of dilators and sponges inserted and the number removed. Evaluates effectiveness of the dilators; to be sure that all sponges and dilators are removed in order to decrease the risk for infection.

Potential Complications of Prostaglandin Cervical Ripening Agents: HYPERSTIMULATION

OF THE UTERUS AND FETAL DISTRESS

Refer to generic collaborative care plan, "Potential Complication: Fetal Compromise," which begins on p. 27 in Chapter 3.

Focus Assessments

- Review history prior to administration of cervical ripening agent. Ensures that there are no contraindications (e.g., placenta previa, unexplained vaginal bleeding, vasa previa, transverse lie, prior transfundal uterine incision) to the procedure; and to determine if there are conditions that create the need for extra caution (e.g., impaired cardiovascular, hepatic, or renal function; or asthma or glaucoma).
- Monitor for onset of labor. Ensures maternal and fetal well-being and notifies the primary caregiver, should labor occur. Although this treatment is intended to improve the success rate for the induction of labor, in some cases the woman will go into labor after the application of the cervical ripening agent; in that case, oxytocin induction/augmentation may not be needed. If oxytocin is used, it must be with great caution because of the likelihood of uterine overstimulation.
- Assess cervical dilation in 6 hours after insertion of the gel or suppository. If no cervical response and no adverse effects, the doses may be repeated (a maximum of 1.5 mg of dinoprostone can be given in a 24-hr period).
- Obtain a baseline FHR (at least a 20-minute strip) before administration of an oxytocic and then monitor continuously for 1–2 hours thereafter or for 4 hours if UCs occur and continue. FHR pattern reflects fetal status. Continuous FHR is compared to preadministration baseline. Should uterine hyperstimulation occur, decreased blood flow through the placenta will result in fetal asphyxia. Healthcare provider should be notified immediately so that corrective treatment can be implemented, such as subcutaneous terbutaline 1–2 doses to relax the uterus, repositioning the woman, administering IV fluid bolus and oxygen.

Preventive Nursing Activities

- Have the woman remain in a lateral position or supine with hip tilt for 30–60 min after administration of gel; for 2 hrs after administration of a vaginal insert. Minimizes leakage and improves effectiveness. Some healthcare providers allow the woman to eat a small meal if not in labor after the first hour.
- If no signs of labor or fetal distress occur, the woman may be moved to an antepartum unit or sent home. If sent home, instruct to return the next day. If there are no UCs the next day, oxytocin induction will begin.
- If adverse reactions occur (e.g., hyperstimulation, vomiting), notify healthcare provider and remove the gel or

suppository if possible. Inserts made like a tampon are easier to retrieve, but gels may need to be lavaged from the vagina. Prevents maternal and/or fetal injury. If uterine activity has not returned to normal after 10 minutes, then decrease the oxytocin (Pitocin) by half and if no return after another 10 minutes, then discontinue the oxytocin until uterine activity is fewer than 5 contractions in 10 minutes.

Potential Complications of Oxytocin or Misoprostol (Cytotec) Administration: UTERINE HYPERSTIMULATION, WATER INTOXICATION, AND RAPID LABOR

Uterine hyperstimulation may result in placental abruption, uterine rupture, and fetal hypoxia. Rapid labor may result in birth canal lacerations and trauma to the fetus. Also refer to the generic collaborative care plan, "Potential Complication: Fetal Compromise ," beginning on p. 27, in Chapter 3.

Prior to Beginning Oxytocic Administration

- Review maternal history (e.g., pelvic measurements, estimated date of birth, complications of pregnancy, prenatal lab results). Ensures that no contraindications exist for labor induction/augmentation; identifies risk factors for problems that may develop.
- Complete protocols or checklists if required. Some facilities have protocols and checklists that have to be completed prior to the start of oxytocin.
- Review Bishop score. A score of 6 indicates that the cervix is favorable for induction.
- Perform a sterile vaginal exam. If the cervix is soft and at least 50% effaced or dilated to at least 3 cm, it is considered ripe. This means that induction is likely to be successful. This is less important when using a cervical ripening agent because they produce cervical ripening.
- Obtain maternal VSs. Provides a baseline for comparison of subsequent data to evaluate tolerance of medications and labor.
- Apply external monitor and obtain a 15–20-minute FHR reading and NST. Provides a baseline for comparison of subsequent data to evaluate fetal well-being.
- Perform Nitrazine/AmniSure or fern test on vaginal secretions if indicated. Assesses for rupture of membranes.
- Position in side-lying or upright position. Keeps weight of gravid uterus off of abdominal blood vessels and improves venous return to the heart. This helps to ensure adequate placental-fetal blood flow.

Starting the Oxytocin Infusion

- Use a large (at least 18-gauge) IV catheter to start the primary IV. A large-bore catheter is needed in the event of emergency fluid, drug, or blood administration and in case of the need for a surgical birth.
- Administer premixed oxytocin (Pitocin) per protocol (usually 10 U/1,000 ml isotonic electrolyte solution) only with infusion pump. Oxytocin is a high-alert drug for which safety precautions are crucial. Administering via infusion pump allows for precise control of the flow rate and prevents accidental overdose and hyperstimulation of the uterus. Oxytocin is a posterior pituitary hormone that stimulates uterine contractions. The uterus of a pregnant woman is very sensitive to oxytocin, and doses are highly individualized; that is, different women require different blood levels to stimulate UCs. Additionally, the toxic dose is only slightly larger than the therapeutic dose; that is, the blood level that would produce hyperstimulation is only slightly higher than the blood level needed to produce effective UCs. Therefore, it must be used with great care (e.g., in a very dilute solution). Electrolyte solution decreases the likelihood of water intoxication by minimizing the antidiuretic effect of oxytocin. As a safety measure, time label the tubing of each IV mixture.
- Use a two-bag setup; piggyback the oxytocin solution to a primary IV line, close to the insertion site. In case the oxytocin must be discontinued, the primary line will still be available for hydration and other medications.

During the Induction/Augmentation

- Monitor the infusion pump closely, and carefully titrate the drug. Ensures correct dosage. Fluctuations in administration rate may cause undermedication, resulting in ineffective UCs, or overmedication, resulting in uterine hyperstimulation and possible rupture.
- Continuously monitor FHR and document per protocol. Evaluates fetal tolerance of labor. Blood flow to the fetus decreases during UCs, but this is tolerated by a healthy fetus in the presence of a normal labor. However, if hyperstimulation of the uterus occurs, blood flow to the placenta is reduced for longer periods of time, resulting in fetal anoxia, which is reflected by late decelerations, bradycardia, or decreased FHR variability.
- Continuously monitor UCs for frequency, intensity, and resting tone between contractions; palpate if intrauterine pressure catheter (IUPC) is not in place. External monitor does not provide information about the strength of the UCs, only about the duration and frequency. The oxytocin dose is maintained if the IUPC indicates pressures of 40–90 mmHg, UCs are 40–90 sec in duration and 2–3 min in frequency, and cervical dilation occurs at 1 cm/hr in the active phase of labor.

- Assess for nausea, vomiting, headache, dizziness, lethargy, confusion, hypertension, tachycardia and cardiac arrhythmias, peripheral edema, shallow or labored breathing, dyspnea, tachypnea, or change in level of consciousness. These are symptoms of water intoxication, which usually occur only with dosages greater than 20 mU/min. These may also be adverse effects of prostaglandins such as dinoprostone or misoprostol.

- Assess maternal BP and pulse before advancement of the infusion rate. Evaluate for side effects that would preclude advancing the rate. BP may decrease when oxytocin is first administered; it may gradually increase to as much as 30% above baseline. This may be due to the antidiuretic effect of the hormone as well as from anxiety and the discomfort of the UCs.

- Assess UCs and FHR before each increase in the infusion rate. If satisfactory contraction pattern has been established, rate will not need to be increased. If UCs indicate hyperstimulation or if FHR indicates fetal distress, the rate will not be increased and may be decreased or discontinued. If FHR is reassuring and satisfactory labor has not begun, rate will be increased.

- After UCs are established, perform sterile vaginal exams as often as necessary to evaluate labor progress. Evaluates cervical dilation, effacement, and fetal station. Limit vaginal exams only to those absolutely necessary in order to decrease the risk for infection. The frequency of vaginal exams depends on the woman's parity and the characteristics of the UCs. For example, a multipara with strong, frequent UCs will need more frequent exams than a nullipara with mild, brief UCs occurring every 7–8 min.

- Monitor intake and output. Oxytocin, especially at dosages of more than 20 mU/min, is an antidiuretic that acts by decreasing the free water exchange in the kidney and greatly decreasing urine output; decreased output may reflect water retention. Decreased output with a high specific gravity indicates fluid deficit, which may compromise maternal BP and placental circulation.

- After membranes have ruptured, insert (or assist with insertion of) internal fetal electrode and IUPC as needed. Internal electrode provides a more accurate reading of FHR variability. An external monitor does not provide information about the strength/intensity of the UCs; an IUPC is more useful for evaluating intrauterine pressures and the presence of uterine hyperstimulation.

- Administer oxytocin per protocol, usually begin induction at 0.5–2 mU/min and increase the dose 1–2 mU/min at intervals of 15–60 minutes until satisfactory labor is achieved or until a dose of 40 mU/min is reached. The toxic dose of oxytocin is only slightly larger than the therapeutic dose; that is, the blood level that would produce hyperstimulation is only slightly higher than the blood level needed to produce effective UCs. Therefore, it must be increased slowly in order to evaluate the effect of an increase on UCs, and in small increments in order to prevent giving a toxic dose.

- Discontinue the oxytocin immediately and notify the care provider if nonreassuring FHR occurs, intrauterine pressure is greater than 75 mmHg, the uterus does not relax between contractions (does not return to baseline on monitor strip), or UCs are longer in duration than 90 sec or occurring more often than every 2 min. These are signs of uterine hyperstimulation. IV oxytocin is rapid acting and has a half-life of about 3 min. The oxytocin must be stopped immediately to prevent fetal anoxia and uterine rupture.

- Stop the oxytocin and notify the physician immediately if the woman experiences shooting, sharp abdominal pain, stating that "something came loose"; prepare for emergency surgery and birth. A change in the FHR may be the first sign of a uterine abruption or signs of complete uterine rupture; symptoms are less dramatic and develop less rapidly if partial rupture occurs. In this situation UCs will stop; hemorrhage and shock may follow, and the FHR may be absent. This is an emergency, requiring immediate surgery to prevent maternal and fetal death.

- If uterine hyperstimulation occurs, after discontinuing the secondary oxytocin IV line:
  - Reposition the woman on her side or have her lift herself onto her arms and knees (all fours). Improves fetal-placental blood flow.
  - Increase the primary IV rate up to 200 ml/hr, unless contraindicated by symptoms of water intoxication; in which case the IV rate should be reduced to the keep open rate. Provides adequate intravascular volume, supports maternal BP, and ensures blood flow to the fetus; preserves an intravenous route for emergency medications.
  - Administer oxygen by non-rebreather mask at 10 L/min, or per protocol. Because uterine hyperstimulation reduces the amount of blood reaching the fetus, it is important that the blood be as fully saturated with oxygen as possible in order to prevent fetal anoxia.

- If inadequate uterine response is obtained at a dose of 20 mU/min, notify care provider. This may indicate that the induction has failed. If membranes are intact, induction may be discontinued and attempted at a later time; if membranes have ruptured, cesarean birth may be necessary. The care provider may choose to continue increasing the dosage up to 40 mU/min.

INDIVIDUALIZED (NURSING DIAGNOSIS) CARE PLANS

The care plans in this section were developed to address unique patient needs.

Nursing Diagnosis: PAIN[1]

Related Factors: oxytocin-induced UCs (which peak more rapidly than naturally occurring contractions). Refer to the generic NDCP, "Pain,[1]" which begins on p. 18 in Chapter 2.

Nursing Activities and Rationales

Assessments

- Assess UC pattern, cervical dilation, and fetal station before administering analgesics. *Assesses progress of labor. Given too early in labor, analgesics may slow labor progress; given too close to time of the birth, narcotic analgesics can cause respiratory depression in the newborn.*

Independent Nursing Activities

- Provide comfort measures such as damp cloth to forehead, changing damp linens and underpads, repositioning, and frequent mouth care. *Relieves other discomforts, which create stress and increase the perception of pain.*
- Reassure the woman that she is doing well; give positive feedback for her efforts to cope with UCs. *Positive reinforcement helps the woman to relax (tension increases pain).*
- Encourage conscious relaxation between UCs. *Methods include focusing, imagery, effleurage, Lamaze, hypnosis, acupuncture and acupressure, yoga, and music. Prevents fatigue and reduces tension, which increase the perception of pain.*
- Encourage to void at least every 2 hrs. *A full bladder adds to the discomfort and may increase pain.*

Collaborative Activities

- Administer analgesics per order or protocol when labor is established. *Narcotic analgesics alter the perception of pain in the CNS; regional anesthesia prevents pain impulses from ascending through the spinal cord.*

Patient/Family Teaching

- Before starting the oxytocin infusion, explain how the UCs differ from naturally occurring UCs. *This is especially important for labor augmentation when the woman has already experienced some naturally occurring UCs. Prepares woman and partner for short peak-time and allows for more effective coping.*

Nursing Diagnosis: ANXIETY[1]

Related Factors: fear of pain, misinformation from friends/family (old wives' tales), childbirth not proceeding according to expectations, lack of understanding about the need for induction/augmentation, and fear that procedures will harm the fetus. Refer to the generic NDCP, "Anxiety,[1]" which begins on p. 10 in Chapter 2.

Nursing Activities and Rationales

Independent Nursing Actions

- Reassure the woman that the need for induction (or augmentation) is not unusual and that she did nothing to cause the present situation. *The woman may have anticipated a labor and birth without the use of medications. She may feel that the oxytocics and/or analgesics are unnatural and see this as failure on her part. Reassurance and factual information may help decrease her anxiety about her performance.*
- Provide comfort and pain relief measures (pharmacologic and nonpharmacologic) as needed and appropriate to the progress of the labor. *Pain increases the woman's anxiety.*

Nursing Diagnosis: NAUSEA, VOMITING, AND DIARRHEA[1]

Related Factors: side effects of prostaglandins used for cervical ripening or for labor induction/augmentation and water intoxication secondary to high doses of oxytocin.

Goals, Outcomes, and Evaluation Criteria

- Woman reports relief from nausea.

NIC Interventions[2]

Medication Management (2380)—Facilitation of safe and effective use of prescription and over-the-counter drugs.
Nausea Management (1450)—Prevention and alleviation of nausea.
Simple Relaxation Therapy (6040)—Use of techniques to encourage and elicit relaxation for the purpose of decreasing undesirable signs and symptoms such as pain, muscle tension, or anxiety.
Vomiting Management (1570)—Prevention and alleviation of vomiting.

Nursing Activities and Rationales

Assessments

- Monitor subjective feelings of nausea. *Nausea is an adverse effect of prostaglandins; the higher the dose, the more likely it will produce nausea, vomiting, and diarrhea. Nausea may also result from pain and anxiety; it is also a symptom of water intoxication (an occasional adverse effect of oxytocin).*
- Monitor vomiting; record as output. *This is important in evaluating fluid and electrolyte balance and as an indication of the severity of the nausea. GI side effects of prostaglandins are usually mild; however, if they are severe, the procedure (e.g., cervical ripening, labor induction/augmentation) must be discontinued.*

Independent Nursing Activities

- Elevate head of bed or place the woman in a lateral position. To prevent aspiration of vomitus.
- Keep the woman and bedding clean; remove and clean emesis basin immediately. Unpleasant sights, smells, and associations can produce more nausea.
- Apply cool, damp cloth to the woman's wrists, neck, and forehead. Provides distraction and some relief from nausea. Decreasing body temperature can reduce sympathetic nervous system stimulation and decrease nausea.
- Offer cold foods/fluids and foods/fluids with little odor. Warm foods and odors can cause nausea.

Collaborative Activities

- Provide pain control. Pain can cause nausea. Pain activates the sympathetic nervous system resulting in decreased gastrointestinal motility and secretion while at the same time increasing sphincter tone. The vomiting reflex is initiated by a complex set of neural events that occur when afferent receptors are stimulated (by pain) and transmitted to the medulla.

Patient/Family Teaching

- Instruct to use voluntary swallowing and/or deep breathing when nauseated. Suppresses the vomiting reflex.
- Remain on nothing-by-mouth status until vomiting subsides. Presence of food in the stomach can trigger nausea, as can food smells.

▮ *Other Nursing Diagnoses*

- Knowledge deficiency[1] related to lack of prior experience with labor and/or oxytocic induction/augmentation.

ENDNOTES

1. Nursing Diagnoses—Definitions and Classification 2009–2011. Copyright © 2009, 2007, 2005, 2003, 2001, 1998, 1996, 1994 by NANDA International. Used by arrangement with Blackwell Publishing Limited, a company of John Wiley & Sons, Inc. In order to make safe and effective judgments using NANDA-I nursing diagnoses it is essential that nurses refer to the definitions and defining characteristics of the diagnoses listed in this work.
2. Bulechek, G. M., Butcher, H. K., Dochterman, J. M. (2008). *Nursing Interventions Classification* (5th ed). St. Louis, MO: Elsevier, by permission.

REFERENCES

American College of Obstetricians and Gynecologists (ACOG). (2009). *Practice Bulletin No. 107: Induction of Labor, 114*, 386–397.

Robinson, B., & Nelson, L (2008). A review of the proceedings from the 2008 NICHD workshop on standardized nomenclature for cardiotocography. *Reviews in Obstetrics & Gynecology, 1*(4), 186–192.

RESOURCES

Adams, E., & Bianchi, A. (2008). A practical approach to labor support. *Journal of Obstetrical, Gynecological, and Neonatal Nursing, 37*(1), 106–115.

Ambler, P. A. (2007). *Maternal-neonatal facts made incredibly quick.* Philadelphia, PA: Lippincott Williams & Wilkins.

American Academy of Pediatrics and the American College of Obstetricians and Gynecologists. (2007). *Guidelines for perinatal care* (6th ed). Washington, DC: Authors.

American College of Obstetricians and Gynecologists (ACOG). (2009). *ACOG Practice Bulletin Number 106: Intrapartum Fetal Heart Rate Monitoring: Nomenclature, Interpretation, and General Management Principles, 114*(1), 192–202.

American College of Obstetricians and Gynecologists [ACOG]. (2009). *Practice Bulletin No. 107: Induction of Labor, 114*, 386–397.

Beilin, Y., Hossain, S., & Bodian, C. (2003). The numeric rating scale and labor epidural analgesia. *Anesthesia Analog, 96*, 1794–1798.

Bhullar, A., Carlan, J., Hamm, J., Lamberty, N., White, L., & Richichi, K. (2004). Buccal misoprostol to decrease blood loss after vaginal delivery: A randomized trial. *American College of Obstetricians and Gynecologists, 104*(6), 1282–1288.

Brancato, R., Church, S., & Stone, P. (2008). A meta-analysis of passive descent versus immediate pushing in nulliparous women with epidural analgesia in the second stage of labor. *Journal of Obstetrical, Gynecological & Neonatal Nursing, 37*(4), 4–12.

Bulechek, G. M., Butcher, H. K., & Dochterman, J. M. (2008). *Nursing interventions classification (NIC)* (5th ed). St. Louis, MO: Mosby/Elsevier.

Camann, W. (2005). Pain relief during labor. *New England Journal of Medicine, 352*(7), 718–720.

Campbell, D., Lake, M., Falk, M., & Backstrand, J. (2006). A randomized control trial of continuous support in labor by a lay doula. *Journal of Obstetrical, Gynecological, and Neonatal Nursing, 35*(4), 456–464.

Caughey, A. (2009, October). Is there an upper time limit for the management of the second stage of labor? *American Journal of Obstetrics & Gynecology, 337*–338.

Clark, S., Simpson, K., Knox, G., & Garite, T. (2009). Oxytocin: New perspectives on an old drug. *Obstetric Anesthesia Digest, 29*(4), 181.

Figeirredo, B., & Pacheco, A. (2009). Mother-to-infant emotional involvement at birth. *Journal of Maternal Health Child, 13*, 539–549.

Frank, B., Lane, C., & Kokanson, H. (2008). Designing a postepidural fall risk assessment score for the obstetric patient. *Journal of Nursing Care Quality, 24*(1), 50–54.

Gennaro, S., Mayberry, L., & Kafulafula, U. (2007). The evidence supporting nursing management of labor. *Journal of Obstetrical, Gynecological, and Neonatal Nursing, 36*(6), 598–604.

Glantz, J. (2010). Term labor induction compared with expectant management. *Obstetrics & Gynecology, 115*(1), 70–76.

Graham, E., Peterson, S., Christo, D., & Fox, H. (2006). Intrapartum electronic fetal heart rate monitoring and the prevention of perinatal brain injury. *Obstetrics & Gynecology, 108*(3), 656–666.

Hobbins, D. (2004). Survivors of childhood sexual abuse: Implications for perinatal nursing care. *Journal of Obstetrical, Gynecological, and Neonatal Nursing, 33*(4), 485–497.

Hofmeyr, G., Gulmezoglu, A., Novikova, N., Linder, V., Ferreira, S., & Piaggio, G. (2009). Misoprostol to prevent and treat postpartum haemorrhage: A systematic review and meta-analysis of maternal deaths and dose-related effects. *World Health Organization: Bulletin of the World Health Organization, 87*(9), 666–684.

Lothian, J. (2009). Safe, health birth: What every pregnant woman needs to know. *Journal of Perinatal Education, 19*(3), 48–54.

Maccones, G., Hankins, G., Song, C., Haugh, J., & Moore, T. (2008). The 2008 National Institute of Health and Human Development workshop report on electronic fetal monitoring: Update on definitions, interpretation, and research guidelines. *Journal of Obstetrical, Gynecological, and Neonatal Nursing, 37*(5), 510–515.

MacKinon, K., McIntyre, M., & Quance, M. (2005). The meaning of the nurse's presence during childbirth. *Journal of Obstetrical, Gynecological, and Neonatal Nursing, 34*(1), 28–36.

Mahlmeister, L. (2003). Nursing responsibilities in preventing, preparing for, and managing epidural emergencies. *Journal of Perinatal and Neonatal Nursing, 17*(1), 19–32.

Mandel, D., Pirko, C., Grant, K., Kauffman, T., Williams, L., & Schneider, J. (2009). A collaborative protocol on oxytocin administration: Bringing nurses, midwives and physicians together. *Nursing for Women's Health, 131*(6), 480–485.

Moleti, C. (2009). Trends and controversies in labor induction. *American Journal of Maternal/Child Nursing, 34*(1), 40–47.

Murry, M. (2004). Maternal or fetal heart rate? Avoiding intrapartum misidentification. *Journal of Obstetrical, Gynecological, and Neonatal Nursing, 33*(1), 93–104.

Murry, M. (2007). *Antepartal and intrapartal fetal monitoring* (3rd ed.). New York, NY: Springer Publishing Company.

Nagoette, M. (2006). Timing of conduction analgesia in labor. *American Journal of Obstetrics & Gynecology, 194*, 598–599.

N-Dia, Inc. (2009). *AmniSure ROM (rupture of [fetal] membranes) test: Directions for in vitro diagnostic use.* Retrieved from http://www.woongbee.com/0NewHome/AmniSure/pdf/EU.Insert.NDI203REV3.pdf

North American Nursing Diagnosis Association (NANDA). (2009). *Nursing diagnoses classification.* North American Nursing Diagnosis Association. Ames, IA: Wiley Publishing.

Ophir, E., Singer-Jordan, J., Odeh, M., Hirch, Y., Maksimovsky, O., Shaider, O., Yvry, S., Solt, I., & Bronstein, J. (2009). Abnormal placental invasion—a novel approach to treatment, case report and review. *Obstetrical and Gynecological Survey, 64*(12), 811–822.

Parer, J., Ikeda, T., & King, T. (2009). The 2008 National Institute of Child Health and Human Development report on fetal heart rate monitoring. *Obstetrics & Gynecology, 114*(1), 136–138.

Ray, C. L., Audibert, F., Goffinet, F., & Fraser, W. (2009). When to stop pushing: Effects of duration of second-stage expulsion efforts on maternal and neonatal outcomes in nulliparous women with epidural analgesia. *American Journal of Obstetrics & Gynecology, 201*, 361–367.

Rice-Simpson, K., & Creehan, P. (2008). *AWHONN's perinatal nursing* (3rd ed.). Philadelphia, PA: Lippincott Williams & Wilkins.

Roberts, J. (2003). A new understanding of the second stage of labor: Implications for nursing care. *Journal of Obstetrical, Gynecologic, and Neonatal Nursing, 32*(6), 794–801.

Selo-Ojeme, D., Pisal, P., Lawal, O., Rogers, C., Shah, A., & Sinha, S. (2009). A randomized controlled trial of amniotomy and immediate oxytocin infusion versus amniotomy and delayed oxytocin infusion for induction of labor at term. *Obstetrical and Gynecological Survey, 279*, 813–820.

Simpson, K., & James, D. (2005). Effects of immediate versus delayed pushing during second stage labor on fetal well-being. *Nursing Research, 54*(3), 149–157.

Tillett, J. (2007, April–June). Expert opinion: Intermittent auscultation of fetal heartbeat: Can nurses change the culture of technology? *Journal of Perinatal & Neonatal Nursing, 21*(2), 80–82.

Varney, H. (2004). *Varney's midwifery* (4th ed.). Sudbury, MA: Jones & Bartlett.

Whitehead, N., Callaghan, W., Johnson, C., & Williams, L. (2009). Racial, ethnic, and economic disparities in the prevalence of pregnancy complications. *Journal of Maternal Child Health, 13*, 198–205.

8

INTRAPARTUM COMPLICATIONS

Cynthia Waits

DYSTOCIA/DYSFUNCTIONAL LABOR

Dystocia is long, difficult, or abnormal labor. About 8–11% of women with the fetus in normal vertex presentation experience dystocia; it is equally common in first- and second-stage labor and is a leading indicator for primary cesarean births (Ricci & Kyle, 2008). It is of concern because it is fatiguing to both mother and fetus and often requires medical or surgical intervention, which creates additional risk. The risk for fetal death greatly increases when active first-stage labor lasts more than 15 hours. The *Healthy People 2010* initiative's goal is to reduce maternal complications during hospitalized labor and delivery from a baseline of 31.2 per 100 births to a target of 24 per 100 births. As needed, refer to the topics, "Intrapartum Fetal Monitoring," "Amniotomy," and "Induction/Augmentation of Labor," beginning on pp. 242, 246, and 254, respectively, in Chapter 7. Also refer to the topics, "Cesarean Birth," "External Version," and "Forceps- or Vacuum-Assisted Birth," beginning on pp. 277, 295, and 299, respectively, in this chapter.

▌ *Key Nursing Activities*

- Assess for factors that can be a source of dystocia.
- Assess maternal physical and psychologic responses to labor.
- Assess fetal well-being (fetal heart rate [FHR] and pattern, presentation, station, position, status of amniotic membranes).
- Evaluate the status of labor (in terms of fetal descent, cervical effacement and dilation in relation to uterine contractions [UCs], and length of time in labor).
- Assist with and prepare the woman for collaborative interventions (e.g., external cephalic version, oxytocin augmentation of labor).

▌ *Etiologies and Risk Factors*

Dystocia can be caused by any of the following interdependent factors:

- Dysfunctional labor. Abnormal, disorganized UCs; hypertonic UCs that do not cause progress of cervical dilation/effacement; hypotonic UCs. Factors that increase the risk for dysfunctional labor include short stature, obesity, hydramnios, uterine abnormalities, fetal malpresentation or malposition, incorrect timing of analgesia or anesthesia, cephalopelvic disproportion (CPD), overstimulation with oxytocin (causing myometrial fatigue), family history of dystocia, maternal exhaustion, ineffective pushing techniques, maternal age greater than 35 years, gestational age greater than 41 weeks, and chorioamnionitis.
- Fetal causes. Excessive size, multiple gestation, abnormal presentation or position, fetal anomalies (e.g., hydrocephalus). Factors that increase the risk for fetal dystocia include maternal diabetes, obesity, and large size of one or both parents.
- Maternal positioning. Because of the effects of gravity, the mother's position affects the relationship between the UCs and fetal body parts, either facilitating or hindering fetal descent. For example, sitting and squatting facilitate fetal descent during pushing.
- Alterations in pelvic structure. An example of an alteration in pelvic structure would be pelvic contractures that reduce the capacity of the bony pelvis. These may be the result of malnutrition, accidents, congenital abnormalities, or immature pelvic size.
- Psychologic factors. Lack of preparation, anxiety/fear, support system, culture, and past experiences have emotional effects that trigger physiologic responses.

▌ *Signs and Symptoms*

Dysfunctional Labor

- Hypertonic uterine dysfunction. Irregular, uncoordinated, low-amplitude UCs; cervical dilation of 1 cm/hr; or arrest of dilation, usually in latent stage; pain seems out of proportion to intensity of UCs; uterus does not completely relax between UCs (resting tone greater than 15 mmHg per internal uterine pressure catheter [IUPC]); frequently an anxious primigravida.
- Hypotonic uterine dysfunction. Decreased frequency and intensity (less than 30 mmHg per IUPC) of UCs in the active stage; cervical dilation does not progress; commonly caused by CPD and fetal malpositions; hemorrhage following delivery because weak contractions fail to compress blood vessels.
- Inadequate bearing-down efforts. In second stage, voluntary expulsive forces are not strong enough; may not feel the urge to push; may occur because of large amounts of analgesics, anesthesia, maternal exhaustion from a long labor, or inadequate hydration and food intake.

Pelvic Dystocia

- Lack of engagement and fetal descent
- Weak UCs in first stage (occurs with inlet contractures)

Fetal Dystocia

- Lack of fetal descent

- Prolonged second stage, caused by malposition (e.g., persistent occiput posterior occurs in about 25% of all labors)
- Severe back pain
- Breech, face, brow, or shoulder presentation (confirmed by abdominal palpation, vaginal exam, and/or ultrasound)
- Multifetal pregnancy

Diagnostic Studies

- Abdominal palpation. Establishes position and presentation; determines intensity of UCs.
- Vaginal examination. Establishes position, presentation, and cervical dilation and effacement.
- Sonography and/or pelvimetry. Rules out CPD, evaluates fetal presentation and position, and provides information about feasibility of vaginal birth.
- Fetal monitoring. Assesses fetal well-being.

Medical Management

- External cephalic version. Turning the fetus from one presentation to another (e.g., from breech to vertex) by exertion of pressure on the abdomen after administration of a tocolytic.
- Trial of labor (TOL). Allowing 4–6 hrs of spontaneous active labor to assess the safety of a vaginal birth.
- Induction or augmentation with oxytocin. For uterine dysfunction.
- Amniotomy. Augments labor when presenting part is engaged and labor progress has slowed.
- Forceps- or vacuum-assisted birth. Shortens second stage of labor (e.g., because of maternal fatigue or fetal distress).
- Cesarean birth. When vaginal birth is not possible, or for immediate threats to maternal or fetal well-being (e.g., after a failed trial of labor).

Collaborative Problems

Potential Complication of Dysfunctional Labor or Dystocia

- Fetal distress
- Risk for maternal injury (e.g., lacerations, hematomas) or fetal injury (e.g., fractures, anoxia) related to malpresentations, CPD, lack of fetal descent, prolapsed umbilical cord, and use of instruments to facilitate birth

Potential Postpartum Complication of Prolonged Labor

- Infection, postpartum hemorrhage

COLLABORATIVE (STANDARDIZED) CARE FOR ALL WOMEN WITH DYSTOCIA/DYSFUNCTIONAL LABOR

Perform a comprehensive assessment to identify individual needs for teaching, emotional support, and physical care.

Potential Complication of Dysfunctional Labor or Dystocia: FETAL DISTRESS

Refer to the generic collaborative care plan, "Fetal Compromise (Nonreassuring Fetal Heart Rate)," which begins on p. 27 in Chapter 3.

Nursing Diagnosis: RISK FOR MATERNAL AND/OR FETAL INJURY[1]

Related Factors: prolonged labor and/or difficult birth as a result of fetal malpresentations, CPD, lack of fetal descent, prolapsed umbilical cord secondary to lack of fetal engagement, dysfunctional UCs, and use of instruments to facilitate birth. This includes maternal perineal/vaginal/cervical lacerations, fetal/neonatal asphyxia, fetal fractures and soft tissue injury. Refer to "Forceps- or Vacuum-Assisted Birth," beginning on p. 300 in this chapter.

Goals, Outcomes, and Evaluation Criteria

- Woman accomplishes labor without injury or hemorrhage.
- Woman gives birth to an infant without fetal distress or birth injury.

NIC Interventions[2]

Electronic Fetal Monitoring: Intrapartum (6772)—Electronic evaluation of fetal heart rate response to uterine contractions during intrapartal care.

Intrapartal Care (6830)—Monitoring and management of stages one and two of the birth process.

Intrapartal Care: High-Risk Delivery (6834)—Assisting vaginal birth or multiple or malpositioned fetuses.

Labor Induction (6850)—Initiation or augmentation of labor by mechanical or pharmacologic methods.

Medication Administration (2300)—Preparing, giving, and evaluating the effectiveness of prescription and nonprescription drugs.

Medication Management (2380)—Facilitation of safe and effective use of prescription and over-the-counter drugs.

Newborn Monitoring (6890)—Measurement and interpretation of physiologic status of the neonate the first 24 hours after delivery.

Resuscitation: Neonate (6974)—Administering emergency measures to support newborn adaptation to extrauterine life.

Nursing Activities and Rationales

Assessments

- Review history. Family or personal history of dystocia is a risk factor for dystocia in present labor.

- Assess level of fatigue and amount of sleep prior to labor. Extreme fatigue contributes to dysfunctional labor as well as being the result of prolonged labor.
- Assess for factors that can be a source of dystocia (e.g., fear, anxiety, previous labor complications, maternal diabetes, obesity, unfavorable pelvimetry, and fetal anomalies such as myelomeningocele). Aids in planning interventions; interventions vary depending on the cause of the dystocia.
- Review lab data and other diagnostic tests. Evaluates fetal status. For example, ultrasound scanning can identify potential CPD, and fetal scalp pH can identify fetal distress.
- Evaluate status of labor in terms of fetal descent (relationship of fetal presenting part to maternal ischial spines), cervical effacement and dilation in relation to UCs, and length of time in labor. For early recognition and treatment of dystocia. The following patterns are indicators of abnormal labor:
  - Prolonged latent phase (more than 20 hr for nulliparas; more than 14 hr for multiparas)
  - Protracted active phase dilation (less than 1.2 cm/hr for nulliparas; less than 1.5 cm/hr for multiparas)
  - Secondary arrest with no cervical change (2 hrs or more for both nulliparas and multiparas)
  - Protracted descent (less than 1 cm/hr for nulliparas; less than 2 cm/hr for multiparas)
  - Arrest of descent (1 hr or more for nulliparas; 1/2 hr or more for multiparas)
  - Failure of descent (no change during deceleration phase of first stage and during second stage) (Joy, Scott, & Lyon, 2009)
- Monitor for abnormal characteristics of UCs, lack of progress in cervical dilation, or lack of progress in fetal descent and station. See preceding rationale. These are indicators of dystocia and the need for intervention.
- If IUPC not in place, palpate UCs to evaluate intensity. External electronic monitor measures frequency and duration, but not intensity, of UCs. If inserted, evaluate montevideo units (MVUs) for adequate labor.
- Note effacement of cervix, as well as cervical dilation. Cervix must be soft (ripe) in order for dilation to occur.
- During vaginal exams, assess for caput of the fetal vertex. Evaluates progress of labor. If caput is present, as it increases in size it may seem that the head is descending when it actually is not.
- Assess for full bladder or rectum. Prevents the fetus from entering the pelvis.
- Assess for cervical edema. Occurs when cervix is caught between presenting part and symphysis pubis; inhibits complete dilation.
- Palpate abdomen for Bandl's ring. This is a thickened ridge that may develop where the upper and lower uterine segments meet. It occurs in a mechanically obstructed labor

when the lower segment thins abnormally. It may indicate impending uterine rupture.
- If the woman reports severe abdominal pain, assess for fetal distress, vaginal bleeding, and cessation of UCs. Symptoms of uterine rupture or tear, which requires immediate surgical intervention.
- When fetus is in breech presentation or when there is pelvic dystocia, observe for visible cord prolapse when membranes rupture; variable FHR decelerations on monitor strip may also indicate prolapse. Cord prolapse is more likely when the presenting part cannot firmly engage or totally block the cervical os.
- For other assessments (e.g., maternal vital signs [VSs]), refer to the topics, "Normal Labor: First Stage," "Normal Labor: Second Stage," and "Normal Labor: Third Stage," beginning on pp. 221, 232, and 238, respectively, in Chapter 7.

Independent Nursing Actions

- When hypotonic uterine dysfunction occurs:
  - Prepare the woman for ultrasound or X-ray examination and assess FHR, amniotic fluid (if membranes ruptured), and maternal well-being. Identifies or rules out CPD and fetal distress and assists with the decision to augment labor with oxytocin.
  - Assist the woman to ambulate or have her partner do so. Stimulates uterine activity.
  - Assist with a warm bath or shower and administer narcotic analgesics per protocol (e.g., morphine, meperidine, or nalbuphine [Nubain]). Inhibits UCs, reduces pain, and promotes sleep (therapeutic rest). After a 4–6-hr rest period, after relaxation has improved uterine perfusion and energy is restored, the woman will often awaken in active labor with a normal UC pattern.
  - Assist with placement of IUPC. Documents UC intensity and determines if labor is adequate.
- For persistent posterior occiput position:
  - Assist the woman to assume a hands-and-knees position (e.g., kneel and lean over a large birthing ball, the bed, a chair, or an over-bed table). Uses gravity and allows fetal spine to drop toward the woman's anterior abdominal wall and facilitates anterior rotation of fetal head.
  - Have the woman try a squatting position or pelvic rocking. Encourages fetal rotation.
  - Stroke maternal abdomen in the direction that the fetal head should rotate. May stimulate fetus to turn.
  - Have the woman lie on the side toward which the fetus should turn. Makes use of gravity to facilitate rotation.
- Coach the woman to not push but allow the contractions to passively take the baby down until the cervix is completely dilated (known as laboring down). Helps prevent cervical edema, which inhibits complete dilation of the cervix and prevents the mother from resting prior to

pushing. When the baby presses on the pelvic floor, the woman will feel the urge to push.

- If possible, assist the woman to sit or squat during the pushing (second) stage. Makes use of gravity and relationship of maternal and fetal parts to facilitate fetal descent.
- Encourage to void at least every 2 hours and catheterize as needed. Provides room for fetal descent into the pelvis and decreases discomfort during UCs. Also, a full bladder may inhibit UCs.
- Encourage activity unless contraindicated. Maintaining the same position or being confined to bed increases the incidence of dystocia.

Collaborative Activities

- For shoulder or breech presentation, prepare the woman for and assist with external cephalic version. See "External Version," beginning on p. 297 in this chapter.
- For breech presentation, if fetus fails to descend, labor progress ceases, or fetal distress occurs, prepare for cesarean birth. Vaginal birth creates increased risk for injury to the fetal spine, brachial plexus, clavicle, and brain. Because the breech delivers first, prolonged head compression may occur, causing intracranial hemorrhage; prolonged vagal stimulation may cause fetal hypoxia.
- For dysfunctional uterine labor, prepare the woman for and assist with hydrotherapy if available, and prepare the woman for and assist with stripping of membranes or amniotomy and/or oxytocin augmentation of labor (if not contraindicated, e.g., by CPD). See "Amniotomy" and "Induction/Augmentation of Labor," beginning on pp. 246 and 254, respectively, in Chapter 7. An enema may stimulate hypotonic UCs; it also creates more room in the pelvis to allow for fetal descent. Amniotomy stimulates UCs, may enhance cervical dilation by allowing the fetal head to press against cervix, and makes room for the presenting part to engage.
- For second-stage dystocia (e.g., when UCs or voluntary pushing is ineffective), or when fetus fails to rotate from occiput posterior to occiput anterior, prepare the woman for and assist with forceps-assisted birth or vacuum extraction when indicated. Refer to "Forceps- or Vacuum-Assisted Birth," beginning on p. 301 in this chapter.
- When indicated by fetal distress, Bandl's ring, or failure of labor to progress, prepare the woman for and assist with cesarean birth. Refer to "Cesarean Birth," beginning on p. 279, in this chapter.

Patient/Family Teaching

- For hypotonic uterine dysfunction, teach the woman/her partner the technique of nipple stimulation (per order or protocol) prior to starting augmentation with oxytocin. Stimulates UCs by causing release of oxytocin from the pituitary.

▌ Potential Postpartum Complications of Prolonged Labor: INFECTION AND POSTPARTUM HEMORRHAGE

Refer to the generic collaborative care plans, "Potential Complication: Hemorrhage," and "Potential Complication: Infection," beginning on pp. 28 and 29, respectively, in Chapter 3. Also refer to the topics, "Postpartum Hemorrhage" and "Postpartum Infection," beginning on pp. 344 and 347, respectively, in Chapter 10.

INDIVIDUALIZED (NURSING DIAGNOSIS) CARE PLANS

The care plans in this section were developed to address unique patient needs.

▌ Nursing Diagnosis: FATIGUE[1]

Related Factors: energy expended by prolonged first- or second-stage labor and inadequate hydration and food. Also refer to the generic NDCP, "Fatigue,[1]" beginning on p. 14 in Chapter 2.

▌ *Nursing Activities and Rationales*

Assessments

- Assess hydration level and calorie intake (intake and output, moistness of mucous membranes). Insensible fluid loss increases as a result of the increased metabolic rate during labor, so prolonged labor and prescribed nothing by mouth status can result in dehydration. If the woman is on nothing by mouth status, glucose reserves may become depleted, further decreasing available energy for UCs.

Independent Nursing Actions

- For fatigue caused by hypertonic uterine dysfunction, assist with a warm bath or shower and administer narcotic analgesics per protocol (e.g., morphine, meperidine, or nalbuphine [Nubain]). Inhibits UCs, reduces pain, and promotes sleep (therapeutic rest). After a 4–6-hr rest period, the woman will often awaken in active labor with a normal UC pattern.
- Provide pain relief measures. See NDCP, "Back Pain," following; also see generic NDCP, "Pain,[1]" beginning on p. 18 in Chapter 2. Pain relief allows the woman to rest and restores her energy.

Nursing Diagnosis: BACK PAIN (Not a NANDA diagnosis)

Related Factors: pressure of fetal occiput pressing against sacrum secondary to persistent occiput posterior position and obstetric procedures (e.g., low forceps). Refer to the generic NDCP, "Pain,[1]" beginning on p. 18 in Chapter 2.

▮ *Nursing Activities and Rationales*

Patient/Family Teaching

- Teach nonpharmacologic pain relief methods to the woman and her partner. Keeps the partner involved; woman may find interventions by partner to be more supportive and effective than when performed by others.

Independent Nursing Actions

- Apply fist or heel of hand firmly to sacral area during UCs. Counterpressure helps relieve pressure of fetal occiput against sacrum.
- Apply heat or cold applications to sacral area. Provides stimuli to compete with pain stimuli; promotes circulation and muscle relaxation in the area.
- Assist the woman to assume a hands-and-knees position; then the partner or nurse places hands over her gluteal muscles and presses up and inward toward the center of the pelvis during UCs. Produces counterpressure.
- Have the woman assume a sitting position with knees slightly apart and feet flat on floor or stool; partner or nurse cups hands on woman's knees and presses knees straight back toward the woman's hips. Relieves pressure of fetal occiput against sacrum.
- Encourage the woman to sit on a birthing ball. Pelvic rocking opens the pelvis and may be comforting.
- Provide an environment conducive to rest. Conserves energy. Fatigue reduces the woman's ability to cope with UCs and increases perception of pain.
- Listen to the woman's expressions of pain and reassure her that it is not unusual for the occiput posterior position; assure her that she is not overreacting, that the pain is as she perceives it; assure her that the severity of the pain does not indicate immediate danger for her or her baby. Women sometimes become self-critical and wonder if they perceive more pain than they should or they may think that the pain means immediate danger to self or fetus. Accurate information and empathetic listening may help her relax and use breathing and relaxation techniques, thereby reducing the pain.
- Provide measures to relieve anxiety. Anxiety increases the perception of pain.
- Refer to measures for facilitating rotation of the fetal head, in the NDCP, "Risk for Maternal and/or Fetal Injury," beginning on p. 264 in this chapter. If it is possible to rotate the fetus from occiput posterior to occiput anterior, this will remove pressure of the head from maternal sacrum and relieve back pain.

Nursing Diagnosis: ANXIETY/ FEAR[1]

Related Factors: actual or perceived threat to maternal and/or fetal well-being; lack of experience with or information about required interventions; prior negative experiences with labor and birth; fatigue; pain; absence of a support person; restriction of maternal movement; and disappointment and frustration with slow labor progress. Refer to the generic NDCPs, "Anxiety,[1]" and "Fear,[1]" beginning on pp. 10 and 15, respectively, in Chapter 2.

▮ *Goals, Outcomes, and Evaluation Criteria*

- Woman verbalizes understanding of the cause(s) of dystocia.
- Woman verbalizes understanding of necessary procedures and treatments.
- Woman is able to cope with the labor and birth.
- Woman verbalizes increased comfort and decreased anxiety.

▮ *Nursing Activities and Rationales*

Assessments

- Assess anxiety level. Anxiety causes an increase in the levels of stress-related hormones (e.g., β-endorphin, adrenocorticotropic hormone, cortisol, and epinephrine). These hormones act on the smooth muscles of the uterus; increased levels can lead to dystocia by reducing uterine contractility. Stress interferes with adenosine triphosphate synthesis by depleting glycogen stores, reducing the amount of glucose available for energy.

Independent Nursing Actions

- Suggest position changes, if not contraindicated (e.g., left lateral side-lying, high Fowler's, sitting up, rocking in a rocking chair or on a birthing ball, walking, or on knees and leaning on partner or elevated head of bed). Decreases anxiety by relieving muscle tension associated with immobility.
- Assist with warm shower or whirlpool. This is psychologically and physically relaxing.
- Provide quiet environment, soothing music. Decreases unpleasant stimuli that may cause anxiety. If analgesics have been given to a woman with hypertonic UCs, quiet is essential for allowing her to sleep.
- Provide comfort measures such as mouth care, linen changes, and perineal care. Physical comfort measures promote relaxation and feeling of safety.

- Encourage use of learned breathing patterns and relaxation techniques. Provides distraction and promotes relaxation. Prolonged, difficult labor with high levels of anxiety can have adverse psychologic effects on the mother, father, and family.
- Support and encourage the woman and partner in their efforts. Reduces stress and enhances the labor process.
- Encourage activity and position changes as tolerated, unless contraindicated. Activity restrictions and confinement to bed cause psychologic stress, which can compound the physiologic stress of immobility and dystocia. Stress and anxiety can inhibit uterine function and cervical dilation. Anxiety increases the levels of stress-related hormones (β-endorphin, adrenocorticotropic hormone, cortisol, and epinephrine). These hormones reduce the contractility of the smooth muscles of the uterus.
- Do not leave the woman alone; the nurse, partner, or a doula should stay at bedside. Demonstrates caring. A certain amount of dependence occurs normally in labor, and physical presence of a caregiver is reassuring.

Collaborative Activities

- Administer analgesics according to protocol or order. Breaks the pain-anxiety-pain cycle. Pain causes increased anxiety; anxiety increases the perception of pain.

Patient/Family Teaching

- Provide information about the dysfunctional labor pattern, its causes, possible implications for mother and baby, and associated procedures/therapies; discuss advantages and disadvantages of treatment alternatives. Clear, accurate information gives the couple some control over the situation, thereby increasing their ability to cope.

▊ *Other Nursing Diagnoses*

- Risk for Deficient Fluid Volume[1] related to increased metabolic rate, vomiting, diaphoresis, and prescribed nothing by mouth status.
- Ineffective Coping[1] related to anxiety and fear, unrealistic expectations for labor and birth, exhaustion from prolonged labor, insufficient support system, feelings of powerlessness and loss of control, situational crisis, and lack of accurate information.

PRECIPITOUS BIRTH

Precipitous labor is an abnormal labor pattern in which birth occurs within 3 hours of onset. It occurs in about 2% of live births. A *precipitous birth* is one that occurs after a labor of any length; the infant is born rapidly after the cervix is completely dilated, perhaps with only one voluntary push by the mother.

Because some women do not perceive the UCs to be painful and may not even be aware of them, birth may occur at home or en route to the birthing unit. These women have soft perineal tissue that readily stretches, allowing the fetus to descend quickly through the pelvis. Rapid labor and delivery is more likely to occur in grand multiparity or with oxytocin use. In the birthing unit, birth may occur before the physician, nurse practitioner, or midwife is present.

▊ *Key Nursing Activities*

- Identify possible sudden birth and summon additional personnel.
- Promote fetal oxygenation and maternal comfort.
- Proceed in a calm, reassuring manner.
- Identify and prevent complications.
- Summon physician, midwife, nurse practitioner, or hospitalist if applicable.
- Record, at minimum, the following: time of rupture of membranes, amount, color, and odor of amniotic fluid, position of fetus at birth, presence of nuchal cord, time of birth, time of expulsion of placenta, appearance/intactness of placenta, Apgar scores at 1 and 5 minutes, infant's gender, mother's condition, and any medications that were given to the mother or the newborn.

▊ *Etiologies and Risk Factors*

Hypertonic, tetanic UCs cause rapid labor progress (cervical dilation and effacement); along with decreased pelvic resistance and/or a small fetus, fetal descent is rapid, and precipitous birth occurs. Precipitous delivery is more likely to occur with grand multiparity or induction with oxytocin.

Risk Factors

- Hypertonic, tetanic UC pattern from oxytocin or amniotomy
- Large pelvis
- Multiparity
- Preterm or small-for-gestational-age infant
- 40–49 years of age
- Previous precipitous birth
- Family history of precipitous birth

▊ *Signs and Symptoms*

- Lack of awareness that UCs are occurring
- Low back discomfort, not identified as labor
- Nausea and vomiting
- Abrupt onset of frequent, intense UCs, with little uterine relaxation between them
- Rapid cervical dilation and fetal descent
- Urge to bear down (push), with almost simultaneous rectal/perineal bulging and increased vaginal show

▌ *Collaborative Problems*

This section lists potential complications of precipitous labor/birth to the mother and the fetus.

Maternal Complications

- Postpartum hemorrhage from premature separation of the placenta
- Infection
- Uterine rupture
- Lacerations of the perineum, vagina, and cervix from loss of fetal head descent

Fetal Complications

- Hypoxia/anoxia
- Intracranial hemorrhage

COLLABORATIVE (STANDARDIZED) CARE FOR ALL WOMEN HAVING A PRECIPITOUS BIRTH

Perform a comprehensive assessment to identify individual needs for teaching, emotional support, and physical care.

▌ Potential Complication of Precipitous Labor/Birth: POSTPARTUM HEMORRHAGE

Refer to the generic collaborative care plan, "Potential Complication: Hemorrhage," beginning on p. 28 in Chapter 3; refer to "Postpartum: First 4 Hours After Birth (Stage IV Labor)," beginning on p. 307 in Chapter 9; and refer to "Postpartum Hemorrhage," beginning on p. 343 in Chapter 10.

▌ Potential Complication of Precipitous Labor/Birth: INFECTION

Refer to the generic collaborative care plan, "Potential Complication: Infection," on p. 29 in Chapter 3; refer to "Postpartum: First 4 Hours After Birth (Stage IV Labor)," beginning on p. 307 in Chapter 9; and refer to "Postpartum Infection," beginning on p. 347 in Chapter 10.

Preventive Nursing Activities

- If time permits, scrub hands with soap and water and don sterile gloves; if available, place sterile drapes under woman's buttocks. Prevents the introduction of pathogens into the birth canal.

▌ Potential Complications of Precipitous Labor/Birth: UTERINE RUPTURE; AMNIOTIC FLUID EMBOLISM; LACERATIONS OF THE PERINEUM, VAGINA, AND CERVIX; FETAL HYPOXIA/ ANOXIA; INTRACRANIAL HEMORRHAGE

Refer to "Uterine Rupture," beginning on p. 293 in this chapter. Also, for routine assessments (e.g., FHR) and nursing activities, refer to "Normal Labor: Second Stage" and "Normal Labor: Third Stage," beginning on pp. 232 and 238, respectively, in Chapter 7.

NOTE: The rapidity at which labor and birth progress will affect the nurse's ability to perform some of the interventions in this care plan.

Focus Assessments

- Inquire whether the woman has attended childbirth preparation classes or what other preparation she has had. Identifies areas for teaching, e.g., labor process, breathing/ relaxation techniques, so that the woman can cooperate with interventions and reduce the risk of injury.
- Determine fetal position (Leopold's maneuvers). If abnormal fetal presentation or position is found, it is essential to immediately transport the woman to a hospital or birthing unit; or, if in the hospital, to prepare for surgical birth.
- Perform vaginal examination to determine cervical dilation and effacement. Estimates imminence of birth.
- Note history of precipitous birth in woman or family. Identifies risk and enables time to prepare for a rapid labor and delivery.
- Observe for perineal bulging, crowning, rectal distention and passage of feces, and increased vaginal discharge. These signs result from compression of the rectum and perineum by the descending fetal presenting part and indicate imminent birth.
- After crowning, check to see if the amniotic sac is intact. If so, tear it with a clamp or other sharp instrument so the newborn will not breathe in amniotic fluid at its first breath.
- After birth of fetal head, insert a finger in back of the head to check for the umbilical cord. Prevents asphyxiation. If cord is around the neck, the nurse bends the fingers like a hook and pulls the cord over the baby's head. If this cannot be done (e.g., because the cord is tightly looped), place 2 clamps on the cord, cut between clamps, and unwind it. Continue to deliver the head in a downward motion

(external rotation) after suctioning out the mouth and nose, with gentle downward pressure on the side of the infant's head until the anterior shoulder is delivered. The remainder of the infant's body then slides free for the birth. Place the infant in a downward position to suction again if needed. The infant is then placed on a drape or warm blanket on the mother's abdomen. After the cord ceases pulsating, two Kelly hemostat clamps are placed on the cord, followed by the application of the plastic umbilical clamp.

- After placental expulsion, inspect the placenta to see if it is intact. Save it for inspection by the primary caregiver. Retained placental fragments can cause postpartum hemorrhage and infection.
- Following the birth, assess uterine firmness and amount of vaginal bleeding. Massage fundus if necessary to prevent hemorrhage. A contracted uterus compresses the blood vessels at the placental site; if the uterus is not firm, it continues to bleed.
- Inspect perineum for lacerations. In order to institute measures to control bleeding, if needed.

Preventive Nursing Activities

- Have the woman remain in side-lying position, if possible. Improves fetal oxygenation by preventing aortocaval compression, which decreases cardiac output and, thereby, circulation of blood through the placenta to the fetus. Slows fetal descent and minimizes perineal tears.
- Administer oxygen to the mother. Because the uterus relaxes for such a short time between contractions, and because the UCs are so strong, the circulation to the fetus is decreased. It is important that the blood that does reach the fetus be well oxygenated.
- Administer IV fluids per protocol. Maintains blood volume adequate for placental perfusion. See preceding rationale.
- Stop oxytocin if it is being used. Slows the progress of labor by reducing the intensity of the UCs.
- Give tocolytic medication per protocol or order, if there is time. Reduces the intensity and frequency of the UCs.
- When the baby crowns, have the woman pant or breathe rapidly and try not to push. Helps prevent forceful pushing and reduces the degree of lacerations and perineal trauma.
- Apply slight pressure to fetal head with one hand while supporting the perineum with the other; allow the head to be delivered between UCs. When head emerges, provide gentle upward traction to deliver the shoulders. Maintains flexion and slows delivery of the head, reducing perineal tearing and fetal subdural or dural tears that result from change in pressure within the fetal head. The body of the newborn must be supported as it emerges.
- Immediately after birth of the head, suction infant's mouth, throat, and then nasal passages. Suction again after the entire body has emerged. Prevents secretions from being aspirated with the first breath.

- Hold infant with care, to avoid dropping. The infant is covered with vernix and amniotic fluid, and is very slippery.
- Quickly dry and wrap/cover the infant. Prevents heat loss and cold stress.
- When the infant is stable, place it on the mother's abdomen, keeping infant's head slightly lower than the body. Gravity facilitates drainage of fluid and mucus. Weight of the infant on the abdomen helps stimulate UCs and facilitates placental separation and expulsion.
- Do not pull on the cord in an effort to expel the placenta. This may tear and cause hemorrhage.
- Place one hand above the symphysis pubis and maintain gentle, downward traction on the cord; instruct the mother to push. Prevents uterine inversion and expels the placenta.
- Cut the umbilical cord with sterile scissors after clamping with two Kelly clamps/hemostats, and then clamp with sterile clamp, if available. Place clamp about 2 inches from the infant's abdomen. Sterile equipment helps prevent infection; clamp cannot be close to the abdomen because the cord will dry and shrink, making it too tight.
- Put the newborn to breast as soon as possible. Sucking stimulates release of oxytocin from the maternal pituitary gland, stimulating uterine contraction and reducing bleeding from the placental site.
- Clean perineum and area under maternal buttocks. Removes pathogens and medium for their growth.
- If there are perineal lacerations, press a clean perineal pad against the perineum and instruct the woman to press her thighs together. Reduces the amount of bleeding until the physician/midwife can suture.

INDIVIDUALIZED (NURSING DIAGNOSIS) CARE PLANS

The care plans in this section were developed to address unique patient needs.

Nursing Diagnosis: ANXIETY/FEAR[1]

Related Factors: disappointment and fear because the primary care provider is not present; alarm that labor is progressing so rapidly; panic that the mother and the fetus are in danger because the physician/midwife is not present. Refer to the generic NDCPs, "Anxiety[1]" and "Fear,[1]" beginning on p. 10 and 15, respectively, in Chapter 2.

Nursing Activities and Rationales

Independent Nursing Actions

- Keep the woman informed about her labor progress. Helps reduce fear of the unknown; provides a sense of being in control.

- Encourage the partner or family member to remain with the woman; explain how that person can help. Enhances woman's sense of security; the most meaningful, anxiety-relieving support may come from a significant other.
- Assure the woman that you will stay with her. Relieves feelings of fear and abandonment that may occur if primary care provider is not present.
- Remain calm, keep movements unhurried. Implies that the nurse is competent and reassures the woman; if the nurse appears anxious or hurried, this will produce anxiety in the woman.
- After assessments indicate that the newborn is stable, place the baby on the mother's abdomen; allow the father/partner to hold the infant. Promotes parent–infant attachment; reassures the parent(s) that the baby is well and in no immediate danger.

Patient/Family Teaching

- Provide instructions and explanations briefly, in clear, simple language. Most women in this situation are highly anxious; severe anxiety interferes with the ability to process and retain information. In addition, in a rapid labor, the woman is experiencing many physical stimuli, which also interfere with her cognition.

Collaborative Activities

- Direct auxiliary personnel to notify physician/midwife and bring the emergency delivery pack; inform woman/partner that help has been summoned. If not in a birthing unit, ask for help from a bystander or the partner. Nurse must remain with the woman to ensure maternal and fetal safety; however, it is important to summon medical assistance in case complications occur, as well as for maternal reassurance. The woman/partner may feel more secure knowing that the physician/midwife will arrive soon.

▌ Nursing Diagnosis: PAIN[1]

Related Factors: myometrial hypoxia secondary to strong UCs with little relaxation between; insufficient time between UCs for the woman to rest and prepare for the next contraction. Refer to the generic NDCP, "Pain,[1]" beginning on p. 18 in Chapter 2.

Assessments

- Inquire whether the woman has attended childbirth preparation classes or what other preparation she has had. Determines whether she has learned any techniques to cope with the UCs.
- Check for bladder distention. May increase discomfort and cause bladder trauma; encourage the woman to void, as needed.

Independent Nursing Actions

- Ask the support person or, if not in a birthing unit, an apparently competent bystander to assist the woman with breathing and relaxation techniques and perform effleurage. It is difficult to relieve pain during a precipitous labor or birth because UCs are so frequent and intense that the woman has little time between UCs to prepare and cope with the next one (e.g., by using breathing techniques). Also, the nurse may be occupied with other activities in preparation for the birth, and so may not be able to help coach the woman. Narcotic analgesia cannot be given when birth is imminent because of the risk of newborn respiratory depression. Regional anesthesia may not be useful because of the difficulty of administering it during the intense labor and because it will probably not have time to become effective. Effleurage provides cutaneous stimulation, which competes with pain impulses for transmission to the CNS; relaxation techniques may reduce tension and anxiety, thereby decreasing the perception of pain.

INTRAPARTUM PREECLAMPSIA

Approximately 8% of all pregnant women will develop *preeclampsia*, which is defined as the development of gestational hypertension plus proteinuria for the first time after 20 weeks of gestation. In the presence of trophoblastic disease, it can develop before 20 weeks of gestation. Sometimes the first signs of gestational hypertension do not occur until the woman is in labor, and occasionally not until the early postpartum period. BP returns to normal by 12 weeks postpartum. If BP does not return to normal, the woman may have chronic hypertension. *Eclampsia* is the development of seizures or coma in the woman with preeclampsia that cannot be attributed to other causes.

Severe preeclampsia and eclampsia can have serious complications during labor, affecting all cells in all body systems. Symptoms and damage range from mild to life threatening. Some of the effects to the woman can be renal and liver damage, pulmonary edema, congestive heart failure, retinal detachment, thrombocytopenia, oliguria, cerebral hemorrhage, pulmonary embolism, disseminated intravascular coagulation (DIC), abruptio placentae, CNS irritability, seizures, coma, and death. Fetal risks include IUGR, hypoxia, preterm birth, and nonreassuring fetal status related to abruptio placentae, all of which increase the risk for infant mortality.

The HELLP syndrome (hemolysis, elevated liver enzymes, and low platelet count) is one way severe preeclampsia sometimes manifests itself and is an indication of hematologic and hepatic involvement. For antepartum care, refer to " Hypertensive Disorders of Pregnancy," starting on p. 171 in Chapter 6. Also refer to "Normal Labor: First Stage," "Normal Labor: Second Stage," and "Normal Labor: Third Stage," in Chapter 7.

▌ *Key Nursing Activities*

- Review the health history.
- Establish baseline vital signs (especially BP while the woman has been on her left side for at least 15 minutes), weight, and lab results upon admission.
- Provide a quiet environment conducive for rest.
- Monitor for signs of worsening condition or complications of gestational hypertension (headache, visual changes, sudden edema, especially of hands and face, epigastric pain, disorientation, or seizures).
- Monitor FHR.
- Monitor for toxic effects and side effects of MgSO$_4$.

▌ *Etiologies and Risk Factors*

- Maternal age less than 17 years or older than 35 years.
- First pregnancy or a pregnancy with a new partner.
- History of preeclampsia in family or previous pregnancies.
- African American ethnicity.
- Multiple gestation.
- History of preexisting medical condition (chronic hypertension, diabetes or gestational diabetes, lupus or other autoimmune diseases, maternal infection, obesity).
- Low socioeconomic status.

▌ *Signs and Symptoms*

Refer to "Hypertensive Disorders of Pregnancy," beginning on p. 170 in Chapter 6.

▌ *Diagnostic Studies*

- Hourly check of urine for protein and specific gravity test.
- 24-hour urine collection and check for protein and/or creatinine clearance. Detects glomerular damage; 5+ proteinuria indicates a 24-hour protein loss of 5 g or more.
- Complete blood cell count (CBC) or hemoglobin (Hgb), hematocrit (Hct), platelets. Detects hemoconcentration and indicates worsening condition.
- Electrolyte levels. Detects imbalances, especially hypernatremia and hyponatremia.
- Liver function tests and bilirubin. Detects degree of hepatic involvement and progression of disease.
- Blood urea nitrogen, uric acid, and serum creatinine. Assesses for renal function.
- Clotting studies. Assesses for thrombocytopenia or DIC.
- Ultrasound or serial sonography, nonstress tests, biophysical profiles. Tests of fetal well-being.
- Magnesium sulfate (MgSO$_4$) levels. Monitors for therapeutic range and prevents toxic levels.

▌ *Medical Management*

- Good prenatal care and oral hygiene, monitoring and management of preexisting conditions, and adequate nutrition to prevent preeclampsia.

- Compliance with treatment plan to control mild preeclampsia at home.
- Birth of the infant is the only cure for preeclampsia.
- Labor induction by IV oxytocin if there is evidence of fetal maturity and cervical readiness.
- Labor induction or cesarean birth for the woman with severe preeclampsia at 32–34 weeks' gestation.
- In severe cases (i.e., if there are signs of severe preeclampsia with maternal oliguria, renal failure, and signs of the HELLP syndrome) cesarean birth is appropriate regardless of fetal maturity.
- IV MgSO$_4$. Prevents seizure activity; it may also lower BP; may be given with oxytocin. MgSO$_4$ depresses smooth muscles and may diminish UCs, in which case oxytocin is then used to augment labor.
- Oral antihypertensives. Maintains diastolic BP between 90 and 100 mmHg; decreasing the diastolic BP to less than 90 mmHg may decrease uterine blood flow and cause fetal compromise.
- IV antihypertensives. For hypertension unresponsive to oral medication and for hypertensive crisis.
- Bed rest, calm environment, and avoidance of stimulation.
- Calcium gluconate should be available in case the Mg^{++} level becomes toxic. It is an antidote for magnesium.
- Maternal oxygen during labor. May be needed if fetal response to UCs indicates.
- Birth in Sims position or lithotomy position with a wedge under right buttock.
- Invasive hemodynamic monitoring (central venous pressure or pulmonary artery wedge pressure) for eclampsia and sometimes for severe preeclampsia, usually in an intensive care unit setting.
- Betamethasone or dexamethasone if fetus has immature lung profile or is at 34–36 weeks' gestation. Decreases risk for respiratory distress syndrome and necrotizing enterocolitis.
- Fluid and electrolyte replacement. The goal is to correct hypovolemia without causing circulatory overload.
- Sedatives (e.g., diazepam [Valium]). Occasionally given to encourage quiet bed rest or for seizures.
- Furosemide (Lasix). Loop diuretic given for pulmonary edema.
- Digitalis. For congestive heart failure and circulatory failure.
- Dietary modifications. Protein intake between 80 and 100 g/day or 1.5 g/kg/day; sodium intake of less than 6 g/day; non-caffeinated fluids.
- Doppler velocity beginning at 30–32 weeks' gestation. Screens for fetal compromise.

▌ *Collaborative Problems*

Potential Complications of Preeclampsia

- Ineffective tissue perfusion (pulmonary, renal, cerebral, cardiac, hepatic)
- Eclampsia (seizures) and/or coma
- HELLP syndrome (hemolysis, elevated liver enzymes, low platelet count)

- Hemorrhage secondary to placental separation, HELLP syndrome, and/or DIC
- Fetal compromise

Potential Complication of MgSO$_4$ Therapy

- CNS depression

COLLABORATIVE (STANDARDIZED) CARE FOR ALL WOMEN WITH PREECLAMPSIA

Perform a comprehensive assessment to identify individual needs for teaching, emotional support, and physical care.

Nursing Diagnosis: RISK FOR INEFFECTIVE TISSUE PERFUSION (PULMONARY, RENAL, CEREBRAL, CARDIAC, OR HEPATIC)

Refer to the NDCP, "Ineffective Tissue Perfusion (Pulmonary, Cardiovascular, Renal, Cerebral, and Hepatic)[1]" in "Hypertensive Disorders of Pregnancy," beginning on p. 170 in Chapter 6.

Goals, Outcomes, and Evaluation Criteria

- VSs remain within a safe level throughout labor.
- No adventitious lung sounds auscultated.
- Woman reports relief from headaches or visual changes.
- Deep tendon reflexes normal to brisk with no clonus.
- Hct stabilizes.
- Woman is alert and oriented.
- Woman has urinary output of 30 ml/hour or more.

NIC Interventions[2]

Surveillance (6650)—Purposeful and ongoing acquisition, interpretation, and synthesis of patient data for clinical decision making.

Vital Signs Monitoring (6680)—Collection and analysis of cardiovascular, respiratory, and body temperature data to determine and prevent complications.

Nursing Activities and Rationales

Assessments

- Weigh on admission to the hospital; compare with prenatal record for abnormal weight gain pattern. Detects fluid retention and monitors circulation status.
- Monitor BP every 1–4 hours, or more often, as indicated by medication or by the woman's status. Provides information for recognizing progression to severe preeclampsia or eclampsia, and for evaluating results of medications.

- Assess the respiratory rate, rhythm, and depth for ease or difficulty in breathing and for coughing. If pulmonary edema is developing, the woman's respirations will increase as she struggles to get enough oxygen; the rhythm and depth will change, and coughing will occur.
- Auscultate lung sounds over the anterior and posterior chest, including all five lobes. Lung sounds should remain clear to auscultation. Moist crackles and rhonchi are abnormal lung sounds and a sign of pulmonary edema.
- Assess maternal heart rate and pattern. Identifies decreased cardiac perfusion, alterations in fluid volume, alterations in electrolyte levels, and/or renal damage.
- Assess peripheral circulation including edema, skin color, temperature of the extremities, capillary refill time, and peripheral pulses. Determine degree of pitting edema by pressing over bony areas. The peripheral pulse rate should be equal to the apical pulse. Skin color should be without pallor or cyanosis, temperature warm to touch, and capillary refill time less than 3 seconds. Dependent edema is normal in pregnancy; however, edema in nondependent areas such as the face, hands, and sacrum is a sign of gestational hypertension.
- Assess for nausea and vomiting. Signs of preeclampsia.
- Assess for pain. Headaches, especially frontal, are a sign of preeclampsia; epigastric pain is a sign of liver congestion and involvement; edema and decreased perfusion may cause pain and discomfort in other sites. Labor contractions may require pain relief measures because pain can further elevate the BP.
- Insert indwelling catheter and monitor hourly intake and output. Measure every voiding if the woman does not have an indwelling catheter. Output of less than 30 ml/hr (or less than 700 ml in 24 hours) is a sign of renal insufficiency. Intake should correlate with output, taking into consideration the insensible water loss when normal functioning is present. If urine output is insufficient and MgSO$_4$ therapy continues with no change, the woman will develop magnesium toxicity.
- Monitor urine protein hourly or with each voiding. A reading of 3+ or 4+ is a sign of glomerular involvement and severe preeclampsia.
- Assess for signs of CNS irritability (pupil reaction and eye movement, deep tendon reflexes, and clonus). Hyperreactivity and clonus indicate progression to severe preeclampsia.
- Assess for scotomata (dark spots or flashing lights in the field of vision) or other visual changes. These are signs of impending eclampsia.
- Assess for loss of vision (usually temporary). This is a sign of impending cerebral hemorrhage, the most serious complication of eclampsia.
- Assess emotional response and understanding of gestational hypertension and treatments. Identifies woman's coping responses, her level of understanding, and her need for teaching and emotional support.

- Assess fetal heart rate or continuous fetal monitoring if indicated. Detects fetal status.

Independent Nursing Actions

- Assist the woman on bed rest to change her position every 2 hours. Use the side-lying position or supine with a wedge under the back near the kidneys. Changing positions is important to increase blood flow and tissue perfusion. Side-lying prevents aortocaval compression.
- Encourage a high-protein, high-fiber, moderate-sodium diet. Produces less fluid retention while supporting healing and facilitating bowel function.

Collaborative Activities

- Start IV fluids as ordered, with a catheter gauge large enough (16–20 gauge) to give blood, blood products, or fluids if needed. The woman may need blood, blood products, or fluids if her condition worsens. In preeclampsia, the intravascular compartment loses fluid, so hypovolemia can occur very quickly; an IV catheter will be more difficult to insert if this happens. An IV line is also necessary for administration of medications.
- Draw lab specimens as ordered and report adverse findings to the physician. Laboratory tests are used to assist with the diagnosis of preeclampsia, to identify a worsening state, and to monitor for complications. Some lab tests require prompt reporting to the physician for management of the woman.
- Administer medications as ordered, implementing safe techniques and utilizing appropriate nursing interventions. Controls BP and prevents complications. For example, antihypertensive medications require BP monitoring before and after administration. $MgSO_4$ administration requires frequent assessment of the respiratory rate, urinary output of at least 30 ml/hour, the presence of deep tendon reflexes, infusion by an infusion pump piggybacked to mainline fluids, and laboratory tests for therapeutic or toxic levels.
- Administer oxygen if ordered for maternal or fetal needs. Late and variable FHR decelerations are signs of decreased placental perfusion, and the mother may need to change positions and have oxygen.
- Arrange for social services or pastoral care as needed. Provides additional source of support.

Patient/Family Teaching

- Teach the effect of the side-lying position on blood flow and tissue perfusion. The side-lying position keeps pressure from the gravid uterus off the inferior vena cava and aorta. This promotes venous return to the heart and increases cardiac output, thereby promoting maternal and fetal circulation. Understanding may increase compliance and reduce anxiety.
- Teach the importance of rest for improving perfusion to the kidneys. The kidneys are more efficient while a woman is lying down or sleeping. The kidneys require a great deal of blood at all times; while sleeping, the body has a lower blood requirement in other areas of the body, so more blood is available to the kidneys. Central circulation is improved when lying down because blood does not have to work against gravity to return from the periphery to the heart. If the woman understands the importance, she may be more likely to rest.

Potential Complication of PIH: ECLAMPSIA (SEIZURES), COMA

Focus Assessments

- Assess deep tendon reflexes (brachial, wrist, patellar, or Achilles tendons). CNS changes such as headache and hyperreflexia indicate preeclampsia, which may progress to eclampsia.
- Assess for clonus by vigorously dorsiflexing the foot while holding knee in flexed position. This is a sign of CNS irritability. If clonus is present, measure it as 1–4 beats or sustained.
- Monitor for visual disturbances, epigastric pain, vomiting, persistent or severe headache, hyperreflexia, pulmonary edema, or cyanosis. These are signs/symptoms of impending eclampsia.

Preventive Nursing Activities

- Administer $MgSO_4$ by infusion pump, as ordered. Helps prevent seizures by acting on myoneural junction to depress CNS. Administering via pump prevents magnesium from being administered too rapidly, which can result in cardiac dysrhythmias.
- Maintain a calm, quiet, restful environment with low lighting and minimal stimulation if CNS irritability is a potential complication. Helps to prevent seizure activity.
- Allow the woman to watch TV or do other quiet activities. Also, allow significant others at the bedside, but encourage quiet and rest. The woman may become upset and anxious if she cannot have family/partner at the bedside or if she has no activities or distraction.

Potential Complication of PIH: HELLP SYNDROME

Focus Assessments

- Assess for jaundice (although it is not often seen). Hemolysis occurs when red blood cells are damaged during passage through small, damaged blood vessels, resulting in hyperbilirubinemia, especially if liver congestion occurs.

- Assess for epigastric or right upper-quadrant abdominal pain. Associated with liver distention or ischemia, which occur when blood flow is obstructed due to fibrin deposits.
- Assess for nausea, vomiting, malaise, and flulike symptoms. All are symptoms that can occur with HELLP syndrome.
- Assess lab results for thrombocytopenia. A frequent finding in preeclampsia. Platelets aggregate at sites of vascular damage and vasospasm, resulting in platelet count of less than 100,000/mm^3, which is critical.
- Assist with obtaining specimens for a CBC, clotting factors, platelet count, and liver enzymes. HELLP syndrome is diagnosed on the basis of laboratory results rather than clinical symptoms. All women with symptoms of HELLP syndrome should have these tests, regardless of their BP or presence of protein in their urine; a woman with HELLP syndrome may not have symptoms of severe preeclampsia.

Preventive Nursing Activities

- Start IV fluids as ordered with a catheter gauge large enough (16–20 gauge) to give blood or blood products if needed. The woman may need blood or blood products if her condition worsens (e.g., if platelet count is less than 20,000/mm^3). In preeclampsia, the intravascular compartment loses fluid, so hypovolemia can occur very quickly. An IV catheter will be more difficult to insert if this happens. An IV line is also necessary for administration of medications.
- Prepare for immediate birth. Maternal mortality rates as high as 20% may occur with HELLP syndrome. Regardless of gestational age, a woman with true HELLP syndrome should give birth. At 30 weeks' gestation, labor may be induced with oxytocin; prior to that, cesarean birth is indicated.

Potential Complications of PIH: HEMORRHAGE SECONDARY TO PLACENTAL SEPARATION, HELLP SYNDROME, OR DIC

Refer to the generic collaborative care plan, "Potential Complication: Disseminated Intravascular Coagulation" and "Potential Complication: Hemorrhage," beginning on pp. 26 and 28, respectively, in Chapter 3.

Focus Assessments

- Assess for symptoms of preeclampsia. Preeclampsia increases the risk for abruptio placentae; the release of thromboplastin with abruptio placentae predisposes the woman to DIC.
- Assess hourly for vaginal bleeding and/or uterine rigidity. Signs of placental separation.

Preventive Nursing Activities

- Be prepared to administer blood or blood products as ordered utilizing safety precautions. The HELLP syndrome and/or DIC may develop as a result of preeclampsia, and the woman may hemorrhage. Blood products may be needed.

Potential Complication of PIH: FETAL COMPROMISE

Refer to the generic collaborative care plan, "Potential Complication: Fetal Compromise (Nonreassuring Fetal Heart Rate)," beginning on p. 27 in Chapter 3.

Focus Assessments

- Note results of prenatal tests (e.g., NST, amniocentesis). Determines fetal status prior to labor and predicts fetal response to labor and preeclampsia.
- When interpreting FHR pattern, note whether the woman is receiving MgSO$_4$ and/or diazepam (Valium). These medications may decrease FHR variability and cause CNS depression of the newborn.

Preventive Nursing Activities

- Encourage the woman to remain in lateral position or use wedge under right buttock if supine. Increases venous return and promotes optimal blood flow to the placenta by preventing compression of the aorta and inferior vena cava by the gravid uterus.
- Apply internal electrode to fetal presenting part. FHR variability can be more accurately monitored with an internal electrode only if membranes are ruptured.
- Reassure the woman that a pediatrician or neonatal clinical nurse specialist will be present at the delivery. The newborn may require resuscitation or other specialized care at birth.
- Ensure that emergency delivery pack, suction, oxygen, and emergency medications are at bedside or nearby. For immediate use in case of seizure or emergency delivery.

Potential Complications of MgSO$_4$ Therapy: CNS AND NEUROMUSCULAR DEPRESSION AND HYPOTENSION

Refer to the collaborative care plan "Potential Complications of Use of Magnesium Sulfate Therapy" in the care plan on "Hypertensive Disorders of Pregnancy" on pp. 170 in Chapter 6.

INDIVIDUALIZED (NURSING DIAGNOSIS) CARE PLANS

The care plans in this section were developed to address unique patient needs.

Nursing Diagnosis: FLUID VOLUME EXCESS[1] IN THE EXTRACELLULAR TISSUES

Related Factors: fluid shift from the intravascular system to the extracellular tissues; normal physiologic hemodilution of pregnancy; oxytocin administration; and sodium and water retention.

Goals, Outcomes, and Evaluation Criteria

- Electrolytes within a normal range
- Blood urea nitrogen, creatinine, and uric acid remain within a safe range
- Stable BP
- Temperature within normal limits
- Urinary output 30 ml/hour or more
- Lungs clear to auscultation

NIC Interventions[2]

Fluid Management (4120)—Promotion of fluid balance and prevention of complications resulting from abnormal or undesired fluid levels.

Fluid Monitoring (4130)—Collection and analysis of patient data to regulate fluid balance.

Fluid/Electrolyte Management (2080)—Regulation and prevention of complications from altered fluid and/or electrolyte levels.

Nursing Activities and Rationales

Assessments

- Auscultate lungs at least every 8 hours and more frequently if condition is worsening. To assess for crackles or rhonchi that could be a sign of pulmonary edema.
- Assess the woman's weight upon admission to the birthing center or acute care facility and daily at approximately the same time of day and with the same type of apparel. Weight is a good indicator of fluid gains or losses.
- Assess location and extent of edema; measure the degree of the pitting edema if present. Pregnant women normally have dependent edema in their feet and ankles due to the normal physiologic effects of progesterone on the vascular system. Assessing the pretibial area, face, hands, and sacrum if on bed rest provides a better assessment finding. Measuring the pitting with a tape measure objectifies the data and provides more precise information for comparison from one caregiver to another.

- Assess BP and pulse, especially if oxytocin is used to augment labor. The BP elevation that occurs with gestational hypertension may rise even more during labor as a result of anxiety and increased basal metabolic rate. This is even more critical if the woman is receiving oxytocin, because it causes sodium and water retention.
- Assess urine color and amount at least every 2 hours, hourly if on $MgSO_4$. Determines fluid shifts; urine becomes more concentrated as the fluid shifts from the intravascular to extracellular areas. Urinary amounts continue to decrease as glomerular filtration decreases and the kidneys become more ischemic.
- Assess for signs/symptoms of ineffective organ perfusion (e.g., decreased level of consciousness, decreased reflexes, epigastric pain). Progressive edema may reflect organ involvement. Refer to the NDCP, "Risk for Ineffective Tissue Perfusion (Pulmonary, Renal, Cerebral, Cardiac, or Hepatic),[1]" beginning on p. 275 in this chapter.
- Assess the laboratory/diagnostic test reports and inform the provider of abnormal findings. The nurse can help prevent complications for the mother and fetus by knowing the normal ranges for laboratory and diagnostic tests, recognizing changes that indicate the condition is worsening, and reporting promptly to the physician.

Independent Nursing Actions

- Assist the woman to a comfortable position that will decrease edema and promote optimal blood perfusion, on either her left or right side, or place wedge underneath one buttock. Increases venous return and promotes optimal blood flow to kidneys and placenta by preventing compression of the aorta and inferior vena cava by the gravid uterus.
- Provide skin care to edematous areas; avoid placing tape on edematous areas. Edema increases the risk of impaired skin integrity.

Collaborative Activities

- Administer IV fluids as ordered. Even though there is an excess of fluid in tissues, there is an intravascular fluid deficit. If the woman starts to bleed, hypovolemia can occur rapidly due to the low volume in the intravascular system; therefore, it is important to maintain adequate intravascular volume without creating fluid overload.
- Administer medications as ordered. Diuretics are not usually ordered for preeclampsia; however, furosemide (Lasix) may be given if pulmonary edema occurs. Antihypertensive medications and $MgSO_4$ may be ordered. As BP decreases and circulation becomes more normal, kidney function will improve and urine output will increase.
- Insert indwelling urinary (Foley) catheter. For accurate measurement of urine output to monitor fluid status. Also, the woman will probably be on bed rest.

Patient/Family Teaching

- Teach the importance of maintaining intake and output records. Increases the likelihood of the woman's/family's cooperation and, therefore, of obtaining accurate data.
- Teach the importance of urine collection for determining how the woman's condition can be monitored this way. Urine collections are often done to determine amount, creatinine clearance, and proteinuria. Discarding one urinary sample will make the test results inaccurate for a 24-hour measurement period and the test will have to be started over. Time is lost and data that might make the difference for a change in the management of the woman's care would not be available.

Nursing Diagnosis: ANXIETY/ FEAR[1]

Related Factors: unknown and unpredictable outcomes for the fetus, self, and family secondary to gestational hypertension and complications. Use with the generic NDCPs "Anxiety[1]" and "Fear,[1]" beginning on pp. 10 and 15 in Chapter 2.

Nursing Activities and Rationales

Assessments

- Assess whether the woman has had a prior experience with preeclampsia. Enables the nurse to plan necessary teaching and to correct any misconceptions.
- Assess what the woman knows about preeclampsia at this time. Provides a baseline to individualize the teaching plan and eliminate misconceptions. The woman may have received home care before admission, heard reports from others, looked it up on the Internet, or received education regarding it at the practitioner's office.
- Assess the woman's support system by identifying the person she turns to in time of emotional distress. The woman may not have consciously identified the person who helps her the most during time of need. Discussing past crises or emotional upset and having the woman identify the person who usually helps her will confirm for her that the support system is in place.

Independent Nursing Actions

- Use a calm and confident approach. Helps alleviate anxiety transference and instills a sense of control over the situation.
- Listen attentively to what the woman expresses about herself, her condition, and fears. Enables the nurse to understand what the woman fears and institute measures to help her deal with it.

Patient/Family Teaching

- Teach or reinforce the use of relaxation, breathing, and other coping strategies as appropriate for the stage and phase of labor. Helps relieve anxiety by diverting her attention from her fears.

Other Nursing Diagnoses

Also assess for the following nursing diagnoses, which are frequently present with this condition:

- Deficient Knowledge[1] regarding diagnostic tests, treatments, and prognosis for gestational hypertension.
- Pain[1] secondary to gestational hypertension (e.g., headache, epigastric pain, intense UCs secondary to oxytocin administration, placental abruption).

CESAREAN BIRTH

Refer to "Normal Labor: Third Stage," beginning on p. 240 in Chapter 7. For postpartum care, refer to the topic, "Postpartum Care After Cesarean Birth," beginning on page 334 in Chapter 9.

Cesarean birth is the surgical delivery of the fetus through an incision in the abdominal and uterine wall and is the most commonly performed surgery in the United States (Hikel, 2009). Cesarean birth is just as safe as a vaginal delivery (ACOG, 2010). There are two types of cesarean birth—a planned birth, such as a repeat cesarean birth, or unplanned emergent cesarean birth, such as in situations in which the woman is not successful in delivering the fetus vaginally after a long labor leading to a nonreassuring FHR pattern. The woman experiencing a cesarean birth requires delivery and postpartum care, postoperative surgical care, and psychosocial care addressing feelings relative to the mode of delivery.

Key Nursing Activities

- Provide information about procedures.
- Provide emotional support, especially in unplanned cesarean births.
- Involve the partner in the experience to the extent possible.
- Prepare for surgery: insert IV, insert indwelling catheter, perform abdominal skin preparation, administer preoperative medications, check laboratory results, and verify surgical consent.
- Monitor and use medical and surgical asepsis.

Etiologies and Risk Factors

Over one third of the births in the United States are by cesarean section. Cesarean birth may result from maternal, fetal, or placental factors that interfere with or prevent a vaginal birth. No absolute indicators for cesarean birth exist, but most are performed primarily for the benefit of the fetus or as a prophylactic measure to alleviate problems that may occur with a vaginal birth, such as CPD, instead of a trial of labor after cesarean (TOLAC), or by choice. Fetal factors include fetal intolerance to labor; disease or anomaly; malposition or malpresentation; cord prolapse; and macrosomia causing CPD. Maternal indications include hypertensive disorders, diabetes, active herpes genitalia, human papilloma virus that is obstructing the birth canal, and narrow pelvis not allowing descent of the fetus. Placental abnormalities include complete placenta previa or abruptio placenta causing maternal or fetal compromise.

Women older than 35 years have a cesarean birth rate of 30%, almost twice that for teenage women, while the African American rate is 2% more than all other races combined (Fries, 2010). Other women more likely to experience a cesarean birth are those who have private insurance, are of a higher socioeconomic status, or give birth in a private hospital. Fear of medical malpractice is another reason why cesarean birth is sometimes performed. As a rule, nurse midwives usually have a much lower rate of cesarean sections due to the number of low-risk women for whom they care and their continual support during labor.

Signs and Symptoms

Subjective. Maternal statements of exhaustion or inability to push.
Objective. Failure to progress, defined as descent of the fetus of less than 1 cm/hr in the primigravida, and 2 cm/hr in the multipara, and/or failure to dilate at least 1.2 cm per hour in the primigravida and 1.5 cm per hour in the multipara. Fetal intolerance to labor, defined as late or severe variable decelerations, no variability (flat baseline), fetal heart rate less than 110 beats per minute with less than average variability, or pH below 7.25. Fetal malposition, such as a transverse arrest. Fetal malpresentation, such as breech, shoulder, or face.

Diagnostic Studies

Diagnostic studies vary with the condition creating the need for cesarean birth. Some studies are routinely performed for all surgeries, as well (e.g., CBC, blood type and cross-match). The following are some examples:

- Preoperative CBC. Routine preoperative study.
- Urinalysis. Routine preoperative study.
- Coagulation profile that includes prothrombin time and partial thromboplastin time. Detects coagulation abnormalities.
- Serum electrolytes and Ph. Determines acid-base balance prior to surgery.
- Blood type and cross-match. Routine preoperative study.
- Serology, rapid plasma reagin (RPR). Tests for syphilis.
- Rapid beta Streptococcus. Identifies need for prophylactic antibiotics.
- Ultrasound. Establishes fetal position, presentation, gestational age, and placental location.
- Biophysical profile. Determines fetal well-being.
- Nonstress test. Determines fetal well-being.
- Amniocentesis. Determines fetal lung maturity if there is questionable gestational age.

- Postoperative CBC. Determines the effect of the blood loss.

Medical Management

The following represent intrapartal management. For postpartum medical management, see "Postpartum Care After Cesarean Birth," beginning on page 334 in Chapter 9.

- Intravenous fluids. For hydration and provides route for administration of medications and blood, if needed.
- Indwelling urinary catheterization. Facilitates monitoring of intake and output; keeps bladder empty to protect from inadvertent incision.
- Abdominal skin preparation. Removes pathogenic organisms.
- Sodium citrate and citric acid (Bicitra). Reduces the likelihood of serious pulmonary damage; this nonparticulate antacid is given prior to a cesarean birth to neutralize gastric secretions in case of aspiration.
- Metoclopramide (Reglan). Enhances gastric emptying and prevents nausea and vomiting.
- Cimetidine (Tagamet). Decreases gastric acid production.
- General anesthesia usually used in emergency situations; otherwise, regional anesthesia (either spinal or epidural).
- Preferably nothing by mouth or ice chips only. Keeps stomach contents to a minimum to prevent aspiration of stomach contents during or after surgery.
- Preoperative antibiotics different from those used for group B Streptococcus.

Collaborative Problems

Potential complications of cesarean birth include the following:

- Hemorrhage
- Thrombophlebitis
- Pulmonary embolism
- Incision and/or puerperal infection or dehiscence
- Urinary tract infection
- Maternal injury (e.g., aspiration, trauma)

COLLABORATIVE (STANDARDIZED) CARE PLAN FOR ALL WOMEN HAVING A CESAREAN BIRTH

Perform comprehensive assessment to identify individual needs for teaching, emotional support, and physical care.

Potential Complication of Cesarean Birth: HEMORRHAGE

Also use with the generic collaborative care plan, "Potential Complication: Hemorrhage," beginning on p. 28 in Chapter 3.

Focus Assessments

- Before surgery, determine if the woman gave informed consent and had all questions answered. Ensures the woman was informed of risks and benefits of the procedure in terms she understood as explained by the healthcare provider.
- Before surgery, remove nail polish from fingernails and toenails. Allows for viewing nail beds to assess circulatory status.
- Estimate blood loss or note the blood loss estimated by the anesthesia care provider. Establishes a baseline related to blood loss during surgery and recovery, for use in planning postpartum care.
- Monitor BP, heart rate, and respirations before, during, and after surgery and anesthesia. This is usually the responsibility of the anesthesiologist during surgery. Epidural and spinal anesthesia are particularly likely to cause hypotension in pregnant women because they relax smooth muscles in the blood vessels, thereby reducing BP. In pregnant women, peripheral vasoconstriction is the primary regulator of BP; when this regulator is blocked by anesthesia, the backup physiologic mechanisms are not adequate to maintain the BP. Excessive blood loss causes changes in VSs, which include hypotension due to decrease in circulating blood volume; tachycardia due to the heart's attempt to pump the available blood faster to nourish the body's organs; and initially tachypnea due to the respiratory system's compensation of the developing metabolic acidosis, and later bradypnea as the respiratory system begins to lack adequate oxygen to perform the function of breathing.
- Insert indwelling urinary catheter prior to surgery. Keeps the bladder empty, preventing bladder injury during surgery; allows for assessment of adequate kidney perfusion by monitoring urine output. The woman will be confined to bed after surgery until the epidural anesthesia wears off and she regains use of her legs.
- While woman is still in the operating room, assess uterine tone frequently. After birth, a contracted myometrium constricts the blood vessels at the placental site, preventing bleeding. Relaxation causes spurting of blood from the spiral arteries. Uterine atony is the most common cause of postpartum hemorrhage.
- Place sequential compression devices on the woman's legs as soon as she is placed on the operating room table prior to the epidural. Prevents blood stasis, which contributes to hypotension during spinal or epidural anesthesia.
- Assess lochial flow while the woman is still in the operating room and evacuate the vaginal vault prior to moving off the operating room table. Heavy lochial flow immediately after delivery is related to uterine atony or cervical or vaginal lacerations. Frequent monitoring of lochia is required to determine the amount of blood loss and whether it may

be due to atony (dark red in color) or laceration (bright red in color). During the postpartum period, more than one pad saturated per hour indicates excessive blood loss (one pad = 100 cc).
- Inspect abdominal dressing (saturated or oozing with blood). Circle and date/time drainage area with pen. Indicative of bleeding from the surgical site. A thick abdominal dressing is applied during surgery; unless it is saturated or soiled, it is not usually removed for 24–48 hours. After the woman is transferred to the recovery room and to the postpartum area, the circle allows other nurses to see how much bleeding has occurred in a given time.
- Note prenatal and intrapartum Hct levels. Provides a baseline for postpartum evaluation. Hct of 33% or more in the postpartum period usually indicates maternal tolerance of blood loss.
- Monitor urinary output. Less than 30 ml/hr indicates decreased kidney perfusion, which stimulates the renin-angiotension mechanism, thereby conserving vascular fluid.

Preventive Nursing Activities

- Provide IV fluids, as ordered. Ensures sufficient volume before surgery and during postpartum period. Prolonged labor before surgical birth contributes to hypovolemia. IV fluids expand the volume of circulating fluid, compensating for the relaxation of blood vessels caused by regional anesthesia (epidural or regional block is usually used unless there is an emergency, and then general anesthesia is more likely). Also provides a route for medication administration.
- Place a wedge under the woman's hip prior to surgery or adjust operating table to slant slightly to one side. Position must allow access to the abdomen for surgery; however, it is important to keep the fetus and uterus off the inferior vena cava, ensuring adequate venous return. Obstruction of the vena cava by the gravid uterus (when in supine position) can cause a 50% decrease in cardiac output.
- Administer blood replacement, as necessary. Replaces volume and oxygen-carrying capacity of the blood.
- Administer oxytocin (Pitocin), methylergonovine (Methergine), or carboprost tromethamine (Hemabate) immediately after birth, as ordered. Prevents hemorrhage by contracting the myometrium, compressing the exposed blood vessels at the placental site.

Potential Complication of Cesarean Birth: THROMBOPHLEBITIS

Refer to "Thromboembolic Disease," beginning on page 350 in Chapter 10. Nursing activities in this section are for intrapartum;

however, thrombophlebitis is usually an antepartum or a postpartum complication. It would be unusual to first recognize it during the intrapartum stage.

Focus Assessments

- Assess for positive Homan's sign. Provides baseline for evaluation during postpartum period. Complaints of calf pain with dorsiflexion of the foot may occur with deep vein thrombus.
- Assess for presence of redness; warmth; and painful, palpable lumps on legs. Provides baseline for evaluation during postpartum period. These are signs of superficial thrombophlebitis.
- Assess for varicose veins. Predisposes to thrombophlebitis by creating stasis of blood in the peripheral veins, allowing formed elements to settle out of the central flow and adhere to vessel walls.
- Assess history of previous venous thrombus. Identifies woman at higher risk for recurring thrombus.
- Assess IV fluid intake and adequacy of hydration (e.g., skin turgor). Establishes hydration status so that treatment can be initiated to compensate for the decrease in plasma volume that occurs after delivery through diaphoresis and diuresis. Dehydration contributes to sluggish circulation, which enhances thrombus formation.

Preventive Nursing Activities

- Report history of long labor or operative delivery to the receiving nurse when the woman is transferred from operating area. Clotting factors and plasma fibrinogen increase during pregnancy, which places the woman at high risk for development of thrombophlebitis. Immobility caused by a lengthy labor or an operative delivery increases formation of thrombi due to pooling and stagnation of blood in the lower extremities.
- Assist to ambulate as soon as condition is stable. If the woman is unable to ambulate, initiate active range of motion exercises. Prevents deep vein thrombus. Early ambulation prevents stagnation of blood in the lower extremities. Women will not usually be ambulatory for several hours postoperatively because of residual effects of the regional anesthesia; however, active range of motion during the recovery period promotes blood circulation by causing muscular contractions in the legs.
- Keep sequential compression devices on woman's legs until ambulating. Remove every 8 hours to inspect skin. Promotes venous return from the legs, decreasing stasis-induced thrombophlebitis. Removing sequential compression devices allows for inspection of skin for edema or other alterations.
- If there is time before the birth (e.g., for a planned cesarean birth), teach the woman about postoperative turning, coughing, and deep breathing measures. These measures improve oxygenation and circulation and help to prevent stasis in the peripheral blood vessels.

▌Potential Complication of Cesarean Birth: PULMONARY EMBOLISM

For focus assessments and postpartum care, refer to the collaborative care plan, "Potential Complication of Thrombophlebitis: Pulmonary Embolism," which begins on p. 352 in Chapter 10.

Focus Assessments

- Assess respiratory symptoms (e.g., dyspnea, tachypnea, pleuritic pain, cough, hemoptysis, rales). These are symptoms of pulmonary embolism (occlusion or infarction of the pulmonary circulation).
- Assess mental status (e.g., anxiety, syncope). May result from systemic hypotension and/or hypoxia, as well as from the unexpected and uncomfortable symptoms.
- Assess for cardiac symptoms (e.g., tachycardia, hypotension). The occlusion causes hypoxic vasoconstriction and pulmonary edema, thereby decreasing pulmonary-cardiac circulation and, subsequently, cardiac output.
- Assess integument (e.g., peripheral or central cyanosis). This is related to hypoxia.
- Assess for fever greater than 37°C (98.6°F). Indicates that the thrombus has caused infarction. Infarction (ischemia followed by necrosis) causes an inflammatory reaction, which results in increased temperature.
- Assess vital signs and oxygen saturation levels. Changes, especially in oxygen saturation levels, indicate hypoxia.

Preventive Nursing Activities

- Institute preventive measures. The best way to treat thrombophlebitis is to prevent it. If thrombophlebitis occurs, early treatment (including bed rest) may prevent dislodging of the thrombus into the circulation.
- Administer IV fluids, as ordered. Increases vascular volume and decreases likelihood of venous stasis. Helps prevent thrombophlebitis; if thrombophlebitis occurs, helps prevent clot extension. The woman will be on nothing by mouth status before and after surgery.
- Encourage use of sequential compression stockings or thrombo embolic deterrent (TED) hose while the woman is on bed rest. Promotes venous return from the legs, decreasing stasis-induced thrombophlebitis. These are more frequently ordered for women who have varicose veins.
- Ensure proper application and fit of elastic stockings. If stockings are too tight, they can actually impede circulation; if they are too loose, they are not effective. Correct measurement is the key to appropriate fitting of stockings.
- Encourage active and passive range of motion exercises while the patient is on bed rest. Promotes venous return from the legs, decreasing stasis-induced thrombophlebitis.

- Do not pad or prop pillows under knees. Pressure interferes with venous return from the legs, creating stasis.
- Instruct the woman not to cross her legs. Interferes with venous return from the legs, creating a risk for thrombophlebitis.
- Instruct the woman to make frequent position changes (at least every 2 hours) when sitting or lying for prolonged periods. Prevents venous stasis.

Potential Complications of Cesarean Birth: INCISION INFECTION AND/OR PUERPERAL INFECTION

Use with the generic collaborative care plan, "Potential Complication: Infection," beginning on p. 29 in Chapter 3. Also refer to the generic NDCP, "Risk for Infection,[1]" beginning on p. 21 in Chapter 2.

Focus Assessments

- Review history for preexisting infections and risk factors (e.g., diabetes, sexually transmitted infections). Determines level of risk and individualizes interventions.
- Note time that membranes ruptured. The longer the time from ROM to birth, the higher the risk of chorioamnionitis.
- Monitor sterile technique of all care providers. Ensures that sterile technique is observed.

Preventive Nursing Activities

- Observe sterile technique for invasive procedures such as vaginal exams, IV insertion, and insertion of indwelling urinary catheters. Prevents introduction of pathogens directly into the body.
- Perform preparation of abdominal area according to agency protocol (this may include shaving the abdomen and the mons). Removes microorganisms from the skin, preventing their introduction into the surgical incision.
- Provide surgical gown and mask for the partner, according to agency protocol. Prevents introduction of pathogens into the operating room.
- Perform perineal cleansing from front to back. Prevents introduction of *Escherichia coli* from anal area into the vagina and urinary meatus.
- Administer parenteral antibiotic preoperatively, as indicated. Antibiotics may be ordered to prevent an infection (especially if there is prolonged ROM) or to treat an existing infection.
- During antepartum period, encourage the woman to eat a diet high in protein, vitamin C, and iron. Enhances wound healing.

- Perform good hand washing and teach the woman, family, and visitors to wash their hands frequently. Removes pathogens on hands that can cause infections.

Potential Complication of Cesarean Birth: URINARY TRACT INFECTION

Use with the generic collaborative care plan, "Potential Complication: Urinary Tract Infection," beginning on p. 33 in Chapter 3, and the generic NDCP, "Risk for Infection,[1]" beginning on p. 21 in Chapter 2.

Focus Assessments

- Note the appearance of urine in indwelling catheter drainage tubes. Cloudiness is a sign of infection.

Preventive Nursing Activities

- Observe sterile technique for insertion of indwelling urinary catheter. Prevents introduction of pathogens directly into the bladder.
- Perform perineal cleansing from front to back. Prevents introduction of *E. coli* from anal area into the vagina and urinary meatus.

Potential Complication of Cesarean Birth: MATERNAL INJURY (E.G., ASPIRATION, TRAUMA)

Focus Assessments

- Determine whether the woman is wearing contact lenses and whether she has dental bridges or crowns. In case intubation and general anesthesia are required, reduces chance of injury.
- Ask time and content of last food and drink. Eating prior to surgery increases the risk of vomiting and aspiration; may preclude use of general anesthesia.
- After insertion of indwelling urinary catheter, monitor urine output. Reflects hydration level, kidney perfusion (and, therefore, circulatory adequacy); blood-tinged urine may indicate surgical trauma to bladder or ureter.

Preventive Nursing Activities

- Remove contact lenses, dentures, and jewelry. Tape rings if the woman does not wish to remove them. Reduces risk of injury.
- Ensure that suction and resuscitation equipment are available and functioning. For emergency use, in case

the woman vomits or other complications occur. Check equipment daily and record to maintain safely working equipment.

- Ensure that the woman remains on nothing by mouth status prior to surgery. Decreases the risk of vomiting and aspiration.
- Count instruments and sponges accurately, according to agency protocol. Ensures that nothing is accidentally left inside the woman's abdomen.
- Use approved transport devices when moving the woman. Prevents injury to the woman.

Nursing Diagnosis: ANXIETY[1]

Related Factors: unplanned or emergency cesarean birth, unfamiliar environment, and procedures. Use with the generic NDCP, "Anxiety,[1]" beginning on p. 10 in Chapter 2.

NIC Interventions[2]

Cesarean Section Care (6750)—Preparation and support of patient delivering a baby by cesarean section.

Nursing Activities and Rationales

Assessments

- Note whether cesarean birth was planned or unplanned. Even a planned surgical birth can create anxiety; however, with an unplanned cesarean, the couple has no time for emotional preparation.

Independent Nursing Actions

- Use touch, speak slowly, and remain calm. Communicates care and concern for the woman; prevents transmission of anxiety to the woman/couple.
- Maintain eye contact during preoperative procedures and surgery. Presence of caregivers wearing masks may be anxiety producing. Eye contact provides support.
- Include the woman/partner in discussions/conversations in the operating room. Ignoring the woman is depersonalizing and can increase anxiety.
- Urge the primary support person to remain with the woman as much as possible, if this is culturally acceptable and agreed to by the anesthesia care provider. Provides continuing emotional support.
- Provide the couple some private time if there is time before the birth. Gives them time to think about new information, gather their resources, and find effective coping strategies.
- Stay with the woman if her partner is not there or has to leave. Prevents feelings of abandonment and increased anxiety.

- If the birth is an unplanned cesarean birth, emphasize the positive aspects of the situation (e.g., a normal FHR, good nutritional status of the mother). Provides hope for a good outcome; reduces perception of threat.

Patient/Family Teaching

- Provide essential information about pre- and intraoperative procedures and sensations the woman may be experiencing. Verbal communication is important; silence can be frightening. Anticipatory guidance helps decrease anxiety. The woman may be anxious about sensations she is experiencing (e.g., the coldness of solutions used to prepare the abdomen, the pressure during the actual birth of the infant, the presence of unfamiliar equipment and masked/gowned personnel, the bright lights).

Nursing Diagnosis: RISK FOR IMPAIRED PARENT–INFANT/ CHILD ATTACHMENT[1]

Related Factors: emergency or unplanned cesarean birth; unfamiliar environment of the operating room; and preparations and equipment for surgery. Use with the generic NDCP, "Risk for Impaired Parent–Infant/Child Attachment,[1]" which begins on p. 19 in Chapter 2.

Goals, Outcomes, and Evaluation Criteria

- Parent(s) speak positively about the fetus and anticipate her/his birth.
- Parent(s) refer to the fetus as "her" or "him" or by a name they have chosen.

NIC Interventions[2]

Environmental Management: Attachment Process (6481)— Manipulation of the patient's surroundings to facilitate the development of the parent–infant relationship.

Nursing Activities and Rationales

Assessments

- Assess level of childbirth preparation. Determines whether lack of information may be contributing to any anxiety. Anxiety can interfere with attachment process.
- Assess age, ethnicity, degree of acculturation, use of personal space, and communication patterns. Provides data for meeting psychosocial needs. The amount of early physical contact desired is different among cultures.
- Observe for parent behaviors that indicate bonding (e.g., talking to the fetus, talking positively about the baby). Identifies emerging problem so that interventions can begin immediately.

- Assess the couple's perception of the birth experience, noting the circumstances surrounding the cesarean birth. A positive birth experience facilitates attachment.
- Assess for parental behaviors that indicate that they have not begun to attach to the fetus, (e.g., lack of interest in the birth, calling the fetus "it"). Parents who feel a loss from not experiencing a vaginal delivery need an opportunity to deal with those feelings before they are ready and prepared to begin the attachment process with their newborn. The cesarean birth experience may produce feelings of inadequacy and may require additional time for attachment to begin.
- Assess anxiety level. Anxiety can interfere with attachment.

Independent Nursing Actions

- In emergency situation, stay with the woman, offer reassurance, use touch. Relieves anxiety, which can interfere with her positive experience of the birth.
- When starting maternal IV, use tubing long enough to allow for freedom of movement. Enables the woman to hold and examine the infant after the birth.
- Limit number of people present prior to surgery, considering the parents' preferences. Provides a peaceful environment, limits stimuli that may provoke anxiety.
- If the father chooses not to be in the delivery room, allow him to be nearby, where he can hear the newborn's first cry; encourage him to carry the infant to the nursery for the initial assessment; and involve him in care of the woman in the recovery room to the extent possible. Facilitates attachment by increasing his involvement in the experience.
- Place the infant in the mother's arms following birth or in her arms when transporting to the recovery area. Provide opportunity for parent(s) to see and hold the baby immediately after birth. Perform as many assessments or interventions as possible with the infant on the mother's body or being held. Early physical contact promotes maternal and paternal attachment. Newborns have highly developed senses that allow them to actively participate in interactions from birth. Keep in mind that the physical condition of the mother and infant is the first priority.
- Keep parent(s) informed of the care that is being given to the newborn at birth. If possible, position the infant warmer so that the parents can see the newborn while care is given. Recovering mother and baby together is best when feasible. Birth is an emotionally charged time for all members of the family. As they express joy and pride, their feelings of accomplishment strengthen family bonds.
- Encourage early breastfeeding, e.g., during the recovery period. Promotes attachment. Stimulates maternal release of prolactin, which initiates the onset of lactation.
- Encourage parents to do whatever they feel comfortable doing in the way of holding and caring for the newborn. Some want immediate time; others may prefer to wait until the recovery period, when the infant is clean and dry. The parents' wishes should be supported to the extent that physical status allows.
- Encourage the mother to room in with her infant after the recovery period and as soon as she is able to care for the baby. Provides the parents with increased opportunities to interact with their infant and participate in reciprocal attachment behaviors.
- Encourage the parents to verbalize their feelings related to the birth experience, including any disappointments. So that those areas may be addressed. Feelings related to disappointment may interfere with successful attachment.

INDIVIDUALIZED (NURSING DIAGNOSIS) CARE PLANS

The care plans in this section were developed to address unique patient needs.

■ Nursing Diagnosis: ACUTE PAIN[1]/ DISCOMFORT

Related Factors: procedures, such as insertion of intravenous catheter and epidural or spinal catheter. Incisional pain may occur, rarely, as a result of incomplete epidural/spinal anesthesia; the woman having an unplanned cesarean birth because of intrapartum complications (e.g., dystocia) may be experiencing uterine contractions prior to administration of regional anesthesia.

Use with the generic NDCP, "Pain,[1]" beginning on p. 18 in Chapter 2. During the preoperative and intraoperative periods, the woman is more likely to experience discomfort; acute pain is more likely to occur in the postoperative/postpartum period.

■ *NIC Interventions[2]*

Cesarean Section Care (6750)—Preparation and support of patient delivering a baby by cesarean section.

■ *Nursing Activities and Rationales*

Assessments

- Palpate the bladder for distention. Prior to administration of anesthesia, this may be a source of discomfort.
- Assess the patient for evidence of muscular aches and pains. These can occur from being in one position for long periods of time.

Independent Nursing Actions

- Position the woman in a comfortable position, usually lateral recumbent, using pillows for support of back and legs. Muscle strain and lying in an uncomfortable position contribute to pain/discomfort.

- Maintain a quiet environment. Enhances rest and comfort and decreases anxiety.
- If there is time, teach the patient use of deep breathing exercises, relaxation techniques, and distraction. Assists with pain reduction postoperatively.
- Relieve anxiety as possible. Anxiety increases tension, which increases pain.

Patient/Family Teaching

- Explain the reasons for the pain the woman experiences. Enhances understanding and cooperation with methods for pain relief.
- Answer questions about anesthesia and medications that are available for relief of postoperative pain. Provides opportunities for the woman to participate in her plan of care.

Collaborative Activities

- Administer preoperative medications as ordered (e.g., sedatives). Potentiates the action of anesthetics; relieves anxiety, which can increase perception of pain.

Nursing Diagnosis: SITUATIONAL LOW SELF-ESTEEM[1]

Related Factors: the perception that the birth experience represents failure at a major life event; inability to deliver the infant vaginally, therefore not having a normal birth; the loss of control that frequently accompanies the emergency nature of some cesarean birth experiences; and change in body image.

▍ *Goals, Outcomes, and Evaluation Criteria*

- Woman verbalizes acceptance of self and own limitations.
- Woman expresses satisfaction with performance during the birth experience.
- Woman participates in making decisions about care.
- Woman maintains eye contact.

▍ *NIC Interventions[2]*

Cesarean Section Care (6750)—Preparation and support of patient delivering a baby by cesarean section.
Family Integrity Promotion: Childbearing Family (7104)—Facilitation of the growth of individuals or families who are adding an infant to the family unit.
Self-Esteem Enhancement (5400)—Assisting a patient to increase his/her personal judgment of self-worth.

▍ *Nursing Activities and Rationales*

Assessments

- Assess the woman's/couple's perceptions about cesarean birth, noting the circumstances surrounding the birth process. Assess the couple's feelings, anxieties, and role in the birth experience, including cultural influences on their perceptions. Assists the nurse in identifying a potential for self-concept disturbance during the postpartum period. Women who have an unplanned cesarean birth and general anesthesia have more negative perceptions of the birth experience than do women who have a vaginal delivery or a planned cesarean delivery.
- Emphasize the positive aspects of the experience. Assists the couple to not place blame or experience guilt for not undergoing a vaginal delivery. Parents may grieve the loss of an anticipated vaginal delivery.
- Assess the couple's usual coping strategies. Provides a baseline regarding past successful coping mechanisms. Building upon the couple's strengths will facilitate the integration of the cesarean birth experience in a positive manner.

Independent Nursing Actions

- Support the woman's partner and help him to share in the birth as he would in a vaginal birth, to the extent that this is culturally acceptable to the couple. Encourages perception of the event as a birth rather than a surgery. Presence and support of the partner helps the woman to respond positively to the experience, even though the birth may not occur as she had planned. The partner can help the woman recall the birth experience later; in a crisis situation, memory lapses are common.
- If the partner is not allowed or chooses not to be present in surgery, provide progress reports for him as much as possible. Relieves anxiety and helps him to remain involved.
- Provide choices in care when possible (e.g., choice of site for IV). Enhances sense of control over the situation.
- If the woman wears glasses, be sure they accompany her or her significant other to the operating room. Enables her to see the infant at birth.

Patient/Family Teaching

- Explain that it is normal to feel disappointed when birth does not occur as planned. The couple needs to understand that their feelings of failure related to the inability to deliver their newborn vaginally are expected. Once the nurse initiates the discussion, the couple will feel more comfortable in discussing the events that led to the cesarean delivery, recognizing that they did not cause the need for the cesarean birth. Their self-esteem will be enhanced and they will be able to focus on the positive outcome of the delivery.
- Reinforce that cesarean birth is, indeed, childbirth and not just a surgery. Use terms such as cesarean birth rather than cesarean section. Reassures the woman that her experience was not flawed or lacking in any way. The woman may feel that the cesarean birth is unnatural and may feel inadequate for not being able to give birth vaginally (i.e., normally).

VAGINAL BIRTH AFTER CESAREAN

Vaginal birth after cesarean (VBAC) is considered safe (ACOG, 2010). There are many factors as to why healthcare practitioners may or may not advise a trial of labor (TOL) after a cesarean. Because indications for primary cesarean birth (e.g., breech presentation, fetal intolerance to labor) do not necessarily recur, it may be possible to have a safe and successful birth with subsequent pregnancies. Except for a few special concerns, care is the same as the standardized intrapartum care for all women is. Refer to all of Chapter 7 for care of the woman during labor and birth.

Key Nursing Activities

- Provide encouragement and promote self-efficacy regarding the ability to achieve vaginal birth.
- Institute continuous electronic fetal and uterine monitoring in active labor.
- Provide venous access (e.g., saline lock) during active labor, per order or protocol.
- During TOL, evaluate for active labor (adequate UCs, engagement and descent of presenting part, and dilation and effacement of cervix).
- Observe for maternal or fetal complications; if complications occur, notify physician and institute emergency interventions.

Guidelines for Attempting VBAC

The following are recommended ACOG guidelines when contemplating VBAC (ACOG, 2010).

- Women with one prior low transverse uterine incision may be counseled and encouraged to attempt labor and VBAC.
- A woman with two or more previous cesarean births may attempt VBAC if she's had a prior vaginal delivery. The risk for uterine rupture is, however, greater for women with two previous cesarean births than for women with one previous cesarean birth.
- VBAC is contraindicated in women with a classic (vertical) or T-shaped uterine incision.
- The woman should have a clinically adequate pelvis and no other uterine scars.
- A physician must be immediately available throughout active labor to monitor labor and perform emergency cesarean birth if needed.
- There is insufficient data to determine risk of VBAC for women who have had external version, multiple gestation, breech presentation, large fetus (more than 4,000 g), or previous myomectomy.

Diagnostic Studies

- Sonography and/or maternal pelvimetry prior to TOL. Rules out CPD.
- Other antepartum tests to establish maternal and fetal well-being (e.g., CBC, blood type and screen). Refer to "Antepartum Fetal Monitoring and Diagnostic Tests," beginning on p. 60 in Chapter 4.

Medical Management

- Provide a 4–6-hour TOL and attempt vaginal birth if TOL indicates that it is safe and likely to be successful.
- Use oxytocin with caution, if necessary to augment labor.
- Prostaglandin preparations are contraindicated because of high risk of uterine rupture.
- Heparin or saline lock (or other venous access device).
- Clear liquids, or nothing by mouth if at higher risk (e.g., more than one previous cesarean).
- Continuous electronic fetal monitoring.
- Intrauterine pressure catheter or fetal electrode (if at higher risk).

Collaborative Problems

Potential Complications of VBAC

- Hemorrhage
- Rupture at site of uterine scar

COLLABORATIVE (STANDARDIZED) CARE FOR ALL WOMEN HAVING VBAC

Perform a comprehensive assessment to identify individual needs for teaching, emotional support, and physical care.

Potential Complication of VBAC: HEMORRHAGE

Refer to the generic collaborative care plan, "Potential Complication: Hemorrhage," beginning on p. 28 in Chapter 3, and "Postpartum Hemorrhage," beginning on p. 343 in Chapter 10.

Potential Complication of VBAC: RUPTURE AT SITE OF UTERINE SCAR

Refer to "Uterine Rupture," beginning on p. 293 in this chapter.

INDIVIDUALIZED (NURSING DIAGNOSIS) CARE PLANS

The care plans in this section were developed to address unique patient needs.

Nursing Diagnosis: ANXIETY/FEAR[1]

Related Factors: excitement at the opportunity to experience labor and vaginal birth; concern about the possible failure of the TOL and the need for a repeat cesarean birth; fear of harm to self and fetus (e.g., uterine rupture); and having heard old wives' tales such as, "Once a cesarean, always a cesarean." Refer to the generic NDCPs, "Anxiety[1]" and "Fear[1]" beginning on pp. 10 and 15, respectively, in Chapter 2.

Nursing Activities and Rationales

Independent Nursing Actions

- Pay careful attention to the woman's psychologic needs during the TOL. Anxiety can inhibit the release of oxytocin, thus decreasing the UCs and possibly leading to failure of the TOL.
- Support women in their decision for TOL. Fosters trust in caregivers.
- Reiterate that VBAC is safe. Evidence supports a very low complication rate of less than 1% from VBAC (Gregory, Fridman, & Korst, 2010). The woman may have heard the outdated saying, "Once a cesarean, always a cesarean."
- Present VBAC in a positive way, but acknowledge that a cesarean may be needed. Providing realistic information promotes trust. The couple may be excited at the opportunity to experience labor and birth, but they need time to prepare for the possibility that the birth may not proceed as hoped for/anticipated.
- Encourage the couple to discuss previous labor (cesarean) experience. It is helpful for the woman/couple to express feelings of failure and loss of control, as well as to express concern about how they will manage during the present labor and birth.
- If TOL does not proceed to vaginal birth, encourage the woman to express her feelings about having another cesarean birth. After being reassured that vaginal birth is safe and possible, the woman/couple may be disappointed or feel that they have failed. It is important to family well-being that they feel satisfied with their participation in the birth experience. Women may suppress emotions ranging from a sense of failure to anger or betrayal when they are unable to have a vaginal birth (Meddings, MacVane Phipps, Haith-Cooper, & Haigh, 2007).
- Reassure the woman that bonding with the newborn will be successful no matter how the delivery occurs. Helps alleviate fears about delayed bonding following cesarean birth.

INTRAUTERINE FETAL DEATH

Intrauterine fetal death (IUFD) is death of a fetus that occurs at 20 weeks' gestation or later, before the onset of labor. At less than 20 weeks' gestation the loss is considered to be an abortion or miscarriage. Some states within the United States have an additional birth weight requirement in addition to the 20 weeks' gestation or longer for defining fetal death.

Spontaneous labor usually occurs within 2 weeks after IUFD. However, if prolonged retention of the fetus occurs after death, the degenerating tissues release thromboplastin into the maternal bloodstream, activating the extrinsic clotting system. This triggers the formation of multiple small blood clots, depleting fibrinogen and factors V and VII. Fibrinogen levels begin falling 3 to 4 weeks after death of the fetus.

Key Nursing Activities

- Provide emotional support to the family.
- Facilitate grieving.
- Assess for complications (DIC and infection).

Etiologies and Risk Factors

The cause of the IUFD is often unknown. The current rate in the United States is 6.4/1,000 live births with over half of all intrauterine deaths occurring before 28 weeks' gestation (Tempfer et al., 2009). Etiologies may be of maternal, placental, umbilical cord, or fetal origin. Maternal causes include diabetes, hypertension, preeclampsia, eclampsia, infections, and isoimmunization. Placental and umbilical cord problems include abruptio placentae, placenta previa, umbilical cord compression, and prolapse. Congenital malformations (fetal origin causes) account for about 35% of all fetal deaths (MacDorman & Kirmeyer, 2009).

Signs and Symptoms

Subjective. Mother reports absence of fetal movement or a decrease in the signs and symptoms of pregnancy.
Objective. Absence of fetal heart tones, ultrasonography reveals an absence of fetal heart and body movement.

Diagnostic Studies

- Abdominal ultrasonography. Detects the absence of fetal heart and body movement; detects overriding of fetal cranial bones.
- Maternal estriol levels. A decrease is a sign of IUFD.
- Fibrinogen levels. Establishes fetal demise. Level falls 3–4 weeks after the death of the fetus and continues to drop to dangerous levels unless treatment is instituted.
- Hgb, Hct, CBC, on admission. As a baseline, and to evaluate ability to tolerate bleeding; also assesses for infection.
- Platelet count, fibrinogen level, prothrombin time, and partial thromboplastin time. Identifies risk for hemorrhage and/or DIC.

Medical Management

- Provide factual information.
- Type and cross-match for two or three units of blood upon admission.

- Confirm the fetal demise.
- Delivery of the demised fetus before complications can result (before fibrinogen levels fall dangerously). If the woman is in labor at the time of the fetal death, delivery is the choice of action. If other complications are not present, she may choose to wait for labor to occur spontaneously.
- Use of laminaria or other osmotic dilators when the cervix is not soft and ready to dilate.
- Vaginal prostaglandin E_2 (PGE2) suppositories may be used for induction of labor.
- Oral misoprostol 400 μg every 4 hours may be used to induce labor.
- IV oxytocin to induce labor, in conjunction with cervical ripening methods as needed.
- Determine cause of death if possible by doing the following:
  - ▶ Examine fetus for gross abnormalities.
  - ▶ Send placenta to pathology.
  - ▶ Cultures, X-rays, photographs, and/or autopsy, as indicated.
  - ▶ Review prenatal record and maternal and family history.
  - ▶ Other lab tests as needed.

▌ *Collaborative Problems*

Potential Complications of IUFD

- Maternal infection
- Disseminated intravascular coagulation (DIC)
- Psychic trauma

COLLABORATIVE (STANDARDIZED) CARE FOR ALL WOMEN EXPERIENCING INTRAUTERINE FETAL DEATH

Perform a comprehensive assessment to identify individual needs for teaching, emotional support, and physical care. For general care during labor, refer to "Normal Labor: First Stage," "Normal Labor: Second Stage," and "Normal Labor: Third Stage," beginning on pp. 223, 234 and 240, respectively, in Chapter 7.

▌ Potential Complication of IUFD: MATERNAL INFECTION

Refer to the generic collaborative care plan, "Potential Complication: Infection," beginning on p. 29 in Chapter3; and the generic NDCP, "Risk for Infection,[1]" beginning on p. 21 in Chapter 2.

Focus Assessments

- Monitor labor progress. Prolonged labor increases the likelihood of infection.
- Assess for signs of preexisting infections upon admission (foul or abnormal vaginal discharge, pain, burning or frequency of urination, elevated WBC count 15,000/ mm³ or more, and temperature higher than 100.4°F, or 38.6°C). If fetal death has occurred, infection may already be present.
- Assess for ROM and note the time, amount, color, and odor of the fluid. The greater the length of time from ROM to birth, the greater the risk for infection.

Preventive Nursing Activities

- Limit the number of visitors present during the labor and birth, if possible. The woman with an IUFD is already at higher risk for an infection due to her condition. Visitors bring microorganisms into the labor and delivery area, although immediate family members usually do not pose a risk. The more people present, the greater the risk for infection.
- Maintain hydration during the labor and birth. Hydration of cells is important in preventing infection. Hydration is essential for waste product removal from cells and elimination by the kidneys.

▌ Potential Complication of IUFD: DISSEMINATED INTRAVASCULAR COAGULATION

Refer to the generic collaborative care plan, "Potential Complication: Disseminated Intravascular Coagulation," and "Potential Complication: Hemorrhage," beginning on pp. 26 and 28, respectively, in Chapter 3.

Focus Assessments

- Assess and report the laboratory findings, e.g., fibrinogen levels; normal fibrinogen level during pregnancy is 450 mg/dl. Clinically significant coagulopathy occurs when levels fall to less than 100 mg/dl.

Preventive Nursing Activities

- Use 16- or 18-gauge catheter when starting IV. This is large enough for administration of blood or blood components and for rapid administration of fluids to restore volume in the event of hemorrhage.
- Draw or confirm that lab personnel have drawn blood for prothrombin time and partial thromboplastin time; report findings promptly to physician, even when in normal range. Determines whether DIC is occurring; information is needed for medical decision making.

INDIVIDUALIZED (NURSING DIAGNOSIS) CARE PLANS

The care plans in this section were developed to address unique patient needs.

Nursing Diagnosis: DEFICIENT KNOWLEDGE[1]

Related Factors: lack of knowledge of or experience with induction of labor to deliver the fetus, causes of fetal death, or possible complications of fetal death (e.g., DIC). Refer to the generic NDCP, "Deficient Knowledge,[1]" beginning on p. 13 in Chapter 2.

Goals, Outcomes, and Evaluation Criteria

- Woman acknowledges that the diagnostic tests indicate fetal demise.
- Woman verbalizes understanding of the labor plan for delivery.
- Woman verbalizes understanding of potential complications of IUFD.

NIC Interventions[2]

Infection Protection (6550)—Prevention and early detection of infection in a patient at risk.
Teaching: Disease Process (5602)—Assisting the patient to understand information related to a specific disease process. The fetal demise is not a disease state, but complications can arise from the condition.

Nursing Activities and Rationales

Assessments

- Assess prior experience with or knowledge of IUFD. In order to individualize care, the nurse must know about prior experiences and coping methods used.
- Determine whether the woman/family have attended childbirth education classes or experienced another pregnancy or birth. If the IUFD occurred soon after 20 weeks' gestation, the woman and family might not have attended childbirth classes yet. Assessing their knowledge is a starting point for providing information on the labor and delivery process and coping techniques, as necessary.
- Assess type of pain management to be used. Allows nurse to discuss patient's desire for pain relief because labor induction is painful. It also allows choices during this difficult time.
- Assess prior experience with or knowledge of postpartum self-care. The woman will have a postpartum recovery period similar to all women giving birth.
- Assess experience with or knowledge of DIC. Allows for individualization of teaching plan. DIC is one of the complications that can occur from this condition.

Patient/Family Teaching

- Explain the nursing care for the situation and why it is important that the fetus be delivered. The physician informs the woman and family regarding the fetal demise and complications that can arise from her condition. They

may seek reassurance from the nurse on the course of action (induction of labor).
- Explain what to expect for the management of the labor and delivery. The woman may not have started her childbirth education series, and this may be a first labor experience. Even if she has given birth previously, she may not be familiar with oxytocin induction, which is often needed.

Nursing Diagnosis: GRIEVING[1]

Related Factors: normal response to the actual loss of the fetus, the lifestyle associated with having the child; loss of the parental role; and grief for the loss to the siblings and to the extended family.

Goals, Outcomes, and Evaluation Criteria

- Woman identifies the people who provide the most emotional support.
- Woman expresses feelings about the loss to significant other, support persons, and healthcare providers.
- Woman progresses through the stages of grief and loss without dysfunctional grieving.

NIC Interventions[2]

Active Listening (4920)—Attending closely to and attaching significance to a patient's verbal and nonverbal messages.
Emotional Support (5270)—Provision of reassurance, acceptance, and encouragement during times of stress.
Grief Work Facilitation: Perinatal Death (5294)—Assistance with the resolution of a perinatal loss.
Support System Enhancement (5440)—Facilitation of support to patient by family, friends, and community.

Nursing Activities and Rationales

Assessments

- Assess support system already in place for the mother and father. Identifies those family members who are available to provide support or identifies the lack of family support so that appropriate referrals can be made.
- Assess the stages of grieving for the mother, father, and significant others. Helps the nurse determine if they are in a normal grieving pattern. It also helps to explain their behavior. There are specific interventions that are helpful in each stage of the grieving process.
- Assess for any previous fetal loss experiences. Enables the nurse to individualize interventions for the family.
- Ask what actions the mother and family wish to take with this fetus (their child). It may be necessary to make suggestions. The mother and family may want to hold, cuddle, stroke, dress, rock, talk, sing, baptize, undress, take pictures, and/or make preparations for a funeral. These will be the only moments with this child and what they do during

this time can have an effect on their healing process and whether they attempt to try another pregnancy. It may not occur to them that these activities are possible for them.

- Identify with the mother personal coping strategies she has used in the past. Coping strategies that have been successful before will probably be helpful during the grieving process.
- Make referrals to support groups and mental health practitioners as needed. The mother/family may need help with the grieving process.
- Initiate bereavement care according to hospital policy. This is a guideline for the nursing staff to follow to be sure all aspects of care are carried out and to meet state and governing body recommendations.

Independent Nursing Actions

- Ensure that the woman and family are offered the choice of being on the maternity unit or other unit after delivery. Although labor and postpartum nurses are probably best prepared to support parents who have had a fetal loss, some parents find it too painful to be on a unit where they must see parents with healthy newborns, at least so soon after their loss.
- Facilitate open communication between the physician, mother, father, and other family members. Be aware that the woman/family may not actually accept that the fetus is dead until the birth occurs. Denial is a common early response in the grieving process.
- Caregivers must recognize that the grieving process is ongoing. A set protocol for fetal or neonatal deaths should be in place at the hospital or birthing center, to include the following:
  - Clean the baby, wrap in a clean, dry blanket, comb the hair, and see if the mother and father would like to see and hold their baby. Prepare infant for viewing.
  - Ask if the family has a name for their baby. If so, refer to the baby by that name.
  - Collect pictures, a lock of hair, the linens that touched the baby, armband, and stocking cap, and give to the mother. If she is not ready to receive them, provide written information about hospital policy for keeping such items and how they may be obtained at a later date if desired. Research shows that families need pictures and memories of their baby. Anything that can connect them to this baby will become very important. A clear picture, such as digital photo, is preferred. This is all they will ever have to remember that child. It helps to make the experience real for them and the people who will share these memories. Grieving theory indicates that the birth must first be integrated as a reality before grieving can be resolved.
- Try to have all the paperwork signed at once, so there's no need to keep going back to the woman/family with one more thing. Reduces sources of stress for the family.

- Try to arrange for the same nurse to provide care to the woman and family. Once rapport and trust have been established, a relationship develops. The nurse providing care during the labor and birth has had adequate time to develop a strong bond. It would be of great benefit for the woman and family to have this nurse participate in their care during the duration of the hospital stay.
- Nurses coming into contact with the mother and family need to acknowledge the loss that has occurred. A statement such as, "I understand you've had a loss" may initiate discussion. "I'm here for you if you would like to talk" is another way to initiate discussion. Pulling up a chair and sitting alongside the woman and giving her full attention is also helpful. Not acknowledging the loss lessens the significance of the loss to the woman. She needs for the nursing staff to acknowledge her loss, allow her to vent her feelings, reassure her it is normal to cry and that it is part of the grieving process, and comfort her.
- Coordinate with other members of the collaborative team to provide similar care, pastoral care, and bereavement care. Prevents the woman/family from receiving mixed messages from different persons/groups.
- Recall the dos and don'ts of caring for these families:
  - Do listen to families vent their feelings. Repeating their story facilitates healing.
  - Assist the mother to create memories. Facilities healing and closure.
  - Use symbols as angels, candles, stars, and hearts. Helps bring meaning to the parents.
  - Allow the parent to parent. This is a lifelong role, even though the child died.
  - Express to the parents that grief does not go away and life will never be the same. Conveys that grief is normal and acceptable regardless of when it occurs.
  - Explain that holidays and anniversaries exacerbate feelings of grief. Allows parents to appreciate that this is a normal reaction.
  - Let the mother make her own decisions. Allows a sense of control because she knows what is best for her.
  - Share and clarify information, including autopsy. Prevents misunderstanding of information and allows opportunity for questions.

Collaborative Activities

- Check to see that the practitioner or practitioner's staff has informed the hospital admissions and nursing staff of the fetal demise, or the need to confirm a fetal demise, before the woman's admission. Prevents inappropriate comments and questioning regarding the pregnancy.

Patient/Family Teaching

- Teach regarding ultrasonography to assess for fetal heart and body movement. Understanding may reduce fear and anxiety. It helps to have the ultrasonography as soon as possible once the decision is made that it is necessary.

- Teach regarding the plans for labor and delivery of a demised fetus. Information reduces fear of the unknown and helps the woman and family to actively participate as much as possible. This may help in resolving grief, by resolving denial.

- Explain burial options to family (i.e., private funeral home versus hospital or county burial). Familiarize yourself with the options available in your community. Information helps the family in decision making and helps restore a sense of control.

- It may be necessary to reexplain information regarding these and other topics to family members. Because of grief, stress, and anxiety, the woman may not absorb all the information herself; some family members may not have been present when information was shared.

Nursing Diagnosis: SITUATIONAL LOW SELF-ESTEEM[1]

Related Factors: feelings of guilt that the woman or her partner caused the loss in some way, feelings of unworthiness to have a child and be a parent, feelings of poor self-worth in general, role changes, questioning if the role of mother or father will be attained, blaming oneself for the loss, and guilt regarding the ambivalence experienced with the pregnancy.

Goals, Outcomes, and Evaluation Criteria

- Woman makes decisions about her self-care and other activities of daily living.
- Woman uses effective coping strategies to help her with the loss.
- Woman openly communicates regarding the loss of the fetus and her role in life with that loss.
- Woman demonstrates acceptance of self.
- Woman and family openly communicate their loss to each other.
- Woman makes decisions regarding funeral arrangements, memorial service, and burial.

NIC Interventions[2]

Anticipatory Guidance (5210)—Preparation of patient for an anticipated developmental and/or situational crisis.

Coping Enhancement (5230)—Assisting a patient to adapt to perceived stressors, changes, or threats that interfere with meeting life demands and roles.

Decision-Making Support (5250)—Providing information and support for a patient who is making a decision regarding health care.

Self-Esteem Enhancement (5400)—Assisting a patient to increase his/her personal judgment of self-worth.

Nursing Activities and Rationales

Assessments

- Assess feelings about self. Listen carefully to the words the woman uses to express her feelings. Any mention of guilt, blaming self for the cause, or saying she should have done this or that differently are expressions of self-blame and poor self-esteem.

Independent Nursing Actions

- Promote positive comments about the self. The woman needs to focus on the positive, not the negative. Negative self-talk lowers self-esteem.

- Identify with the mother what she is going to do in the next 4 hours that will have a positive effect on her versus a negative effect. An example of a positive activity would be completing her daily hygiene measures.

- Set mutual easily attainable goals. Meeting the goals and expectations of others will help promote self-esteem.

Collaborative Activities

- Provide pain medication, postpartum treatments, and activity within the orders provided by the physician. Even though there is not a live baby, the woman undergoes the same physiologic (e.g., hormonal) changes as any other woman who has given birth. The postpartum recovery will depend on the whether the woman had a full-term delivery, 20-week delivery, an episiotomy, etc. The woman carrying a fetus to term may have an episiotomy, which requires treatments. Uterine cramping may be uncomfortable in the multipara and pain medication may be necessary. Being uncomfortable may add to her poor feelings about herself.

Patient/Family Teaching

- Teach that resolution of grief will take time and that each day is a new day upon which to focus. The woman will always feel like she is not getting better if she has unrealistic goals that she cannot meet. She can do something each day to feel better about herself.

Nursing Diagnosis: INTERRUPTED FAMILY PROCESSES[1]

Related Factors: crisis with the intrauterine death/loss of the fetus/future child/mother role/father role/grandparent role; poor communication between the mother and family members, depression and the effects upon their roles in the family, and inability to fulfill their parental roles with their other children.

Goals, Outcomes, and Evaluation Criteria

- Woman identifies and uses the support system within the family and community.
- Woman acknowledges the crisis and accepts changes of the family roles.
- Family members visit in the hospital, listen to the woman and her partner, and offer support.
- Family members provide care for the distressed members in the family and assist with responsibilities.

NIC Interventions[2]

Coping Enhancement (5230)—Assisting a patient to adapt to perceived stressors, changes, or threats that interfere with meeting life demands and roles.

Family Integrity Promotion (7100)—Promotion of family cohesion and unity.

Family Process Maintenance (7130)—Minimization of family process disruption effects.

Family Support (7140)—Promotion of family values, interests, and goals.

Nursing Activities and Rationales

Assessments

- Assess the family structure and the members within the family. The nurse needs to understand who makes up the family before approaching the members for assistance. Family members are basically whomever the woman designates as a family member.
- Assess the stages of grieving exhibited by the family members. Helps the woman understand reactions that are being exhibited by individual family members.

Independent Nursing Actions

- Establish rapport and trust with the woman and family. Establishing rapport and trust is always the first step in the nurse–patient relationship and provides the foundation upon which that relationship is built.
- Provide a calm, supportive, and accepting environment. The family has many painful emotions. The environment should provide a sense of calmness where the family can focus on what is important to them. A chaotic or noisy environment causes anxiety and decreases coping abilities.
- Encourage the family to express feelings. The family needs to share their feelings because this event affects the family and not just one individual. The mother has lost her child, the grandmother has lost her grandchild, etc.
- Make provisions for a family member to stay in the room with the mother if she wishes. Most of the time the father of the baby will want to remain in the room with the mother. Regardless of who remains with the mother, the nurse continues to listen, be present, and provide emotional support.

- Encourage the family to help care for the mother while in the hospital and make suggestions for ways they can help when she goes home. Helps the family feel that they have a role and can help in some way. Fosters the woman's feelings of being supported by her family.
- Listen attentively to the woman and family's expression of feelings. Enables advocacy for the woman. The woman and family may have special requests that are extremely important for them to have peace or closure. The nurse may be able to make accommodations if these are expressed and understood.
- Arrange for a private room, flexible family visitation times, and refreshments for the family, if possible. The family needs privacy to share their feelings. Flexible visitation times accommodate important family members who work unusual hours or out-of-town guests. A cup of coffee, glass of water, tea, or juice from the nurse conveys caring and facilitates better communication.

Collaborative Activities

- Arrange for social service consult or recommend family support group referrals. The nurse needs to inform the primary care provider as to how the family is coping with the loss and may need to request outside intervention especially upon discharge. How the woman perceives this experience will have an impact on the decision to attempt another pregnancy and/or to parent other children.

Patient/Family Teaching

- Teach the family about the stages of grieving and loss. Emphasize how each family member will progress through the stages at different times and in different ways. Reinforce the importance of recognizing that each is grieving in her/his own way and to look for ways to understand and support one another. It is distressing for families when one is displaying anger while another member is displaying acceptance, for example; understanding why each person reacts they way he/she does will help family members be more supportive of one another.

Nursing Diagnosis: SPIRITUAL DISTRESS[1]

Related Factors: feelings of anger because the baby has been taken from the woman and her partner and they have lost their role and relationship with that child, confusion and questions about the meaning of the event, such as, "Why did this happen to us?" They might also question why this would happen to someone so innocent as a baby, as in, "Why would God do such a thing?" The event is also a challenge to their belief/values system.

Goals, Outcomes, and Evaluation Criteria

Woman/partner/family:

- Seek an understanding of the experience.
- Participate in spiritual rituals that are important to them.
- Display love and caring for each other.
- Demonstrate coping techniques.

NIC Interventions[2]

Hope Instillation (5310)—Facilitation of the development of a positive outlook in a given situation.

Spiritual Growth Facilitation (5426)—Facilitation of growth in the patient's capacity to identify, connect with, and call upon the source of meaning, purpose, comfort, strength, and hope in his/her life.

Spiritual Support (5420)—Assisting the patient to feel balance and connection with a greater power.

Nursing Activities and Rationales

Assessments

- Assess the impact of the loss on spiritual beliefs. Communication regarding the couple's spiritual beliefs helps to confirm the importance of this pregnancy/child/loss.
- Assess the woman's and family's acceptance of the loss. Although denial is a normal part of grieving, it is difficult to move forward if the woman and family are in a state of denial. The denial has to be dealt with first. While the woman is in labor there may still be hope that everyone is wrong about the fetal death. Usually seeing, holding, and touching the baby will dispel denial.

Independent Nursing Actions

- Listen for cues regarding spiritual distress and methods of practice for the woman/family's beliefs. There are various ways of practicing beliefs. Do not generalize or make assumptions; but listen and identify how the family members feel in this situation.
- Encourage relationships with the significant other and family members. How the significant other feels is very important to the woman. Fathers usually experience loss in a different way than the woman, who has a physical and mental connection to the fetus. The more involved the father has been in the pregnancy, the more he may feel this loss. This is a time when they need to support and provide hope for each other in order to strengthen family bonds.
- Demonstrate caring and comfort when providing care (e.g., touch, eye contact). Caring and support are essential for healing. The woman and family need recognition that they have suffered a loss and that it is meaningful for them and others.
- Encourage the woman to participate as much as possible in her own care. This focuses the woman on the present,

which will facilitate hope for tomorrow. Passiveness displays signs of losing hope and giving up.

- Convey acceptance for preferred religious/spiritual practices; discuss the couple's spiritual needs with them. Some families feel baptism is important immediately; prayers, songs, providing the baby with a rosary, special clothing, and a funeral or memorial service may be planned.
- Inquire if the woman and family would like to pray, if they would like the nurse to pray, if they prefer to wait for other family members, or to call their pastor or contact hospital ministries for prayer. Giving options allows them to choose what is appropriate for them and informs them the nurse is willing and available to assist in the manner they choose and that it is important to the hospital staff that their needs are met.
- Display empathy and focus on the woman's and family's feelings. Empathy conveys understanding of how they feel in this situation. It is tempting to talk about one's own experiences but the focus should not be on the nurse. Crying with the family shows that the nurse cares and understands the loss. Touch is extremely helpful when demonstrating empathy.

Collaborative Activities

- Arrange for social service consult or make recommendations for support group interventions. A physician's order may be necessary for social service consult or approval to recommend a support group for continued care for after the woman leaves the hospital. It is unrealistic to think that grief, spiritual distress, etc. will be resolved by discharge, and the woman and family need to have options for further help.
- Provide a follow-up call at set intervals. Demonstrates caring, assists parents at handling the situation, and helps them to move on.

Patient/Family Teaching

- Teach about community support groups, to inquire within their church if they have a support group, and to recognize it takes time to deal with the loss and the meaning of the loss within their values and beliefs. Hospital care provides a supportive environment, hopefully tangible memories, and empowerment for the woman and family to seek continued assistance from their faith and support services as needed upon returning home to their daily lives.
- Inform the family of the hospital chapel and services within the hospital. The chapel can be a place for solitude and family togetherness during the acute crisis.

Other Nursing Diagnoses

Also assess for the following nursing diagnoses, which are frequently present with this condition.

- Powerlessness[1] related to the fetal demise, hospitalization, possible cesarean delivery, and potential complications from the fetal demise.

- Compromised individual or Family Coping[1] related to the loss associated with the fetal demise and poor communication among the mother, father, and other family members, inability to concentrate or focus on the family, family being in different stages of grieving, and separation from family and support system at a time of desperate need.
- Complicated Grieving[1] related to unresolved feelings of grief from the fetal loss, remaining in one stage of grieving (denial, anger, or depression) and not being able to move on to the next, unresolved guilt over the loss, loss of self-esteem, feelings of despair, the change in the relationship with the significant other, and grieving the loss of not being able to get their life back on track again.

UTERINE RUPTURE

Uterine rupture is rare, occurring in only about 1 in 1,500 to 2,000 or 0.07% of pregnancies (Nahum & Pham, 2010). Uterine rupture represents an acute, potentially life-threatening source of hemorrhage from separation of the scar from a previous cesarean delivery, trauma, or other anomaly of the uterus. Uterine rupture is a dangerous complication for women attempting labor after cesarean delivery. A *complete rupture* extends through the uterine wall into the peritoneal cavity, myometrium, or broad ligament. An *incomplete rupture* extends into the peritoneum but not into the peritoneal cavity, or broad ligament. Uterine rupture necessitates immediate surgery. Fetal mortality can reach 80%, and maternal mortality can reach 50–75%, thus early identification and intervention are essential.

■ Key Nursing Activities

- Prevention is the best treatment, so careful assessment for at-risk women is essential.
- If rupture occurs:
  - ▶ Start IV fluids, administer oxygen, and call for help.
  - ▶ Prepare for blood transfusion.
  - ▶ Prepare for immediate surgery.
- Be prepared for maternal and/or fetal death.

■ Etiologies and Risk Factors

- Separation of the scar (uterine dehiscence) from a previous cesarean birth.
- Uterine trauma (e.g., accidents, surgery, blunt trauma from motor vehicle accidents, battery, falls, and gunshot or knife wounds).
- Congenital anomalies of the uterus.
- Overstimulation with oxytocin/hyperstimulation/hypertonus.
- Overdistended uterus (e.g., multifetal gestation).
- External or internal version (due to abnormal fetal lie).
- Malpresentation.
- Difficult forceps-assisted birth.
- Multigravida.
- Prostaglandin preparations.

- Previous termination of pregnancies.
- Trial of labor after cesarean.
- Obstructed labor.
- Vigorous pressure on the uterus at birth.

■ Signs and Symptoms

Signs and symptoms vary with the extent of the rupture, which may be silent or dramatic.

Incomplete Rupture

Subjective. Possibly no pain, especially if regional anesthesia is being used; feelings of faintness; increasing abdominal tenderness.

Objective. FHR may or may not show late decelerations, decreased variability, tachycardia, or bradycardia; vomiting; hypotonic UCs (after the rupture); lack of labor progress. Late signs include signs of hypovolemia (e.g., hypotension and increased pulse rate) and absence of fetal heart tones.

Complete Rupture

Subjective. Sudden, sharp, shooting pain; acute abdominal and shoulder pain; statement that "Something came loose," or "Something tore," or "Something gave way"; if the woman is in labor, UCs stop and pain is relieved.

Objective. Hypovolemic shock (initial change in vital sign pattern, hypotension, tachypnea, pallor, cool, clammy skin, vomiting, tachycardia); tense, rigid uterus; rigid abdomen from intra-abdominal bleeding; fetal parts may be palpable through the abdominal wall; absent FHR if the placenta separates.

■ Diagnostic Studies

- Type and cross-match (should already have been done before labor).
- FHR monitoring.
- Electronic monitoring and palpation of UCs.
- Rupture confirmed only when surgery is performed and uterus is visible.

■ Medical Management

Medical management depends on the severity of the rupture.

- Small rupture. Laparotomy and birth, repair of the laceration, and blood transfusions.
- Complete rupture. Hysterectomy, birth, and blood replacement.

■ Collaborative Problems

Potential Complications of Uterine Rupture

- Pulmonary embolism
- Hypovolemic shock
- Fetal mortality

COLLABORATIVE (STANDARDIZED) CARE FOR ALL WOMEN EXPERIENCING UTERINE RUPTURE

Perform a comprehensive assessment to identify individual needs for teaching, emotional support, and physical care.

Potential Complications of Uterine Rupture: PULMONARY EMBOLISM, HYPOVOLEMIC SHOCK, AND FETAL MORTALITY

Refer to the generic collaborative care plan, "Potential Complication: Hemorrhage," which begins on p. 28 in Chapter 3.

Focus Assessments

- Before labor, review history for factors that place the woman at risk for uterine rupture. See "Etiologies and Risk Factors," preceding. Allows the nurse to identify women who need careful assessment during labor for uterine rupture. The most important nursing care is the prevention of uterine rupture.
- For women who have risk factors and all women having oxytocin induction/augmentation, institute continuous electronic monitoring of FHR and uterine contractions (UCs); assess frequency, duration, and intensity of UCs. Identifies symptoms early so that treatment can be initiated.
- For women who have risk factors and all women having oxytocin induction/augmentation of labor, if intrauterine pressure catheter (IUPC) is not being used, palpate UCs frequently. Identifies uterine hyperstimulation or hypertonus, which can precede uterine rupture. External monitor does not provide data about the intensity of the UCs.
- Be alert for subjective symptoms of uterine rupture. See "Signs and Symptoms," preceding. Enables emergency treatment. Fetal and maternal mortality are high for uterine rupture.
- If subjective symptoms occur, confirm by assessing for objective signs. See "Signs and Symptoms," preceding. Provides complete information upon which to base nursing and medical decisions/interventions.
- When rupture occurs, obtain maternal VSs (BP, pulse, respirations, pulse pressure); observe for other symptoms of hypovolemic shock (restlessness, apprehension, pallor, and cool and clammy skin). When bleeding occurs, the BP falls in response to loss of fluid volume. Heart rate and respirations increase in an effort to compensate for hypovolemia.
- Note FHR. Nonreassuring FHR or absence of FHR confirms uterine rupture and the necessity for immediate surgery.

- Be alert for complaint of chest pain. This is a symptom of pulmonary embolism. Medium to large size emboli cause severe pain related to tissue hypoxia secondary to arterial occlusion.
- For women undergoing trial labor after cesarean section, observe closely for complaints of sharp or stabbing pain in the area of prior incision, vaginal bleeding, blood-tinged urine, ascending station of the fetal presenting part, and hypovolemia. These findings indicate uterine rupture.

Preventive Nursing Activities

- Before labor, be sure that a type and screen has been done. Hemorrhage is common, and blood transfusion is often needed to treat/prevent hypovolemia.
- Report signs and symptoms of uterine rupture immediately to physician/midwife; call for help; do not leave the patient. This is an obstetric emergency and it must be evaluated and treated immediately, if suspected, in order to prevent maternal and fetal death.
- Start or increase IV fluids. Provides intravenous access for fluid administration to prevent hypovolemia until blood replacement can be initiated and ensures rapid administration of volume expanders and blood products to maintain circulating volume as needed.
- Obtain blood immediately. Transfusion will probably be needed to restore both volume and blood formed elements (e.g., RBCs, WBCs, platelets).
- Administer oxygen per protocol or order. When circulating volume is low, inadequate oxygen reaches maternal and fetal tissues via the blood. It is important that the blood that does reach the tissues carries as much oxygen as possible in order to prevent damage to major organs.
- Prepare the woman and family for immediate surgery according to agency protocol and ensure surgery team is standing by (e.g., insert an indwelling urinary catheter, transport the woman to the operating room). This is an emergency situation. At minimum, a laparotomy will be performed to deliver the infant and repair the laceration. If complete rupture has occurred, a hysterectomy will be performed.
- Provide information about spiritual support services available in the agency; have another team member stay with the family, if possible, or suggest that the family contact their own spiritual adviser. Fetal and maternal mortality are high in this condition. The nurse will be busy providing for the mother's physical needs and may not be available to provide emotional/spiritual support for the family.
- Provide additional reassurance and support, frequent observation of maternal-fetal status, and continuous fetal monitoring for women undergoing a trial of labor after a cesarean section. They are at increased risk for uterine rupture because of previous uterine incision.

Other Nursing Diagnoses

Also assess for the following nursing diagnoses, which are frequently present with this condition.

- Anxiety/Fear[1] related to realistic concern for maternal and fetal safety/survival.
- Risk for spiritual distress[1] related to questioning of beliefs and values secondary to maternal or fetal death or injury.

EXTERNAL VERSION

Version is a procedure used to change fetal presentation (i.e., turn the fetus in utero) by manipulation, using gentle, constant pressure on the maternal abdomen. *External cephalic version (ECV)* changes fetal presentation from breech or shoulder to cephalic by external manipulation of the mother's abdomen. Version is successful about 60% of the time. Version is also used successfully in changing 3–4% of breech positions in term pregnancies. The need for emergency intervention (e.g., cesarean birth) occurs in less than 1–2% of cases, and the fetal death rate is 1 per 5,000 external cephalic attempts.

Key Nursing Activities

- Reinforce the healthcare provider's explanation about the procedure and ensure informed consent.
- Assess for contraindications to version (previous cesarean section, uterine anomalies, CPD, placenta previa, multiple gestation, and oligohydramnios).
- Obtain baseline FHR, ultrasonography, and NST prior to procedure.
- Administer medications if ordered or prepare equipment if epidural is planned.
- Monitor maternal and fetal response to preprocedure medication and the procedure.
- Provide aftercare instructions.
- Administer Rh immune globulin if mother is Rh negative.

Etiologies and Risk Factors

Etiologies and risk factors are not applicable.

Signs and Symptoms

Signs and symptoms are not applicable. Criteria that should be met before performing ECV include:

- Single fetus (in breech or shoulder presentation)
- Fetal breech not engaged
- Adequate amount of amniotic fluid
- Reactive NST
- Fetus is at 36 or more weeks' gestation

Diagnostic Tests

- FHR and NST prior to procedure. Establish fetal well-being.

- Leopold's maneuvers. Determine fetal presentation.
- Ultrasound. Assesses amount of amniotic fluid, confirms fetal presentation, identifies IUGR and/or fetal malformations, and locates the placenta and position of the umbilical cord.
- Tests, as needed, to identify maternal problems/contraindications such as PIH, diabetes, and placenta previa.
- Ongoing FHR monitoring.

Medical Management

- Confirm the need for ECV.
- Epidural anesthesia or spinal anesthesia may be used. Evidence suggests equivocal ECV success rates (Sullivan et al., 2009).
- Rule out absolute contraindications to ECV, including:
  - ▶ IUGR. If fetus is stressed; amniotic fluid may be decreased.
  - ▶ Ruptured membranes. Results in inadequate amniotic fluid or possible prolapsed cord.
  - ▶ Multifetal gestation. Fetuses can become entangled during ECV.
  - ▶ Major fetal abnormality.
  - ▶ Abnormal FHR. Fetus may not tolerate procedure; other action may need to be taken, e.g., cesarean birth.
  - ▶ Presence of a condition that dictates a cesarean birth (e.g., placenta previa).
  - ▶ Maternal problems such as gestational hypertension, cardiac disease, or gestational diabetes requiring insulin.
- Use caution in the presence of relative contraindications, including:
  - ▶ Previous cesarean birth. Scarring increases the risk of uterine tearing.
  - ▶ Nuchal cord. Cord may tighten around fetal neck during procedure.
  - ▶ Oligohydramnios. Increases risk of umbilical cord compression; makes turning difficult.
  - ▶ Establish intravenous line. Enables administration of medications if complications occur.
- IV ritodrine (subcutaneous terbutaline is the choice of IV drugs), or IV MgSO$_4$ if β-mimetic agents are contraindicated. Relaxes the uterus, which decreases pain and increases the likelihood of successful version.
- Perform procedure in birthing unit, rather than outpatient setting. In case further intervention, such as cesarean birth, is needed.
- Discontinue procedure if fetal head is moved to a head-down position, two attempts have been made, maternal or fetal problems occur, or the woman indicates that the procedure is too painful or stressful to continue.
- Vaginal examination. Determines cervical dilation and fetal descent.

Collaborative Problems

- Potential complication of ECV: Fetal distress
- Potential complication of ECV: Rh sensitization
- Potential rare complication of ECV: Femur fracture

- Potential complication of β-mimetic tocolytic agents: Tachycardia, dysrhythmias, myocardial ischemia, and pulmonary edema

NOTE: Continuous administration of β-mimetics can also cause hyperglycemia and hyperinsulinemia; however, that is extremely unlikely with the one-time dose given for ECV. Therefore, urine and blood glucose are not routinely checked after this procedure.

COLLABORATIVE (STANDARDIZED) CARE FOR ALL WOMEN HAVING EXTERNAL CEPHALIC VERSION

Perform a comprehensive assessment to identify individual needs for teaching, emotional support, and physical care.

Potential Complication of ECV and/or β-Mimetic Tocolytic Agents: FETAL COMPROMISE

Refer to the generic collaborative care plan, "Potential Complication: Fetal Compromise (Nonreassuring Fetal Heart Rate)," beginning on p. 27 in Chapter 3.

Focus Assessments

- Ask if the woman has had food or fluids within the preceding 8 hours. An empty stomach prevents vomiting and possible aspiration. Should maternal or fetal complications occur, cesarean birth may be necessary. Also, nausea and vomiting can occur because of the stress of the procedure or as a side effect of tocolytic medications.
- Obtain a 20-min baseline FHR and NST prior to the procedure. Establishes fetal well-being and provides a baseline for postprocedure comparison.
- Monitor FHR during the procedure and for 1–2 hr after. Evaluates fetal tolerance of the procedure and of tocolytic agents.

Preventive Nursing Activities

- Teach the woman to monitor for UCs after dismissal. ECV may stimulate labor.
- Teach the woman how to count fetal movements after dismissal. Advise her to call her healthcare provider if there are fewer than 10 movements in 3 hours, if there are no movements in the morning, or if there are no movements at all. Helps the woman assess fetal viability. Absence of fetal movement or decreased movement may indicate fetal distress.
- If there is significant FHR bradycardia or decelerations, call it to the attention of the care provider and initiate

intrauterine resuscitation. If signs of fetal distress occur, the procedure should be discontinued.
- After a successful procedure, it may be necessary to hold the fetus in the new presentation until the tocolytic is out of the mother's system and the uterus regains tone. Prevents the fetus from turning again to breech or shoulder presentation.

Potential Complication of ECV: RH SENSITIZATION

Focus Assessments

- Review records and ask the woman whether she is Rh negative. Determines whether there is a risk for sensitization. The manipulation of the fetus can cause fetomaternal bleeding.
- Observe for vaginal bleeding after the procedure. This could signal placental separation or the beginning of labor. Also signals increased risk for sensitization.

Preventive Nursing Activities

- Administer anti-D immunoglobulin per order or protocol. Prevents sensitization if the fetus is Rh positive and fetomaternal bleeding occurs. Rh immune globulin prevents the mother from forming antibodies against the fetal blood cells.

Potential Complications of β-Mimetic Tocolytic Agents: TACHYCARDIA, DYSRHYTHMIAS, MYOCARDIAL ISCHEMIA, AND PULMONARY EDEMA

NOTE: These complications are dose related and are usually seen with continuous administration of tocolytic drugs. For ECV, a one-time dose is given, so there is no need to continue monitoring for side effects and complications once the medication has cleared the mother's bloodstream.

Focus Assessments

- Assess BP, pulse, and respirations every 15 min. Determines presence of side effects (tachycardia) and complications.
- Assess for chest pain, shortness of breath, crackles, rhonchi. These are symptoms of pulmonary edema. Chest pain might also indicate myocardial ischemia. Note: These are very unlikely with a one-time dose.
- Assess for tremors, headache, nausea and vomiting, flushing, and palpitations. Although these are not

complications, they are side effects that may occur from β-mimetic tocolytic agents.

Preventive Nursing Activities

- Notify primary care provider if mother's heart rate is greater than 120 beats/min. Allows procedure to be postponed until side effect is relieved. The procedure is stressful and can cause dangerous dysrhythmias.

INDIVIDUALIZED (NURSING DIAGNOSIS) CARE PLANS

The care plans in this section were developed to address unique patient needs.

▌ Nursing Diagnosis: PAIN[1]

Related Factors: forceful manipulation of the fetus through the abdomen and movement of the fetus within the uterus. Refer to the generic NDCP, "Pain,[1]" which begins on p. 18 in Chapter 2.

▌ *Goals, Outcomes, and Evaluation Criteria*

- Woman is free of pain (which can necessitate stopping the procedure).

▌ *Nursing Activities and Rationales*

Assessments

- Be alert for and inquire about maternal signs of discomfort during the procedure. The procedure may cause discomfort and should be stopped if the woman feels the discomfort is too great.

Independent Nursing Actions

- Warm the gel that is spread over the mother's abdomen before the procedure. Cold gel may cause abdominal muscles to tense, making the procedure more difficult and painful.

Collaborative Activities

- Administer IV ritodrine or subcutaneous terbutaline per order or protocol. These β-mimetic agents relax the uterine smooth muscle and make version easier, thereby enhancing the mother's comfort during the procedure.

Patient/Family Teaching

- Explain, prior to the ECV, that the procedure may be uncomfortable or even painful, but that if the pain is too great, she can direct the physician to stop the procedure. Anticipatory guidance allows for a sense of control and lessens anxiety, which increases the perception of pain.

▌ *Other Nursing Diagnoses*

Also assess for the following nursing diagnoses, which are frequently present with this condition.

- Anxiety/Fear[1] related to (1) the possibility that the procedure may fail and cesarean birth will be necessary, (2) complications that may result because of the procedure, and (3) anticipation of pain.

AMNIOINFUSION

Amnioinfusion is a procedure used during labor, by which warmed sterile normal saline or lactated Ringer's solution is introduced into the uterus transcervically through an IUPC to replace lost or absent amniotic fluid volume and to dilute impurities in the amniotic fluid, e.g., meconium. When there is a small amount of amniotic fluid, the umbilical cord can easily become compressed during UCs or fetal movement. This decreases blood flow to the fetus and is evidenced by variable FHR decelerations. The goal is to minimize or prevent adverse fetal effects such as umbilical cord compression or meconium aspiration. Studies support the use of amnioinfusion as safe and effective in resolving FHR decelerations (Choudhary, Bano, & Ali, 2009).

▌ *Key Nursing Activities*

- With the mother's permission, perform a vaginal examination to rule out cord prolapse, determine cervical dilation, effacement, station, status of membranes, and presentation.
- Ask the woman to position herself for placement of a fetal scalp electrode and IUPC.
- Monitor VSs, UCs (including resting tone), and associated maternal discomfort.
- Assess for increased uterine tone and abdominal overdistension.
- Observe for improvement in FHR pattern, using continuous electronic fetal heart rate monitoring. Administer bolus fluid per order or protocol; monitor continuous flow rate, if applicable.
- Explain the need to be on bed rest.

▌ *Etiologies and Risk Factors*

Indications for amnioinfusion include the following:

- Oligohydramnios (e.g., as a result of placental insufficiency, postmaturity, or ROM).
- Presence of nonperiodic (variable) FHR decelerations, not corrected by maternal position changes because of cord compression or nonreactive NST.
- Preterm labor with premature rupture of membranes.
- Medium to heavy meconium staining. (Although recent studies did not support amnioinfusion as a method to reduce the risk for aspiration syndrome or perinatal death [Simpson & Creehan, 2008], it may help dilute the fluid and decrease the incidence of meconium below the infant's vocal cords.)

Contraindications include:

- Ominous FHR patterns (e.g., lack of variability, rate of more than 180 bpm in absence of maternal fever)
- Vaginal bleeding (suspected placenta previa or placental abruption)
- Cord prolapse
- Uterine hypertonicity
- Nonvertex position
- Uterine anomaly
- Multiple gestation
- Fetal anomalies incompatible with life
- Chorioamnionitis
- Any situation in which placement of an IUPC is contraindicated or not advisable
- Impending delivery

Signs and Symptoms

- Variable FHR decelerations
- Small amount of amniotic fluid on sonogram
- Meconium-stained amniotic fluid on ROM

Medical Management

- Rupture membranes, if necessary, to place IUPC.
- Administer normal saline or lactated Ringer's solution via infusion pump with a dual lumen intrauterine catheter through an IUPC. Commonly, 300–800 ml fluid bolus is infused at 10–15 ml/min until decelerations diminish, with additional fluid bolus administered as needed. A continuous flow rate of 3 ml/min may be used, or the two methods may be used in combination.
- When treating decelerations, start amnioinfusion before FHR pattern becomes ominous because it takes about 30 min to increase the amniotic fluid volume.
- Carefully monitor uterine activity noting if increased uterine resting pressure is higher than the preinfusion baseline. Attempt to maintain uterine pressure at less than 25 mmHg.
- If fetal status does not improve, prepare for immediate cesarean birth.

Collaborative Problems

Potential Complications of Amnioinfusion

- Uterine overdistention
- Increased uterine tone
- Ascending infection
- Fetal bradycardia (if solution is colder than room temperature)

COLLABORATIVE (STANDARDIZED) CARE FOR ALL WOMEN UNDERGOING AMNIOINFUSION

Perform comprehensive assessment to identify individual needs for teaching, emotional support, and physical care.

Potential Complications of Amnioinfusion: UTERINE OVERDISTENTION AND INCREASED UTERINE TONE

Focus Assessment

- Assess frequency and intensity of UCs continually during the procedure. Detects overdistention and/or increased uterine tone (which will cause a high reading on the IUPC).
- To check the true uterine resting tone, discontinue the amnioinfusion. When fluid is being infused, the resting tone will appear higher than normal because of the resistance to outflow and turbulence at the end of the catheter.
- Monitor FHR continuously for a decrease in the frequency and intensity of variable decelerations. Evaluates amnioinfusion improvement of fetal status.
- Monitor output of fluid and record to avoid iatrogenic polyhydramnios. Can occur if the fetal head is pressed closely against the cervix. Too much fluid may result in maternal symptoms of shortness of breath, hypotension, or tachycardia. It is important to maintain accurate fluid intake and output.

Preventive Nursing Activities

- Administer fluid bolus per order or protocol; carefully monitor continuous flow infusion. Prevents uterine overdistention.
- If FHR pattern does not begin to improve within 30 minutes of amnioinfusion, prepare for cesarean birth. It takes about 30 minutes to increase the amniotic fluid volume enough to relieve pressure on the umbilical cord. If FHR does not become reassuring, immediate cesarean birth may be necessary.
- Warm saline solution with fluid warmer before administration. Prevents creating more stress for the fetus, especially for the preterm or small-for-gestational-age fetus.

Potential Complication of Amnioinfusion: ASCENDING INFECTION

Refer to the generic NDCP, "Risk for Infection,[1]" beginning on p. 21 in Chapter 2, and the generic collaborative care plan, "Potential Complication: Infection," beginning on p. 29 in Chapter 3.

INDIVIDUALIZED (NURSING DIAGNOSIS) CARE PLANS

This section contains care plans that were developed to address unique client needs.

Nursing Diagnosis: DEFICIENT KNOWLEDGE[1] (OF REASONS FOR AMNIOINFUSION AND OF RISKS AND BENEFITS)

Related Factors: lack of preparation for labor complications (such as umbilical cord compression), as well as misinformation and lack of information about amnioinfusion. See the generic NDCP, "Deficient Knowledge,[1]" beginning on p. 13 in Chapter 2.

▌ *Nursing Activities and Rationales*

Patient/Family Teaching

- Explain the need for amnioinfusion; explain that FHR pattern may mean that the cord is compressed and how amnioinfusion can help that condition. Information provides a sense of control and removes fear of the unknown.
- Tell the woman that the procedure should not be uncomfortable. Alleviates fear of pain.
- Explain the need to remain on bed rest during the procedure. Bed rest is necessary in order to administer the fluids and to monitor UCs and FHR. Knowledge of need may improve compliance and reduce anxiety.
- Explain how her self-care needs (e.g., hygiene, toileting, keeping the bed dry) while she is on bed rest can be met. Removes a source of anxiety. Explain that she can use a bedpan, or that an indwelling catheter can be inserted if she is allowed to do so.
- Explain that the FHR will not improve immediately. Reduces fear. It takes about 30 min to increase the amniotic fluid volume, so improvement in FHR will take a little longer than that.
- Explain that you will monitor the FHR and her UCs carefully during and after the procedure. Reassures her that she and the fetus will not be harmed by the procedure.
- Inform the woman of the possibility of cesarean birth if FHR does not improve after amnioinfusion. Anticipatory guidance allows the woman and her partner time to prepare and cope with the possibility that the birth may not proceed as they had anticipated.

▌ *Other Nursing Diagnoses*

Also assess for the following nursing diagnoses, which are frequently present with this condition:

- Anxiety/Fear[1] related to unknown outcome of labor, fear of harm to self and/or fetus, and unfamiliarity with amnioinfusion.

FORCEPS- OR VACUUM-ASSISTED BIRTH

Forceps or vacuum extractor is used to apply traction to the fetal head during birth to assist fetal descent and/or rotate the fetal head from occiput posterior or occiput transverse to the occiput anterior position. In the United States, vacuum extraction is slightly more common than forceps-assisted birth. A vacuum extractor is a cup-shaped instrument that uses suction to grasp the fetal head. Forceps are curved metal instruments with two blades that lock in the center. Today only about 4–8% of births are assisted with these instruments. There are many types, each with special functions. There are three categories of forceps application, according to the location of the fetal head at the time of application. They are:

1. *Outlet forceps.* Fetal skull has reached the perineum and scalp is visible between UCs and rotation does not exceed 45 degrees.
2. *Low forceps.* Leading edge of fetal skull at +2 station or below, but not on the pelvic floor with rotation greater than 45 degrees.
3. *Mid forceps.* Fetal head is engaged, but is higher than +2 station (e.g., +1, 0).

▌ *Key Nursing Activities*

- Obtain instruments and urinary catheter.
- Place woman in lithotomy position.
- Assess, record, and report FHR before forceps are applied; monitor throughout procedure.
- Coach woman to not push during forceps application.
- Be prepared for immediate cesarean birth if vacuum or forceps fail.
- Following birth, observe mother and infant for trauma.

▌ *Risk Factors*

Asian women are 63% more likely to have operative delivery than Caucasian women; African American women are 40% less likely to have operative delivery than Caucasian women. The following variables increase the likelihood that a woman will need operative birth (either forceps- or vacuum-assisted or cesarean):

- Older than 35 years
- Height less than 4 feet, 11 inches (150 cm)
- Pregnancy weight gain of more than 33 lb (15 kg)
- Smoker
- Gestational age greater than 41 weeks
- Epidural anesthesia
- Presence of dystocia
- Abnormal FHR tracing

▌ *Indications for Forceps- or Vacuum-Assisted Birth*

Instrumental (operative) birth is used in second-stage labor when any condition threatens the mother or fetus and can be relieved by birth, and when vaginal birth can be accomplished quickly without undue trauma. Indications include the following:

- Maternal indications. Exhaustion, inability to push effectively (failure to progress in second stage), effects of regional anesthesia on motor innervations (and pushing ability), previous spinal cord injury, cardiac or pulmonary disease, and intrapartum infection.

- Fetal indications. Prolapsed cord, placental abruption, and nonreassuring FHR patterns, abnormal position or immaturity.

Contraindications to Forceps- or Vacuum-Assisted Birth

Cesarean birth is preferred if a more rapid birth is needed than can be accomplished with forceps or vacuum extractor (e.g., severe fetal compromise, maternal pulmonary edema), or if forceps or vacuum extraction would be too traumatic (e.g., a high fetal station or cephalopelvic disproportion). *Relative contraindications* to vacuum extraction include face or breech presentation, gestation less than 35 wks, previous fetal scalp blood sampling, and suspected fetal macrosomia.

Medical Management

- Ensure that the cervix is completely dilated.
- Ensure vertex presentation and location (station) of fetal head and ensure that the head is engaged.
- Type of pelvis must be identified, and there must be no CPD.
- Catheterize. Provides more room in the pelvis and limits bladder trauma.
- Position and station known.
- Clinically adequate pelvis known.
- Rupture membranes, if necessary. Allows access to fetal head.
- Administer adequate anesthesia. Usually a pudendal or epidural block; midforceps may require epidural or general anesthesia.
- Episiotomy. Provides room for instruments and fetal head.
- Empty rectum. Allows room for descent of fetal head.
- With vacuum extraction, traction is applied and the woman is coached to bear down. If rapid descent of the fetus does not occur, the procedure is stopped and cesarean birth is performed.

Collaborative Problems

Potential complications of forceps- or vacuum-assisted birth include those outlined in this section.

Maternal

- Vaginal laceration or hematoma, periurethral lacerations, extension of episiotomy into the anus
- Hemorrhage
- Infection

Fetal

- Anoxia/hypoxia
- Bradycardia, marked tachycardia
- Prolonged severe variable decelerations or late decelerations

Infant

- Ecchymoses, facial and scalp lacerations or abrasions, facial nerve injury, caput succedaneum, cephalhematoma

(and subsequent hyperbilirubinemia), chignon (at application area of vacuum extractor), intracranial hemorrhage, subgaleal hematomas (occurs when emissary veins are damaged and blood accumulates in the potential space between the galea aponeurotica and periosteum of the skull [Simpson & Creehan, 2007]), retinal hemorrhage, and hyperbilirubinemia.

COLLABORATIVE (STANDARDIZED) CARE FOR ALL WOMEN HAVING FORCEPS- OR VACUUM-ASSISTED BIRTH

Perform a comprehensive assessment to identify individual needs for teaching, emotional support, and physical care.

Potential Complications (Maternal) of Forceps- or Vacuum-Assisted Birth: VAGINAL LACERATION OR HEMATOMA, BLADDER INJURY, PERIURETHRAL LACERATIONS, AND EXTENSION OF EPISIOTOMY INTO THE ANUS

Focus Assessments

- Monitor UCs and FHR once forceps have been applied and advise provider when UC is present. As a rule, the provider applies traction only during a contraction.
- Observe for trauma during the immediate and subsequent postpartum period:
  - Bright red, continuous bleeding that occurs even when the uterus is contracted. Bleeding is a symptom of vaginal wall laceration.
  - Severe and unrelenting pain, edema, and/or discoloration of labia and perineum. These are signs of vaginal hematoma.
  - Urine retention. Palpate bladder and assess voiding. Urine retention may result from bladder or urethral injuries/edema. (See the generic NDCP, "Urinary Retention,[1]" beginning on p. 22 in Chapter 2.)

Preventive Nursing Activities

- Catheterize per order or protocol prior to application. Prevents trauma to bladder; makes room for descending fetal presenting part and for forceps.

- Encourage to use breathing techniques while forceps are being applied. Prevents pushing during application of forceps.

Potential Complication (Maternal) of Forceps- or Vacuum-Assisted Birth: POSTPARTUM HEMORRHAGE (FROM LACERATIONS OR UTERINE ATONY)

Refer to the generic collaborative care plan, "Potential Complication: Hemorrhage," beginning on p. 28 in Chapter 3.

Potential Complications (Maternal) of Forceps- or Vacuum-Assisted Birth: INFECTION DURING THE POSTPARTUM PERIOD

Refer to the generic collaborative care plan, "Potential Complication: Infection," beginning on p. 29 in Chapter 3, and the generic NDCP, "Risk for Infection,[1]" beginning on p. 21 in Chapter 2.

Potential Complications of Forceps- or Vacuum-Assisted Birth: ANOXIA/HYPOXIA, FACIAL AND SCALP LACERATIONS OR ABRASIONS, FACIAL NERVE INJURY, CAPUT SUCCEDANEUM, CEPHALHEMATOMA, CHIGNON, AND INTRACRANIAL HEMORRHAGE

Refer to "Newborn Care: First 4 Hours," and "Newborn Care: 4 Hours to 2 Days," beginning on pp. 369 and 376, respectively, in Chapter 11.

Focus Assessments

- Assess, record, and report FHR before forceps are applied. Ensures that fetal status does not require immediate

cesarean birth; provides baseline by which to evaluate fetal well-being during procedure.
- Assess FHR every 5 min or by continuous electronic fetal heart rate monitoring and report rate less than 100 bpm. Determines fetal tolerance of procedure; if FHR drops, the provider typically removes and reapplies the forceps.
- Observe for mild (not below 100 beats/min) fetal bradycardia when traction is applied. This results from head compression and is transient.
- Assess the newborn for the following:
  - Retinal hemorrhages. Can occur from pressure to the head, especially if birth was achieved rapidly.
  - Facial skin abrasions. These allow entry of microorganisms.
  - Cerebral edema. This can occur from traumatic birth.
  - Facial asymmetry (that is most obvious when infant cries). This suggests facial nerve injury.

Preventive Nursing Activities

During labor, provide nursing activities to minimize factors that increase the risk of operative/instrumental birth, as described in the following lists.

For Dystocia/Dysfunctional Labor

- Change maternal position, encourage ambulation, assist with pelvic rocking, use of birthing ball, have the woman empty bladder frequently. Refer to the topic, "Dystocia/ Dysfunctional Labor," beginning on p. 265 in this chapter.

For FHR Abnormalities

- Encourage ambulation, position changes, left lateral position. Provide adequate hydration and monitor to detect early FHR changes. Be prepared for cesarean birth within 10 minutes. Refer to "Dystocia/Dysfunctional Labor," beginning on p. 265 of this chapter. If good application or suction cannot be obtained, or if no descent occurs with application of traction, immediate cesarean birth will likely be necessary to prevent harm to mother and fetus.

For the Newborn

- Keep skin abrasions clean. Removes and prevents growth of pathogens.
- No treatment is needed for facial bruising. Cold is not used for newborns because of the risk of hypothermia. See Chapter 12.
- Document detailed description of wounds. Provides baseline for later comparison.

INDIVIDUALIZED (NURSING DIAGNOSIS) CARE PLANS

This section includes care plans developed to address unique patient needs.

Nursing Diagnosis: DEFICIENT KNOWLEDGE[1] (OF PROCEDURE AND/OR SEQUELAE TO MOTHER/INFANT)

Related Factors: unanticipated need for instrumental birth and unfamiliarity with forceps and vacuum-extraction procedures. Refer to the generic NDCP, "Deficient Knowledge,[1]" beginning on p. 13 in Chapter 2.

Goals, Outcomes, and Evaluation Criteria

- Woman remains in control and able to cooperate during the procedure.
- Woman expresses understanding of the nature of any fetal trauma (e.g., caput, chignon, abrasions) that occurs.

Nursing Activities and Rationales

Patient/Family Teaching

- Explain the procedure and what the woman can expect to feel. Relieves fear and anxiety that occur in an unexpected, unfamiliar, and threatening situation. With adequate anesthesia, she should feel pressure, but no pain. If she is to have general anesthesia, explain that as well.
- Explain that the forceps are safe for the baby, that they fit like two tablespoons around an egg; or explain how the vacuum extractor works. Alleviates fear at the appearance of the instruments.
- Advise the woman that she will be expected to pant and blow while forceps are being applied. Decreases the urge to push during the contraction, so that good application can be obtained.
- Following the birth, explain any marks on the baby or other apparent injuries. For example, explain that the infant's skin is delicate, so pressure of the forceps has caused minor bruising (or a little scrape) that usually goes away without treatment; or explain that the chignon, which occurs with vacuum extraction, will disappear within 2 or 3 days. Information decreases anxiety.
- While the woman is in the hospital, point out improvements in the baby's appearance as they occur (e.g., bruises fade, caput recedes, abrasions heal). Provides reassurance that the infant is indeed well.

Nursing Diagnosis: PERINEAL PAIN (POSTPARTUM)

Related Factors: trauma secondary to instrumental birth, e.g., bruising, hematomas, and lacerations. Refer to the generic NDCP, "Pain,[1]" beginning on p. 18 in Chapter 2.

Goals, Outcomes, and Evaluation Criteria

- Woman ambulates satisfactorily after administration of analgesics.
- Woman is able to obtain adequate rest and sleep, uninterrupted by pain.
- Woman is free of pain, which can interfere with mother–infant bonding.

Nursing Activities and Rationales

Assessments

- Assess ability to ambulate and perform self-care measures. Perineal hematomas and bruising can cause enough pain to interfere with ambulation and activities of daily living.
- Observe interactions with infant. Ensures that bonding is occurring and that pain is not interfering with the woman's ability to care for and interact with the infant. (See Chapter 12.)

Independent Nursing Actions

- Apply ice pack to perineum during the first 12 hours after birth. Reduces pain by numbing the area; helps limit edema formation in the perineum.
- After the first 12 hours postbirth, use warm, moist packs or sitz bath. Reduces pain and promotes healing by increasing circulation to the affected area and aiding in resolution of edema and bruising.

Collaborative Activities

- Administer prescribed analgesics at least 30 minutes prior to activity. Ensures adequate pain relief so that activities are not inhibited by pain.
- Report instrumental delivery to postpartum nurses or oncoming shift. Ensures continuity of care and prevents further complications from the maternal injuries.

Other Nursing Diagnoses

Also assess for the following nursing diagnoses, which may be present:

- Anxiety/Fear[1] related to lack of previous experience with procedure.
- Risk for Infection[1] related to trauma. See the generic NDCP, "Risk for Infection,[1]" which begins on p. 21 in Chapter 2.

ENDNOTES

1. Nursing Diagnoses—Definitions and Classification 2009–2011. Copyright © 2009, 2007, 2005, 2003, 2001, 1998, 1996, 1994 by NANDA International. Used by arrangement with Blackwell Publishing Limited, a company of John Wiley & Sons, Inc. In order to make safe and effective judgments using NANDA-I nursing diagnoses it is essential that nurses refer to the definitions and defining characteristics of the diagnoses listed in this work.
2. Bulechek, G. M., Butcher, H. K., Dochterman, J. M. (2008). *Nursing Interventions Classification* (5th ed). St. Louis, MO: Elsevier, by permission.

REFERENCES

American College of Obstetricians and Gynecologists (ACOG). (2010, August). Practice bulletin #115, vaginal birth after previous cesarean delivery. *Obstetrics & Gynecology, 116*(2 Pt 1), 450–463.

Bulechek, G. M., Butcher, H. K., & Dochterman, J. M. (2008). *Nursing interventions classification (NIC)* (5th ed.). St. Louis, MO: Mosby/Elsevier.

Choudhary, D., Bano, I., & Ali, S. M. (2009, August 14). Does amnioinfusion reduce caesarean section rate in meconium-stained amniotic fluid? *Archives Gynecology and Obstetrics.* Retrieved from http://www.springerlink.com/content/w1201160q5675253/

Fries, K. (2010). African American women & unplanned cesarean birth. *American Journal of Maternal Child Nursing, 35*(2), 110–115.

Gregory, K.D., Fridman, M., & Korst, L. (2010, August). Trends and patterns of vaginal birth after cesarean availability in the United States. *Seminars in Perinatology, 34*(4), 237–243.

Hikel, K. (2009). The real risk for cesareans: An expert interview with Pamela K. Spry, BSN, MS, PhD. *Medscape.com Ob/Gyn & Women's Health Care.* Retrieved from http://www.medscape.com/viewarticle/706095

Joy, S., Scott, P. L., & Lyon, D. (2009, August). Abnormal Labor. eMedicine from WebMD. Retrieved from http://emedicine.medscape.com/article/273053-overview

MacDorman, M. F., & Kirmeyer, S. (2009). Fetal and perinatal mortality, United States, 2005. *National Vital Statistics Reports.* Hyattsville, MD: National Center for Health Statistics. 57(8).

Meddings, F., MacVane Phipps, F., Haith-Cooper, M., & Haigh, J. (2007). Vaginal birth after caesarean section (VBAC): Exploring women's perceptions. *Journal of Clinical Nursing, 16*, 160–167.

Nahum, G. G., & Pham, K. Q. (2010, May 12). Uterine rupture in pregnancy. *eMedicine.com.* Retrieved from http://emedicine.medscape.com/article/275854-overview

North American Nursing Diagnosis Association. (2009). *Nursing diagnoses classification.* North American Nursing Diagnosis Association. Ames, IA: Wiley Publishing.

Oregon Evidence-based Practice Center. (2010, March). Vaginal birth after cesarean: New insights. *Evidence Report/Technology Assessment.* AHRQ Publication No. 10-E001, U.S. Department of Health and Human Services. Retrieved from http://www.ahrq.gov/downloads/pub/evidence/pdf/vbacup/vbacup.pdf

Ricci, S., & Kyle, T. (2008). *Maternity and pediatric nursing.* Philadelphia, PA: Lippincott Williams & Wilkins.

Simpson, K., & Creehan, P. (2008). *AWHONN's perinatal nursing* (3rd ed.). Philadelphia, PA: Lippincott Williams & Wilkins.

Sullivan, J. T., Grobman, W. A., Bauchat, J. R., Scavone, B. M., Grouper, S., McCarthy, R. J., & Wong, C. A. (2009) A randomized controlled trial of the effect of combined spinal-epidural analgesia on the success of external cephalic version for breech presentation. *International Journal Obstetric Anesthesia, 18*(4), 328–334.

Tempfer, C., Brunner, A., Bentz, E. Lanager, M., Reinthaller, A., & Hefler, L. (2009). Intrauterine fetal death and delivery complications associated with coagulopathy: A retrospective analysis of 104 cases. *Journal of Women's Health, 18*(4), 469–474.

RESOURCES

Brass, E. (2010). Thrombocytopenia in pregnancy. *Postgraduate Obstetrics & Gynecology, 30*(4), 1–8.

Buley, K. (2010). Puzzling out preeclampsia. *Nursing Made Incredibly Easy, 8*(2), 20–29. doi: 10.1097/01.NME.0000368747.44795.7a

Capitulo, K. (2004). Perinatal grief online. *Maternal Child Nursing, 29*(5), 305–311.

Caughey, A. (2009). Informed consent for a vaginal birth after previous cesarean delivery. *Journal of Midwifery & Women's Health, 54*(3), 249–253.

Chancellor, J., & Thorp, J. (2008). Blood pressure measurement in pregnancy. *British Journal of Obstetrics and Gynecology, 115*(9), 1076–1077.

Chhabra, S., Dargan, R., & Nasare, M. (2007, May). Antepartum transabdominal amnioinfusion. *International Journal of Gynaecology and Obstetrics, 97*(2), 95–99.

Clark, S., Belfort, M., Dildy, G., & Meyers, J. (2008). Reducing obstetric litigation through alterations in practice patterns. *Obstetrics and Gynecology, 112*(6), 1279–1283.

DeBackere, K., Hill, P., & Kavanaugh, K. (2008). The parental experience of pregnancy after perinatal loss. *Journal of Obstetric, Gynecologic & Neonatal Nursing, 37*(5), 525–537.

DiMarco, M., Menke, E., & McNamara, T. (2001). Evaluating a support group for perinatal loss. *Maternal Child Nursing, 26*(3), 135–140.

Ekelin, M., Crang-Svalenius, E., Nordstrom, B., & Dykes, A. (2008). Parents' experiences, reactions, and needs regarding a nonviable fetus diagnosed at a second trimester routine ultrasound. *Journal of Obstetric, Gynecologic & Neonatal Nursing, 3*(4), 446–454.

Gamble, J., Creedy, D., McCourt, C., Weaver, J., & Beake, S. (2007). A critique of the literature on women's request for cesarean section. *Birth, 34*(4), 331–340.

Georges, I., Kehdy, E., Ghanem, J., El-Rahi, C., & Nakad, T. (2006). Rupture of uterine scar 3 weeks after vaginal birth after cesarean section (VBAC). *Journal of Maternal-Fetal and Neonatal Medicine, 19*(6), 371–373.

Gootscholten, K., Kok, M., Guid, O., Mol, B., & Van der Post, J. (2008). External cephalic version-related risks: A meta-analysis. *Obstetrics & Gynecology, 112*(5), 1143–1151.

Hashima, J., & Guise, J. (2007, May). Vaginal birth after cesarean: A prenatal scoring tool. *American Journal of Obstetrics & Gynecology,* e22–e23.

Heazell, A., & Froen, J. (2008). Methods of fetal movement counting and the detection of fetal compromise. *Journal of Obstetrics and Gynaecology, 28*(2), 147–154.

Humburg, J., Ladewig, A., Hoesli, I., & Holzreve, W. (2009). Recurrent postpartum urinary retention: A case report. *Journal of Obstetrics and Gynecology, 35*(2), 368–371.

Korteweg, F., Erwich, J., Holm, J., Ravise, J., Van der Meer, J., Veeger, N., & Timmer, A. (2009). Diverse placental pathologies as the main cause of fetal death. *Obstetrics & Gynecology, 114*(4), 809–817.

Lang, C., & Landon, M. (2010). Uterine rupture as a source of obstetrical hemorrhage. *Clinical Obstetrics and Gynecology, 53*(1), 237–251.

Lowdermilk, D. L., Perry, S. E., & Bobak, I. M. (2007). *Maternity & women's health care* (9th ed.). St. Louis, MO: Mosby.

Lowe, N. (2007). A review of factors associated with dystocia and cesarean section in nulliparous women. *Journal of Midwifery & Women's Health, 52*(3), 216–228.

Martin, J. (2002). *Intrapartum management modules: A perinatal education program* (3rd ed.). Philadelphia, PA: Lippincott Williams & Wilkins.

McKinney, E. S., & Murray, S. S. (2009). *Foundations of maternal-newborn nursing* (5th ed.). Philadelphia, PA: W. B. Saunders.

Nolan, A., & Lawrence, C. (2009). A pilot study of a nursing intervention protocol to minimize maternal-infant separation after cesarean birth. *Journal of Obstetric, Gynecologic & Neonatal Nursing,38*(4), 430–441.

O'Grady, J. P., & Taugher, C. (2008, August 21). Vacuum extraction. *eMedicine.com.* Retrieved from http://emedicine.medscape.com/article/271175-overview

Olagundoye, V., Black, R., & MacKenzie, Z. (2008). Impact of the severity of fetal distress on decision-to-delivery intervals for assisted vaginal delivery. *Journal of Obstetrics and Gynaecology, 28*(1), 51–55.

Papp, S., Dhaliwal, G., Davies, G., & Borschneck, D. (2004). Fetal femur fracture and external cephalic version. *Obstetrics and Gynecology, 105*(3), 1154–1156. doi: 10.1097/01.AOG.0000157032.81436.c6

Peters, R. (2008). High blood pressure in pregnancy. *Nursing for Women's Health, 12*(5), 412–421.

Pillitteri, A. (2010). *Maternal & child health nursing: Care of the childbearing and childrearing family* (6th ed.). Philadelphia, PA: Lippincott Williams & Wilkins.

Pinettte, M., Kahn, J., Gross, K., Wax, J., Blackstone, J., & Cartin, A. (2004). Vaginal birth after cesarean rates are declining rapidly in the rural state of Maine. *Journal of Maternal, Fetal and Neonatal Medicine, 16,* 37–43.

Pongsatha, S., & Tongson, T. (2004). Therapeutic termination of second trimester pregnancies with intrauterine fetal death with 400 micrograms of oral misoprostol. *Journal of Obstetrics and Gynecology, 30*(3), 217–220.

Roehrs, C., Masterson, A., Alles, R., Witt, C., & Rutt, P. (2008). Caring for families coping with perinatal loss. *Journal of Obstetric, Gynecologic & Neonatal Nursing, 37*(6), 631–639.

Sibony, O., Alran, S., & Qury, J. (2006). Vaginal birth after cesarean section: X-ray pelvimetry at term is informative. *Journal of Perinatal Medicine, 34,* 212–215.

Singla, A., Yadav, P., Vaid, N. B., Suneja, A., & Faridi, M. M. (2010). Transabdominal amnioinfusion in preterm premature rupture of membranes. *International Journal of Gynaecology and Obstetrics, 108*(3),199–202.

Sinha, P., & Langford, K. (2009). Forceps delivery in 21st century obstetrics. *Internet Journal of Gynecology & Obstetrics, 11*(2), 9. Retrieved from http://www.ispub.com/journal/the_internet_journal_of_gynecology_and_obstetrics/volume_11_number_2_6/article_printable/forceps-delivery-in-21st-century-obstetrics.html

Ward, S., & Hisley, S. (2009). *Clinical pocket companion for maternal-child nursing care.* Philadelphia, PA: F.A. Davis Company.

Winstein, K. (2009, January 7). Early C-section risks, study finds: Elective procedures increase complications for infants when done before 39 weeks. *Wall Street Journal,* D1. Retrieved from http://online.wsj.com/article/SB123138530855663493.html

Xu, H., Wei, S., & Praser, W. (2008). Obstetric approaches to the prevention of meconium aspiration syndrome. *Journal of Perinatology, 28,* S14–S18. doi:10.1038/jp.2008.145

Yeomans, E. (2010). Operative vaginal delivery. *Obstetrics & Gynecology, 115*(3), 645–653.

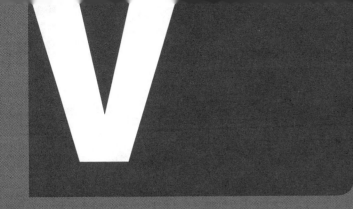

POSTPARTUM CARE

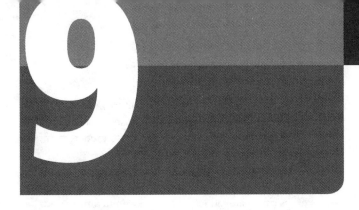

NORMAL POSTPARTUM CARE

Judith J. Hilton

POSTPARTUM PERIOD: FIRST 4 HOURS AFTER BIRTH (FOURTH STAGE OF LABOR)

The fourth stage of labor refers to the first 4 hours following birth. It is a time of elation and excitement for the new mother, but she may also be exhausted. The mother holds her infant for the first time and is encouraged to initiate breastfeeding. During this time the physiologic changes that occurred in pregnancy begin to reverse, and the maternal organs start readjusting to the nonpregnant state.

Key Nursing Activities

- Monitor for complications, especially postpartum (PP) hemorrhage and urinary retention
- Promote parent–child attachment
- Initiate breastfeeding if not contraindicated
- Encourage rest
- Monitor and control pain
- Transfer from recovery care to PP or mother–baby care after 1 or 2 hours if VSs are stable, uterus is firm, and lochia flow is small to moderate in amount (follow agency protocol).

Etiologies and Risk Factors

There are no risk factors for the fourth stage of labor because it is a normal process. The etiology is the birth of the infant.

Signs and Symptoms

A variety of normal behaviors and symptoms may occur. The mother may be thirsty, fatigued, excited, or unable to sleep. Mild uterine cramping and fairly heavy lochia rubra are normal. Symptoms such as a boggy uterus, bladder distention, excessive perineal bruising, and lacerations of the perineum and birth canal indicate problems rather normal postpartum recovery.

Diagnostic Studies

- Urinalysis. May be ordered to detect proteinuria or infection. Because autolysis occurs to return the uterus to its prepregnant size, it is normal to have a urine protein of 1+ during the first 2 postpartum days.
- White blood cell count. May be ordered to assess for infection; normal values of 20,000 to 25,000/mm^3 are common during the first 1–2 postpartum weeks.
- Hemoglobin (Hgb) and hematocrit (Hct). Assess for excessive blood loss and/or anemia. Hgb and Hct may be difficult to evaluate in the first 48–72 hours after birth because of the changing blood volume and greater loss of plasma volume than in red blood cells (Blackburn, 2007). A decrease of two percentage points from the admission Hct indicates a blood loss of about 500 ml (James, 2008).

Medical Management

- Prevention of complications (e.g., infection, urinary retention, hematoma, hemorrhage)
- Control of pain through:
  - Oral narcotic analgesics (e.g., acetaminophen [Tylenol] with codeine)
  - Nonsteroidal anti-inflammatory analgesics (NSAIDs; e.g., naproxen [Anaprox])
  - Topical antiseptic or anesthetic ointments or sprays

Collaborative Problems

Note: Two nursing diagnoses are included because they should be a part of the standardized care for all postpartum women.

Potential Complications of first 4 hours after birth (Stage IV labor)

- Postpartum hemorrhage
- Trauma to perineum and birth canal (e.g., hematoma, lacerations, bruising)
- Infection
- Urinary retention
- Risk for impaired parent/infant/child attachment[1]
- Risk for injury[1]: falls

COLLABORATIVE (STANDARDIZED) CARE FOR ALL NORMAL POSTPARTUM WOMEN DURING THE FIRST 4 HOURS AFTER BIRTH

Perform a comprehensive assessment to identify individual needs for teaching, emotional support, and physical care.

Potential Complication of Postpartum Period (Fourth Stage of Labor): POSTPARTUM HEMORRHAGE

Also see the generic collaborative care plan, "Potential Complication: Hemorrhage," beginning on p. 28 in Chapter 3.

Focus Assessments and Rationales

- Identify risk factors for PP hemorrhage (e.g., long labor, multiparity, large baby, manual removal of adherent placenta, previous history of PP hemorrhage, excessive uterine manipulation). Hemorrhage is the most common threat during the immediate postpartum period. If risk factors are present, an individualized nursing care plan should be instituted for the woman (e.g., Risk for Fluid Volume Deficit[1]).

- Assess fundal height, position, and tone every 15 min for the first hour; then every 30 min for 1 hour; then hourly (or according to agency protocol). Establishes position and firmness of uterus. Fundus should be firm. When contracted, the interlacing fibers of the myometrium compress blood vessels at the placental site to keep them from bleeding and allow clotting to begin. If the fundus is higher than normal and not in the midline, the urinary bladder may be full or clots may be present within the uterus; these can interfere with uterine contraction.

- Monitor lochia on same schedule as fundal assessments. Identifies abnormal bleeding. Observe for color and amount, presence of clots and odor, and pooling or clots on woman's sheets or buttocks. Normally lochia trickles from the vagina as the uterus contracts. Gushing may occur briefly as the uterus contracts with massage. Spurting, bright red blood indicates cervical or vaginal tears or uterine atony.

- Palpate the bladder. A full bladder (palpable above the symphysis pubis) can displace the fundus and interfere with uterine contraction.

- Assess urine output. At birth, the prenatal tendency to retain fluid reverses. Increased renal blood flow results in diuresis.

- Assess blood pressure (BP) on same schedule as fundal assessment. Hypotension can occur from hypovolemia secondary to hemorrhage. Orthostatic hypotension can occur from splanchnic engorgement following birth. For the most accurate reading, BP checks should be done with the woman in the same position each time. The preferred position is supine (London, Ladewig, Ball, Bindler, & Cowen, 2010).

- Assess heart rate on same schedule as fundal assessment. Stroke volume, cardiac output, and heart rate, which are increased during pregnancy, may remain increased or may decrease following birth as blood that was shunted through the uterus and placenta returns to the maternal circulation. A rapid pulse may indicate hypovolemia secondary to hemorrhage, as the body attempts to compensate for a decreasing BP.

- Institute pad count. Detects hemorrhage secondary to uterine atony or vaginal/uterine lacerations. Excessive bleeding exists if pads are saturated within a 15-min time period.

- Monitor Hgb and Hct levels. Aids in estimating amount of blood loss. If Hgb is 10 mg or less or Hct is 30% or less, the woman will not tolerate blood loss well.

Preventive Nursing Activities

- If bladder is palpable above symphysis pubis and woman cannot void, notify the care provider and insert urinary catheter. A full bladder can cause uterine atony.

- Notify care provider if blood loss is excessive and/or if there are other signs of hemorrhage (e.g., hypotension, tachycardia, narrow pulse pressure). Ensures that medical intervention is obtained, if needed.

- If the woman had intravenous (IV) fluids during labor, keep the IV line open for 1–2 hours after birth, or until condition is stable (or according to order or agency protocol). Ensures ready access for administering fluids, emergency medications, and/or blood should hemorrhage occur. Normally no more than 400 ml of fluid is lost during birth.

- Massage the fundus if boggy. Stop massaging when uterus becomes firm. Prevents excessive bleeding and promotes evacuation of blood clots. Massage stimulates uterine contractility, and when performed every 10–15 minutes for the first hour following birth, it reduces the incidence of PP hemorrhage. As the interlacing uterine muscles contract, uterine blood vessels are compressed, which helps control bleeding. Blood clots that are not expelled can prevent uterine contraction. Excessive uterine massage, however, can cause muscle fatigue and loss of contractility.

- Encourage and assist with breastfeeding as soon as possible after the birth and at any time uterine atony is present, taking the mother's wishes and needs into consideration. The baby's sucking stimulates the posterior pituitary to release oxytocin, which causes uterine contraction. The mother may be too fatigued to breastfeed, however, and in some cultures, breastfeeding is not started until milk production begins.

- Administer oxytocin at birth per protocol, and again during the PP, if uterus does not stay firm. See "Normal Labor: Third Stage," beginning on p. 238 in Chapter 7.

Potential Complication of Postpartum Period (Fourth Stage of Labor): TRAUMA TO

THE PERINEUM AND/OR BIRTH CANAL (E.G., HEMATOMA, LACERATIONS, OR BRUISING)

Focus Assessments and Rationales

- Review labor and birth records for presence of risk factors (e.g., forceps-assisted birth, precipitous labor, long second stage). If the woman is at higher than normal risk for trauma to the perineum, she may require more than the usual standardized care; if so, an individualized nursing diagnosis care plan should be instituted.
- Assess perineum and episiotomy every 15 min for the first hour; then every 30 min for 1 hour; then hourly (or according to agency protocol). Establishes the presence of edema, hematoma, lacerations, ecchymoses, or loss of approximation of episiotomy edges. Edema may cause the episiotomy edges to separate.
- Assess for signs of unrepaired laceration. A slow trickle of bright red blood in the presence of a firm uterus may indicate an unrepaired laceration of the vagina or cervix.
- Assess for severe perineal pain or intense pressure. These are symptoms of hematoma formation, which may require surgical intervention. Pain is caused by tissue hypoxia secondary to pressure of blood accumulation within the tissues. Pain is determined by the woman stating her comfort level on a scale of 1–10 with 10 indicating severe pain.
- Monitor heart rate and BP. Elevated heart rate and decreasing BP in the presence of a firm uterus and no visible excess blood loss may be signs of hematoma formation resulting from blood loss from the vascular compartment into the tissues.

Preventive Nursing Activities

- Apply an ice pack to the perineum, leaving on for 15–20 minutes and off for 15–20 minutes alternating. Decreases the formation of edema and ecchymoses by constricting local blood vessels and facilitating clotting. This tends to limit the size of the hematoma, pressure caused by the hematoma, and subsequent pain. If local cold is applied for more than 20 min, reflex vasodilation may occur and it will not be effective.

Potential Complication of Postpartum Period (Fourth Stage of Labor): INFECTION

See the generic collaborative care plan, "Potential Complication: Infection," beginning on p. 29 in Chapter 3.

Focus Assessments and Rationales

- Review labor and birth records for preexisting infections or exposure to infectious organisms. Signs and symptoms of

a new infection will occur slowly, probably not earlier than 24–48 hours after birth. However, the nurse must be aware of preexisting infections during the first 4 hours to provide necessary interventions and be alert for complications.
- Assess for elevated temperature. Elevated maternal temperature may occur following childbirth due to dehydration and the physical demands of labor (Cunningham et al., 2010).

Preventive Nursing Activities

- Provide frequent pad changes and perineal care, using front-to-back techniques, until the woman is able to care for herself. Removes the warm, moist medium for growth of pathogens and avoids transferring *Escherichia coli* from the rectum to the vagina and urinary tract.

Potential Complication of Postpartum Period (Fourth Stage of Labor): URINARY RETENTION

Refer to the NDCP, "Urinary Retention,[1]" beginning on p. 22 in Chapter 2.

Focus Assessments and Rationales

- Monitor intake and output, including IV fluids. Establishes the presence of urine outflow obstruction or renal complications. Urine output should approximate intake. At birth of the baby, the prenatal tendency to hold fluids in the tissues reverses. At the same time, renal plasma flow remains elevated for several days, resulting in rapid bladder filling. In addition, the woman may have received IV fluids during labor. If edema prevents the bladder from emptying, distention may occur quickly.
- Ask the woman whether she feels the sensation of the need to void. If she is still having residual effects from an epidural anesthetic, she may not feel the sensation of fullness.
- Note time of first voiding after birth of infant. Woman should void within 8 hours after birth.
- Assess temperature and other indications of hydration (e.g., skin turgor). Determines that lack of urine output is not caused by dehydration. Mild temperature elevation occurs with dehydration.
- Monitor woman's ability to empty the bladder completely. Detects full bladder, which can interfere with uterine contractions. After emptying, the bladder should not be palpable and the uterine fundus should be firm.

Preventive Nursing Activities

- If the woman has not voided, at least once an hour, encourage her to try to void. Establishes the adequacy of urine output and assesses the woman's ability to void and fully empty her urinary bladder.

- If there is no nausea, offer clear fluids; encourage the woman to sip on fluids often. Establishes that failure to void is not caused by inadequate intake. A great deal of fluid is lost during labor and birth, both because of blood loss and metabolic demands.
- Initiate measures to promote voiding as needed:
  - If the woman is unable to void in sitting position, have her stand over the commode or try to void while she is in the shower. Because of urethral and perineal edema, the usual voiding position may not be as effective.
  - Run water in the bathroom while the woman attempts to void. Sensory stimuli and the power of suggestion may promote voiding.
  - Stroke the inner aspect of the woman's thigh. May stimulate sensory nerves and promote micturition reflex.
  - Place the woman's hand in warm water while she tries to void. May prompt voiding by the power of suggestion.
  - Provide a sitz bath if available and instruct to try to void in the sitz bath. Warm water may relax the perineum and decrease edema.
- If the bladder is palpable above the symphysis pubis, catheterize according to order or agency protocol. See the generic NDCP, "Urinary Retention,[1]" beginning on p. 22 in Chapter 2.

Nursing Diagnosis: RISK FOR IMPAIRED PARENT–INFANT/ CHILD ATTACHMENT[1]

See the generic care plan: "Risk for Impaired Parent–Infant/Child Attachment,[1]" beginning on p. 19 in Chapter 2. Also refer to the NDCP, "Risk for Impaired Parent–Infant/Child Attachment,[1]" which begins on p. 232 of the topic, "Normal Labor: Second Stage," in Chapter 7.

Nursing Diagnosis: RISK FOR INJURY (FALLS)[1]

Related Factors: exhaustion, orthostatic hypotension, blood loss, side/prolonged effects of epidural anesthesia, etc.

▋ *Signs and Symptoms*

Signs and symptoms of risk for injury by falls are not applicable. Presence of signs/symptoms indicates an actual, not a potential, problem.

▋ *Goals, Outcomes, and Evaluation Criteria*

- Woman describes side effects of regional anesthesia.

- Woman uses call bell when needing assistance.
- Woman follows selected risk control strategies (e.g., does not get out of bed without help).
- Woman uses personal support systems to control risk.

▋ *NIC Interventions[2]*

Postanesthesia Care (2870)—Monitoring and management of the patient who has recently undergone general or regional anesthesia.

Postpartal Care (6930)—Monitoring and management of the patient who has recently given birth.

Risk Identification (6610)—Analysis of potential risk factor, determination of health risks, and prioritization of risk reduction strategies for an individual or group.

▋ *Nursing Activities and Rationales*

Assessments

- Review records for amount of blood lost during the birth and for Hgb level. Anemia and blood loss decrease the number of RBCs available to deliver oxygen to the brain, thereby predisposing the woman to syncope.
- Monitor spinal/epidural anesthesia level. Determines the need for safety measures. The woman should be able to raise her legs, raise her buttocks off the bed, and have no feelings of numbness or tingling before being allowed to attempt ambulation with assistance.
- Assess level of consciousness. Determines the degree of sedation and when to allow increased activity level. The woman receiving general anesthesia or narcotic analgesics should be fully awake, oriented to time, person, and place before being allowed to attempt ambulation with assistance. Note: It is unlikely that a normal postpartum woman will have had general anesthesia, although it is sometimes used if an emergency birth is necessary.

Independent Nursing Actions

- Assist with the first ambulation. When first changing from supine to upright position, orthostatic hypotension may occur.
- Postpone shower or sitz bath until after recovery period, if possible. If one is necessary, accompany the woman the first time. In addition to orthostatic hypotension, the warmth of the shower or sitz bath may cause vasodilation and subsequent dizziness.
- If dizziness/syncope occurs, help the woman to lie flat or sit on a chair or the floor with her head between her knees. Uses gravity to promote circulation to the brain.
- Keep an ammonia ampule ready for use when helping with ambulation. If the woman becomes dizzy or faint, inhaling the ammonia may be helpful.

Patient/Family Teaching

- Teach the woman the need for seeking assistance before getting out of bed. In the first few hours after birth, the woman is fatigued and may not have full motor control of her legs because of regional anesthesia. Many women do not ambulate during this 4-hour period. Their understanding that they are at increased risk for falls and injury may ensure their compliance with asking for assistance (e.g., to go to the bathroom).

- Teach the woman how to use call light. Ensures that the woman knows how to secure assistance if she needs to urinate or ambulate.
- Encourage the woman to get out of bed slowly. Helps prevent orthostatic hypotension.

INDIVIDUALIZED (NURSING DIAGNOSIS) CARE PLANS

The care plans in this section were developed to address unique patient needs.

■ Nursing Diagnosis: PAIN[1]

Related Factors: uterine contractions, episiotomy, hematoma, perineal edema and bruising, bladder distention, and hemorrhoids. See the generic NDCP, "Pain,[1]" beginning on p. 18 in Chapter 2.

■ *Nursing Activities and Rationales*

Assessments

- Assess episiotomy/laceration/incision for evidence of bleeding/hematoma formation. Increased bleeding and swelling at site of episiotomy/laceration/incision increase pain and discomfort. Early recognition of bleeding or swelling allows for early interventions to prevent worsening of the pain.
- Assess for urinary retention. A full bladder adds to the discomfort the woman may be experiencing and may cause uterine atony.

Independent Nursing Actions

- Ensure adequate fluid intake. Facilitates healing. Dry tissues and mucous membranes do not heal well and place the woman at increased risk for infection and increased pain.
- Apply ice pack to perineum immediately after birth, then leave on for 15–20 min and off for 15–20 minutes. Cold provides local anesthesia and causes local vasoconstriction and helps to prevent perineal edema. This helps to limit the discomfort of episiotomy and/or hemorrhoids. If cold is applied for longer than 20 min, reflex vasodilation will occur and the ice pack will not be effective.
- Provide information about care and what to expect over the next 24 hours. Information relieves anxiety, which may decrease the perception of pain.

- Encourage the woman to talk about the birthing experience. Helps relieve tension, which may decrease pain. It also distracts from pain.
- Provide comfort measures such as perineal care, clean gown and linens, and mouth care. Provides comfort, enhances feelings of well-being.
- Provide warm blankets, if woman is experiencing chills/tremors; reassure her that chills/tremors are common, normal, and will last only a short while. Relieves physical discomfort and anxiety, which increase the perception of pain.
- While woman is still experiencing effects of epidural anesthesia, reposition her frequently. Improves circulation, prevents discomfort of tissue hypoxia. The limited ability to move her legs may interfere with the woman's ability to change positions.
- Encourage rest and sleep between assessments. Exhaustion from labor and birth interfere with the ability to cope with pain/discomfort.

Patient/Family Teaching

- If pain is severe, encourage to use breathing and relaxation techniques learned for labor. Provides distraction and enhances sense of control.

■ *Other Nursing Diagnosis*

Also assess for the following nursing diagnosis, which is frequently present with this condition.

- Anxiety[1] related to lack of experience, lack of support, lack of information, misinformation, or lack of confidence in parenting skills/abilities.

POSTPARTUM PERIOD: DAYS 1–2

During the first 1–2 days following birth, the woman experiences many changes. The physiologic changes that occurred in pregnancy begin to reverse, and the maternal organs start readjusting to the nonpregnant state. It is a time of elation and excitement for the new mother, but she may also be exhausted. The first-time mother must learn to care for herself and her infant and adjust to her added responsibilities. For other mothers it is a time of adjustment to the new infant and return to care of self and other children. Although the potential complications remain the same as during the recovery period (stage IV labor), the nursing focus shifts from physical care to teaching for self-care.

■ *Key Nursing Activities*

- Monitor for and prevent complications
- Facilitate breast- or bottle feeding
- Promote comfort
- Encourage family bonding
- Teach regarding self-care, infant care, and home care

Etiologies and Risk Factors

There are no risk factors because this is a normal process. Etiologies include vaginal birth or cesarean birth.

Signs and Symptoms

A variety of normal behaviors and symptoms may occur.

- During the first 2 hours following birth, the woman experiences lochial flow about that of a heavy menstrual period. The flow should steadily decrease after that time. Lochia rubra (consisting mainly of blood) usually persists for 3–4 days; however, lochia serosa (a pale, thinner pink or brown discharge) is sometimes seen on days 1 and 2 PP.
- The uterus should remain firm and be about 1 cm above the umbilicus within 12 hours following birth. Typically it descends 1–2 cm every 24 hours.
- As the woman begins to lose the excess tissue fluid that accumulated during pregnancy, profuse diaphoresis and diuresis (resulting in urinary urgency and frequency) occur during the first 2–3 days. This is further stimulated by decreased estrogen levels and the reduction in venous pressure in the lower extremities after the birth of the baby.
- Breast tenderness may occur by the second or third day, when milk production begins.
- Symptoms such as afterpains, perineal and rectal pain/discomfort, and fatigue are common, but mild problems that occur in the postpartum period.
- Temperature may rise to 38°C (100.4°F) after childbirth from fluid loss during labor and the birth process and the physical demands of labor (Cunningham et al., 2010). Temperature should return to normal after 24 hr.

Diagnostic Studies

- Urinalysis. May be ordered to determine the presence of infection (bacteria, increased WBCs).
- White cell count. May be ordered to determine the presence of infection (normal values of 20,000–25,000/mm^3 are common during the first one to two PP weeks).
- Hgb and Hct. Determines return to normal or abnormal values that may indicate excessive blood loss and/or anemia. Hgb and Hct may be difficult to evaluate in the first 48–72 hours after birth because of the changing blood volume and greater loss of plasma volume than of red blood cells. A decrease of two percentage points from the admission Hct indicates a blood loss of 500 ml (James, 2008). Values should approximate prelabor values within 6 weeks PP. As the extracellular fluid accumulated in pregnancy is excreted, hemoconcentration causes a rise in Hct.

Medical Management

- Monitor lab values for complications, e.g., hemorrhage, hematoma, infection, thrombophlebitis.
- Rubella vaccine if titer is less than 1:8, indicating no immunity.

- Rho(D) immune globulin (RhoGAM) for Rh-negative women who give birth to Rh-positive infants.
- Review hepatitis B status.
- Oral analgesics, e.g., acetaminophen (Tylenol), acetaminophen with codeine, NSAIDs, topical analgesics/antiseptics, e.g., witch hazel pads for episiotomy.
- Oxytocic medications for heavy bleeding, e.g., oxytocin (Pitocin), methylergonovine (Methergine), prostaglandin F$_{2a}$, (Hemabate [US]/Prostin 15/M [Canada]).
- Stool softeners, e.g., docusate sodium (Colace).
- Vitamin and iron supplements.

Collaborative Problems

Note: Four nursing diagnoses are included in the following list because they should be a part of the standardized care for all postpartum women even though they are not, by definition, collaborative problems.

Potential Complication of Days 1–2 of Postpartum Period

- Postpartum hemorrhage
- Trauma to perineum and birth canal (e.g., hematoma, lacerations, bruising)
- Puerperal infection
- Urinary retention
- Thrombophlebitis
- Risk for impaired parent/infant/child attachment[1]
- Readiness for enhanced family coping[1]
- Risk for constipation[1]
- Health-seeking behaviors[1]

STANDARDIZED CARE FOR ALL NORMAL POSTPARTUM WOMEN DURING DAYS 1–2

Perform a comprehensive assessment to identify individual needs for teaching, emotional support, and physical care.

Potential Complication of the Postpartum Period Days 1–2: POSTPARTUM HEMORRHAGE

See the generic collaborative care plan, "Potential Complication: Hemorrhage," beginning on p. 28 in Chapter 3, and the collaborative care plan for "Postpartum Hemorrhage," beginning on p. 308 in the preceding topic, "Postpartum Period: First 4 Hours After Birth (Fourth Stage of Labor)." Care for this potential problem is essentially the same on days 1 and 2, except that monitoring is less frequent than during the first 4 hours, and teaching for self-care becomes more important.

Focus Assessments and Rationales

- Monitor vital signs every shift. Detects signs of hemorrhage such as tachycardia, hypotension, poor skin turgor, or dry mucous membranes. These are, however, not the most immediate signs of blood loss.
- Monitor lochia for color and amount at least once per shift. Identifies normal progression of lochia from rubra to serosa. The reappearance of bright red blood after rubra lochia has ceased is a sign of active bleeding.
- Assess fundal height and tone every shift. Determines position and firmness of uterus. Fundus should remain firm and recede (involute) approximately one fingerbreadth each day. Displacement of the fundus, which is normally in the midline, indicates the presence of a full urinary bladder, which may cause uterine atony.
- Pad count, if heavier than normal bleeding occurs. Determines the presence of abnormal bleeding. Estimates of bleeding are based on amount of blood in centimeters on pad within 1 hour (i.e., scant is less than 2.5 cm, light is less than 10 cm, moderate is less than 15 cm, and heavy is one pad saturated within an hour).

Preventive Nursing Activities

- Teach signs and symptoms of postpartum hemorrhage. The woman who recognizes signs and symptoms of uterine bleeding will access treatment earlier than one who does not.
- Administer oxytocic medications as ordered if excessive bleeding persists and monitor uterine tone and lochia. These drugs stimulate uterine contractions to control postpartum uterine atony.

Potential Complication of Postpartum Period Days 1–2: HEMATOMA

See collaborative care plan for "Trauma to the Perineum and/or Birth Canal (e.g., Hematoma, Lacerations, Bruising)," beginning on p. 308 in the topic, "Postpartum Period: First 4 Hours After Birth (Fourth Stage of Labor)," preceding in this chapter.

Focus Assessments and Rationales

- Assess episiotomy, lacerations once per shift for edema and excessive bruising. Detects presence of pelvic or vulvar hematomas. Large areas of bluish-colored skin, tenderness, or pain are indications of hematoma.
- Assess level of pain. Pain is the most common symptom of hematomas; however, a subperitoneal hematoma may not be painful and the initial symptom may be shock. Most vulvar hematomas will be visible. The woman's comfort level should be less than 3 on a scale of 1–10.

Potential Complication of Postpartum Period Days 1–2: INFECTION (E.G., EPISIOTOMY, BREASTS, AND PUERPERAL)

See the generic NDCP, "Risk for Infection,[1]" beginning on p. 21 in Chapter 2; the generic collaborative care plan, "Potential Complication: Infection," beginning on p. 29 in Chapter 3; and the collaborative care plan, "Infection," beginning on p. 309 in the topic, "Postpartum Period: First 4 Hours After Birth (Fourth Stage of Labor)," earlier in this chapter.

Focus Assessments and Rationales

- Monitor VSs once per shift. Detects presence of infection. Temperature higher than 101°F (38.3°C) is indicative of infection. Temperature elevations above 100.4°F on two occasions within the first 10 postpartum days may also indicate infection. Heart rate and respirations increase as fever increases, due to increased metabolic rate caused by the fever.
- Assess episiotomy site once per shift. Redness, swelling, increased pain or purulent drainage may indicate the presence of infection. These signs may not become apparent until after the first 24 hours after birth. Third- and fourth-degree lacerations increase the risk for infection.
- Assess level of pain. Increased pain after pain has been controlled or the continuation of uncontrolled pain may indicate a localized infection, which can become systemic if not recognized and treated.
- Assess lochia once per shift. Foul-smelling lochia is an indication of infection. Early detection may prevent localized infection from becoming systemic.
- Assess fundus once per shift. A uterus that is very tender or remains boggy (does not contract well) may indicate retained tissue or uterine infection. Uterus should be 1–2 cm (about 1 fingerbreadth) lower in the abdomen each day.
- Check labor record for risk factors (e.g., premature rupture of membranes, prolonged labor, frequent vaginal examinations). Determines if special risk for infection exists and special interventions needed.
- Examine nipples for cracks, redness, or soreness. Nipple cracks provide a portal of entry for pathogens, predisposing the woman to mastitis.

Preventive Nursing Activities

- Use good hand-washing techniques. Prevents transmission of microorganisms from dirty to clean areas of breasts or perineum or from nurse to woman.
- Teach and encourage perineal care several times each day and after voiding or defecation; teach to change pads at least every 3–4 hours. Promotes healing and prevents

infection. Use of a perineum bottle or sitz bath three to four times each day increases circulation to the area, which promotes healing and removes microorganisms from episiotomy/lacerations, vagina, and cervix.

- Teach to cleanse perineum from front to back. Prevents the spread of fecal contaminants and other bacteria to the episiotomy/laceration or vagina.
- Teach nipple care (e.g., do not use soap; when infant is breastfeeding, break suction with index finger before removing baby from the breast). Soap dries the nipples and contributes to cracking. Breaking suction prevents trauma.
- Provide dietary information, especially regarding foods high in protein, vitamin C, and iron. Protein and vitamin C are necessary for healing and tissue regeneration. Iron is necessary for hemoglobin synthesis and is also necessary for healing.
- Encourage fluid intake of up to 2,000 ml/day. Helps increase urine production and prevents urinary stasis; urinary stasis predisposes to UTI.

Potential Complication of Postpartum Period Days 1–2: URINARY RETENTION[1]

See the generic NDCP, "Urinary Retention,[1]" beginning on p. 22 of Chapter 2; also see the collaborative care plan, "Potential Complication of Postpartum Period: Urinary Retention,[1]" beginning on p. 309 in the topic, "Postpartum Period: First 4 Hours After Birth (Fourth Stage of Labor)," previously in this chapter.

Note: Bladder or urethral edema or trauma to the urinary meatus may inhibit voiding postdelivery. Because increased renal blood flow continues, diuresis begins within 12 hours following birth and continues for about a week, increasing urine output.

Focus Assessments and Rationale

- Assess for signs of bladder infection. Frequency, urgency, and burning on urination may indicate bladder infection. Stasis of urine, as in bladder retention, provides a medium for growth of pathogens. Differentiate burning on urination from pain during voiding, when urine comes in contact with perineal lacerations/episiotomy.

Preventive Nursing Activities

- Monitor infusion of intravenous fluids, if any. Most women will not have an IV after the first 12 hours postpartum. However, for those who do, too rapid infusion of fluids may cause rapid filling of the bladder and increase distention when the woman is not voiding well.
- Continue hourly assessments until the woman voids. If she does not void by 6–8 hours after birth, or if the bladder is distended on palpation, catheterize per order or

protocol. Relieves discomfort of a full bladder, prevents bladder injury, and prevents uterine atony and possible hemorrhage.

- Once the woman has voided, monitor her ability to completely empty the bladder. Urinating small amounts at frequent intervals may be an indication of either urinary retention or bladder infection. Residual amounts greater than 100 ml are an indication of inadequate emptying.
- Once the woman has voided, encourage her to void at least once per hour for a few hours, and then at least every 4 hr thereafter. Helps reestablish normal urinary patterns during early postpartum period, especially following general anesthesia or trauma to the urethra or meatus. After the woman is voiding in adequate amounts and emptying her bladder, time periods between voidings can be extended.
- Teach to perform Kegel exercise several times daily. Helps recover and maintain tone of pubococcygeal muscle and prevents stress incontinence.

Potential Complication of Postpartum Period Days 1–2: THROMBOPHLEBITIS

Refer to the generic NDCP, "Ineffective Peripheral Tissue Perfusion,[1]" beginning on p. 18 in Chapter 2; also see the NDCP, "Ineffective Tissue Perfusion (Peripheral),[1]" which begins on p. 352 in "Thromboembolic Disease" in Chapter 10.

Focus Assessments and Rationales

- Review the woman's records for risk factors for thrombophlebitis (e.g., varicose veins, multiparity, history of venous thrombosis). The presence of risk factors significantly increases the woman's likelihood of developing thrombophlebitis. If the woman has risk factors, an individualized NDCP should be instituted so that special monitoring and preventive actions can be taken.
- Perform test for Homan's sign. The presence of pain when the woman's foot is dorsiflexed is a sign of deep vein thrombosis.

Preventive Nursing Activity

- Encourage ambulation as soon after birth as possible. Contraction and relaxation of muscles during ambulation promotes venous return and prevents stasis of blood in dependent veins. Most women are ambulatory on postpartum days 1 and 2. Ambulation can begin as soon as the VSs are stable, fundus is firm, bleeding is not heavy, and there are no residual effects of epidural anesthesia.

Nursing Diagnosis: READINESS FOR ENHANCED FAMILY COPING[1]

Related Factors: needs and goals being met, performing adaptive tasks, and coping effectively.

Goals, Outcomes, and Evaluation Criteria

Family members will:

- Verbalize/demonstrate desire to integrate infant into family structure.
- Demonstrate support for one another.
- Participate in decision making.
- Work together to meet agreed-upon goals.
- Perform expected roles.
- Express commitment to one another.

NIC Interventions[2]

Family Integrity Promotion (7100)—Promotion of family cohesion and unity.

Family Integrity Promotion: Childbearing Family (7104)—Facilitation of the growth of individuals or families who are adding an infant to the family unit.

Family Support (7140)—Promotion of family values, interests, and goals.

Nursing Activities and Rationales

Assessments

- Assess maternal behaviors. Determines if alterations that require intervention are present. Behaviors that indicate attachment include the mother holding the infant closely or in the en face position or talking to and admiring the infant.
- Assess relationship with significant other. Determines if alterations are present that need intervention. Behaviors that indicate coping include positive conversations between the couple, both parents wanting to be involved in the infant's care, absence of arguments or withdrawn behavior, willingness to discuss concerns, etc.
- Assess support system. Determines the availability of family members who can offer physical and emotional support. If the partner is absent or if the relationship is not secure, other support systems may be necessary, such as grandparents or community resources.

Independent Nursing Actions

- Encourage the woman to include immediate family in planning for newborn. Family members who feel that they are needed and appreciated are more likely to become involved in the care of the infant when needed and offer emotional support to the mother/parents.

Patient/Family Teaching

- Explain normal variations for newborn's appearance. Decreases fears regarding normalcy of the infant. Conditions such as molding, caput succedaneum, and mottling may cause the mother fear and anxiety if she does not understand that they are temporary conditions and do not mean that the infant will not grow or develop normally.
- Teach regarding physical and emotional changes associated with postpartum. Decreases anxiety and fear of the unknown by preparing the couple for changes that may occur. Expected alterations are easier to cope with than those that are unexpected since they may be interpreted as being abnormal.
- Teach regarding the need for integrating siblings into care of the infant. Older siblings may feel left out or unwanted when a new baby arrives. Including them when caring for the infant when feasible helps them feel wanted and will facilitate their acceptance of a new family member.
- Teach parents that sibling jealousy is normal. Parents may feel that their child/children are acting out abnormally and punish the older sibling, which may interfere with the older sibling's ability to accept the new family member.
- Teach parents to encourage older siblings to verbalize feelings of fear/jealousy. Allows older siblings to identify their fears and concerns about being abandoned or neglected and allows parents to correct misconceptions and provide emotional support during the adjustment period.

Nursing Diagnosis: RISK FOR CONSTIPATION[1]

Related Factors: fear of painful defecation because of episiotomy and/or hemorrhoids. Refer to the generic NDCP, "Constipation,[1]" beginning on p. 11 in Chapter 2.

Goals, Outcomes, and Evaluation Criteria

- Woman will have soft, formed stool by day 3 postpartum.

Nursing Activities and Rationales

Assessments

- Assess the woman's bowel sounds. Determines if peristalsis has returned to normal following birth and/or anesthesia.
- Palpate for diastasis recti. If the two rectus muscles along the median line of the abdominal wall are separated (as sometimes happens from stretching of the muscles during pregnancy), bearing down efforts will be less effective.
- Assess stools for color, consistency, amount, and frequency. Hard, formed stools are an indication of inadequate intake of fluid and/or fiber, both of which are needed for normal bowel elimination.

Independent Nursing Actions

- Suggest that the woman who has an episiotomy or hemorrhoids take an analgesic 30–60 minutes before defecation and use local anesthetic creams/sprays or witch hazel pads afterward. Alleviates some of the pain of defecation and the fear of painful defecation. Helps the woman relax her perineum to facilitate defecation.

Patient/Family Teaching

- Teach the effects of pain medication and iron supplements. Narcotic analgesics decrease motility of the gastrointestinal tract and increase the risk for constipation. Iron also predisposes to constipation. The woman who understands this can compensate for its effects by increasing her intake of fluids and fiber.

Nursing Diagnosis: HEALTH-SEEKING BEHAVIORS[1]

There are no related factors since Health-Seeking Behaviors[1] is a wellness diagnosis.

Goals, Outcomes, and Evaluation Criteria

- Woman asks questions about health/health promotion.
- Woman implements strategies to eliminate unhealthy behaviors.
- Woman seeks information about infant immunizations.
- Woman seeks information about caring for infant and meeting infant's health needs.

NIC Interventions[2]

Family Integrity Promotion: Childbearing Family (7104)— Facilitation of the growth of individuals or families who are adding an infant to the family unit.

Health Education (5510)—Developing and providing instruction and learning experiences to facilitate voluntary adaptation of behavior conducive to health in individuals, families, groups, or communities.

Health System Guidance (7400)—Facilitating a patient's location and use of appropriate health services.

Immunization/Vaccination Management (6530)—Monitoring immunization status, facilitating access to immunizations, and provision of immunizations to prevent communicable diseases.

Nursing Activities and Rationales

Assessments

- Assess knowledge of rubella titers and Rho(D) immune globulin (RhoGAM). Determines the need for teaching and further intervention.

- Assess readiness for learning. The woman who asks questions and is free of pain or excessive anxiety is generally ready to learn. Women who are not ready to learn are not as likely to retain information as well as those who are ready to learn.
- Assess phase of maternal adjustment to parental role. The three phases of adjustment are characterized by dependent, dependent-independent, and interdependent behavior. In Rubin's framework, they are referred to as taking in and taking hold (Sleutel, 2003). Because the first 24 hours may be a time of excitement and preoccupation with the new role, the mother's perceptions may be narrowed, so information may need to be repeated.

Independent Nursing Actions

- Encourage the woman to see her healthcare professional for any healthcare concerns. Ensures timeliness of treatment for any problems that occur following the birth process and decreases fears related to misinformation.
- Encourage the woman to make and keep an appointment for a postpartum exam. Traditionally, this is 4–6 weeks after birth.

Collaborative Activities

- Administer rubella vaccine before discharge if titers are 1:8 or lower. Prevents fetal anomalies in future pregnancies. Women who have not had rubella or who are not serologically immune may contract rubella during a future pregnancy.
- Assess for allergies to eggs or feathers before administering rubella vaccine. If allergy is present, withhold vaccine to prevent allergic or anaphylactic reaction.
- Instruct to avoid pregnancy for 3 months after receiving rubella vaccine. If necessary and appropriate, send woman home from hospital with some form of contraception. Rubella is teratogenic to the fetus.
- Administer Rho(D) immune globulin (RhoGAM) to Rh-negative women who have given birth to an Rh-positive infant. Administration of Rho immune globulin within 72 hours after birth suppresses the immune response and prevents maternal sensitization and incompatibility with fetus in future pregnancies. Rho(D) immune globulin (RhoGAM) can be given up to 2 weeks postpartum, but it may be less effective than when given within 72 hours after birth.

Patient/Family Teaching

- Explain rubella titers and immunization recommendations; review side effects and risks; provide written information. Increases the woman's understanding of the need for adequate antibody titers to prevent fetal anomalies from occurring in future pregnancies and to alleviate misconceptions and fears.
- Explain Rh factors and Rho(D) immune globulin (RhoGAM) administration to Rh-negative mothers.

Increases what the woman understands about the need for protecting future pregnancies from Rh incompatibilities and to alleviate misconceptions and fears.

Nursing Diagnosis: RISK FOR IMPAIRED PARENT–INFANT/ CHILD ATTACHMENT[1]

See the generic NDCP, "Risk for Impaired Parent–Infant/Child Attachment,[1]" beginning on p. 19 in Chapter 2. Also refer to the NDCP, "Risk for Impaired Parent–Infant/Child Attachment" beginning on p. 232 of "Normal Labor: Second Stage," in Chapter 7.

▌ *Nursing Activities and Rationales*

Assessments

- Inquire about the parenting/emotional support that the woman and her partner received from their own parents. The way in which one is parented strongly influences one's ability to parent as an adult. Those who have had positive parenting role models are more likely to adjust to the demands of parenting.
- Assess the relationship between the woman and her partner. A good relationship with open communication is important in learning to parent.

Independent Nursing Actions

- Encourage rooming in, if it is available in the agency. Facilitates attachment by allowing mother, infant, and other family members privacy for interaction.

Collaborative Activities

- Provide follow-up home visits at 1 week and again at about 4 weeks, especially if the family is at risk for attachment problems. It is difficult to make a thorough assessment of bonding, which occurs gradually, in the acute care agency because of the limited amount of time the nurse can spend with the family.

INDIVIDUALIZED (NURSING DIAGNOSIS) CARE PLANS

This section includes care plans that were developed to address unique patient needs.

▌ Nursing Diagnosis: PAIN[1]

Related Factors: episiotomy/lacerations, breast/nipple soreness, afterpains, and hemorrhoids. See the generic NDCP, "Pain,[1]" beginning on p. 18 in Chapter 2. Also refer to NDCP, "Pain,[1]" beginning

on p. 311 in "Postpartum Period: First 4 Hours After Birth (Fourth Stage of Labor)," in this chapter.

▌ *Nursing Activities and Rationales*

Assessment

- Assess understanding of afterpains. Determines if teaching is needed in order to enhance woman's comfort and decrease her anxiety.

Independent Nursing Actions

- After the first 24 hours, discontinue ice to perineum and encourage sitting in a tub of warm water or a sitz bath for episiotomy and/or hemorrhoid pain. Ice is not effective in preventing edema after 24 hours. At that time it is better to use warmth to create local vasodilation and promote blood and lymph flow through the area to help resolve existing edema.
- For afterpains, encourage the woman to lie on her abdomen. Promotes warmth and helps to relax abdominal muscles; provides competing stimuli.
- Administer nonsteroidal anti-inflammatory analgesic (e.g., naproxen sodium [Anaprox] at least 30 min before the mother breastfeeds. The baby's sucking causes the posterior pituitary to release oxytocin, which stimulates uterine contractions and intensifies afterpains. NSAIDs block naturally produced prostaglandin synthesis, interfering with uterine contractility; they also act peripherally as analgesics to modify pain.

Collaborative Activities

- For episiotomy/lacerations/hemorrhoids, teach to apply anesthetic cream or spray to perineum, sparingly, 3–4 times per day. Provides local anesthesia.
- Teach to use witch hazel pads after voiding or defecation. For cooling, astringent effect.

Patient/Family Teaching

- Teach the woman about afterpains. Increases the woman's understanding of the cause of her discomfort. Afterbirth pains are cramping sensations caused by the uterus as it contracts following birth.
- Teach to contract gluteal muscles when sitting down, and to sit on a hard, not a soft, padded chair. Prevents direct pressure on perineum.
- Teach to lie on her side. Prevents pressure on episiotomy.

▌ Nursing Diagnosis: RISK FOR DEFICIENT FLUID VOLUME[1]

Related Factors: decreased oral fluid intake and postpartum diuresis/diaphoresis. See the NDCP, "Risk for Deficient Fluid

Volume,[1]" which begins on p. 226 in the topic, "Normal Labor: First Stage," in Chapter 7.

Nursing Diagnosis: RISK FOR INEFFECTIVE BREASTFEEDING[1]; OR EFFECTIVE BREASTFEEDING[1]

Related Factors: risk for ineffective breastfeeding: lack of prior experience due to the current condition being the woman's first pregnancy or first lactation experience or due to severe anxiety or depression. *Related Factors:* effective breastfeeding: infant gestational age greater than 34 weeks, normal infant oral structure, maternal confidence, basic breastfeeding knowledge, and normal breast structure.

Goals, Outcomes, and Evaluation Criteria

- Woman recognizes early hunger cues of infant.
- Woman expresses comfort of position during nursing.
- Woman assists infant with proper alignment and latch-on.
- Infant has regular and sustained suckling/swallowing at the breast.
  - Infant is content after feeding.
  - Woman verbalizes satisfaction with the feeding process.
  - Infant has adequate elimination patterns for his or her age.

NIC Interventions[2]

Breastfeeding Assistance (1054)—Preparing a new mother to breastfeed her infant.

Nursing Activities and Rationales

Assessments

- Assess knowledge of breastfeeding (e.g., positioning, latching on, and infant sucking and swallowing). Determines the educational needs of the mother in order to plan teaching.
- Assess infant's maturity level and gestational age. Determines variations that may impede infant's ability to suck or latch on to the breast.
- Observe infant's ability to suck. Determines if infant is obtaining adequate milk to meet nutritional needs. Premature infants may have a poor suck reflex, which places them at increased risk for nutrition deficit.
- Monitor infant's ability to grasp the nipple correctly and latch on. The ability of the baby to latch on depends on the size of the baby's mouth and the size of the mother's nipple and areola. The baby's mouth should cover the entire nipple and approximately 2–3 cm around the nipple. The baby's nose, cheeks, and chin will be in contact with the breast when the baby is latched on correctly.
- Monitor infant for smacking or clicking noises when breastfeeding. These sounds may indicate that the baby is not correctly latched on. The baby should be removed from the breast and latch-on reattempted.
- Assess mother for pain when infant sucks. May indicate that the infant is not correctly latched on, which may result in nipple soreness. Bruising and blistering of the nipples may develop if nipple rubs against the roof of infant's mouth (Riordan & Wambach, 2010).
- Assess for milk let-down. Ensures that infant is receiving milk. Signs of milk let-down include tingling sensation in the nipples, uterine cramping, leakage from the opposite breast, change in baby's suck from quick to slower, drawing pattern, and audible infant swallowing.

Independent Nursing Actions

- Encourage rooming in (keeping the baby in the mother's room). Provides opportunity for the mother to learn to recognize feeding cues.
- Before discharge, be sure the parents are knowledgeable about breastfeeding and know when to contact the care provider. Breastfeeding does not necessarily come naturally. Parents should view breastfeeding as a learning process.

Patient/Family Teaching

- Instruct mother on proper positioning; help position baby as needed. Makes mother aware that effective breastfeeding depends on proper technique. The position in which the mother feels most comfortable and allows the baby to latch on is the correct position. This may include the football hold, cradle, modified cradle, or across-the-lap positions.
- Instruct on proper nipple care, including how to prevent nipple soreness. Use of soaps and alcohol can dry out nipples, cause cracking, and increase pain and soreness. A well-fitting supportive bra worn continuously for at least 72 hours following birth enhances comfort, especially when engorgement is present.
- Instruct mother how to burp the newborn; demonstrate as needed. Makes mother aware of techniques to enhance infant feeding and comfort and prevent accumulation of air in the baby's stomach. Ingested air decreases space for milk and may cause stomach or intestinal cramping.
- Teach the mother to feed baby on cue and to not limit the duration of feedings; the baby is finished when the suck/swallow pattern has slowed, the breast is soft, and the baby seems content. Incorrect positioning, latching on, and removing from the breast causes sore nipples. The length of time a feeding lasts has no effect on soreness. Some babies may complete a feeding in 5–10 minutes; others may require up to 45 min. The average time is 15 min per breast.
- Show the mother how to wake a sleepy baby (e.g., remove clothing except for diaper; massage the chest and back, apply a cool cloth to the baby's face, talk to the baby). Newborns sleep a great deal and might not, at first, awaken for a feeding in time to avoid becoming hypoglycemic.

Newborns should feed at least every 3 hours (8–12 feedings in 24 hours).

Nursing Diagnosis: DEFICIENT KNOWLEDGE: SELF-CARE[1]

Related Factors: being a primigravida and lack of previous experience. See the generic NDCP, "Deficient Knowledge,[1]" beginning on p. 13 in Chapter 2.

Goals, Outcomes, and Evaluation Criteria

- Woman describes routine postpartum assessments.
- Woman expresses understanding of physiologic changes of postpartum.
- Woman performs her own perineal care.
- Woman describes signs and symptoms of postpartum complications.
- Woman describes and uses comfort measures for common postpartum discomforts.

NIC Interventions[2]

Postpartal Care (6930)—Monitoring and management of the patient who has recently given birth.

Nursing Activities and Rationales

Assessments

- Assess knowledge of routine postpartum care. Determines the need for teaching regarding postpartum care, complications that need to be monitored for, and infant care.
- Assess readiness to learn. Determines if the woman is ready and capable of learning. A prolonged or difficult labor may leave the woman fatigued and unable or unwilling to learn new skills. Uncontrolled pain limits the woman's ability to concentrate and learn.

Independent Nursing Actions

- Discuss plans for birth control or refer for birth control counseling. An unplanned pregnancy that occurs before healing has fully occurred may jeopardize the physical well-being of the mother. The woman should understand that breastfeeding is not a reliable source of contraception.
- Encourage to perform activities of daily living as tolerated. Activity enhances self-esteem, prevents complications such as constipation and thrombophlebitis, and helps build physical stamina following the birth process and allows the mother to perform self- and infant care more easily.

Collaborative Activity

- Refer to or suggest appropriate community resources (e.g., La Leche League, visiting nurse services, Women, Infants, and Children (WIC) nutritional program, community health department). Provides support for adapting to parenting.

Patient/Family Teaching

- Teach normal physical and emotional changes that take place during the postpartum period. Prepares the woman for changes that she will undergo and helps her differentiate normal changes from those that are abnormal and need to be reported. Knowledge decreases fears and helps prepare the woman for self-care at home. Emotions tend to be labile during the postpartum period, so realizing that this is normal may help the woman to cope and not be overwhelmed by her fluctuating emotions and the demands of new roles/responsibilities.
- Teach the symptoms that should be reported to the care provider. Foul-smelling lochia, fever, malaise, a return of bright red bleeding, or depression are all signs of problems that should be evaluated quickly rather than waiting for the scheduled 4- or 6-week visit.
- Discuss the need for postpartum exercises; provide written instructions; help devise a schedule. Exercises improve circulation and help the abdominal muscles regain their tone. It will help the woman regain her prepregnant figure and enhance feelings of well-being.
- Teach about home care, including breast care, perineal care, lochial progression, nutrition, the need for sleep and rest, use of sitz baths, signs of complications, etc. Prepares the woman to assume her own care when discharged; to help prevent complications such as mastitis, wound infection, nutritional or fluid deficits, or fatigue; and facilitates healing and return of well-being.
- Explain the need for keeping follow-up appointments with healthcare provider. Helps ensure that the woman will be evaluated for healing and a return to her prepregnant state.
- Explain the need for abstaining from sexual intercourse for 6 weeks or until after her 6-week follow-up examination. Prevents infection. The cervix remains open and the lining of the uterus is not well healed until around 6 weeks. Sexual intercourse during this time period increases the woman's risk for infection.

Nursing Diagnosis: DEFICIENT KNOWLEDGE, INFANT CARE[1]

Related Factors: primipara status and lack of previous experience. See the generic NDCP, "Deficient Knowledge,[1]" on p. 13 in Chapter 2. For more details on infant care, see Chapter 11, *Normal Newborn Care.*

Goals, Outcomes, and Evaluation Criteria

- Woman describes normal infant characteristics.

- Woman demonstrates infant safety practices including cardio-pulmonary resuscitation.
- Woman demonstrates proper bathing, dressing, and feeding techniques.

■ NIC Interventions[2]

Infant Care (6820)—Provision of developing appropriate family-centered care to the child under 1 year of age.

■ Nursing Activities and Rationales

Assessments

- Assess knowledge of infant bathing, dressing, and diapering. Determines level of knowledge and how to proceed with teaching regarding infant care.
- Assess/observe ability to perform infant bathing, diapering, cord care, cardiopulmonary resuscitation. Determines the need for additional teaching, demonstrations, or practice before the woman is discharged to home with the expectation that she can adequately and safely care for her newborn infant.
- Observe response to infant cues. Ensures that infant needs such as feeding, comforting, bathing, and diapering are met.
- Assess parent–infant attachment. Determines the need for intervention. The woman who does not attach to her infant will most likely be unable to identify and meet the infant's needs.

Independent Nursing Actions

- Provide positive feedback when care is carried out correctly. Praise and positive reinforcement help build self-confidence and ensure that the behaviors will be repeated.
- Involve partner/family in care of the newborn. Family members who are included and feel valued can offer valuable emotional support to the mother and help with physical care of the infant if the mother becomes fatigued or overwhelmed.

Collaborative Activity

- Refer to community resources as appropriate. First-time mothers, in particular, may feel the need for additional support until they become comfortable with caring for their newborn. They may be unaware of community resources or services that are available to them.

Patient/Family Teaching

- Teach cardiopulmonary resuscitation, bathing, cord care, circumcision care, and diapering. Helps ensure safe and effective home care of the infant and to make sure that the infant's physical and emotional needs will be met.
- Teach the need for well-baby checkups. Helps ensure the health and well-being of the infant, which includes absence of infection (cord), adequate nutrition, growth and development within developmental standards, and ensure early detection of complications that may retard growth or development.

■ Other Nursing Diagnoses

Also assess for the following nursing diagnoses, which are frequently present with this condition:

- Sleep pattern disturbance[1] related to changing hormone levels, excitement, anxiety, and pain.
- Risk for ineffective coping[1] (individual or family) related to unrealistic expectations of infant or parental role, inadequate support system, and overwhelming demands of the parenting role.

POSTPARTUM PERIOD: FIRST HOME VISIT

The first home visit by a nurse helps bridge the gap between hospital care and home care. It allows mothers to return home earlier and may reduce the need for rehospitalization or nonessential healthcare visits. Often new mothers have many questions after they return home. The nurse can offer emotional support, assess for problems, provide additional teaching, and decrease stress on new families. The home visit should be planned and well organized. Usually, personal contact is made before the woman is discharged from the birthing center and agrees to the visit. Prior to the visit, the nurse should review the discharge summary and any other pertinent inpatient records, including physicians' orders; this helps to provide continuity of care. The nurse should also obtain directions and/or a map to the family's home.

■ Key Nursing Activities

- Assess for complications.
- Assess ability of mother to care for infant.
- Assess mother's self-care abilities.
- Assess for indications of successful/unsuccessful transition.
- Teach regarding self-care, infant care, well-baby follow-up, and postpartum follow-up care.

■ Etiologies and Risk Factors

Risk factors and etiologies include short maternity stay, follow-up after cesarean birth, postpartum complications, and insecurity in newly assumed role as parent.

■ Signs and Symptoms

See "Postpartum Period: Days 1–2," beginning on p. 311 in this chapter.

■ Diagnostic Studies

Diagnostic studies are not usually a part of the PP home visits for the normal PP woman.

▌ *Medical Management*

- Refer to "Postpartum Period: Days 1–2," beginning on p. 311 of this chapter. Medical management during this period is a continuation of that begun during the inpatient stay.
- The woman may be given a prescription for combination analgesics (such as acetaminophen [Tylenol] with codeine) but more often will be advised to use over-the-counter, nonnarcotic analgesics.
- The woman will probably continue topical analgesics/antiseptics (e.g., witch hazel pads) for episiotomy care for a few days.
- Vitamin and iron supplements are usually continued at least until the 4- to 6-week follow-up visit.

▌ *Collaborative Problems*

Note: One nursing diagnosis is included in this section because it should be a part of the standardized care for all postpartum women even though it is not, by definition, a collaborative problem.

Potential Complications of Postpartum Period: First Home Visit

- Delayed postpartum hemorrhage
- Puerperal infection, urinary tract infection, mastitis
- Thrombophlebitis
- Postpartum depression
- Risk for impaired parent–infant/child attachment[1]

COLLABORATIVE (STANDARDIZED) CARE FOR ALL NORMAL POSTPARTUM WOMEN, FIRST HOME VISIT

Perform a comprehensive assessment to identify individual needs for teaching, emotional support, and physical care.

▌ Potential Complication of Postpartum Period First Home Visit: DELAYED POSTPARTUM HEMORRHAGE

See the generic collaborative care plan, "Potential Complication: Hemorrhage," beginning on p. 28 in Chapter 3; and the collaborative care plan, "Postpartum Hemorrhage" beginning on pp. 308 and 312 in the preceding topics, "Postpartum Period: First 4 Hours After Birth (Fourth Stage of Labor)" and "Postpartum Period: Days 1–2," in this chapter. Care for this potential problem is essentially the same at the first home visit, except that by that time, hemorrhage is more likely to occur as a result of retained placental fragments than from uterine atony; and nursing care

focuses on follow-up evaluation and reinforcing teaching that was done in the inpatient setting.

Focus Assessments and Rationales

- Assess VSs, fundal height, and lochia. Identifies any signs/symptoms of hemorrhage. Subinvolution of the uterus may indicate retained placental fragments, which can cause delayed postpartum hemorrhage.

Preventive Nursing Activity

- Remind the woman to call her care provider if lochia becomes bright red or if it has a foul odor. Bright red lochia is a sign that hemorrhage may be occurring; foul odor indicates infection, which can delay healing and lead to hemorrhage.

▌ Potential Complication of Postpartum Period First Home Visit: PUERPERAL INFECTION, URINARY TRACT INFECTION, AND MASTITIS

See the generic NDCP, "Risk for Infection,[1]" beginning on p. 21 in Chapter 2; the generic collaborative care plan, "Potential Complication: Infection," beginning on p. 29 in Chapter 3; the generic collaborative care plan, "Urinary Tract Infection," beginning on p. 33 in Chapter 3, and the collaborative care plans, "Infection," beginning on p. 309 and "Infection (e.g., Episiotomy, Breasts, and Puerperal)," beginning on p. 313, in the topics, "Postpartum Period: First 4 Hours After Birth (Fourth Stage of Labor)" and "Postpartum Period: Days 1–2," respectively, in this chapter.

Focus Assessments and Rationales

- Assess temperature and advise the woman to take her own temperature if she does not feel well. Also assess her ability to take her temperature. Detects presence of infection. Temperature greater than 101°F (38.3°C) is indicative of infection. Temperature elevations greater than 100.4°F on two occasions within the first 10 postpartum days may also indicate infection.
- Assess episiotomy site. Redness, swelling, increased pain or purulent drainage may indicate infection. These signs may not become apparent until the first home visit.
- Assess fundal height and lochia. A uterus that is very tender or boggy (does not contract well) may indicate retained tissue or uterine infection. Foul-smelling lochia is an indication of infection. Early detection may prevent localized infection from becoming systemic.
- Examine nipples for cracks, redness, or soreness. Nipple cracks provide a portal of entry for pathogens, predisposing the woman to mastitis. Sore nipples may cause the

woman to limit the infant's feedings, resulting in incomplete emptying.

- Assess hand-washing techniques and perineal care. Determines the need for reteaching.
- If any symptoms of infection are present, obtain appropriate cultures (e.g., lochia, nipple discharge, urine, episiotomy drainage). Identifies causative organism so that specific antibiotic treatment can be given.

Preventive Nursing Activities

- Discuss air drying the nipples and advise to not use plastic-lined nursing pads. Prevents skin breakdown; decreases moisture, which provides growth medium for pathogens.
- Review signs and symptoms of UTI. Facilitates prompt treatment when infection is present. Frequency, urgency, and dysuria are classic symptoms of cystitis; fever, hematuria, and suprapubic pain may indicate ascending infection.
- Teach signs and symptoms of mastitis (flulike symptoms such as fever and chills; localized breast pain; a hot, reddened, wedge-shaped area on the breast, usually in the upper outer quadrant of the breast). Helps the woman differentiate between breast engorgement, which she can self-treat, and mastitis, which requires medical attention.
- Teach methods for relieving breast engorgement (e.g., ice packs to the breasts, 15 min on and 45 min off, large bags of frozen peas or corn can be used; place fresh cabbage leaves inside the bra; mild analgesic; having the infant nurse). Engorgement can lead to inadequate emptying of the breasts, predisposing to mastitis. If used continuously, ice can cause rebound engorgement.

▌Potential Complication of Postpartum Period First Home Visit: THROMBOPHLEBITIS

Refer to the generic NDCP, "Ineffective Peripheral Tissue Perfusion,[1]" beginning on p. 18 in Chapter 2; see the collaborative care plan, "Potential Complication of Postpartum Period Days 1–2: Thrombophlebitis," beginning on p. 314 in the topic, "Postpartum Period: Days 1–2" in this chapter; and see the NDCP, "Ineffective Tissue Perfusion (Peripheral),[1]" beginning on p. 352 in "Thromboembolic Disease" in Chapter 10.

Preventive Nursing Activities

- Provide information. Advise the woman to contact care provider if she experiences (1) pain and tenderness in her lower legs and/or warmth, redness, and hardness over a vein; or (2) if there is pain on dorsiflexion of her foot, unilateral leg pain or calf tenderness, a localized area that is hot to touch, or pallor and/or swelling of the lower leg. (1) These are signs/symptoms of superficial thrombophlebitis. (2) These are signs/symptoms of deep vein

thrombosis. Teaching helps ensure that she will recognize a developing problem and seek medical help before complications develop.

▌Potential Complication of Postpartum Period First Home Visit: POSTPARTUM DEPRESSION

See "Postpartum Depression," beginning on p. 359 in Chapter 10.

Focus Assessments and Rationales

- Assess infant's sleep pattern and maternal fatigue level. Most mothers experience an emotional letdown in the early postpartum period. This is exaggerated by fatigue and sleep deprivation.
- Assess for emotional lability—crying easily for no apparent reason, a let-down feeling, fatigue, insomnia, restlessness, headaches, anxiety, sadness, and anger. These are symptoms of postpartum blues, a common psychologic response that seems to peak around the 5th postpartum day. Postpartum blues, experienced by 75–80% of women, are usually mild and short term (lasting 2 wks or less), but must be differentiated from the more severe postpartum depression.

Preventive Nursing Activities

- Advise the woman to nap when the baby naps, go to bed early, and let friends and family know if she is not rested enough for visitors. Fatigue from around-the-clock demands of the new baby can intensify the feelings of depression.
- Assure her that the blues are normal and common. Relieves guilt and anxiety.
- Advise her to take time for herself (e.g., go for a walk; take a hot bath while others care for the baby). The mother may feel a loss of the support and attention she received while pregnant. Doing something for herself can relieve some tension and promote feelings of self-worth.
- Teach to differentiate blues and postpartum depression, and to notify care provider promptly if the following occur:
  - Worsening of sleep disturbance.
  - Loss of appetite.
  - Increased intensity of depression, thoughts about incompetence as a parent, fears for the baby, and suicidal thoughts.
  - Fatigue that continues to the point of interfering with functioning.
  - Withdrawal and social isolation while feeling emotionally unsupported.
  - Perceiving the baby as demanding and burdensome.
  - Feelings of failure, overwhelming guilt, loneliness, and low self-esteem. These are all signs of PPD, which should

be promptly reported so that treatment can be implemented to prevent damage to the mother/infant relationship, or even physical danger to the mother and baby.

- Provide a screening tool such as "Am I Blue?" (Johnson & Johnson, 1996) to assess the level of postpartum blues. May help the woman to decide when to seek help.

Nursing Diagnosis: RISK FOR IMPAIRED PARENT–INFANT/CHILD ATTACHMENT[1]

See the generic NDCP, "Risk for Impaired Parent–Infant/Child Attachment,[1]" beginning on p. 19 in Chapter 2. Also refer to the NDCP, "Risk for Impaired Parent–Infant/Child Attachment,[1]" beginning on p. 236 in "Normal Labor: Second Stage," in Chapter 7.

Nursing Activities and Rationales

Assessment

- Observe parent/infant interactions. Determines whether bonding has progressed since the assessments that were made in the inpatient setting. Bonding may occur over a period of time. Also, if the mother becomes fatigued or ill after returning home, this can have a negative effect on attachment that was evaluated as satisfactory in the inpatient setting.

INDIVIDUALIZED (NURSING DIAGNOSIS) CARE PLANS

This section includes care plans that were developed to address unique patient needs.

Nursing Diagnosis: PAIN[1]

Related Factors: episiotomy/lacerations, breast/nipple soreness, breast engorgement, and hemorrhoids. See the NDCP, "Pain,[1]" beginning on p. 18 in Chapter 2. Also refer to the NDCP, "Pain,[1]" beginning on p. 317 in "Postpartum Period: Days 1–2" in this chapter.

Goals, Outcomes, and Evaluation Criteria

- Woman describes and uses self-care methods for relieving pain/discomfort.

Nursing Activities and Rationales

Assessments

- Ask the woman what medications and pain-relief measures she is using. Determines if teaching is needed in

order to enhance comfort; to ensure that medications are being used correctly.
- Assess infant who is breastfeeding for proper latch-on and duration of breastfeeding. Proper latch-on may lessen discomfort due to breastfeeding. If smacking or clicking sound occurs, remove infant and reattempt latch-on.

Independent Nursing Actions

- Show the woman how to fold a towel and make a sitz bath in the bathtub; stress that the tub should be cleaned before and after the sitz bath. Relieves episiotomy pain; cleanliness will help prevent episiotomy or vaginal infections.
- Encourage the woman to attend breastfeeding classes, especially when difficulty is encountered. Breastfeeding classes teach proper breastfeeding techniques for promoting successful breastfeeding. Use of correct techniques will lessen the discomfort and make breastfeeding more enjoyable.

Patient/Family Teaching

- Teach proper positioning of infant for breastfeeding. Proper positioning decreases breast discomfort and facilitates the ability of the infant to receive milk without ingesting excess air.
- Teach methods for relieving breast engorgement (e.g., ice packs to the breasts, 15 min on and 45 min off, large bags of frozen peas or corn can be used; place fresh cabbage leaves inside the bra; mild analgesic; having the infant nurse; removing milk by manual expression or with a breast pump). Engorgement can lead to inadequate emptying of the breasts, predisposing to mastitis. If ice is used continuously, it can cause rebound engorgement. The exact mechanism of action of cabbage is unknown, but it is thought to occur from the effect of natural estrogens contained in cabbage. Analgesics relieve descomfort.
- If nipples are cracked or sore, advise to limit breastfeeding to 5 min on each breast, beginning on the less tender side. Feedings can be gradually increased by 1–2/min per day. Reduces trauma to the nipple. The baby sucks hardest during the first 5 min of feeding, so it helps to begin with the less tender nipple. However, limiting sucking can cause engorgement and decrease the milk supply.
- Review teaching performed in inpatient setting, as needed. The excitement and fatigue associated with childbirth make it difficult to retain information received during the first few postpartum days.

Nursing Diagnosis: RISK FOR IMBALANCED NUTRITION: LESS THAN BODY REQUIREMENTS[1]

Risk Factors: deficient knowledge of calories and nutrients needed for lactation, lack of time and energy to prepare and eat a proper diet, deliberate calorie reduction in an effort to return to prepregnant weight, and lack of appetite.

Goals, Outcomes, and Evaluation Criteria

- Woman gradually returns to prepregnant weight.
- Woman's dietary intake is adequate for tissue repair and lactation (if appropriate).
- Woman reports taking prescribed vitamin, iron, and other supplements.

NIC Interventions[2]

Nutritional Counseling (5246)—Use of an interactive helping process focusing on the need for diet modification.

Nutritional Monitoring (1160)—Collection and analysis of patient data to prevent or minimize malnourishment.

Teaching: Prescribed Diet (5614)—Preparing a patient to correctly follow a prescribed diet.

Nursing Activities and Rationales

Assessments

- Assess eating habits prior to and during pregnancy; ask about dietary intake for past 24 hours. Determines the need for additions to or changes in present diet in order to meet the needs for tissue repair and lactation (if relevant).
- Evaluate current weight, weight during pregnancy, and ideal weight for height (body mass index). Average weight loss at delivery is 10–12 lb. During the first 2 postpartum weeks, the woman usually loses about 5 lb more.
- Review hemoglobin and hematocrit; assess for pallor and fatigue. Assesses for anemia. Reduced Hgb can slow the healing process.
- Assess ability to meet nutritional needs. Financial, knowledge, and cultural issues may interfere with adequate nutrition.
- Assess food preparation techniques. Some cooking methods cause nutrient loss (e.g., vitamins are lost when vegetables are cooked in a large amount of water; undercooking meats and eggs increases the risk of bacterial and parasitic infections).
- Assess cultural preferences and beliefs about food. Enables the nurse to offer alternative foods to meet dietary needs.

Independent Nursing Actions

- Help the woman to plan a diet that includes a wide variety of foods, especially fresh and lightly processed foods. Stressing variety is a more positive approach than condemning junk food and is more likely to encourage compliance with a diet containing necessary nutrients.
- When planning with the woman, consider lifestyle influences and food preferences (e.g., for fast food). Increases the likelihood of compliance with the suggested diet.

Collaborative Activities

- Refer to the Women, Infants, and Children (WIC) program and/or the food stamp program, as needed. These programs provide nutrition services for those who qualify. WIC provides vouchers for selected foods (e.g., eggs, cheese, milk, juice, and fortified cereals) for pregnant and lactating women at nutritional risk.
- Refer for nutritional counseling, if necessary. May be necessary in order to meet individual needs. For example, women with limited income may need help in planning meals using protein sources other than meat (e.g., beans, cheese, and peanut butter).

Patient/Family Teaching

- Teach the basic food groups (following MyPyramid); stress the need for protein, calories, vitamin C, and calcium. A well-balanced diet would ensure that the woman is getting the necessary nutrients. Eating a variety of foods, from each of the food groups, helps insure a balanced diet. MyPyramid is a useful teaching tool because it is easy to understand and use without special nutrition knowledge.
- Teach caloric requirements. For nonlactating women, calorie requirements are the same as before pregnancy; a reduction of 300 kcal/day along with moderate exercise should result in weight loss to prepregnant weight. Lactating women need about 500–800 more kcal/day than their nonpregnant intake (at least 1800 kcal/day).
- Explain the need for vitamin and calcium supplements. For lactating women, needs for protein, calcium, and vitamins B and C are similar to or slightly higher than during pregnancy; this covers the amount of nutrients released in the milk and the mother's needs for tissue maintenance. It is especially important that calcium intake be adequate; supplemental calcium may be needed if the woman does not consume enough dietary calcium. Protein is needed to promote tissue healing and regeneration. Vitamin C is needed for cell wall synthesis and iron absorption. Supplemental iron may be given for a short while to compensate for the blood lost during birth, but overall iron requirements are the same as for the nonpregnant state.

Nursing Diagnosis: DEFICIENT KNOWLEDGE: SIGNS OF MATERNAL COMPLICATIONS[1]

See the NDCP, "Deficient Knowledge: Self-Care,[1]" beginning on p. 319 in "Postpartum Period: Days 1–2," in this chapter. Also see the generic NDCP, "Deficient Knowledge,[1]" beginning on p. 13 in Chapter 2.

Nursing Activities and Rationales

Assessments

- Assess level of knowledge of normal physiologic changes that occur in the first week and subsequent weeks postpartum. Enables planning for necessary teaching.

Patient/Family Teaching

- Review normal physiologic changes that occur in the first week and subsequent weeks postpartum, as needed. Helps the woman differentiate between normal changes and those that may indicate complications.
- Review the signs and symptoms of puerperal infection, mastitis, urinary tract infection, delayed postpartum hemorrhage, and thrombophlebitis, as needed. The excitement and fatigue associated with birth make it difficult to retain information received in the inpatient setting.

Nursing Diagnosis: RISK FOR INEFFECTIVE BREASTFEEDING; OR EFFECTIVE BREASTFEEDING

See the NDCP, "Risk for Ineffective Breastfeeding[1]; or Effective Breastfeeding,[1]" beginning on p. 318 in "Postpartum Period: Days 1–2" in this chapter.

Nursing Activities and Rationales

Assessments

- Assess mother's intake of fluids. Adequate fluid intake is essential to support lactation. If she is not thirsty and if her urine is clear to light yellow, she is probably drinking enough. Most lactating/breastfeeding women find that they drink 2–3 quarts of fluid per day.
- Assess dietary intake. The woman needs 200–500 extra calories per day to provide adequate nutrients for the baby and to protect her body stores. Regardless of her diet, however, the composition of the milk will vary only a little. If calories are severely restricted, milk supply may decrease.
- Weigh the infant. Determines the adequacy of the feedings. If baby is feeding well and having good urine output (6–8 wet diapers per 24 hours), but not gaining enough weight, it may be that the mother is switching to the second breast too soon and not emptying the first breast. Infant should gain 15–30 g/day after the milk is in, and should regain birth weight by 10–14 days.
- Determine whether the mother's milk is in. This usually occurs on the 3rd or 4th postpartum day.
- Assess breastfeeding technique. Nipple soreness may develop from faulty latch-on. Nipples may become bruised or blistered due to rubbing against the roof of the infant's mouth (Riordan & Wambach, 2010).

Independent Nursing Actions

- Encourage the father, children, and other family and friends to help with household chores and caring for other children. Provides time for the mother to rest; fatigue has a negative effect on lactation.

Collaborative Activity

- Provide information about La Leche League, peer counseling support groups such as those offered through WIC, and lactation consultants in hospitals or physicians' offices. The mother needs a list of resources she can call for help with breastfeeding concerns.

Patient/Family Teaching

- Suggest that the mother keep a drink within reach during feedings. Facilitates adequate fluid intake. Otherwise, a busy mother may not take time to drink enough.
- Explain the importance of adequate rest, especially during the first 2 postpartum weeks; suggest sleeping when the baby sleeps. Fatigue and stress can interfere with milk production and let-down.
- Advise to not use breast creams routinely; lanolin is safe to use on dry or sore nipples (unless the mother is allergic to wool). Some contain alcohol, which may dry the nipples; others contain vitamin E, which may be toxic to the infant if enough is consumed.
- If the mother needs breast support, advise not to wear an underwire bra and be sure the bra does not bind. Encourage to breastfeed at least once a day without a bra. Poorly fitting or underwire bras may cause clogged milk ducts. Breastfeeding without a bra will allow all milk ducts to empty completely.
- Advise that breastfeeding is not an effective method of contraception. Prevents an unplanned pregnancy. Although breastfeeding does delay the return of ovulation and menstruation, ovulation can occur before the first menstrual period, so it is unreliable as a contraceptive method.
- Caution that smoking may decrease the milk supply; advise to not smoke within 2 hrs before feeding and to not smoke in the same room with the infant. Over time, the effect of nicotine on the milk ejection reflex can decrease milk production. The infant should be protected from secondhand smoke.
- If the mother chooses to drink alcohol, advise her to have only one drink and to consume it immediately after a feeding. Excessive amounts can have serious effects on the baby and can affect the mother's milk ejection reflex.
- Advise to avoid caffeine (which is found in coffee, tea, chocolate, and many soft drinks). Only 1% of the ingested caffeine gets into the breast milk; however, the infant

cannot excrete the caffeine well, so it accumulates in the infant's system and can cause irritability and poor sleeping.

- Advise to not use a pacifier until breastfeeding is well established. The newborn needs to learn the association between sucking and satiation. Pacifier use has been associated with early termination of breastfeeding (Walker, 2007).

Nursing Diagnosis: HEALTH-SEEKING BEHAVIORS[1]

Related Factors: there are no related factors because this is wellness diagnosis.

Goals, Outcomes, and Evaluation Criteria

- Woman verbalizes understanding of need for maintaining follow-up care for self and infant.
- Woman seeks information about maintaining health of self and baby.
- Woman reports performance of health screenings.
- Woman participates in an exercise program.
- Woman reports attempts to balance work and child care with exercise and leisure.
- Woman maintains a healthy diet.

NIC Interventions[2]

Exercise Promotion (0200)—Facilitation of regular physical exercise to maintain or advance to a higher level of fitness and health.

Health Education (5510)—Developing and providing instruction and learning experiences to facilitate voluntary adaptation of behavior conducive to health in individuals, families, groups, or communities.

Teaching: Individual (5606)—Planning, implementation, and evaluation of a teaching program designed to address a patient's particular needs.

Nursing Activities and Rationales

Assessments

- Assess level of knowledge regarding health-promoting behaviors during postpartum period. Determines learning needs; the woman must have information about health promotion in order to engage in healthy behaviors.
- Monitor nutritional status and weight. Indicators of normal postpartum progression and adequate nutrition to support healing allow for adequate breastfeeding and obtainment of prepregnancy weight without compromising the woman's or newborn's health. Women who breastfeed may require up to 1,000 additional calories per day to adequately provide for their own and their infant's nutritional needs.

- Monitor vital signs and physical symptoms. Indicators of overall postpartum well-being. Decreased urinary output, fever, peripheral edema, puffy eyes, and elevated blood pressure are indications of complications that require further evaluation and possible intervention.
- Assess activity tolerance, family responsibilities, fatigue and ability to care for newborn. Identifies any problems with sleep and rest or role transition so that appropriate interventions can be planned. (See the generic NDCPs, "Activity Intolerance[1]" and "Fatigue,[1]" beginning on pp. 9 and 14, respectively, in Chapter 2.)

Independent Nursing Actions

- Develop good rapport with patient. Promotes emotional comfort and security, enhancing open communication.

Patient/Family Teaching

- Teach potential harmful effects of alcohol and drug use, including over-the-counter medications, on newborn. Breastfeeding mothers need to understand the effects of medications on their infants. However, the mother should not be unduly concerned about taking commonly prescribed analgesics, which are considered relatively safe for breastfeeding mothers. Mothers should be encouraged to talk to their practitioner about any drugs they are using and possible effects on the newborn.
- Discuss schedule of office visits for mother and baby. The first postpartum visit is typically 4–6 weeks following the birth. Infants are seen within the first month after birth. Women must be aware of the need for keeping scheduled appointments in order to monitor growth and development of the infant and initiate immunizations. Women will be monitored for progression of postpartum recovery and any complications that may have developed.
- Encourage the woman to get adequate sleep and rest. Offer ideas, such as napping immediately after feeding the infant, when infants usually sleep, or scheduling rest periods at frequent intervals until normal energy levels return. Adequate rest is necessary in order to meet the increased metabolic needs created by lactation and healing. Eight hours of uninterrupted sleep per night is ideal, but if the infant wakes frequently, this may not be possible.
- Encourage the partner to participate in nighttime care of the infant. Affords the woman an occasional night of uninterrupted sleep.
- Provide oral and written information on dietary requirements; advise against weight-reduction diets while breastfeeding. Sufficient calories and nutrients are needed to provide adequate quantities of milk necessary to support infant growth and development.
- Encourage a gradual return to normal activities and participation in an exercise program, including Kegel exercises. Exercise improves muscle tone and when balanced with rest, improves strength, well-being and appearance, and

prevents excessive fatigue from immobility. Kegel exercises help women regain perineal muscle tone that may have been lost during the stretching and tearing of childbirth. Kegel exercises also help women retain bowel and bladder control in later life.

- Teach regarding care of the newborn, as needed. For details, refer to the topic, "Newborn Care: 4 Hours to 2 Days," beginning on p. 376 in Chapter 11.

Nursing Diagnosis: RISK FOR INEFFECTIVE SEXUALITY PATTERN[1]

See the NDCP, "Ineffective Sexuality Pattern[1]" in "Postpartum Period: Weeks 1–6," beginning on p. 332 in this chapter.

Nursing Activities and Rationales

Patient/Family Teaching

- Advise that sexual activity can be resumed when the woman is comfortable and vaginal flow has stopped. This is usually at 4–6 weeks PP, although some women may feel comfortable enough to resume sexual activity between 3 and 4 weeks. This allows time for bleeding to stop, the cervix to close, and healing to occur.
- Advise to use contraception. Breastfeeding is not a reliable contraceptive; the woman could become pregnant prior to the first return check-up (at 4–6 weeks). Such an early pregnancy would place undue stress on the woman's body.

Nursing Diagnosis: READINESS FOR ENHANCED FAMILY COPING[1]

See the NDCP, "Readiness for Enhanced Family Coping[1]" in "Postpartum Period: Weeks 1–6," beginning on p. 330 of this chapter.

Nursing Diagnosis: CONSTIPATION[1]

Related Factors: inadequate fiber intake, insufficient fluid intake, sedentary lifestyle or inadequate physical activity, stress or anxiety, neglect in establishing or maintaining regular times for defecation, pain or fear of pain, or oral iron supplements. The new mother may be too tired and overwhelmed with demands of infant care to drink adequate fluids, to prepare and consume a proper diet, or to obtain adequate exercise. She may experience stress and anxiety

regarding her abilities to fulfill the maternal role and conflicting family roles (e.g., as wife). The infant's needs may interfere with her establishing regular times for defecation. At the time of the first home visit, she may still be experiencing painful defecation secondary to episiotomy and/or hemorrhoids; and she is probably taking oral iron supplements. Nursing activities, to be successful, should focus on ways to relieve the mother's anxieties, on ways to provide adequate rest, and on relief of episiotomy pain. It is not adequate to merely provide information about dietary fiber and fluids. Refer to the generic NDCP, "Constipation,[1]" beginning on p. 11 in Chapter 2.

Nursing Diagnosis: DISTURBED SLEEP PATTERN[1]

Related Factors: the mother's discomforts and the demands of infant care, depression, and anxiety, especially if the baby is difficult to comfort. See the generic NDCP, "Sleep Deprivation or Disturbed Sleep Pattern,[1]" beginning on p. 21 in Chapter 2.

Nursing Activities and Rationales

Assessments

- Assess fatigue level. The amount of sleep a person requires varies with lifestyle, health, and age. Fatigue is common in the postpartum period.
- Discuss family members' responsibilities and the family's daily routine. Determines who is available to help, at what times, and engages them in problem solving about times she may be able to rest. Sharing household tasks will reduce the woman's responsibility for them and help to conserve her energy.

Independent Nursing Actions

- Urge the father or other family member to provide infant care at night, occasionally. Allows the mother an occasional night of uninterrupted sleep.
- Advise to limit the number of visitors and activities for the first few weeks. Conserves energy.

Patient/Family Teaching

- Explain ways to modify the infant's sleep-wake cycles. For example, if the infant is sleeping during the day and waking at night, wake her/him every 3–4 hours during the daytime and try to stimulate him or her to stay awake. When the infant wakes at night, leave her/him alone for a few minutes before responding to the cries. It takes about 5–6 weeks to regulate the infant's sleep-wake cycle so that she/he sleeps longer stretches of time at night and is awake more during the day.
- Suggest that the woman nap when the infant is sleeping. Helps the woman obtain needed rest.

POSTPARTUM PERIOD: WEEKS 1–6

The mother continues to experience physical and emotional changes throughout the 6 weeks following birth. During this time she learns to care for herself and her infant as independently as possible. Toward the end of the 6-week time period, the woman will have made numerous role and family adjustments in order to incorporate the new infant into the family.

■ Key Nursing Activities

- Monitor for complications.
- Provide teaching to support self-care.
- Facilitate adjustment to parenting.
- Encourage family bonding.

■ Etiologies and Risk Factors

Risk Factors do not apply because this is a normal process. Etiology is birth of the infant.

■ Signs and Symptoms

Common discomforts, such as fatigue, breast engorgement, and episiotomy pain should gradually subside as the body returns to the prepregnant state and adjusts to postpartum changes. The following changes occur:

- Involution of the uterus, through autolysis, returns the uterus to a nonpregnant state. At 1 week the uterus weighs about 500 g; by the 9th postpartum day, it should not be palpable abdominally; at 6 weeks it weighs 50–60 g.
- Lochia rubra lasts for about 3 days; lochia serosa lasts until about day 10, when it changes to lochia alba. Lochia alba, a whitish discharge, may continue up to and beyond 6 weeks.
- Menstruation may resume at 4–5 weeks postpartum (later in lactating women).
- Vaginal mucosa is atrophic and dries in the lactating woman due to reduced estrogen levels.
- Episiotomy healing should be complete in 2–3 weeks.
- Hemorrhoids usually decrease in size by the end of the 6-week period.
- Breast tenderness does not usually persist after lactation is well established.
- In nonlactating women, the breasts return to prepregnant size and are soft and nontender.

■ Diagnostic Studies

- CBC. Assesses for anemia. Hgb and Hct should return to prepregnant levels (i.e., 12–16 g/dl and 37–47%).
- Papanicolaou smear. Screens for cervical cancer and human papillomavirus.
- Urinalysis. Assesses for the presence of urinary tract infection.

■ Medical Management

- Women who have had an uncomplicated vaginal birth are scheduled for a routine follow-up examination usually at PP week 6. Ensures that physiologic and emotional adjustments have been made successfully and that no complications are occurring.
- Prenatal vitamins may be prescribed.
- Lactating women may require supplemental calcium.
- Bimanual examination of the uterus may be done. Ensures that involution is complete.
- Subinvolution of the uterus may be treated by dilation and curettage or oral ergonovine and antibiotics. Prevents late postpartum hemorrhage. Treatment depends on cause. Dilation and curettage is done to remove retained placental fragments. Research suggests that curettage may traumatize the implantation site and increase bleeding but is necessary when bleeding is severe (Cunningham et al., 2010). Ergonovine and antibiotics are used when subinvolution is caused by infection.

■ Collaborative Problems

Note: Two nursing diagnoses are included here because they should be a part of the standardized care for all postpartum women; they are not, strictly speaking, collaborative problems because they are not physical complications, and because nurses can perform independent actions for their treatment.

Potential Complications of Postpartum

- Subinvolution of the uterus and/or delayed postpartum hemorrhage
- Infection
- Risk for impaired parenting[1]
- Risk for imbalanced nutrition[1]

COLLABORATIVE (STANDARDIZED) CARE FOR ALL NORMAL POSTPARTUM WOMEN AT WEEKS 1–6

Perform a comprehensive assessment to identify individual needs for teaching, emotional support, and physical care.

■ Potential Complication of Postpartum Period Weeks 1–6: UTERINE SUBINVOLUTION AND/OR DELAYED POSTPARTUM HEMORRHAGE

See the generic collaborative care plan, "Potential Complication: Hemorrhage," beginning on p. 28 in Chapter 3, and the collaborative care plan, "Potential Complication of Postpartum Period: Postpartum Hemorrhage," beginning on p. 308 in "Postpartum Period: First 4 Hours After Birth (Fourth Stage of Labor)," in this chapter.

Focus Assessments and Rationales

- Ask the woman to describe her lochia. Lochia flow gradually subsides and changes in color. Within 10 days after the birth, the lochia turns yellow to white (lochia alba) and diminishes in amount, although scant flow may continue up to 6 weeks. Lochia rubra occurring 3–4 weeks following birth may be caused by complications such as endometriosis, infection, or retained placental fragments. If the woman fails to progress to alba within 2 weeks, subinvolution may be the cause.
- Assess fundal height and tone. Determines the stage of uterine involution. The fundus is normally between the symphysis pubis and the umbilicus by the 6th day following birth and is no longer palpable by the 9th or 10th day. Infection or retained placental fragments are risk factors for subinvolution (failure of uterine involution). This, in turn, can cause late postpartum hemorrhage.
- Ask the woman how many vaginal pads she uses each day. Assesses for progression or recurrence of uterine bleeding. The number of pads saturated within a day should gradually decrease throughout the 6 weeks following birth.

Preventive Nursing Activities

- Monitor Hgb and Hct. Determines the presence of anemia related to continual postpartum bleeding.
- Encourage prenatal vitamins with iron regimen. Restores hemoglobin to prepregnancy levels and delivery levels and prevents the development of anemia.
- Encourage diet high in protein and iron. Prevents the development of anemia secondary to excessive blood loss.

▌Potential Complication of Postpartum Period: INFECTION

See the generic NDCP, "Risk for Infection,[1]" beginning on p. 21 in Chapter 2; the generic collaborative care plan, "Potential Complication: Infection," beginning on p. 29 in Chapter 3; the generic collaborative care plan, "Urinary Tract Infection," beginning on p. 33 in Chapter 3; the collaborative care plan, "Infection (e.g., Episiotomy, Breasts, and Puerperal)," beginning on p. 313 in "Postpartum Period: Days 1–2," and "Puerperal Infection, Urinary Tract Infection, and Mastitis" beginning on p. 321 in "Postpartum Period: First Home Visit," in this chapter.

▌Nursing Diagnosis: RISK FOR IMPAIRED PARENT–INFANT/ CHILD ATTACHMENT[1]

See the generic NDCP, "Risk for Impaired Parent–Infant/Child Attachment,[1]" beginning on p. 19 in Chapter 2; also refer to the NDCP, "Risk for Impaired Parent–Infant/Child Attachment,[1]" beginning on p. 232 in "Normal Labor: Second Stage," in Chapter 7; also see the NDCP, "Risk for Impaired Parent–Infant/Child Attachment,[1]" beginning on p. 317 in "Postpartum Period: Days 1–2," in this chapter.

▌Nursing Activities and Rationales

Assessments

- Assess the woman's physiologic adjustments and recovery. By the 6th postpartum week or even sooner, parent–infant attachment should be strong. However, if the mother is having physical problems, this can have a negative impact on attachment.
- Continue to assess bonding behaviors through interview and observation. Lack of reciprocal interaction (e.g., mother missing infant cues, infant not responding to mother) indicates lack of attachment and requires prompt intervention.
- Inquire about parents' concerns about infant behaviors and their parenting skills. Verbalizing concerns helps to relieve anxiety. Also provides an opportunity to reinforce their positive parenting behaviors and to review previous teaching about infant behaviors.

Collaborative Activities

- Provide follow-up home visits at 1 week and again at about 4 weeks, especially if the family is at risk for attachment problems. Bonding occurs gradually. Because of the limited amount of time the nurse can spend with the family in the acute care agency, it is difficult to make a thorough assessment of bonding.
- Assess mother for signs and symptoms of postpartum depressed mood and/or postpartum major mood disorder. Postpartum depression may affect bonding. Postpartum depression occurs in 4.5–28% of postpartum women (Doucet, Dennis, Letourneau, & Blackmore, 2009). Most affected women think their symptoms are normal for new mothers and do not seek medical attention (Driscoll, 2008).
- If serious problems are suspected or there is evidence of possible abuse or neglect, notify the authorities. Special evaluation is needed to determine interventions needed for the safety of the infant.

▌Nursing Diagnosis: RISK FOR IMBALANCED NUTRITION: LESS THAN BODY REQUIREMENTS[1]

Refer to the NDCP, "Risk for Imbalanced Nutrition: Less Than Body Requirements,[1]" beginning on p. 323 in the topic, "Postpartum Period: First Home Visit," in this chapter.

INDIVIDUALIZED (NURSING DIAGNOSIS) CARE PLANS

This section includes care plans that were developed to address unique patient needs.

Nursing Diagnosis: INTERRUPTED BREASTFEEDING[1]

Related Factors: mother's return to work, abrupt weaning of infant, maternal illness or medications, and infant illness.

Goals, Outcomes, and Evaluation Criteria

- Woman explains benefits of continuing breastfeeding.
- Woman safely collects and stores breast milk.
- Woman recognizes signs of reduced milk supply.
- Woman verbalizes knowledge of the weaning process.

NIC Interventions[2]

Bottle Feeding (1052)—Preparation and administration of fluids to an infant via a bottle.

Emotional Support (5270)—Provision of reassurance, acceptance, and encouragement during times of stress.

Lactation Counseling (5244)—Use of an interactive helping process to assist in maintenance of successful breastfeeding.

Lactation Suppression (6870)—Facilitating the cessation of milk production and minimizing breast engorgement after giving birth.

Nursing Activities and Rationales

Assessments

- Discuss the woman's need/desire to return to work. Determines if interventions to support breastfeeding are necessary.
- Assess woman's desire to continue or discontinue breastfeeding. Assists with planning interventions to support continued breastfeeding or weaning, as the woman chooses. There are many reasons why a woman may not want or have the ability to continue breastfeeding, such as lack of infant growth or the mother's desire or need to return to work. Once reasons are identified, misconceptions can be corrected or alternatives found that may allow the woman to continue breastfeeding if she wishes.
- Identify support system for maintaining lactation. The amount of support influences the woman's desire to continue breastfeeding.
- Assess adequacy of woman's milk supply. Helps determine if the infant's nutritional needs are being met. Infrequent breastfeeding because of working may cause milk production to decrease, adversely affecting the nutrition of the infant.

- Teach regarding availability of assistance. Guidance can be sought through the Le Leche League and lactation consultants.

Independent Nursing Actions

- During lactation suppression, encourage the use of intermittent ice packs to breasts. Cold decreases discomfort associated with breast engorgement during lactation suppression by decreasing circulation and milk production.
- During lactation suppression, encourage woman to place cabbage leaves inside her bra. Decreases discomfort of breast engorgement. The exact mechanism of action is unknown, but it is thought to occur from effect of natural estrogens contained in cabbage.

Collaborative Activities

- Advise to take a prescribed mild analgesic, as needed. Decreases the discomfort caused by breast engorgement during lactation suppression.

Patient/Family Teaching

- If the woman desires to continue feeding human milk while she is at work, teach her how to use a breast pump. Allows for continued feeding of human milk to the infant while preventing breast tissue damage or contamination of human milk.
- Teach how to store and warm human milk. Prevents contamination of the milk or bacterial growth and subsequent illness of the infant.
- Suggest that the woman practice a few weeks before returning to work—using the breast pump and gradually begin to give the baby a bottle during her normal work hours. Familiarizes the infant with the bottle, making the change less traumatic for both. Also allows her to freeze and stockpile milk for use when she returns to work. She can breastfeed before and after work and use formula or stored human milk during work hours.
- Teach the need for wearing a well-fitted support bra when attempting lactation suppression. Decreases breast discomfort during the process of lactation suppression.
- When the woman is attempting lactation suppression, teach to avoid stimulating the breasts. Nipple stimulation, warm running water directed at the breast, breast pumping, or infant sucking will stimulate the production of milk and increase the risk for breast engorgement when the infant is not nursing to empty the breasts.

Nursing Diagnosis: READINESS FOR ENHANCED FAMILY COPING[1]

Related Factors: needs being sufficiently gratified and adaptive tasks effectively addressed to enable goals of self-actualization to surface.

▋ *Goals, Outcomes, and Evaluation Criteria*

- Family enables member role flexibility (e.g., members share care of infant).
- Family members take part in decision making (e.g., about mother returning to work).
- Parent(s) express satisfaction with the progress being made to integrate the infant into the family.

▋ *NIC Interventions[2]*

Family Integrity Promotion: Childbearing Family (7104)— Facilitation of the growth of individuals or families who are adding an infant to the family unit.

*Parenting Promotion (8300)—*Providing parenting information, support, and coordination of comprehensive services to high-risk families.

▋ *Nursing Activities and Rationales*

Assessments

- Assess family structure and cultural background. These factors affect the ability to adapt and the amount/type of support available. For example, it may be more difficult for a single parent to adapt if single parenting is not culturally acceptable in her social setting; and an extended family may provide more support than a nuclear family. In a blended family, in which the newborn may be a half-sibling or a step-sibling, there are added pressures on the mother to accommodate the needs of all family members.
- Explore how the woman/couple has coped with stressors and life changes in the past. People tend to use the same coping strategies over and over. Identifying strategies that were successful in the past enables the woman/couple to choose those strategies and avoid strategies that did not work as well.
- Monitor couple's relationship to one another following birth of baby. Identifies family structure and situation in order to determine if interventions are needed. A strong partner relationship will facilitate transition to parenthood, whereas a problematic relationship will hamper the transition process.
- Assess knowledge of woman/partner regarding integration of baby into the family unit. Determines what teaching is needed and how to proceed with teaching regarding changing family roles, expectations, etc. Effective planning requires identification of the needs and problems that may arise as they assume responsibility for their newborn.
- Assess support system (e.g., family members, friends, housekeeper, babysitter). New parents often experience stress and anxiety when they bring a newborn home. A strong support system eases the transition to parenthood. Parents without support systems are likely to experience greater anxiety, frustration, and insecurity and take longer to adapt to their new roles.

- Identify family's interaction system. Determines how the family reacts to the needs and concerns of its members in order to identify possible obstacles to transitioning into the parental role or strengths.
- Assess siblings' response to the baby. Siblings might be resentful of the attention the parents give the new baby, and they may act out or demonstrate regressive behaviors (e.g., a potty-trained sibling may wet or soil him/herself).
- Assess perception of ability and comfort with assuming roles as parents. Transition to the role of parent requires flexibility, acquisition of new skills, and realistic expectations of their infant and their ability to care for and nurture the infant. Inaccurate perceptions or discomfort with their skills and abilities may make the transition to parenthood more stressful than it would be otherwise.

Independent Nursing Actions

- Reinforce positive parenting behaviors. Encourages positive behaviors, builds self-confidence and self-esteem as the couple learns new skills and adapts to caring for their infant independently.
- Assist the couple to set realistic goals for themselves and the family. Unrealistic goals may require the couple to expend energy that would be better used for coping and adjusting to changes in family dynamics.
- Help the couple to identify problems they can anticipate for the family during the coming months. In order to provide anticipatory guidance, clarify misconceptions, and engage in effective problem solving.
- Provide a telephone number for someone who is available 24 hours a day. Provides a feeling of security. New parents need 24-hour access to healthcare advice in the early postpartum period; crises, problems, and questions can arise at any time of the night or day.

Collaborative Activities

- Refer to counseling, as appropriate. Counseling may help improve family interactions, assist couple to develop coping strategies, and provide an opportunity to ventilate their frustrations or anxiety as they adjust to their new roles. Couples may need to be reassured that seeking counseling is not a sign of weakness or failure on their part.
- Teach regarding the availability of community resources (e.g., La Leche League, parenting classes) and provide written materials for later use. The couple may be unaware of community resources available to them. Women who are adjusting to the physiologic and psychologic changes occurring during the postpartum period will not remember all teaching that was provided. Written materials regarding community resources can be referred to later as needed.

Patient/Family Teaching

- Encourage to seek support and take time away from the newborn during the adjustment period. Facilitates successful transition to the parental role. Parents often need permission to leave their newborn with grandparents or others even for short periods of time, even though it is needed for them to renew their own relationship and care for other siblings. A rested, nonfrustrated parent makes the transition to parenthood more readily than one who is anxious or overwhelmed.

- Reassure the couple that it is normal to feel inadequate and stressed during the role transition, especially for first-time parents. Enhances feelings of self-worth. Parents sometimes believe that parenting should come naturally. When they find parenting difficult, they may mistakenly believe that this is because of their own shortcomings and that other parents are better parents.
- Explain that it usually takes 5 or 6 weeks for a family to adjust to the birth of a baby; however it can occasionally take longer. Reassures the family that their experience is normal and restores self-esteem. Provides information so that if they are still stressed and overwhelmed after 3 or 4 months, they will know to seek help.
- Explain that it is normal for siblings to act out or have behavior changes. This usually reflects their feelings of resentment and frustration over the decreased attention they receive after the birth of the baby. Understanding that the behaviors are normal allows the parents to be more understanding and strengthen ties with the children.
- Help the couple to prioritize tasks and arrange their schedule so they can spend time alone with each of the other children. Helps foster the successful integration of other children into the family unit and prevent them from feeling left out, neglected, or jealous of the newborn. Helps the siblings to feel more secure and fosters coping.

Nursing Diagnosis: INEFFECTIVE SEXUALITY PATTERN[1]

Related Factors: postpartum physiologic changes/discomforts, adjustment to new role as parents, impaired relationship with partner, fatigue, lack of knowledge about body changes, lack of privacy, demands of infant, and fear of pregnancy.

Goals, Outcomes, and Evaluation Criteria

- Couple discusses the effect the birth has had on their relationship.
- Couple expresses satisfaction with sexual relationship.
- Woman expresses satisfaction with body appearance.
- Woman makes adjustment to changes in physical appearance.
- Woman verbalizes understanding that some changes of pregnancy are reversible.
- Woman verbalizes self-worth.

NIC Interventions[2]

Body Image Enhancement (5220)—Improving a patient's conscious and unconscious perceptions and attitudes toward his/her body.

Postpartum Care (6930)—Monitoring and management of patient during postpartum to prevent complications of postpartum condition and promote a healthy outcome for both mother and infant.

Sexual Counseling (5248)—Use of an interactive helping process focusing on the need to make adjustments in sexual practice or to enhance coping with a sexual event/disorder.

Nursing Activities and Rationales

Assessments

- Assess current and past sexual patterns and practices. Facilitates care planning and teaching individualized to specific needs and expectations.
- Assess woman's relationship with partner. Identifies strengths in the couple's relationship that will allow them to continue with or rebuild a satisfactory sexual relationship, or identifies problems that interfere with their sexual relationship. With the added responsibilities of a newborn infant, a couple with a stressful or weak relationship may find it difficult to return to their former sexual functioning.
- Assess understanding of contraception. Determines the need for further teaching. Compliance with any contraceptive method will be increased if the couple participates in choosing a method that is convenient and acceptable to them. Pregnancy may occur before onset of menses, even if the woman is breastfeeding. Oral contraceptives are the most effective method, but they are contraindicated for some women (e.g., those who are breastfeeding, those with diabetes or a history of thrombophlebitis). The couple may choose to be abstinent; use the rhythm method; or use foams, condoms, and/or gels. If the woman has been using a diaphragm, it should be refitted following the birth of the baby.
- Assess the woman's perception of self, including body image; determine partner's perception as well. Identifies potential obstacles to the woman's regaining her positive feelings of sexuality. The changes associated with pregnancy or lactation can cause the woman to feel unattractive or undesirable, which may negatively affect her desire and ability to respond sexually. For example, the partner may not see her, or she may not see herself, as physically attractive if she is lactating or if her body has not returned to its prepregnant shape. Identification of these feelings/concerns allows for individualized care planning.
- Assess the woman's/partner's sleeping patterns and energy levels. Fatigue, discomfort, and even the presence of the baby may interfere with the ability to initiate or respond sexually.

Independent Nursing Actions

- Establish trust. Women are often reluctant to discuss their concerns about sexuality. Trust increases comfort and allows for enhanced communications.
- Initiate the topic of sexual adjustment; do not wait for the woman to ask questions. Many new parents are eager for information but are reluctant to bring up the subject of sexuality and sexual functioning. If the nurse introduces the topic, it lets the woman know that resuming sexual activity is a legitimate concern and that the nurse is willing to answer questions.
- Discuss sexual concerns in a relaxed, accepting, and matter-of-fact manner. Places the woman at ease and facilitates communication. Sexuality is a private matter that many people have difficulty discussing.
- Provide privacy. Demonstrates respect for the person, which facilitates open communication.
- Encourage to express concerns and fears. Assists the nurse with identification of specific problems for which care planning is necessary.
- Encourage woman to dress, apply makeup, etc. A new mother may become easily fatigued and feel no need to dress or apply makeup. Sexual attractiveness has a strong emotional component. Women who feel good about themselves are more likely to feel good about their sexuality. Dressing, applying makeup, etc., enhances the woman's self-image, contributes to her feelings of self-worth and attractiveness, and may increase her physical attractiveness to her partner.

Collaborative Activity

- Refer for counseling, if needed. A couple who cannot achieve sexual satisfaction may have deeper relationship problems and need help to establish open communication and trust.

Patient/Family Teaching

- Teach the woman and her partner about physiologic changes following birth and their effect on sexual drive and response. Prepares them for changes the woman may experience. For the first 2–3 months following birth, women may experience increased arousal time, decreased intensity, and reduced strength of orgasm due to reduced estrogen levels.
- Suggest that the couple plan their lovemaking soon after feedings if the woman is breastfeeding. Orgasm may stimulate the let-down reflex, causing milk to leak from the breasts. Intercourse may be more pleasurable between feedings, when the breasts are not full or leaking.
- Prepare the couple for the possibility that the male partner may have difficulty achieving an erection. The partner, too, may be fatigued from the demands of his new role. Additionally, much sexual desire is psychologic and visual. If

the male sees his partner as a mother, he may have difficulty reacting sexually to her as a woman. Or he may not find her postpartum body as physically attractive as previously.
- Teach the woman how to control discomfort with intercourse (dyspareunia) initially. Sexual activity can be safely resumed before the traditional 6-week checkup because the risks for hemorrhage and infection are minimal by 2 weeks after birth, unless the woman has been instructed otherwise by her practitioner. A water-soluble lubricant (or contraceptive creams or jellies) may be needed to counter vaginal dryness. The side-lying or female-on-top position allows the woman to control the depth of penile penetration while vaginal tissues are tender.
- If necessary, teach alternatives to penis–vagina intercourse for achieving orgasm (e.g., cunnilingus, masturbation, mutual stroking of genitalia); be aware that one or both partners may find such alternatives unacceptable. Achieves sexual gratification until penile penetration can be achieved without discomfort.
- Teach the woman the relationship between contraception and lactation. Women sometimes feel sexually aroused when breastfeeding their infants; consequently they frequently resume sexual activity earlier than nonbreastfeeding women. It is important that women understand that breastfeeding may delay the onset of menses but does not guarantee that pregnancy will be avoided. A woman who engages in unprotected sex is at increased risk of becoming pregnant earlier than she planned.

Nursing Diagnosis: DISTURBED BODY IMAGE[1]

Related Factors: unrealistic expectations, incorrect belief that all body changes are permanent, lack of acceptance of body changes that are permanent.

Goals, Outcomes, and Evaluation Criteria

- Woman acknowledges and accepts changes in body.
- Woman identifies personal strengths.
- Woman devises and follows a realistic plan to improve appearance (e.g., begins a program of exercise and diet, pays attention to grooming).
- Woman expresses satisfaction with body appearance and function.

NIC Interventions[2]

Body Image Enhancement (5220)—Improving a patient's conscious and unconscious perceptions and attitudes toward his/her body.
Coping Enhancement (5230)—Assisting a patient to adapt to perceived stressors, changes, or threats that interfere with meeting life demands and roles.

Self-Esteem Enhancement (5400)—Assisting a patient to increase his/her personal judgment of self-worth.

Nursing Activities and Rationales

Assessments

- Assess the woman's verbal and nonverbal responses to her body. Determines whether interventions are needed to enhance body image. The woman's perceptions of changes in her body may be realistic, exaggerated, or even imagined.
- Assess woman's expectations for regaining prepregnant body appearance. If the woman expected to regain her body shape/appearance right away, she may become depressed when this does not occur. If the woman and/or partner place much emphasis on appearance, this can precipitate grief and perhaps even a crisis.
- Monitor the frequency of statements of self-criticism. Evaluates level of self-esteem.

Independent Nursing Actions

- Actively listen to the woman's concerns about her body and acknowledge that her concerns are legitimate. Promotes trust and open communication.
- Assist in identifying positive aspects of her body and realistic expectations for returning to the prepregnant state. Unrealistic expectations will result in disappointment and loss of self-esteem.
- Encourage the woman to maintain her usual daily grooming routine (e.g., applying makeup, styling her hair). Promotes viewing herself as attractive.
- Help the woman choose attractive, loose-fitting clothing. Helps make weight gain and loss of muscle tone less obvious until prepregnant contours are achieved.
- Help to plan a realistic exercise routine. Facilitates regaining of lost muscle tone and burning of excess calories.
- Help to plan a well-balanced weight-loss diet for the non-lactating woman. Following birth, a woman retains about half the weight over 24 lbs (11 kg) gained during pregnancy. This must be lost by diet and exercise. When dietary and lifestyle changes start during the prenatal period, excessive weight gain during pregnancy can be prevented (Asbee et al., 2009).
- Encourage the lactating woman not to diet until she stops breastfeeding. Caloric restriction my result in inadequate milk production; however, because of the number of calories required for milk production, many lactating women find that they lose weight even without trying to follow a weight-loss diet.
- Suggest to the partner that he pay special attention to the woman (e.g., with time, attention, cards). If the woman feels he is interested in her, she will feel more positive about herself and her attractiveness.
- Encourage the partner to not joke or comment negatively about the woman's appearance. Negative comments and jokes reinforce her feelings of unattractiveness, and contrary to what he might think, they do not provide motivation for change.

Patient/Family Teaching

- Provide information about body changes that are permanent and those that can be affected by diet and exercise. Information is needed in order for the woman to have realistic expectations and avoid disappointment. It takes about 6 weeks for the abdominal muscles and uterus to return to the prepregnant state. Linea nigra, darker pigmentation of the areola, and coarser hair may not change after birth.

Other Nursing Diagnoses

Also assess for the following nursing diagnoses, which are frequently present with this condition:

- Constipation[1] related to lack of exercise and/or inadequate fluids and fiber in the diet.
- Risk for impaired parenting[1] related to inadequate support from partner/family, unrealistic expectations, stresses of role changes, lack of role models, family problems (e.g., financial difficulties).
- Sleep deprivation/disturbed sleep pattern[1] related to frequent waking of newborn throughout the night, anxieties about added responsibilities of parenthood, postpartum discomforts.

POSTPARTUM CARE AFTER CESAREAN BIRTH

Cesarean birth refers to birth of the infant through a surgical incision into the uterus. A planned cesarean birth is a scheduled birth, whereas an unplanned cesarean is an emergency. A cesarean birth may be the optimal choice when either the mother or fetus is threatened, although the mother may grieve the loss of the experience of giving birth in the traditional manner. The woman undergoing cesarean birth will receive the usual postpartum care as well as postoperative care. For general, nonsurgical, postpartum care, refer to the following topics:

- "Postpartum Period: First 4 Hours After Birth (Fourth Stage of Labor)," beginning on p. 307 in this chapter
- "Postpartum Period: Days 1–2," beginning on p. 311 in this chapter
- "Postpartum Period: First Home Visit," beginning on p. 320 in this chapter
- "Postpartum Period: Weeks 1–6," beginning on p. 328 in this chapter

The care plans in this topic outline the care needed after cesarean birth that is over and above that outlined in the aforementioned topics.

Key Nursing Activities

- Monitor for complications, especially surgical wound infection, postpartum hemorrhage, and urinary retention.
- Promote parent–infant attachment.
- Initiate breastfeeding, if not contraindicated.
- Encourage rest.
- Monitor and control pain.
- Transfer from recovery care to postpartum or mother–baby care after 1 or 2 hours (follow agency protocol) if VSs are stable, uterus is firm, and lochia flow is small to moderate in amount, and the woman is recovered from effects of anesthesia.

Etiologies and Risk Factors

Etiologies and risk factors include surgical birth of the infant.

Signs and Symptoms

Symptoms are similar to those of the woman giving vaginal birth, except for the surgical wound. The mother may be thirsty, fatigued, excited, or unable to sleep following recovery from anesthesia. Surgical incision pain, mild uterine cramping, and fairly heavy lochia rubra are normal (although amount of flow may sometimes be less than it would be after a vaginal birth). Symptoms such as wound swelling or purulent drainage, boggy uterus, and bladder distention indicate problems rather than normal postpartum recovery.

Diagnostic Studies

- Urinalysis. Detects proteinuria or infection or is done after removal of urinary catheter.
- White cell count. May be ordered to detect infection (normal values of 20,000–25,000/mm³ are common during the first 1–2 postpartum weeks).
- Hgb and Hct. Detects excessive blood loss and/or anemia; Hgb and Hct may be difficult to evaluate in the first 48–72 hours following birth because of the changing blood volume and greater loss of plasma volume than in RBCs; decrease of two percentage points from the admission Hct indicates a blood loss of about 500 ml (James, 2008).
- Wound culture. If symptoms are present, identifies infection of draining surgical wound.

Medical Management

Medical management is the same as for vaginal birth, except for the following:

- Patient-controlled analgesia morphine or meperidine (Demerol). Controls pain during first 24 postoperative hours.

- Epidural narcotics. Control pain during first 24 postoperative hours.
- Antiflatulent agents and rectal tube. Relieve abdominal distention.
- Intravenous infusion low rate for 24 hours. Replaces fluid losses and supports renal function and urine output.
- Indwelling urinary catheter for 24 hours or until woman is ambulatory.

Collaborative Problems

Potential Complications of Cesarean Birth

- Postpartum or surgical hemorrhage
- Infection: UTI, mastitis, puerperal, incision
- Thrombophlebitis

Potential Complications of Epidural Anesthesia and/or Analgesia

- Urinary retention
- Itching
- Nausea and vomiting
- Respiratory depression

COLLABORATIVE (STANDARDIZED) CARE FOR ALL WOMEN EXPERIENCING CESAREAN BIRTH

Perform a comprehensive assessment to identify individual needs for teaching, emotional support, and physical care.

Potential Complication of Cesarean Birth: POSTPARTUM OR SURGICAL HEMORRHAGE

See the generic collaborative care plan, "Potential Complication: Hemorrhage," beginning on p. 28 in Chapter 3. In addition to the interventions performed after a vaginal birth, those discussed in this section apply to cesarean birth.

Focus Assessments and Rationales

- Assess surgical dressing every 15 min for first hour; then every 30 min for 1 hour; then hourly (or according to agency policy). Dressing applied in surgery is not removed for the first 24 hours. The first sign of incision hemorrhage is the appearance of blood on the dressing. Vital signs change only after significant blood loss.

Preventive Nursing Activity

- If there is blood on the dressing, mark the edges of the drainage with a pen and mark the time. Facilitates the determination of how fast bleeding is occurring.

Potential Complication: INFECTION (UTI, MASTITIS, PUERPERAL, INCISION)

See the generic NDCP, "Risk for Infection,[1]" beginning on p. 21 Chapter 2; see the generic collaborative care plan, "Potential Complication: Infection," beginning on p. 29 in Chapter 3; and see the topic, "Surgical Procedures," beginning on p. 134 Chapter 5. In addition to the interventions performed after a vaginal birth, those in this section apply to cesarean birth.

Focus Assessments and Rationales

- Inspect (and teach woman to inspect) abdominal incision for redness, swelling, separation of edges, and drainage. Detects wound infection. Erythema, warmth, and mild swelling at the incision site are normal and indicate that the inflammatory response is providing hemostasis and collagen synthesis for healing. An expanding area of erythema, increased warmth, and swelling and continued or escalating pain indicate infection. Infection prolongs the inflammatory response, inhibits deposition of collagen fibers, and interferes with healing, which can lead to wound dehiscence.
- Assess for urinary retention. An indwelling urinary catheter may remain in place for 24 hours. Once the catheter is removed, the woman normally voids with 4–6 hours. If voiding does not occur, the bladder is palpated for distention. See the generic NDCP, "Urinary Retention,[1]" beginning on p. 22 in Chapter 2.
- Assess color of urine. Tea or cola colored urine may indicate bleeding due to surgical trauma to the ureters and needs to be reported immediately.

Preventive Nursing Activity

- Before discharge, teach the woman to notify her healthcare provider if any of the following signs occur: temperature greater than 38°C (100.4°F), painful urination, lochia heavier than a normal period, wound separation, redness or oozing at incision site, or severe abdominal pain. Facilitates immediate treatment of infection and bleeding.

Potential Complication of Cesarean Birth: THROMBOPHLEBITIS

Refer to the generic NDCP, "Ineffective Peripheral Tissue Perfusion,[1]" beginning on p. 18 in Chapter 2; also see the NDCP, "Ineffective Tissue Perfusion (Peripheral),[1]" beginning on p. 352 in "Thromboembolic Disease," in Chapter 10. In addition to the interventions performed after a vaginal birth, those in this section apply to cesarean birth.

Focus Assessments and Rationales

- Assess for deep vein thrombosis. Perform check for Homans' sign by supporting leg and dorsiflexing the foot. Calf pain is a positive sign of deep vein thrombosis; however, it is present only in about 35% of patients. The absence of pain does not rule out the presence of deep vein thrombosis.
- Ask woman about heavy feeling, throbbing, or tight sensations in her calf, especially with activity. These are signs that often accompany deep vein thrombosis.

Preventive Nursing Activities

- Until effects of epidural anesthesia wear off, reposition the woman every hour. Prevents stasis in the legs, which may be immobile as a result of the anesthetic.
- Encourage use of elastic stockings. Prevents stasis of blood in lower extremities by promoting venous blood flow and preventing bulging of lower leg veins.
- Assist with progressive ambulation as soon as vital signs are stable, pain is controlled, and motor control of the legs is present. Ambulation, with support, should occur within 24 hours, often as early as 4 or 5 hours after birth, to prevent venous stasis in the legs.
- Maintain adequate hydration. Hydration prevents increased viscosity of blood, which increases the risk for decreased blood flow and thrombus formation.

Potential Complications of Epidural Anesthesia and/or Analgesia: URINARY RETENTION, ITCHING, NAUSEA AND VOMITING, AND RESPIRATORY DEPRESSION

Refer to the topic, "Epidural Anesthesia/Analgesia," beginning on p. 248 in Chapter 7.

INDIVIDUALIZED (NURSING DIAGNOSIS) CARE PLANS

The care plans in this section were developed to address unique patient needs.

Nursing Diagnosis: Pain[1]

This section discusses pain related to surgical incision, uterine cramping, and intestinal gas. See the generic NDCP, "Pain,[1]" beginning on p. 18 in Chapter 2.

Nursing Activities and Rationales

Assessments

- Assess for incision pain. Determines the intensity of pain and the effectiveness of administered narcotic analgesics.
- Assess nonverbal cues regarding pain response. Many women do not complain of pain even though they are experiencing pain. Nonverbal cues such as grimacing, crying, withdrawn behavior or reluctance to move or interact with the newborn may indicate pain. Pain must be controlled because it affects mobility and bonding with the newborn.
- Assess bowel sounds at least once per shift; ask the woman to inform you if she passes flatus. Determines whether peristalsis has returned postoperatively. Loss of peristalsis increases the accumulation of intestinal gas, which increases pain. Peristalsis generally returns within 72–96 hours following general anesthesia.
- Assess abdomen for distention and pain. These are signs of intestinal gas buildup, which accompanies decreased peristalsis secondary to anesthesia and decreased activity. A distended abdomen places pressure on the incised muscles, which increases pain.
- Assess tip of epidural catheter when removed. If the woman is receiving epidural analgesia, the catheter will be removed about 24 hours following the cesarean birth. It is essential to check the catheter tip, which is color coded, to make sure the catheter is removed intact. If the tip is missing, it has been sheared off into the epidural space and may require surgery for removal.
- Differentiate incisional pain from afterpains (uterine cramping). NSAIDs (e.g., ibuprofen [Motrin]) may be more effective for cramping than a narcotic because of their prostaglandin-inhibiting action. Prostaglandins cause the uterus to contract.

Independent Nursing Actions

- Encourage the woman to ask for pain medication before pain becomes severe. Pain is easier to control before it becomes severe. Higher doses of analgesics are required to inhibit the perception of pain when it is severe. Severe pain also induces anxiety, which in turn contributes to the pain cycle and makes pain more difficult to control.
- Until effects of anesthesia wear off, help with position changes at least hourly. Prevents venous stasis, pressure on bony prominences and enhances comfort. Repositioning may relax abdominal muscles, which helps reduce the sensation of pain.
- Assist with progressive ambulation as soon as vital signs are stable, pain is controlled, and motor control of the legs is present. Ambulation, with support, should occur within 24 hours, often as early as 4 or 5 hours after birth, to stimulate peristalsis.
- Suggest that the woman try rocking in a rocking chair if gas pains are present. For relief of pain. A rocking motion stimulates peristalsis without placing stress on the suture line.

Collaborative Activity

- If epidural anesthesia was used, epidural narcotics can be given in the recovery period. Provides pain relief for approximately 24 hours.

Patient/Family Teaching

- Teach the woman how to use a patient-controlled analgesia pump if available. Patient-controlled analgesia allows the woman to control the frequency with which she receives medication for pain. She should be encouraged to self-administer medication often enough so that pain does not become severe. A woman whose pain is well controlled is able to ambulate and initiate self-care earlier than one who does not gain good control of her pain.
- Teach what to expect following cesarean birth. The woman who is well prepared for the postoperative period adapts better than the woman who is anxious because she does not know what to expect. Anxiety contributes to pain.
- Demonstrate how to splint the incision when moving about in bed or ambulating. Facilitates movement and coughing by decreasing tension on the incised muscles.
- Explain the need for taking nothing by mouth until bowel sounds are present and for avoiding carbonated beverages. Carbonated beverages cause intestinal gas.

Nursing Diagnosis: DEFICIENT KNOWLEDGE: SELF-CARE[1]

Related Factors: lack of prior experience with cesarean birth. See the generic NDCP, "Deficient Knowledge,[1]" beginning on p. 13 in Chapter 2.

Goals, Outcomes, and Evaluation Criteria

- Woman verbalizes understanding of postoperative incisional care.
- Woman demonstrates postoperative self-care.
- Woman coughs and deep breathes every 2 hours.
- Woman gradually resumes self-care without pain or fatigue.

NIC Interventions[2]

Postanesthesia Care (2870)—Monitoring and management of the patient who has recently undergone general or regional anesthesia.

Postpartum Care (6930)—Monitoring and management of the patient who has recently given birth.

▌ *Nursing Activities and Rationales*

Assessments

- Assess level of consciousness and ability to ambulate. Determines the woman's ability to ambulate, turn, and respond to stimuli following spinal, epidural, or general anesthesia and narcotic analgesia. Recovery from anesthesia varies among women, placing them at risk for falls if they are not fully awake, able to move all extremities, and alert prior to ambulation. Uncontrolled pain inhibits the ability to ambulate and increases her risk of falling.

- Assess ability and readiness to resume activities of daily living. Women vary in the amount of time required to resume self-care. Some women will be fatigued and sleepy while others will be excited and ready to assume activities of daily living. Women are frequently the best judge of their bodies and abilities and what they are ready to do following surgical birth.

- Assess lung sounds, abdomen, and surgical incision. Detects postoperative complications including atelectasis, pneumonia, paralytic ileus, or wound infection. As with any abdominal surgery, the woman undergoing cesarean birth is at increased risk for the usual postoperative complications.

Patient/Family Teaching

- Teach deep breathing exercises and/or use of incentive spirometer. Helps prevent atelectasis or pneumonia. Deep breathing ventilates the lower lungs and prevents alveolar collapse. It also enhances the expectoration of secretions. Trapped secretions provide an excellent medium for bacterial growth and increase the risk for pneumonia.

- Teach to call for assistance prior to ambulating. Reduces the woman's risk for falls, especially if not fully awake following general anesthesia, unable to freely move both lower extremities or taking pain medications.

- Encourage to report pain, especially when not well controlled. Determines the effectiveness of prescribed medications in controlling pain so that alternative interventions can be planned. Women who are in pain are less likely or able to resume self-care or care of their newborn.

- Teach regarding what to expect during normal postpartum and postsurgical period. Decreases anxiety by reducing fear of the unknown. The woman who knows what to expect has an increased feeling of control and is better able to adjust to her new situation. Fear produces anxiety, which increases pain and may prevent the woman from resuming self-care.

- Teach care of surgical incision. Decreases fear and anxiety related to home care of surgical incision. Incisions closed with sutures or staples are usually kept covered for 24–48 hours to prevent introduction of pathogenic organisms. Thereafter, the wound edges are closed and there is no need for a dressing. Showering is permitted as long as wound edges are well approximated.

- Teach the need for follow-up to remove sutures/staples. Sutures/staples are generally left in place from 5 to 7 days following cesarean birth. By then, collagen fibers have been deposited and there is little risk for wound edge separation (dehiscence).

- Teach signs and symptoms that need to be reported. Temperatures up to 38.5°C (101.3°F) for 48–72 hours following surgery are anticipated due to the inflammatory response. Fever continuing beyond 72 hours or spiking in the early evening is an indication of infection and needs to be reported. The incision should be free of redness, swelling, pain, or drainage, and edges should remain well approximated. The woman who understands what to report is more likely to do so when abnormalities occur.

- Teach to avoid lifting more than 10 pounds for 6 weeks. Lifting increases intraabdominal pressure and places stress on internal suture line, which can predispose the woman to development of incisional hernia in the future.

- Teach to place infant in the football hold for breastfeeding. Prevents pressure on the surgical incision and increased pain. The woman who is in pain may not want or be able to breastfeed her infant.

- Teach woman regarding perineal and breast care. See the topics, "Postpartum Period: Days 1–2" and "Postpartum Period: Weeks 1–6," beginning on pp. 311 and 328, respectively, in this chapter. Breast care does not differ for women undergoing vaginal and cesarean birth. Perineal care is similar in regard to lochia, but episiotomy/lacerations do not exist with cesarean birth. Fundal involution occurs the same for both types of birth.

- Teach the need for balancing rest with activities/care of the newborn. Women need to realize that they have undergone major surgery and their energy stores will be reduced. Balancing rest with essential activities and infant care prevents fatigue and allows healing to occur.

▌ Nursing Diagnosis: DISTURBED BODY IMAGE[1]

Related Factors: incision and perceived loss of physical attractiveness. Refer to the NDCP, "Disturbed Body Image,[1]" beginning on p. 333 in "Postpartum Period: Weeks 1–6," in this chapter.

▌ *Goals, Outcomes, and Evaluation Criteria*

- Woman freely verbalizes feelings and concerns regarding incision.
- Woman makes positive statements about herself.

▌ Nursing Activities and Rationales

Assessments

* Assess feelings about surgical incision. Determines if woman has negative feelings about herself that may interfere with her recovery, ability to resume self-care or care of her infant, or place her at risk for postpartum complications such as depression. The extent of response to the incision is related more to the value or importance the woman places on it than to the actual appearance of the incision itself.
* Assess the impact of the change in body appearance. The woman's developmental stage affects her reactions to changes in body appearance. Adolescents and young adults may be affected by a change in appearance more than older women since they are at the stage when developing social and intimate relationships is very important.
* Assess for behaviors that indicate positive or negative integration of body change. Behaviors may take the form of self-critical remarks, failure to look at the incision, totally ignoring it, or becoming preoccupied with it. Positive behaviors indicate progress toward self-acceptance whereas negative behaviors indicate the need for intervention.

Independent Nursing Actions

* Acknowledge that negative feelings about incision are normal. Reassures the woman that her feelings are normal and that changes in body appearance or function can precipitate grieving. Some women must be reassured that grieving for their previous appearance is okay.
* Encourage to verbalize her concerns and to ask questions. Some women may view their scars as mutilating and a threat to their sexual attractiveness. Verbalization helps the woman place her situation in perspective with everything else that is going on in her life and allows the nurse to correct misconceptions that may be anxiety producing.

Patient/Family Teaching

* Teach about surgical incision care. Increases the woman's understanding about how the incision will heal and look after it is healed and to involve her in care of her incision. Beauty and freedom from scars and blemishes are an important aspect of American society. Women who look at and participate in their own care are more likely to integrate their bodily appearance into their self-concept in a positive manner.

▌ Nursing Diagnosis: RISK FOR COMPLICATED GRIEVING[1]

Related Factors: inability to deliver vaginally, as well as unmet expectations for labor and birth.

▌ Goals, Outcomes, and Evaluation Criteria

* Woman uses coping mechanisms effectively.
* Woman identifies members of her support system.
* Woman freely expresses her feelings and concerns.

▌ NIC Interventions[2]

Cesarean Section Care (6750)—Preparation and support of patient delivering a baby by cesarean section.

Postpartum Care (6930)—Monitoring and management of the patient who has recently given birth.

▌ Nursing Activities and Rationales

Assessments

* Assess for behaviors that indicate grief. Identifies the need for planning and intervention. Women who undergo cesarean birth may have feelings of fear, disappointment, frustration, anger, or loss of self-esteem due to their inability to give birth as they had hoped and anticipated. They are less likely to breastfeed and may have delayed ability to verbalize positive feelings about the birth process or their newborn.
* Assess for available support systems. The woman may need reassurance from her partner and other members of her support system in order to adjust to her loss. Women with readily available support systems are likely to adjust more quickly than those who do not have a support system.

Independent Nursing Actions

* Encourage to perform activities of daily living as tolerated. Facilitates increased activity. Decreased activity causes fatigue and may contribute to grief and feelings of decreased self-worth.
* Encourage partner to assist with care when feasible. Involvement of the partner is affirming to the relationship and may help the woman progress through the grief process.
* Offer reassurance that vaginal birth is possible following cesarean birth. Reasons for the primary cesarean birth, such as dystocia, breech presentation, or fetal distress, are not necessarily recurring problems; therefore, the woman may be able to undergo vaginal birth in the future. This knowledge may help the woman adapt more successfully to this cesarean birth.

Patient/Family Teaching

* Teach that grief is a normal response. The woman may not understand that what she is feeling is a normal response, which may delay her recovery. She may need to be reassured that it is okay to grieve. The ability to grieve allows the individual to heal emotionally and adjust to her loss in a positive manner.

Nursing Diagnosis: RISK FOR IMPAIRED PARENT–INFANT/CHILD ATTACHMENT[1]

See the generic care plan, "Risk for Impaired Parent–Infant/Child Attachment,[1]" beginning on p. 19 in Chapter 2. Also refer to the NDCP, "Risk for Impaired Parent–Infant/Child Attachment,[1]" beginning on p. 232 of the topic, "Normal Labor: Second Stage," in Chapter 7.

Nursing Diagnosis: BREASTFEEDING (EFFECTIVE OR INEFFECTIVE)[1]

Refer to the NDCP, "Risk for Ineffective Breastfeeding;[1]" or "Effective Breastfeeding,[1]" beginning on p. 318 of the topic "Postpartum Period: Days 1–2," in this chapter.

Nursing Activities and Rationales

Assessment

- Assess for breastfeeding effectiveness. Helps ensure that the infant receives adequate nutrition without producing increased pain for the mother. The woman with a surgical incision may be reluctant to breastfeed or might discontinue breastfeeding before her infant has received adequate milk due to increased pain or discomfort.

Patient/Family Teaching

- Teach positions that facilitate breastfeeding without increasing pain. Alternate positions for breastfeeding do not increase pain at the surgical incision. Options include side lying, the football hold (infant's body beneath and supported by the mother's arm and the infant's head at the breast), or sitting with the infant resting on a pillow. All of these positions allow for effective feeding without placing pressure on the abdomen.
- Teach to use patient-controlled analgesia to reduce pain during breastfeeding. Women are often concerned about use of narcotics for pain control and their effect on the newborn, and therefore do not self-administer adequate analgesics. Narcotics do pass with human milk; however, the small doses delivered by patient-controlled analgesia pumps do not normally have an adverse effect on the newborn and they significantly enhance the woman's comfort, making breastfeeding more effective physiologically and psychologically.

Other Nursing Diagnoses

Also assess for the following nursing diagnoses, which are frequently present with this condition:

- Fatigue.[1] See the generic NDCP, "Fatigue,[1]" beginning on p. 14 in Chapter 2.
- Disturbed Sleep Pattern.[1] See the generic NDCP, "Sleep Deprivation or Disturbed Sleep Pattern,[1]" beginning on p. 21 in Chapter 2.

END NOTES

1. Nursing Diagnoses—Definitions and Classification 2009–2011. Copyright © 2009, 2007, 2005, 2003, 2001, 1998, 1996, 1994 by NANDA International. Used by arrangement with Blackwell Publishing Limited, a company of John Wiley & Sons, Inc. In order to make safe and effective judgments using NANDA-I nursing diagnoses it is essential that nurses refer to the definitions and defining characteristics of the diagnoses listed in this work.
2. Bulechek, G. M., Butcher, H. K., Dochterman, J. M. (2008). *Nursing Interventions Classification* (5th ed). St. Louis, MO: Elsevier, by permission.

REFERENCES

Asbee, S., Jenkins, T., Butler, J., White, J., Elliot, M., & Rutledge, A. (2009). Preventing excessive weight gain during pregnancy through dietary and lifestyle counseling. *Obstetrics and Gynecology, 1113,* 305–312.

Blackburn, S. (2007). *Maternal, fetal, and neonatal physiology: A clinical perspective* (3rd ed.). Philadelphia, PA: Saunders.

Bulechek, G. M., Butcher, H. K., & Dochterman, J. M. (2008). *Nursing interventions classification (NIC)* (5th ed.). St. Louis, MO: Mosby/Elesevier.

Cunningham, F., Leveno, K., Bloom, S., Hauth, J., Rouse, D., & Spong, C. (2010). *Williams obstetrics* (23rd ed.). New York, NY: McGraw-Hill.

Doucet, S., Dennis, C., Letourneau, N., & Blackmore, E. (2009). Differentiation and clinical implications of postpartum depression and postpartum psychosis. *JOGGN, 38*(3), 269–279.

Driscoll, J. (2008). Psychological adaptation to pregnancy and postpartum. In K. R. Simpson & P. A. Creehan (Eds.). *AWHONN Perinatal nursing* (3rd ed., pp. 78–87). Philadelphia, PA: Lippincott Williams & Wilkins.

James, D. (2008). Postpartum care. In K. R. Simpson & P. A. Creehan (Eds.), *AWHONN Perinatal nursing* (3rd ed., pp. 473–526). Philadelphia, PA: Lippincott Williams & Wilkins.

Johnson & Johnson. (1996). *"Am I Blue?" Compendium of postpartum care.* Skillman, NJ: Johnson & Johnson Consumer Products.

London, M., Ladewig, P., Ball, J., Bindler, R., & Cowen, K. (2010). *Maternal & child nursing care* (3rd ed.). New York, NY: Pearson.

North American Nursing Diagnosis Association. (2009). *Nursing diagnoses classification*. North American Nursing Diagnosis Association (NANDA). Ames, IA: Wiley Publishing.

Riordan, J., & Wambach, K. (2010). *Breastfeeding and human lactation* (4th ed.). Sudbury, MA: Jones & Bartlett.

Sleutel, M. R. (2003). Intrapartum nursing: Integrating Rubin's framework with social support theory. *Journal of Obstetric, Gynecologic, & Neonatal Nursing, 32,* 76–82. doi: 10.1177/0884217502239803

Walker, M. (2007). International breastfeeding initiatives and their relevance to the current state of breastfeeding in the United States. *Journal of Nurse-Midwifery & Women's Health, 52*(6), 549–555.

RESOURCES

Moore, E., Anderson, G., & Bergman, N. (2007). Early skin-to-skin contact for mothers and their healthy infants. *Cochrane Database of Systematic Reviews.*

Poggi, S. (2007). Postpartum hemorrhage and the abnormal puerperium. In A. H. DeCherney, L. Nathan, T. M. Goodwin, & N. Laufer (Eds.), *Current obstetric & gynecologic: Diagnosis & treatment* (10th ed., pp. 477–497). New York, NY: Lange Medical Books/McGraw-Hill.

Uterine massage for preventing postpartum hemorrhage. *Cochrane Database of Systemic Reviews* (3).

Wilson, B., Shannon, M., & Shields, K. (2010). *Nurse's drug guide 2010.* Upper Saddle River, NJ: Pearson Education.

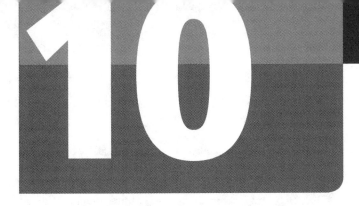

POSTPARTUM COMPLICATIONS

Carol J. Green

POSTPARTUM HEMORRHAGE

Postpartum bleeding is a significant cause of maternal mortality and morbidity affecting 4–6% of births (Francois & Foley, 2007). Hemorrhage following birth is defined as bleeding that exceeds 500 ml for a vaginal birth or 1,000 ml for a cesarean birth. *Primary* (or early) *postpartum hemorrhage* occurs within the first 24 hours following birth. *Secondary* (or late) *postpartum hemorrhage* occurs from 24 hours to 6 weeks after birth (ACOG, 2006). Blood loss is estimated at birth by comparing the admission hematocrit (Hct) level with that obtained on the first postpartum day. A 10% drop in Hct suggests hemorrhage.

▮ Key Nursing Activities

- Recognize risk factors for postpartum hemorrhage.
- Recognize early signs of postpartum hemorrhage (boggy fundus, infection, etc.).
- Collect data to determine the cause of bleeding.
- Institute measures to prevent bleeding.
- Initiate early treatment for bleeding.
- Provide emotional support and information.
- Teach strategies to minimize bleeding when the woman returns home following birth.

▮ Etiologies and Risk Factors

The most frequent cause of postpartum hemorrhage is uterine atony. The uterus must remain contracted after birth to control bleeding from the placental attachment site. If the uterus relaxes, bleeding will occur. Factors that prevent uterine contraction and retraction include:

- Overdistention due to polyhydramnios, multifetal pregnancy, large-for-gestational-age infant, fetal or uterine structural abnormality.

- Poor contractility related to prolonged labor, oxytocin inducted/augmented labor, medications (e.g., magnesium, general anesthesia, nonsteroidal anti-inflammatory drugs), endometritis, chorioamnionitis.
- Retained tissues including retained placental fragments, placenta previa, placenta accrete, and retained blood.
- Other causes of postpartum hemorrhage such as lacerations, incisions, trauma, hematomas, uterine rupture, uterine inversion, subinvolution, blood coagulation and/or platelet defects/problems, fetal death, mediolateral episiotomy, history of postpartum hemorrhage, uterine infection, use of forceps, or intravaginal manipulation.

Signs and Symptoms

Subjective. Thirst, lightheadedness, feeling faint, fatigue, anxiety.

Objective. Increased capillary refill time longer than 3 seconds; pale skin color; change in the level of consciousness; dry mucous membranes; boggy fundus that does not contract with massage; heavy, bright red bleeding; continuous bright red bleeding; large blood clots; normal vital signs at the onset; tachycardia; decreased blood pressure (BP); narrowing of pulse pressure; tachypnea; oliguria; signs of shock (profound hypotension; anuria; absence of bowel sounds; cold, clammy skin; and shallow, rapid respirations); and DIC (refer to the generic collaborative care plan, "Disseminated Intravascular Coagulation," beginning on p. 26 in Chapter 3).

Diagnostic Studies

- Complete blood count (CBC) with platelet count. Determines the degree of hemorrhage; initially, the Hgb does not accurately reflect degree of blood loss.
- Fibrinogen. Detects clotting abnormalities.
- Prothrombin time and activated partial thromboplastin time. Detect clotting abnormalities.
- D-dimers (fibrin degradation fragment). Helps rule out or detect hypercoagulability.
- Blood type and cross-match. Ensures availability of blood if needed.
- Clot observation test. Allows for quick determination of blood-clotting ability.
- Serum electrolytes. Detects electrolyte imbalances.
- Arterial blood gases. Assesses for oxygenation in presence of shock.
- Ultrasonography. May establish the presence of retained placenta.

▮ Medical Management

- Uterine compression and/or massage. Expresses clots from the uterus and facilitates uterine contraction and retraction.
- Indwelling urinary catheter if needed. Prevents distended urinary bladder and facilitates measurement of output.
- Intravenous fluid resuscitation (e.g., crystalloids). Supports circulating volume until bleeding is stopped.

- Blood replacement (e.g., packed RBCs; platelets; fresh, frozen plasma) if blood loss is greater than 2,000 ml or patient experiencing shock symptoms. Restores circulating volume and oxygen-carrying capacity (Smith & Brennan, 2009).
- Pitocin (oxytocin) 10–40 U in 1,000 ml lactated Ringer's solution or normal saline or oxytocin 10 U intramuscularly (IM). Stimulates uterine contraction.
- Ergonovine or methylergonovine (Methergine) 0.2 mg IM, every 2–4 hours. Stimulates uterine contractions (contraindicated in women with BP elevation). Methylergonovine may be given orally after initial hemorrhage is controlled.
- Carboprost tromethamine (Hemabate [United States]/ Prostin 15/M [Canada]), IM. Contains 15-methyl prostaglandin F_2 alpha, which stimulates uterine contraction; may also be given directly into the myometrium to control postpartum hemorrhage.
- Misoprostol (Cytotec, PGE_1). Single dose 800–1,000 mcg given rectally to induce or augment uterine contractions.
- Manual examination of uterus. Detects retained placental fragments and the cause of the bleeding.
- Uterine packing.
- Surgical procedures (e.g., hysterectomy).

▌ Collaborative Problems

Potential Complications of Postpartum Hemorrhage

- Hypovolemic shock
- Disseminated intravascular coagulation

Note: This problem is combined with the nursing diagnosis, "Deficient Fluid Volume,[1]" in this care plan.

COLLABORATIVE (STANDARDIZED) CARE FOR ALL WOMEN WITH POSTPARTUM HEMORRHAGE

Perform a comprehensive assessment to identify individual needs for teaching, emotional support, and physical care.

▌ Nursing Diagnosis: DEFICIENT FLUID VOLUME[1]

Related Factors: excessive blood loss secondary to uterine atony, lacerations, incisions, coagulation defects, retained placental fragments, and hematomas.

See the generic collaborative care plan, "Hemorrhage," beginning on p. 28 in Chapter 3.

▌ Goals, Outcomes, and Evaluation Criteria

- Woman is oriented to person, place, and time.

- Woman has moist mucous membranes and elastic skin turgor.
- Woman is free from thirst.
- Woman's VSs are at or near baseline.
- Woman's capillary refill is less than 3 seconds.
- Woman has light yellow urine and amount consistent with diuresis and intake.
- CBC, Hgb, and Hct are consistent with the amount of blood lost during birth process.
- Uterus remains contracted or contracts readily with massage
- Lochia is small to moderate in amount and decreases as healing occurs.
- Coagulation studies are within normal limits.

▌ NIC Interventions[2]

Bleeding Reduction: Postpartum Uterus (4026)—Limitation of the amount of blood loss from the postpartum uterus.

Blood Products Administration (4030)—Administration of blood or blood products and monitoring of patient's response.

Fluid Management (4120)—Promotion of fluid balance and prevention of complications resulting from abnormal or undesired fluid levels.

Shock Management (4250)—Facilitation of the delivery of oxygen and nutrients to systemic tissue with removal of cellular waste products in a patient with severely altered tissue perfusion.

Hypovolemia Management (4180)—Expansion of intravascular fluid volume in a patient who is volume depleted.

▌ Nursing Activities and Rationales

Assessments

- Assess for risk factors upon admission to postpartum unit. Identifies women who are at risk for loss of fluid volume so that it can be incorporated into their plans of care.
- Perform a comprehensive postpartum assessment involving all the body systems. Establishes a baseline of woman's overall well-being or identifies problems that may be present, which is used for later comparison.
- Monitor BP. Changes in BP pattern often precede hypotension related to blood loss. Because of the body's compensatory mechanisms, as much as 1,000 ml of blood loss may occur before hypotension develops.
- Monitor temperature. Normal body temperature may be as high as 100.4°F (38.0°C) during the first 24 hours postpartum. Temperature increases with fluid volume loss.
- Monitor heart rate and respirations. Mild increases in heart rate and respirations may occur from the stress of birth; however, a consistently elevated heart rate is an indication of hypovolemia. Tachycardia and tachypnea may not occur until a large volume loss (greater than 1,000 ml) has occurred.
- Assess capillary refill time; mucous membranes for color and hydration; skin turgor; urine amount, color, and concentration; and the color of nail beds. Detects patterns or

trends that suggest that shock from blood loss is developing, which may include a drop in BP or change in BP pattern, tachycardia, tachypnea, thirst, restlessness, decreased urine output, etc.

- Assess type and amount of bleeding. Assess perineal pads and perineum every 10–15 minutes for the first hour or until stable, every 30 minute for 2nd hour or after 1 hour of being stable. After two 30-minute stable checks, assess every 4 hours for 24 hours, then every 8 hours until discharge or condition changes. This provides an estimate of blood loss and helps with identification of source or cause of bleeding. Hourly pad saturation or visual leakage of bright blood from the vagina is an indication of hemorrhage.
- Assess uterine fundus for firmness and placement. Use the same schedule as previous nursing activity, assessing for bleeding. Determines if uterus is relaxed or boggy. Uterine contraction is necessary to control bleeding. Uterine displacement occurs from filling with blood and/or clots or bladder distention.
- Assess for both fluid volume deficit and fluid volume excess during treatment for the deficit. Fluid volume excess can occur from fluid replacement, causing fluid volume overload.

Independent Nursing Actions

- Apply an ice pack to fundus, hematoma, or laceration. Ice produces localized vasoconstriction, which decreases blood flow and helps control bleeding.
- Massage relaxed or boggy uterus and express blood and clots, if present. Massaging the uterus stimulates contraction, which reduces bleeding. Uterine relaxation can occur when the uterus is excessively massaged. Once it is firm, discontinue uterine massage for several minutes. Retained clots prevent the uterus from contracting fully.
- Monitor and report laboratory findings (e.g., CBC, Hgb, Hct, serum electrolytes, coagulation studies) to care provider. Medical care decisions are based on these data.
- Promote an empty bladder through voiding or catheterization. A distended bladder can displace the uterus to the side, predisposing to uterine atony and making uterine massage difficult.
- Measure and record intake and output. Detects changes that indicate hypovolemia. Fluid intake should normally approximate output. Blood is shunted away from the kidneys during periods of hypovolemia, which reduces urinary output. Decreased output (less than 30 ml/hr) is an indication of hypovolemia and/or inadequate fluid volume replacement.
- Promote bedrest if heavy bleeding is occurring, limit activity, and elevate legs 20–30 degrees. Decreases metabolic demands on the body, increases venous blood return to the heart, protects blood flow to vital organs, and maintains the woman's safety.

- Remain with the woman experiencing heavy bleeding until she is stable. Shock is an emergency situation that can develop rapidly from hemorrhage. Heavy bleeding may be an indication of hemorrhage.
- Encourage newborn contact with mother and promote breastfeeding within the first 2 hours. Contact immediately after birth with the newborn who makes sucking sounds on his or her fists, cries, or breastfeeds causes the release of oxytocin in the mother's body, helping the uterus to contract and remain contracted during this time of high risk for hemorrhage.

Collaborative Activities

- Administer oxygen as ordered and/or mechanical ventilation if necessary. Oxygen and/or mechanical ventilation may be necessary if blood loss is so excessive that it prevents adequate tissue perfusion to major organs.
- Maintain patent IV access site with a large-bore intravenous catheter until patient is stable. Fluids will need to be rapidly infused if hypovolemic shock occurs. Packed RBCs are highly viscous and require a 16–18 gauge catheter for rapid infusion.
- Administer fluid and electrolytes as ordered. Helps to reestablish fluid balance and prevent hypovolemic shock, dehydration, and electrolyte imbalances. Crystalloid fluid replacement maintains intravascular volume and prevents hypovolemia.
- Administer packed RBCs or other blood products as prescribed. Prevents hypovolemic shock by replacing blood volume or blood components and oxygen-carrying capacity.
- Administer medications (oxytocin, methylergonovine maleate) as prescribed and adhere to nursing implications for the drug; monitor for the desired action and any side effects. Oxytoxics increase contractility of the uterus and decrease or stop hemorrhage when uterine atony is the causative factor. Monitor BP prior to the administration of methylergonovine; it is contraindicated if BP is elevated.

Patient/Family Teaching

- Teach the woman how to palpate the fundus, where it should be located, and the need for it to remain contracted. Helps the woman understand how to monitor her own uterus so that the nurse can be summoned if she feels her uterus becoming boggy or soft.
- Teach the woman about the type and amount of lochia. Ensures that the woman will recognize excessive bleeding and report it immediately whether she is in the birthing unit or at home.
- Teach the woman to call for assistance when ambulating. Weakness, hypotension, lightheadedness, and fatigue may occur secondary to blood loss, placing the woman at increased risk for falls.

INDIVIDUALIZED (NURSING DIAGNOSIS) CARE PLANS

This section includes care plans that were developed to address unique patient needs.

Nursing Diagnosis: FEAR[1]

Related Factors: threat to physical well-being (because of hemorrhage), deficient knowledge of treatment measures for hemorrhage, and the powerlessness experienced in the hospital environment. See the generic NDCPs, "Anxiety[1]" and "Fear,[1]" beginning on pp. 10 and 15 in Chapter 2.

Nursing Activities and Rationales
Assessments

- Assess reaction to postpartum hemorrhage and correct any misconceptions. Helps establish a baseline for care planning. Education helps corrects misconceptions and often reduces fear and anxiety about the unknown.
- Assess whether the woman is capable of following directions. Blood loss interferes with the woman's ability to think clearly, which is frightening to the woman. Fear can alter the woman's ability to comprehend or follow directions accurately.
- Assess the woman's ability to participate in activities of daily living. Fear may impede the woman's ability to meet her own needs or focus on what needs to be done.

Independent Nursing Actions

- Support the woman's use of healthy defense mechanisms. Use of healthy defense mechanisms can help the woman and family cope with the situation.

Collaborative Activities

- Administer prescribed medications and monitor for desired and adverse effects. Antianxiety agents may be prescribed to promote relaxation and comfort if the woman's fear is excessive or interferes with her ability to cope with her situation. If they do not produce desired effects, alternative interventions should be considered.

Nursing Diagnosis: PAIN[1]

Related Factors: uterine contractions, uterine massage, and expression of clots, distention from blood between uterine wall and placenta, episiotomy, trauma, and surgical interventions. See the generic NDCP, "Pain,[1]" beginning on p. 18, Chapter 2.

Nursing Activities and Rationales
Assessments

- Observe for verbal and nonverbal cues of discomfort, including facial grimacing, movement, and guarding.

Allows the nurse to detect pain even when the woman is not verbally complaining of pain or discomfort.
- Assess family support systems. Culture and family have a significant impact on how an individual perceives and deals with pain. The pain experience may be greater in the absence of support systems.

Collaborative Activities

- Select and administer pain medication as prescribed after assessing the woman's health status. Evaluate the effectiveness of the medication and any adverse effects. More than one type of analgesic may be prescribed. The nurse and patient will decide which medication is best suited for the type of pain the woman is experiencing.

Patient/Family Teaching

- Stress the importance to the woman of verbalizing when she has pain and requesting interventions as necessary. Supports active participation in obtaining pain relief and allows for better pain control.
- Teach the woman to request pain medication before the pain is severe and to allow time for her particular type of pain medication to become effective. Taking the medication before the pain is severe allows for more effective pain control. IV medications work almost immediately, IM injections require 20–30 minutes, and oral medications may take 30–45 minutes to become effective.

Nursing Diagnosis: RISK FOR IMPAIRED PARENT–INFANT/CHILD ATTACHMENT[1]

Related Factors: interruption of the bonding process secondary to maternal hemorrhage; lack of early parent–infant contact because of the mother's fatigue from postpartum hemorrhage, or from medical interventions associated with postpartum hemorrhage. See the generic NDCP, "Risk for Impaired Parent–Infant/Child Attachment,[1]" beginning on p. 19 in Chapter 2.

Nursing Activities and Rationales
Assessment

- Assess prenatal record to see if mother sought care early in the pregnancy, attended scheduled visits, attended education sessions, and gained weight according to the expected weight gain pattern. Determines the presence of risk factors that may affect the parent–infant/child bonding experience.
- Note whether the mother calls her newborn by name, asks questions regarding the newborn's condition and location. Indicates the mother's interest in the infant and bonding with her infant.

- Assess mother's bonding with her newborn multiple times once they are reunited; keep in mind the fatigue factor after hemorrhage. Determines if interventions are needed to help the mother attach to her infant.
- Assess whether the mother is attending to the newborn's cues. Indicates mother–infant bonding or lack of bonding if cues are ignored.

Independent Nursing Actions

- Encourage and promote opportunities for the mother to hold her newborn, preferably on her chest skin to skin between the breasts, allowing the newborn to touch the breast with his/her hands. Touch helps establish the bond between mother and infant.
- If the mother is able, encourage breastfeeding for the mother who desires to breastfeed. Helps to establish the bond between mother and infant.
- Reunite mother, infant, and family as soon as she is stable. Early contact fosters mother–infant bonding.

▌ Nursing Diagnosis: DEFICIENT KNOWLEDGE[1]

Related Factors: lack of previous experience with postpartum hemorrhage, self-care, and prescribed medications. Also see the generic NDCP, "Deficient Knowledge,[1]" beginning on p. 13 in Chapter 2.

▌ *Nursing Activities and Rationales*

Assessments

- Assess the woman's knowledge of medication's desired effects and side effects that need to be reported. Determines the woman's knowledge deficits so that teaching plan can be developed.

Independent Nursing Actions

- Encourage frequent rest periods and adequate nighttime sleep. Loss of blood produces fatigue. The woman will need assistance from her partner/family with care of her infant to allow adequate time for sleep and rest while healing occurs.
- Encourage intake of well-balanced diet and at least 64 ounces of fluid each day. Prevents dehydration and facilitates healing.

Patient/Family Teaching

- Teach medication's desired effects, dosage and schedule, and side effects that need to be reported. Informed women are more likely to follow prescribed treatment regimens and recognize and report side effects of medications.
- Teach the woman the signs of infection and the need for

reporting them as soon as noted. Postpartum hemorrhage places the woman at increased risk for infection. If the woman recognizes and reports the signs and symptoms of infection early, it ensures early treatment.

▌ *Other Nursing Diagnoses*

Also assess for the following nursing diagnoses, which are frequently present with this condition:

- Interrupted Breastfeeding[1] related to mother's health state during the postpartum hemorrhage and the fatigue afterward (as a result of anemia), separation from the newborn in the first few hours after birth, and separation from the newborn if rehospitalized with a postpartum hemorrhage.
- Interrupted Family Processes[1] related to change in family roles, inability to assume usual role, and prolonged recovery period.

POSTPARTUM INFECTION

Postpartum infection, defined as fever of 100.4°F (38°C) or greater, includes any infection of the genital canal occurring after the first 24 hours but within 28 days following childbirth, induced abortion, or miscarriage (Ricci, 2009). Most infections occur within 2 weeks following birth but can occur any time until the reproductive organs return to their nonpregnant state, which is 42 days (Aronoff & Zuber, 2008). Postpartum infections are a major source of maternal morbidity and mortality in the world. Endometritis, wound infections, urinary tract infections, mastitis (see "Mastitis," beginning on p. 356 in this chapter), respiratory tract infections, and pelvic cellulitis (parametritis) are examples of postpartum infections.

Note: These care plans are for the woman who has an actual infection. For preventive measures, refer to the generic NDCP, "Risk for Infection,[1]" beginning on p. 21 in Chapter 2 and the generic collaborative care plan, "Potential Complication: Infection," beginning on p. 29 in Chapter 3.

▌ *Key Nursing Activities*

- Assess for risk factors for infection.
- Administer prescribed antibiotics.
- Monitor effectiveness of collaborative management.
- Offer emotional support.

▌ *Etiologies and Risk Factors*

- Streptococcal and anaerobic organisms are the most common infecting pathogens.
- *Staphylococcus aureus* and gonococci are less common but are serious when they occur.
- Concurrent conditions include immunosuppression, diabetes mellitus, malnutrition, anemia, alcoholism, drug dependency, preexisting infection or vaginal infection at time of delivery, or prolonged use of an indwelling urinary catheter.

- Intrapartal risk factors include cesarean or operative delivery, prolonged or difficult labor, prolonged rupture of membranes, internal maternal or fetal monitoring, retained placental fragments, multiple invasive procedures, and postpartum hemorrhage.
- Low socioeconomic status.

Signs and Symptoms

Symptoms vary with the type and location of infection and include subjective and objective symptoms as described next.

Subjective. Anorexia, nausea, fatigue, chills, abdominal tenderness, dysuria, urinary urgency, weakness, and pain.

Objective. Fever (low grade; less than 101.4°F [38.5°C]) is indicative of wound or localized infection; fever greater than 102°F (38.9°C) is indicative of systemic infection; tachycardia; lethargy; foul-smelling lochia; localized erythema; swelling; warmth; tenderness; purulent drainage; wound separation; urinary frequency; changes in urinary color, clarity, and odor; breast swelling; axillary adenopathy.

Diagnostic Studies

- White blood cell count (leukocytosis). WBCs can range from 5,000/mm to 25,000/mm during the postpartum period. The WBC count must be evaluated in relationship to time, previous values, and other signs and symptoms of infection. An increase in WBCs greater than 30% in a 6-hour period is indicative of an infection.
- C-reactive protein. Acute phase protein that denotes active inflammation or infection.
- Cultures (urine, wound, blood, lochia, cervix, uterus). Identifies the causative organism.
- Urinalysis. Determines if the urine is a causative factor for infection.
- Ultrasonography. Confirms the presence of abscess formation or retained placenta.

Medical Management

Endometritis

Endometritis is the most common postpartum infection. Medical management for endometritis includes:

- IV broad-spectrum antibiotics (aminoglycoside, cephalosporin, penicillin, clindamycin)
- Maintenance or restoration of hydration
- Pain control
- Possible incision and drainage of abscess

Wound Infection

- Broad-spectrum antibiotics
- Wound drainage and/or debridement
- Wound cleaning and dressing care
- Possible incision and drainage for abscess

Urinary Tract Infection

- Antibiotics (ciprofloxacin, levofloxacin, trimethoprim-sulfamethoxazole, nitrofurantoin)
- Pain control (urinary analgesics)
- Restoration and maintenance of fluid hydration

Mastitis

See "Mastitis," beginning on p. 356 in this chapter.

- Antibiotic therapy (cephalexin, clindamycin, dicloxacillin)
- Localized heat or cold
- Restoration and maintenance of hydration
- Pain control
- Breast pumping or continued breastfeeding

Collaborative Problems

Potential Complications of Postpartum Infection

- Abscess formation
- Sepsis
- Septic shock

COLLABORATIVE (STANDARDIZED) CARE FOR ALL WOMEN WITH POSTPARTUM INFECTION

Perform a comprehensive assessment to identify individual needs for teaching, emotional support, and physical care.

Potential Complications of Postpartum Infection: ABSCESS FORMATION, SEPSIS, AND SEPTIC SHOCK

See the generic NDCP, "Risk for Infection,[1]" beginning on p. 21 in Chapter 2; the generic collaborative care plan, "Infection," beginning on p. 29 in Chapter 3, and the topics "Vaginal Infections" and "Urinary Tract Infection," beginning on pp. 193 and 195, respectively, in Chapter 6.

Focus Assessments

- Assess for palpable mass at suspected abscess site (may be confirmed by ultrasound). Detects presence of abscess, which may require surgical drainage.
- Monitor for manifestations that warn of sepsis. Fever greater than 102°F (38.9°C), increased lethargy, elevated heart rate and respirations, change in blood pressure pattern or hypotension, or changes in mentation are manifestations of sepsis, which is a potential complication

of infection. Sepsis can lead to septic shock, which is an emergency situation that requires rapid identification and implementation of emergency interventions, fluid volume support, and antibiotic therapy to prevent death.

Preventive Nursing Activities

- Promote good nutrition with foods from all of the food groups following birth. The intake of adequate protein and calories is essential for tissue healing and repair.
- Teach the need to increase fluid intake to 3,000 ml/day. Maintains hydration, prevents dehydration, and helps prevent sepsis.
- Teach and provide perineal hygiene immediately in the postpartum period. Decreases the risk for entrance of pathogenic organisms from incisions, episiotomy, lacerations, or abrasions.
- Teach woman to use a perineum bottle to clean her perineum after each elimination. Demonstrate how to change pads from front to back after elimination. Reduces the risk of fecal contamination of episiotomy or lacerations.
- Teach to use the sitz bath if ordered. Localized heat increases blood flow to the area, which aids in healing and enhances comfort.

INDIVIDUALIZED (NURSING DIAGNOSIS) CARE PLANS

The care plans in this section were developed to address unique patient needs.

Nursing Diagnosis: RISK FOR IMPAIRED PARENT–INFANT/CHILD ATTACHMENT[1]

Related Factors: mother's fatigue from postpartum infection. See the generic NDCP, "Risk for Impaired Parent–Infant/Child Attachment,[1]" beginning on p. 19 in Chapter 2.

Nursing Activities and Rationales

Assessments

- Assess mother's fatigue related to infection. The woman with an active infection who has a fever and is fatigued may be unable to interact with her infant. This can delay the development of initial positive feelings toward the newborn. If identified early, corrective measures can be implemented.
- Assess for indications of bonding multiple times once the mother and infant are reunited, keeping in mind that the mother has an active infection. Determines whether interventions are needed to facilitate mother–infant bonding.

Independent Nursing Actions

- Encourage and promote an opportunity for the mother to hold her newborn preferably when the mother feels the least fatigued. Touch helps establish the bond between mother and infant.
- Encourage breastfeeding for the mother who desires to breastfeed. Helps to establish the bond between mother and infant.
- Reunite mother, infant, and family as soon as she is stable if infectious condition does not require isolation. Early contact fosters mother–infant bonding.
- Suggest doula care if appropriate and available. May facilitate maternal–infant bonding when the woman recovers from infection and is able to fully assume her role as mother.

Nursing Diagnosis: IMBALANCED NUTRITION: LESS THAN BODY REQUIREMENTS[1]

Related Factors: high metabolic demand, anorexia, nausea/vomiting secondary to localized or systemic infection; and possibly related to nothing by mouth status. Refer to the NDCP, "Imbalanced Nutrition: Less Than Body Requirements,[1]" beginning on p. 323 in "Postpartum Period: First Home Visit" in Chapter 9.

Goals, Outcomes, and Evaluation Criteria

- Woman tolerates prescribed diet.
- Woman has moist oral mucous membranes, elastic skin turgor, body mass, and weight is within normal limits.
- Laboratory values (transferrin, albumin, electrolytes) are within normal limits.
- Woman reports adequate energy levels.
- Signs of healing are present (e.g., normal temperature, decreased redness of incision).
- Woman denies anorexia or nausea.

NIC Intervention[2]

Fluid Monitoring (4130)—Collection and analysis of patient data to regulate fluid balance.

Nursing Activities and Rationales

Assessments

- Assess for nausea before bringing in the food tray. If the woman is already nauseated, holding the tray until the nausea passes or antiemetic medication has had an opportunity to decrease the nausea may prevent vomiting.
- Monitor laboratory values (transferrin, albumin, electrolytes). Detects negative nitrogen balance, electrolyte

balance, etc., which reflect nutritional status and directs corrective action.

- Monitor skin turgor, oral mucous membranes for moisture and color, and urinary output and concentration. Detects adequacy of hydration. Decreased intake secondary to nausea, along with elevated temperature, predispose to fluid deficit.
- Monitor dietary intake at all meals and record as percentage eaten, or milliliters if on liquids only. Determines adequacy of nutritional content and calories to support healing.
- Assess how breastfeeding is progressing and if the woman is providing an adequate supply of human milk. Inadequate maternal nutrition can affect milk supply and result in poor nutrition of the infant. Initially, underfed babies cry more and sleep less. However, babies who are chronically undernourished cry less, sleep more, and fail to gain weight.

Independent Nursing Actions

- When possible, encourage the family to bring foods the woman requests or likes. Promotes intake of nutrients. A woman on a regular diet may enjoy food from home or her favorite restaurant while she is recovering from an infection. Also, food has cultural meaning for families and being able to provide nourishment may be significant for them.

Collaborative Activities

- Consult with dietitian to establish protein requirements. Assists with planning for protein replacement. Protein deficiency may be secondary to infection; protein intake may be insufficient because of malaise and anorexia; protein is required for healing.

Patient/Family Teaching

- Teach the woman/family the relationship between good nutrition, wound healing, treating infection, energy, and overall well-being. Active participation by the family is important because the woman will be somewhat dependent until her infection has resolved and she is able to resume self-care and care of her infant. Involvement and information also help to ensure compliance with treatment measures.

▌ Nursing Diagnosis: FEAR[1]

Related Factors: threat to well-being of the woman and infant secondary to the presence of an infection. See the generic NDCP, "Fear,[1]" beginning on p. 15 in Chapter 2.

▌ *Nursing Activities and Rationales*

Assessment

- Assess reaction to presence of infection and correct misconceptions. Establishes a baseline for care planning.

Correcting misconceptions and supplying factual information may reduce fear and anxiety.

▌ Nursing Diagnosis: PAIN[1]

Related Factors: local inflammatory response in tissues. See the generic NDCP, "Pain,[1]" beginning on p. 18 in Chapter 2.

▌ *Nursing Activities and Rationales*

Independent Nursing Actions

- Provide basic comfort measures, such as positioning, maintaining clean and dry linens and gowns, ice packs, cool cloths to the forehead, lip balm or ointment for dry lips, brushing the teeth or rinsing the mouth, or ice chips. Basic comfort measures often provide pain relief without the use of medications. If basic needs are being met, the woman can focus on using relaxation techniques, guided imagery, visualization, and other nonpharmacologic techniques that may also help provide comfort.

▌ *Other Nursing Diagnoses*

Also assess for the following nursing diagnoses, which are frequently present with this condition:

- Activity Intolerance[1] related to fatigue secondary to postpartum infection.
- Risk for Interrupted Family Processes[1] related to change in family roles, inability to assume usual role, or prolonged recovery secondary to postpartum infection.
- Interrupted Family Processes[1] related to client's inability to assume family role secondary to prolonged recovery from infection.
- Interrupted Breastfeeding[1] related to maternal illness.

THROMBOEMBOLIC DISEASE

Thromboembolic disease is a potentially serious complication of the postpartum period, but it can occur in any trimester of pregnancy and is a leading cause of maternal mortality. A *thrombus* is a clot or clots in a blood vessel, caused by inflammation (thrombophlebitis and phlebothrombosis) or partial obstruction. Thrombi can involve *superficial* (the superficial saphenous venous system) or *deep* veins. Pregnancy places a woman at four times the risk for venous thrombosis as nonpregnant women, which most commonly arise in the deep veins of the lower extremities. That risk increases twentyfold during the postpartum period and continues as late as 6 weeks following birth (Brown & Hiett, 2010). Most women develop thromboembolism within the first 2 postpartum weeks. Deep vein thrombosis (DVT) occurs in about 1 in 5,000 postpartum women (Kamaya, Kyung, Benedetti, Chang, & Desser, 2009).

A thrombus may remain asymptomatic but has the potential to dislodge and migrate to the lungs, causing pulmonary embolism and infarction. About 20% of women with DVT develop life-threatening pulmonary embolism (James, Jamison, Brancazio, & Myers, 2006).

Key Nursing Activities

- Early detection and management of venous thrombophlebitis
- Prevention, early detection, and management of DVT
- Pain management
- Maintenance of peripheral tissue integrity

Etiologies and Risk Factors

The following three factors primarily influence the formation of thrombus:

1. Stasis or turbulence of blood flow
2. Endothelial injury
3. Physiologic hypercoagulability related to pregnancy

Antepartum and postpartum thrombus formation is most often caused by venous stasis and hypercoagulation. Risk factors include:

- Pregnancy-related factors. Cesarean birth, normal increases in blood-clotting factors during the postpartum period, progesterone-induced distensibility of veins of the lower extremities during pregnancy, pressure from the fetal head during delivery, multiparity, prolonged bed rest during pregnancy, advanced maternal age, use of oral contraceptives prior to pregnancy.
- Preexisting conditions. Obesity, cardiac disease, systemic lupus erythematosus, sickle cell disease, previous DVT, tobacco use, multiple gestations.

Signs and Symptoms

Subjective. Superficial venous thrombosis: Pain and tenderness in lower extremity. DVT: Unilateral leg pain and calf tenderness (not all women experience pain); positive Homans' sign (pain in calf upon dorsiflexion), although this is not considered a definitive diagnostic sign. Pulmonary embolism: Pleuritic chest pain, apprehension.

Objective. Superficial venous thrombosis: Warmth, redness, and hardness of a vein over the site of the thrombosis. DVT: Fever (up to 40.5°C or 100°F), palpable cord, localized area of extremity hot to touch, pallor and/or swelling of the lower extremity, difference in leg circumference, tachycardia, and hypotension are sometimes present; however, a large clot can be present with only a few symptoms. Pulmonary embolism: Tachycardia, tachypnea, dyspnea, fever, hemoptysis, cyanosis, hypotension, and cardiovascular collapse.

Diagnostic Studies

- Physical examination. May not be a sensitive indicator in the pregnant woman because many of the symptoms occur with pregnancy, e.g., tachycardia, extremity swelling, dyspnea.
- Doppler flow studies with compression ultrasonography. Noninvasive study that shows areas of diminished blood flow or obstruction.
- Impedance plethysmograph. Noninvasive test that detects blood clots in the legs by measuring changes in resistance (impedance) to venous blood flow via electrical monitoring equipment. Repeated testing is required because false negative and positive results are not uncommon.
- Phlebography. Highly sensitive invasive diagnostic study for DVT in which the extent and location of clots are identified under fluoroscopy. Primarily replaced by Doppler ultrasonography but remains the gold standard for diagnosis when noninvasive studies fail to diagnose disease.
- Contrast venography. Invasive diagnostic study that requires use of contrast media that can cause chemical phlebitis; shows areas of diminished flow or obstruction.
- D-dimer. Degradation product of fibrin; low levels help rule out venous thromboembolism.
- Thrombophilia screening. Screens for inherited homeostasis disorders that predispose the woman to clotting events (Brown & Hiett, 2010).
- Perfusion/ventilation scan. Noninvasive study to diagnose pulmonary embolism.

Medical Management

Prevention of venous disorders is the best management strategy.

Superficial Vein Thrombosis

- Nonsteroidal anti-inflammatory agents (for analgesia)
- Rest and elevation of affected leg
- Elastic compression stockings (see "DVT," next list)
- Local application of heat

DVT

- Baseline CBC count, platelet count, prothrombin time, activated partial thromboplastin time, and urinalysis prior to initiation of anticoagulation therapy.
- Anticoagulation therapy. IV heparin initially, followed by subcutaneous heparin, and oral warfarin therapy prior to discharge.
- Serial activated partial thromboplastin time 4 hours after the heparin loading dose and every 4 hours thereafter until stable therapeutic state has been achieved (2.0–3.0 times the control), then daily until IV heparin is discontinued.
- Fibrinolytic agents (for selected patients).
- Bed rest with elevation of the affected leg.
- Antibiotics, if fever persists or septic thrombophlebitis is suspected.
- Analgesic medications for discomfort.
- Elastic stockings correctly fitted and designed so that the pressure gradient decreases from the ankle to thigh without a constricting garter at the top or sequential compression device. Used after symptoms decrease.

■ *Collaborative Problem*

Potential Complication of Thrombophlebitis

- Pulmonary embolism

COLLABORATIVE (STANDARDIZED) CARE FOR ALL WOMEN WITH THROMBOEMBOLIC DISEASE

Perform a comprehensive assessment to identify individual needs for teaching, emotional support, and physical care.

Potential Complication of Thrombophlebitis: PULMONARY EMBOLISM

Focus Assessments

- Assess for signs and symptoms of thrombophlebitis. The best way to prevent pulmonary embolus is to identify and treat thrombophlebitis. If thrombophlebitis occurs, early treatment (including bed rest) may prevent dislodging of the thrombus into the circulation.
- Assess respiratory system (e.g., dyspnea, tachypnea, pleuritic pain, cough, hemoptysis, and rales). These are symptoms of pulmonary embolism (occlusion or infarction of the pulmonary circulation).
- Assess cardiac system (e.g., tachycardia, hypotension). Obstruction of pulmonary blood flow causes vasoconstriction, pulmonary hypoxia, and pulmonary edema. The heart responds by beating faster in an attempt to compensate for the loss of oxygen, ultimately leading to decreased cardiac output.
- Assess integument (e.g., for peripheral or central cyanosis). Peripheral vasoconstriction and central cyanosis occur in response to the body's compensatory response to hypoxia. Blood is shunted away from nonvital to vital organs such as the brain and heart.
- Assess for fever greater than 98.6°F (37°C). Thrombi produce ischemia and subsequent infarction. The death of tissue produces an inflammatory response, leading to elevated WBC counts and fever.
- Review or assist with diagnostic studies, including perfusion/ventilation scans; CBC; electrolytes, enzymes, and arterial blood gas; chest radiograph; electrocardiogram; and pulmonary angiogram. Identifies changes in pulmonary circulation, hypoxemia, pulmonary infiltrates, infarcted or consolidated areas, pleural effusion, electrocardiogram changes, other changes in the pulmonary vascular system, electrolyte imbalances, and leukocytosis.
- Assess mental status (anxiety, syncope). May result from systemic hypotension and/or hypoxia, as well as from the unexpected and uncomfortable symptoms.

Preventive Nursing Activities

- Implement measures to prevent thrombophlebitis. The best way to prevent pulmonary embolus is to identify and treat thrombophlebitis.
- Encourage fluid intake. Increases vascular volume, decreases likelihood of venous stasis, and helps prevent thrombophlebitis. If thrombophlebitis occurs, increased fluid helps prevent clot extension.
- Encourage early ambulation after delivery/cesarean section and develop a walking schedule. Promotes peripheral circulation, decreasing the likelihood of thrombophlebitis, which decreases the risk for pulmonary emboli.
- Encourage use of pneumatic stockings while on bed rest. Promotes venous return from the legs, decreasing stasis-induced thrombophlebitis.
- Encourage active and passive range of motion exercises while on bed rest. Promotes venous return from the legs, decreasing stasis-induced thrombophlebitis.
- Teach the need to avoid applying pressure under the knees (e.g., propping pillows under knees). Pressure interferes with venous return from the legs, creating stasis.
- Ensure proper application and fit of elastic stockings. Stockings that are too tight can actually impede circulation. Stockings that are too loose are not effective.
- Instruct the woman to avoid crossing her legs. It interferes with venous return from the legs, increasing the risk for thrombophlebitis.
- Instruct to make frequent position changes when sitting or lying for prolonged periods. Prevents venous stasis.
- Teach the woman to elevate her legs whenever possible when sitting. Gravity promotes venous return from the legs.
- Teach to avoid garters and knee-high stockings. These physically constrict veins, causing stasis and contributing to thrombophlebitis.
- Discuss the risk of oral contraceptive use related to thrombophlebitis. Estrogen in large doses and in women over the age of 35 is associated with thromboembolic disorders. Even low-dose estrogen is considered a risk factor. Women who have already had a thromboembolic disorder might be advised to consider another form of contraception.

Nursing Diagnosis: INEFFECTIVE TISSUE PERFUSION (PERIPHERAL)[1]

Related Factors: localized venous stasis, obstruction, inflammation, and edema of thrombophlebitis.

▌ Goals, Outcomes, and Evaluation Criteria

- Vital signs remain within normal limits or return to baseline.
- Woman displays adequate circulation compared to unaffected extremity (e.g., normal skin tone for woman, bilaterally equal pulses, bilaterally equal circumferences, intact sensation).

▌ NIC Interventions[2]

Bed Rest Care (0740)—Promotion of comfort and safety and prevention of complications for a patient unable to get out of bed.

Circulatory Care: Venous Insufficiency (4066)—Promotion of venous circulation.

Circulatory Precautions (4070)—Protection of a localized area with limited perfusion.

Positioning (0840)—Deliberate placement of the patient or a body part to promote physiologic and/or psychologic well-being.

Skin Surveillance (3590)—Collection and analysis of patient data to maintain skin and mucous membrane integrity.

▌ Nursing Activities and Rationales

Assessments

- Monitor VSs and be alert for fever. Low-grade and persistent fever indicates inflammation. Fever may indicate septic thrombophlebitis. Septic thrombophlebitis is a serious complication of pyogenic pelvic inflammation.
- Inspect and palpate both thighs and calves for size, temperature, color (pallor), pain, paralysis, paresthesia, and pulses. Provides baseline data for further comparison. Arterial spasm often accompanies venous occlusion. Pain, pallor, paralysis, paresthesia, and diminished or absent pulse indicates severe peripheral circulation dysfunction and requires immediate surgical intervention.
- Monitor serial activated partial thromboplastin time levels for therapeutic range in the woman receiving heparin. Activated partial thromboplastin time levels of 1.5–2.5 times the control value indicate adequate anticoagulation. Overdosing can result in hemorrhage, whereas underdosing will not provide therapeutic benefits.
- Monitor international normalized ratio in the woman receiving warfarin. The therapeutic international normalized ratio level (also known as prothrombin time and pro-time) for treatment of DVT is 2.0–3.0. Overdosing can result in bleeding, whereas underdosing will not provide therapeutic benefits.
- Monitor and report signs of bleeding (e.g., hematemesis, occult or overt blood in stools, hematuria, ecchymosis, excessive or prolonged bleeding from venipuncture sites, petechiae, increased flow of lochia [more than expected for postpartum date]). Signs of bleeding indicate possible overanticoagulation and may pose significant risk of life-threatening hemorrhage.

Independent Nursing Actions

- Maintain bed rest. Bed rest improves venous return from lower extremities because the heart does not have to work against gravity. It also decreases pressure on the peripheral venous system.
- Encourage the woman to change positions frequently while on bed rest. Promotes venous return and prevents stasis of blood in the extremities.
- Remind the woman to avoid placing her knees in a sharply flexed position. This causes pooling of blood in the legs, which increases the risk for thrombophlebitis.
- Elevate the affected extremity without compressing the popliteal area. Gravity provides improved venous return from lower extremities. Compression of the popliteal area can impede venous return, increasing the risk for thrombophlebitis.
- Apply moist heat packs to affected extremity (usually for superficial venous thrombosis). Moist heat helps relieve pain and promotes relaxation and vasodilation. Vasodilation aids in removal of debris from the inflamed area. Care must be taken when testing the temperature before application because the woman is at risk for thermal injury secondary to decreased sensation.
- Encourage fluid intake unless contraindicated. Blood viscosity is increased in states of dehydration. Increased blood viscosity contributes to thrombus formation. Contraindications include fluid restriction for congestive heart failure or renal failure.
- Provide well-fitting, thigh-high elastic stockings. Elastic stockings provide an increasing pressure gradient from ankle to thigh, improving venous return and promoting deep venous flow.

Collaborative Activities

- Administer antibiotics for persistent fever as ordered. Persistent low-grade fever occurs with DVT from inflammation but may also indicate septic thrombophlebitis. Septic thrombophlebitis requires treatment with antibiotic therapy.
- Administer anticoagulants as ordered. Anticoagulants (e.g., heparin, warfarin) prevent further thrombus formation by preventing the conversion of fibrinogen to fibrin, but do not break down existing clots. Administration of anticoagulants may help decrease the occurrence of an embolic event.
- Keep vitamin K and protamine sulfate readily available for injection. Vitamin K is the antagonist for warfarin and protamine sulfate is the antagonist for heparin. Both should be available for administration in the event of anticoagulant overdose or bleeding.

Patient/Family Teaching

- Instruct to report changes in pain and sensation immediately. Increasing pain and decreasing sensation or presence of paresthesia may indicate worsening tissue ischemia.
- Instruct to avoid rubbing the affected area. Rubbing can dislodge the clot, causing it to enter the general circulation and resulting in fatal pulmonary embolization.

Nursing Diagnosis: RISK FOR INEFFECTIVE THERAPEUTIC REGIMEN MANAGEMENT, FAMILY[1]

Related Factors: presence of risk factors such as heparin or warfarin use, lack of information about indications, adverse effects and interactions of medications, or lack of information/understanding about prescribed treatments.

Goals, Outcomes, and Evaluation Criteria

- Woman/family describes dosage, schedule, and adverse effects of prescribed medications.
- Woman/family verbalizes the importance of adhering to prescribed medication regimen.
- Woman/family verbalizes understanding of treatments, e.g., bed rest, compression stockings, heat applications.
- Woman remains free of adverse effects of the treatment regimen.

NIC Interventions[2]

Bleeding Precautions (4010)—Reduction of stimuli that may induce bleeding or hemorrhage in at-risk patients.
Medication Management (2380)—Facilitation of safe and effective use of prescription and over-the-counter drugs.
Teaching: Prescribed Activity/Exercise (5612)—Preparing a patient to achieve and/or maintain a prescribed level of activity.
Teaching: Prescribed Medication (5616)—Preparing a patient to safely take prescribed medications and monitor their effects.
Teaching: Procedure/Treatment (5618)—Preparing a patient to understand and mentally prepare for a prescribed procedure or treatment.

Nursing Activities and Rationales

Assessments

- Assess the woman's and family/caregiver's level of knowledge of prescribed medications and treatments. This information provides a baseline for development of a teaching plan.

Patient/Family Teaching

- Assure the woman on heparin or warfarin that the drug will not affect breastfeeding. Heparin and warfarin are not secreted in human milk and are safe for use during lactation. Consult with the primary healthcare provider regarding recommendations for anticoagulation management during breastfeeding.
- Instruct to avoid the intake of aspirin and aspirin-containing products while on anticoagulation therapy. Use of aspirin in conjunction with anticoagulants may increase the risk for bleeding. Aspirin has antiplatelet effects.
- Instruct the patient on warfarin to take the dose at the same time each day, and to refrain from doubling any missed doses. Consistency of dosing facilitates maintenance of therapeutic ranges and also helps the woman to remember to take her medication. Doubling doses can increase the risk for bleeding.
- Instruct the woman on warfarin therapy to avoid the intake of large amounts of leafy green vegetables because they decrease the effect of the drug. Leafy green vegetables are high in vitamin K. Vitamin K reverses the effects of warfarin.
- Explain the importance of keeping follow-up appointments and inform the woman that her blood will be drawn regularly to ensure that she is taking the correct dose of warfarin. The healthcare provider will monitor the prothrombin time/international normalized ratio to determine if a change in the dose of warfarin is necessary. Initially, her blood will be checked frequently.
- Instruct about the need to use birth control while taking warfarin. Warfarin crosses the placenta and can cause birth defects. If the woman becomes pregnant while taking warfarin, the potential risks and options should be discussed. The risks of estrogen-containing oral contraceptives should be explained. See "Potential Complications: Pulmonary Embolism," beginning on p. 352.
- Teach the woman to recognize and report signs and symptoms of abnormal bleeding. Oozing from the gums, nosebleeds, hematuria, bruising, and frank or occult blood in the stools may indicate overanticoagulation. These signs require immediate medical attention to prevent anemia, excessive bleeding, or hemorrhage.
- Instruct on use of bleeding precautions. The use of a soft-bristled toothbrush, use of electric razors, and avoidance of potentially injurious sports/activities are examples of precautions used to minimize the risk of injury that may result in excessive bleeding.
- Teach the woman how to put on elastic stockings before getting out of bed. When applied correctly, elastic stockings prevent venous congestion/stasis. The woman needs adequate information to perform the task correctly.
- Teach safe administration of warm packs to the affected area. Enhances comfort. The woman needs adequate information to perform the treatment safely and prevent burns.
- Include family member in all teaching. Facilitates maintenance of therapeutic regimen.

INDIVIDUALIZED (NURSING DIAGNOSIS) CARE PLANS

This section includes care plans that were developed to address unique patient needs.

▌ Nursing Diagnosis: PAIN[1]

Related Factors: tissue hypoxia, inflammation, and swelling from thrombophlebitis. Refer to the generic NDCP, "Pain,[1]" beginning on p. 18, Chapter 2.

▌ *Goals, Outcomes, and Evaluation Criteria*

- Woman reports pain decreased to an acceptable level.
- No change in pulse, blood pressure, or respirations (or return to baseline).

▌ *Nursing Activities and Rationales*

Assessments

- Ask the woman about pain-relief measures that have worked in the past and that she prefers; provide information as needed. Allows the woman to have control over her pain and use measures that she feels will benefit her. Often pain control strategies that have been effective in the past will be effective for differing types of pain and new pain situations.
- Observe for nonverbal signs of pain (e.g., tachycardia, tachypnea, hypertension). Pain and the expression of pain are individual responses. Some women may not verbally express pain for a variety of reasons, such as culture or fear of developing narcotic dependence.
- Monitor effectiveness of pain relief measures. Assessment and documentation of response to pain are essential to ensure that the patient's needs are being met. Use the same scale to assess pain levels for consistency in pain evaluation.
- Monitor side effects of pharmacological agents (e.g., respirations, level of consciousness, BP). Close monitoring is needed for the woman who is at risk for pulmonary embolism from thrombophlebitis to create a balance between pain relief and dosages that result in dangerous side effects. Narcotic analgesics may cause decreased level of consciousness, shallow respirations, and hypotension.

Independent Nursing Actions

- Provide basic comfort measures, such as maintaining dry linens, cool cloth to forehead, or lip balm. When basic needs are being met, the woman can focus on relaxation techniques.
- Use a bed cradle to keep sheets and blankets off affected extremity. Provides relief to the sensitive extremity by minimizing contact with linens.
- Apply moist heat packs to affected extremity. Moist heat helps relieve pain and promotes vasodilation. Check the temperature before applying to prevent burns because the woman's sensitivity may be decreased from edema. Avoid placing the weight of the heat pack directly on the extremity because it may impede venous flow.

Collaborative Activities

- Administer analgesics as prescribed. Pain relief increases the woman's ability to cope and comply with the plan of care.

▌ Nursing Diagnosis: ANXIETY[1]

Related Factors: changes in activities of daily living, inability to care for the newborn, and concerns about outcomes of thrombophlebitis. See the generic NDCPs, "Anxiety[1]" and "Fear,[1]" beginning on pp. 10 and 15, respectively, in Chapter 2.

▌ *Goals, Outcomes, and Evaluation Criteria*

- Woman freely discusses concerns with caregivers.
- Woman reports a low level of anxiety.

▌ *NIC Interventions[2]*

Active Listening (4920)—Attending closely to and attaching significance to a patient's verbal and nonverbal expressions of pain.

Anxiety Reduction (5820)—Minimizing apprehension, dread, foreboding, or uneasiness related to an unidentified source of anticipated danger.

Coping Enhancement (5230)—Assisting a patient to adapt to perceived stressors, changes, or threats that interfere with meeting life demands and roles.

Recreation Therapy (5360)—Purposeful use of recreation to promote relaxation and enhancement of social skills.

Simple Relaxation Therapy (6040)—Use of techniques to encourage and elicit relaxation for the purpose of decreasing undesirable signs and symptoms such as pain, muscle tension, or anxiety.

▌ *Nursing Activities and Rationales*

Assessment

- Observe for verbal and nonverbal signs of anxiety. This information provides a baseline upon which to plan nursing interventions and measure their effectiveness. Nonverbal cues may be the first recognized since some patients do not recognize their own anxiety or verbalize it.

Independent Nursing Actions

- Provide time with the woman to explain procedures, offer reassurance, and listen to her concerns. Provide appropriate empathy and emotional support. These interventions often reduce anxiety and facilitate a trusting nurse–patient relationship.

- Ensure the woman has time with her newborn and participates in the baby's care as much as possible. Allowing time for bonding and participation of the mother in the care of the child is important in reducing anxiety.
- Devise a plan of daily activities for the woman and her infant, and allow her as much control as possible. Control reduces anxiety. Concern over the newborn's well-being can be a source of anxiety.
- Allow woman's older children to visit. Concern for her other children's well-being can be a source of anxiety. Allowing visitation is beneficial to both the woman and her children.

Collaborative Activity

- Arrange for diversional activities/occupational therapy when the woman is on bed rest. Provides purposeful and/or enjoyable activity for the woman. This is of particular importance to the woman who may find it difficult to maintain bed rest when bored.

Patient/Family Teaching

- Teach relaxation techniques (e.g., controlled breathing, visualization). Active involvement in relaxation therapy provides the woman with a sense of control and often reduces anxiety.
- Explain the disease process and treatment for thrombophlebitis. Factual information decreases fear of the unknown. Knowledge empowers the woman to actively participate in the planning of her care and management of her disease process.

▌ *Other Nursing Diagnosis*

Also assess for the following nursing diagnosis, which is frequently present with this condition:

- Impaired Home Maintenance[1] related to prescribed activity restriction.

MASTITIS

Mastitis refers to infection and/or inflammation of the breast that may be infective or noninfective. *Noninfective mastitis* relates to breast engorgement from nonexpressed human milk. *Infective mastitis* relates to infection and can lead to breast abscess. Infective mastitis occurs in 1% of women who breastfeed. Symptoms may begin after the 1st week, but more commonly occur between the 2nd and 3rd weeks following birth. Unilateral mastitis is more common than bilateral mastitis.

▌ *Key Nursing Activities*

- Identify signs of mastitis

- Prevent complications
- Offer emotional support
- Enhance comfort

▌ *Etiologies and Risk Factors*

- Noninfective mastitis. Nonexpressed breast milk from incorrect infant positioning or infant attachment for feeding.
- Infective mastitis. *Staphylococcus aureus* (most commonly), *S. epidermidis*, streptococci, and *Candida albicans* (less commonly); bacteria generally invade the breast tissue through cracked or fissured nipples causing infection. The source of the bacteria may be the mouth or nose of the newborn but may also be the hands of the mother or caregivers or the woman's bloodstream. Factors that predispose a woman to mastitis include engorgement; plugged ducts; abrupt weaning; suboptimal feedings; wearing underwire bras or bras that are too tight; sore, cracked nipples; breast trauma; maternal fatigue; and poor maternal nutrition.

▌ *Signs and Symptoms*

Subjective. Infective: Localized tenderness and pain at the site of infection, headache, malaise, anorexia, nausea, flulike symptoms. Mastitis should be suspected in any breastfeeding woman who develops flulike symptoms. *Noninfective:* Mild flulike symptoms.

Objective. Infective: Warm, hard, reddened area at site of infection; fever; vomiting; axillary adenopathy; purulent drainage; cracks or fissures in the nipple. *Noninfective:* Flushing over breast that may or may not be associated with lumps in breast.

▌ *Diagnostic Studies*

- Culture of human milk. Confirms diagnosis and identifies causative organism. A colony count greater than 1,000/ml indicates mastitis.
- CBC with differential. Identifies infection. Leukocytosis greater than 10,000 indicates infection.
- Ultrasound. Confirms presence of abscess.

▌ *Medical Management*

It is important to distinguish noninfective mastitis (inflammation) from infective mastitis (infection) because medical management is different.

Noninfective Mastitis

- Facilitate breast emptying by correcting infant positioning and attachment
- Analgesics
- Localized heat or cold
- Frequent breastfeeding or decompression

Infective Mastitis

- Antibiotic therapy (e.g., penicillinase-resistant antibiotics such as cephalosporin, dicloxacillin)

- Pain control
- Localized heat or cold
- Increased fluid intake (2–3 liters)
- Frequent breastfeeding or decompression
- Incision/drainage if abscess is present

Collaborative Problems

- Abscess formation
- Systemic infection

COLLABORATIVE (STANDARDIZED) CARE FOR ALL WOMEN WITH MASTITIS

Perform a comprehensive assessment to identify individual needs for teaching, emotional support, and physical care.

Potential Complications of Mastitis: ABSCESS FORMATION AND SYSTEMIC INFECTION

Focus Assessments

- Assess for palpable mass at suspected abscess site (may be confirmed with ultrasound). Establishes presence of abscess. Abscesses are localized collections of pus within breast tissue. Ducts are distended from the accumulation of WBCs and retained milk. The central core of the abscess may be necrotic and contain creamy, yellowish exudate. Surgical incision and drainage are necessary to remove necrotic tissue and exudate and allow drainage of bacteria and WBCs.
- Assess for systemic infection. The high concentration of pathogens within an abscess can readily enter the blood and lymphatic systems, causing systemic infection and sepsis. Fever, tachycardia, increased or uncontrolled pain, purulent drainage, and lethargy are signs of systemic infection. Sepsis exists when the pathogen enters the bloodstream and produces bacteremia. Untreated or inadequately treated bacteremia predisposes the woman to septic shock.
- Assess for fatigue and other infections. Fatigue causes stress, which suppresses immune function. Infections increase the demands on the immune system. Both of these predispose the woman to development of mastitis if not already present.

Preventive Nursing Activities

- Teach and provide perineal hygiene. Decreases the risk for contamination of breasts with pathogenic organisms from incisions, episiotomy, lacerations, or abrasions. The mother may be the source of infection due to changing perineal pads and performing perineal care.
- Teach proper hand washing prior to feeding infant or touching breasts. Hand washing is the most effective means of removing microorganisms and preventing contamination of the breasts. Touching the breasts or infant, especially around the mouth prior to breastfeeding, can be a source of contamination if hands are not thoroughly washed.
- Teach the importance of changing nursing pads when wet. Prevents bacterial growth. A warm, damp environment and the presence of milk are excellent media for bacterial growth. Frequent changing of pads decreases the risk for infection.
- Teach the importance of completely emptying breasts via breastfeeding or pump. If the woman has nipple soreness, she may be tempted to skip a feeding or stop feeding before breasts are empty. However, breast engorgement and milk stasis contribute to development of noninfective mastitis, which can result in infective mastitis. Therefore, emptying the breasts is an important preventive measure.
- Administer and monitor effectiveness of antibiotic therapy. Inhibits pathogenic growth and prevents development of systemic infection. Mastitis should begin to resolve within 48 hours following initiation of antimicrobial therapy.
- Teach to avoid wearing tight bras or those with underwires. Reduces pressure on breasts, which may interfere with complete emptying of mammary ducts and decreases the risk for mastitis.
- Encourage breastfeeding or breast pumping. Reduces risk for abscess formation. Breastfeeding should occur from both breasts to ensure emptying and prevent abscess formation. If breasts are too sore for breastfeeding, encourage pumping.
- Teach the importance of maintaining antibiotic schedules at home. If treated with antibiotics early, mastitis generally resolves within 2 days. Compliance with drug schedules helps maintain therapeutic blood levels of antibiotics necessary to eliminate the infectious organism completely. The woman who understands the importance of taking medications as prescribed is more likely to comply.
- Teach signs and symptoms that need to be reported and importance of follow-up if infection continues. Mastitis generally occurs after the woman is discharged from the acute setting; therefore, she must be prepared to monitor and report her own condition so that early intervention can be provided.

INDIVIDUALIZED (NURSING DIAGNOSIS) CARE PLANS

The care plans in this section were developed to address unique patient needs.

Nursing Diagnosis: INTERRUPTED BREASTFEEDING[1]

Related Factors: pain and breast abscess.

Goals, Outcomes, and Evaluation Criteria

- Woman explains benefits of continuing breastfeeding.
- Woman verbalizes signs of inadequate emptying of breasts.
- Woman verbalizes signs of abscess formation.

NIC Interventions[2]

Bottle Feeding (1052)—Preparation and administration of fluids to an infant via a bottle.

Emotional Support (5270)—Provision of reassurance, acceptance, and encouragement during times of stress.

Lactation Counseling (5244)—Use of an interactive helping process to assist in maintenance of successful breastfeeding.

Nursing Activities and Rationales

Assessments

- Assess woman's pain status. Determines if breast soreness/pain is so severe it will interfere with her desire or ability to continue breastfeeding.
- Assess woman's desire to breastfeed. The woman who has a strong desire to breastfeed her infant is likely to do so in spite of breast soreness or increased pain. The woman who is unsure about breastfeeding may be easily deterred from continuing when pain is severe or surgery for abscess drainage is required.
- Assess infant's weight. It is normal for a newborn to lose a few ounces initially; however, weight loss should not continue if the infant is receiving adequate nutrition. Continued weight loss is an indication of ineffective or interrupted breastfeeding.

Independent Nursing Actions

- Offer emotional support. The woman who is in pain may be discouraged and feel that she has failed as a mother. Reassuring her that she did nothing to cause this condition and that it is temporary may help her cope with treatments and pain until the condition resolves.
- Discourage weaning due to discomfort. Some mothers will decide to stop breastfeeding due to pain. Cessation of breastfeeding while mastitis is present may contribute to pain because of increased breast engorgement. As a result, stasis of milk and reduced expression of milk will occur, all of which contribute to abscess formation. The woman who understands the effects of weaning is more likely to continue breastfeeding.
- Reassure the woman regarding safety of breastfeeding. Women with mastitis should be informed that it is not necessary to discontinue breastfeeding. The infant is not affected by sucking on the involved breast and will not require antibiotic treatment.

Collaborative Activity

- Refer to lactation consultant as appropriate. An acute infection can affect the woman's ability and desire to breastfeed. A lactation consultant may be helpful to the woman who desires to breastfeed but is undergoing pain and fatigue due to infection. A consultant can identify and help correct any incorrect techniques that contributed to the development of mastitis.

Patient/Family Teaching

- Teach to monitor effectiveness of antibiotic therapy. Infection should begin to resolve within 48 hours following initiation of antibiotic therapy. Signs of drug effectiveness include decreased breast swelling and tenderness, decrease in size of palpable mass, decreased discomfort with feeding, absence of fever, etc. Breastfeeding will become less painful as infection subsides.
- Teach to empty breast with each feeding. Prevents stasis of milk, which contributes to abscess formation. Breastfeeding should occur every 2–3 hours. If the woman is too sore to breastfeed, she should express the milk or use a pump to completely empty her breasts to ensure adequate milk production, prevent milk suppression, and facilitate healing.
- Teach to initiate feeding on side without soreness. Feeding on the unaffected side initiates milk ejection on the affected side, which facilitates complete emptying of the affected breast, prevents milk stasis, and facilitates healing.
- Teach the need for maintaining fluid intake of at least 3,000 ml per day. Ensures adequate milk production and prevents milk suppression. Increased milk production helps facilitate breast duct drainage as long as breasts are completely emptied at frequent intervals.
- Teach the benefits of breastfeeding. Women who are in pain may decide to terminate breastfeeding. If they understand the benefits of breastfeeding (enhanced immunity, decreased potential for hypersensitivities, and enhanced nutrition from ideal formula), they may be more inclined to continue breastfeeding.

Nursing Diagnosis: PAIN[1]

See the generic NDCP, "Pain,[1]" beginning on p. 18 in Chapter 2.

Nursing Activities and Rationales

Patient/Family Teaching

- Encourage and teach the use of localized heat/cold. Controls and reduces pain. Heat improves blood flow via vasodilation, improves delivery of WBCs and antibiotics to affected area, promotes removal of waste products and reduces pain by promoting muscle relaxation. Cold reduces blood flow to the affected area, prevents edema, and reduces inflammation, all of which reduce localized pain. The choice to use heat or cold depends on the desired response and actual effect of the localized application.

- Encourage and teach the use of breastfeeding, milk expression, or breast pumping for pain control. Frequent emptying of breast ducts prevents engorgement and stasis of milk, which predisposes to pain and abscess formation. Breastfeeding or pumping should occur every 2–3 hours.

POSTPARTUM DEPRESSION

Postpartum depression is one of three mood disorders that can occur following childbirth. It is a major debilitating disorder affecting 4.5–28% of postpartum women (Doucet, Dennis, Letourneau, & Blackmore, 2009). Postpartum depression (PPD) lies between postpartum blues and postpartum psychosis in severity. *Postpartum blues* are a very mild form of depression. Blues are transient and self-limiting. *Postpartum psychosis* is a severe form of depression involving delusions and hallucinations. It requires psychiatric intervention and can be an indication of bipolar disorder. (Postpartum psychosis is beyond the scope of this care plan. For further information refer to a mental health textbook.) *Postpartum depression* is intense sadness that begins within the first 4 weeks following birth and may continue for as long as a year. Postpartum depression rarely resolves without intervention.

Early recognition and treatment of postpartum depression are essential to protect the safety of and minimize the negative effects to the mother, infant, and family. The mother's inability to interact with her infant negatively affects the infant developmentally and emotionally (Delatte, Cao, Meltzer-Brody, & Menard, 2009) and increases the infant's risk for mental health disorders in later childhood (Pawlby, Sharp, Hay, & O'Keane, 2008).

▍ *Key Nursing Activities*

- Identify signs/symptoms of depression
- Determine risks to infant and mother
- Offer emotional support
- Support parent–infant bonding
- Refer for mental health intervention

▍ *Etiologies and Risk Factors*

The exact cause of PPD is unknown. Significant risk factors include preexisting neurosis or psychosis, history of depression or mood disorders, smoking, low self-esteem, history of childhood sexual abuse, labor/delivery complications for mother or baby, and complicated childbirth (Neiman et al., 2010). Other risk factors include hormonal fluctuations, illness (PIH, diabetes mellitus, thyroid disease), unwanted pregnancy, multifetal pregnancy, fatigue, lack of sleep, financial instability, lack of support from one's partner/family, premature or postmature infant, infant born with a deformity or illness, difficult infant (crying, feeding, etc.), and separation of mother and infant. More than 50% of women who experience postpartum depression will develop depression when they give birth again.

Signs and Symptoms

Subjective. Depressive mood; loss of interest in activities; feelings of being overwhelmed or angry; changes in appetite; decreased energy; feelings of worthlessness or guilt; loss of libido; difficulty concentrating, thinking, or making decisions; suicidal ideation; lack of positive feelings toward the infant; blaming the infant; obsessive thoughts about harming the infant; sleep disturbances; sense of doom; hot or cold flashes; chest pain or discomfort; and dizziness.

Objective. Weight loss or weight gain, crying or uncontrollable sobbing, withdrawn behavior, flat affect, irritability, violent outbursts, panic attacks, rejection of the infant, awkward responses toward infant, abuse of infant, tachycardia, tachypnea, and shaking.

▍ *Diagnostic Studies*

- History. Determines risk factors and past episodes of depression.
- Physical examination. Rules out hormonal imbalances and/or diseases such as anemia, thyroid disease, diabetes mellitus, substance abuse.
- Edinburgh Postnatal Depression Scale. Most widely recognized and used self-report assessment/screening tool that identifies women at risk for PPD. It does not diagnose PPD.
- Postpartum Depression Screening Scale. Self-report screening tool used during postpartum period to identify risk for PPD.
- Postpartum Depression Predictor Inventory-Revised. Identifies women at risk for PPD based on 13 risk factors; promotes dialogue between nurse/provider and woman.

▍ *Medical Management*

- Psychotherapy, cognitive-behavioral therapy
- Medications (antidepressants, anxiolytic agents)
- Electroconvulsive therapy
- Family counseling

▍ *Collaborative Problems*

- Potential complication of postpartum depression: suicide, infant injury, infant death

COLLABORATIVE (STANDARDIZED) CARE FOR ALL WOMEN WITH PPD

Perform a comprehensive assessment to identify individual needs for teaching, emotional support, and physical care.

Nursing Diagnosis: INEFFECTIVE COPING[1]

Related Factors: the birth of the infant and previous history of depression or psychosis.

Goals, Outcomes, and Evaluation Criteria

- Woman reports effective use of coping strategies.
- Woman verbalizes feelings of well-being.
- Woman seeks assistance as needed.
- Woman reports feeling rested.
- Woman performs self-care.
- Woman reports pleasure with performing infant care.

NIC Interventions[2]

Anxiety Reduction (5820)—Minimizing apprehension, dread, foreboding, or uneasiness related to an unidentified source of anticipated danger.

Coping Enhancement (5230)—Assisting a patient to adapt to perceived stressors, changes, or threats that interfere with meeting life demands and roles.

Emotional Support (5270)—Provision of reassurance, acceptance, and encouragement during times of stress.

Mood Management (5330)—Providing for safety, stabilization, recovery, and maintenance of a patient who is experiencing dysfunctional depression or elevated mood.

Support System Enhancement (5440)—Facilitation of support to patient by family, friends, and community.

Nursing Activities and Rationales

Assessments

- Assess for signs of depression. Detects depressive state so that early interventions can be implemented (see objective and subjective signs of depression in "Signs and Symptoms," previously).
- Ask questions about woman's mood. Helps differentiate postpartum blues from postpartum depression. Women cannot be depended upon to voluntarily report changes in their feelings or mood even if they recognize it themselves. Asking leading questions about sleep, energy levels, and ability to concentrate helps differentiate postpartum blues from PPD.
- Monitor for fatigue, changes in self-care, or decreased activity. Fatigue is a significant risk factor for PPD, which may lead to inability or disinterest in caring for self or overall decreased activity.

Independent Nursing Actions

- Reassure the woman that many women experience what she is feeling. The woman may feel that she is the only person who has negative thoughts about herself or her infant or who feels no joy at giving birth. Recognizing that she is not unusual or being judged negatively may increase her willingness to answer questions honestly and openly.
- Encourage a well-balanced diet. Nutritional deficits can contribute to feelings of depression and fatigue.
- Encourage rest periods and provide periods of uninterrupted sleep. Fatigue and sleep disturbances are risk factors for depression and may exacerbate symptoms and suicidal ideation.
- Encourage participation in exercise program. Exercise stimulates endorphin production and may enhance emotional well-being and counteract depression.
- Encourage family participation in care of the infant and other children. Depression alters the ability of the mother to care for her infant and other children and increases her stress level and fatigue. The help of other family members relieves pressure on the mother and allows her to take care of herself.
- Offer support to the partner. Helps the partner cope with the woman's depression and meet his own needs. The partner often feels frustrated, blamed, neglected, or confused. Providing opportunities for the partner to verbalize his concerns and feelings allows the nurse to correct misconceptions and reassure him that his partner's recovery is possible and likely.
- Reassure the family that PPD is a temporary situation in most cases. Understanding that improvement is likely in the future may help the family cope with their current situation. Depression may continue for up to a year, but with early treatment, it may resolve much earlier.

Collaborative Activities

- Refer to available community resources as appropriate. Helps the family cope with their current situation by facilitating their access to agencies such as child care, home health aides, homemaker services, support groups, meal programs, counseling. The family may be unaware of community resources available to them.
- Refer for mental health treatment. Women with severe depression should be referred for immediate mental health intervention to protect the safety of both the mother and infant.

Patient/Family Teaching

- Teach partner/family signs and symptoms to report. Ensures early treatment of PPD. Women generally leave the hospital prior to developing signs and symptoms of PPD; therefore, the partner/family should be taught how to recognize signs of depression and the importance of reporting signs of depression to the healthcare provider immediately. Early intervention facilitates early resolution and may prevent injury to the mother, infant, and other children.
- Teach the woman the need for maintaining medication dosages and schedules. Antidepressant drugs may

take several weeks to reach therapeutic levels; thereafter, adherence to dosages and schedules is essential to maintain effectiveness of pharmacologic intervention. Antidepressant drugs elevate mood and increase the capacity for coping with stress.

- Teach the woman about medication use and breastfeeding. The risks and benefits of antidepressant medication use while breastfeeding must be considered and discussed with the woman by the provider. Breastfeeding is generally avoided during peak dosages of antidepressant medications. Thereafter, infants must be monitored to determine medication effects and determine whether bottle feeding must replace breastfeeding while the woman is on medication.
- Teach use of relaxation and other coping strategies. Decreases stress and increases the ability to cope with current situation. Strategies that have been successful in the past are likely to be successful to some degree even when the woman is depressed.
- Teach woman/partner/family regarding electroconvulsive therapy when treatment modality is used. Electroconvulsive therapy may be needed when depression is resistant to medications or psychotherapy and the woman is at significant risk of causing injury to herself or her infant. Electrical current precipitates convulsions that change chemical reactions in the brain and may relieve resistant depression.

Nursing Diagnosis: RISK FOR SUICIDE[1]

Related Factors: prenatal depression, stressed relationships, lack of social support, illness, stress, history of depression or psychosis, multiparity, inadequate nutrition, fatigue, decreased self-esteem, and immaturity.

▌ *NIC Interventions[2]*

Anxiety Reduction (5820)—Minimizing apprehension, dread, foreboding, or uneasiness related to an unidentified source of anticipated danger.

Behavior Management: Self Harm (4350)—Helping a patient to manage negative behavior.

Coping Enhancement (5230)—Assisting a patient to adapt to perceived stressors, changes, or threats that interfere with meeting life demands and roles.

Crisis Intervention (6160)—Use of short-term counseling to help the patient cope with a crisis and resume a state of functioning comparable to or better than the precrisis.

Mood Management (5330)—Providing for safety, stabilization, recovery, and maintenance of a patient who is experiencing dysfunctional depression or elevated mood.

▌ *Nursing Activities and Rationales*

Assessments

- Monitor for comments indicating suicidal ideation. Comments such as, "I'm worthless" or "They'd all be better off without me," are suggestive of suicidal ideation in a depressed individual and warrant further investigation or intervention to prevent suicide attempt.

Independent Nursing Actions

- Establish a trusting relationship. Creates a therapeutic environment in which the woman feels safe. The woman who feels safe is more likely to verbalize her thoughts and feelings, including plans for suicide.
- Encourage verbalization of fears, thoughts, and plans. Women who think about suicide may verbalize their plans or intentions. Spending time with the depressed woman and encouraging her to express her thoughts may make it possible for her to talk about her feelings regarding her infant and suicide.
- Ask the woman if she has a plan for suicide. Determines if the woman is planning on committing suicide. If the woman expresses feelings about suicide, it is essential that she be queried about a plan. Women who have formulated a plan of action for suicide are at significantly increased risk of following through with their plan since they have thought their decision through to the end.

Collaborative Activities

- Report suicidal ideation immediately. The woman who is thinking about suicide is highly likely to attempt suicide. It must be reported immediately so that protective actions can be taken to safeguard her.
- Encourage increased exercise. Exercise has been shown to decrease depression in many instances, including PPD.

Patient/Family Teaching

- Teach family to monitor for signs of suicide ideation. Helps prevent suicide attempts. Family members are the ones most likely to recognize the first intentions of the woman to commit suicide. They need to know how to recognize signs of suicide ideation and when and how to notify healthcare providers.

Nursing Diagnosis: RISK FOR OTHER-DIRECTED VIOLENCE[1]

Related Factors: feelings of inadequacy or self-worth, multiple births, ill infant, stress, or history of depression.

▌ *Goals, Outcomes, and Evaluation Criteria*

- Woman displays absence of dependent abuse.

- Woman reports absence of threats of dependent abuse.
- Woman reports feelings of violence to healthcare provider.
- Woman seeks assistance as needed.
- Woman controls behaviors that could lead to violence toward dependents.

▌ NIC Interventions[2]

Abuse Protection Support (6400)—Identification of high-risk, dependent relationships and actions to prevent further infliction of physical or emotional harm.

Abuse Protection Support: Child (6402)—Identification of high-risk, dependent child relationships and actions to prevent possible or further infliction of physical, sexual, or emotional harm or neglect of basic necessities of life.

Coping Enhancement (5230)—Assisting a patient to adapt to perceived stressors, changes, or threats that interfere with meeting life demands and roles.

Crisis Intervention (6160)—Use of short-term counseling to help the patient cope with a crisis and resume a state of functioning comparable to or better than the precrisis.

Mood Management (5330)—Providing for safety, stabilization, recovery, and maintenance of a patient who is experiencing dysfunctional depression or elevated mood.

▌ Nursing Activities and Rationales

Assessments

- Assess for history of previous PPD or inability to care for newborn due to depressive episode. Determines if a protective plan for the infant is warranted. Women who have experienced PPD with previous births are at increased risk for depression with each successive birth.
- Monitor mother–infant interactions. Detects alterations that require intervention. The inability to care for or disinterest in her infant may cause feelings of guilt or worthlessness, which may contribute to the woman's thoughts of suicide or need to harm the infant. PPD can have significant negative effects on the infant that may persist into childhood.
- Monitor infant for signs of inadequate nutrition/hydration. Prevents infant nutritional deficits due to mother's lack of interest in feeding her infant. Many women are able to care for their infants adequately even though they find no joy in doing so. However, others are unable to care for their infants at all due to the severity of their depression.
- Ask the woman if she has thoughts about injuring her baby. Determines risk to the infant. The depressed mother may be obsessively thinking of harming her infant. The infant at least risk for harm is the one whose mother has no thoughts or plans for injuring the infant. The woman who has thought about harming her infant (or other dependent children), has considered a specific method (e.g., suffocating, drowning.) for doing so, has that method available to

her, and has a detailed plan that is highly lethal is at greatest risk for harming her infant. Protective interventions need to be implemented immediately to safeguard the infant or other dependents.

Collaborative Activities

- Contact social services/family members immediately when a child or infant is identified to be at risk for injury. Children who are at risk for injury should be removed from the home immediately to protect their safety. Inpatient hospitalization may be required for treatment of women whose depression progresses to psychosis.

Patient/Family Teaching

- Teach the partner to report increased signs or symptoms of infant neglect immediately. Prevents harm to the infant and other dependent children. Worsening of symptoms may indicate ineffectiveness or noncompliance with medication dosages or schedules, or worsening of depression, both of which place dependent children at increased risk for harm.
- Teach woman the need for complying with prescribed medications. The woman may become frustrated if she does not start to feel better immediately, which can lead to greater stress and increased risk for the infant. She needs to understand that it may take up to 4 weeks for medications to reach therapeutic levels and begin to alter her depression.
- Encourage partner/family to be involved in care of the infant. Protects the infant from harm, relieves the mother from the stressors of caring for the infant, and facilitates parent–infant attachment and infant growth and development.

INDIVIDUALIZED (NURSING DIAGNOSIS) CARE PLANS

The care plans in this section were developed to address unique patient needs.

▌ Nursing Diagnosis: SLEEP PATTERN DISTURBANCE[1]

See the generic NDCP, "Sleep Deprivation or Disturbed Sleep Pattern,[1]" beginning on p. 21 in Chapter 2.

▌ Nursing Activities and Rationales

Assessments

- Assess effects of prescribed medications on woman's sleep pattern. Some antidepressant medications enhance sleep while others are energizing. Energizing medications are best taken in the morning, while sleep-enhancing drugs are best taken at night. The practitioner should be notified if medications are altering the woman's sleep patterns so that adjustments in schedules can be made if needed to facilitate sleep.

Independent Nursing Actions

- Encourage reporting of mood changes that alter sleep patterns. Sleep disturbances are a common sign of depression. When the woman is unable to sleep it increases her fatigue, inability to care for herself or her baby, and decreases her ability to cope with stress, infant care, and additional responsibilities.
- Encourage the woman to ask partner/family to care for infant when rest or sleep is needed. Provides the woman a full night's sleep or periods of uninterrupted rest.

Nursing Diagnosis: RISK FOR IMPAIRED PARENT–INFANT/CHILD ATTACHMENT[1]

See the generic NDCP, "Risk for Impaired Parent–Infant/Child Attachment,[1]" beginning on p. 19 in Chapter 2.

Nursing Activities and Rationales

Assessments

- Assess history. Determines if the infant is at risk. When a previous child has been removed from the home due to neglect secondary to PPD, this infant is at increased risk for neglect, abuse, or impaired attachment.
- Monitor mother's reaction to infant. Determines if attachment is or is not occurring so that corrective interventions can be planned and implemented. Depression may interfere with bonding. Lack of eye contact, disinterest in holding or caring for the infant, lack of cuddling or talking to the infant are signs of impaired attachment.
- Assess woman's ability to care for and meet needs of infant. Identifies the need for care planning. Some depressed women are able to provide physical care to their infant but not emotional care and love; others are unable to provide any care or love whatsoever. PPD can have significant negative effects on the infant that may persist into childhood if not identified and addressed.

Independent Nursing Actions

- Involve partner/family in care of infant. Relieves pressure on mother and facilitates parent–infant attachment and infant growth and development.

Nursing Diagnosis: SITUATIONAL LOW SELF-ESTEEM[1]

Related Factors: PPD, feelings or fear of failure, and inability to react to, love, or care for the infant.

Goals, Outcomes, and Evaluation Criteria

Woman and/or partner (family):

- Verbalize personal strengths.
- Accept positive comments from others.
- Function in roles perceived as important.

NIC Interventions[2]

Coping Enhancement (5230)—Assisting a patient to adapt to perceived stressors, changes, or threats that interfere with meeting life demands and roles.

Mood Management (5330)—Providing for safety, stabilization, recovery, and maintenance of a patient who is experiencing dysfunctional depression or elevated mood.

Self-Esteem Enhancement (5400)—Assisting a patient to increase his/her personal judgment of self-worth.

Nursing Activities and Rationales

Assessments

- Assess the woman's perception of self. Determines if the woman's self-perception is negative or positive (e.g., she has exhibited expressions of shame, worthlessness, inability to care for infant). Lack of self-esteem and anger turned toward self contribute to depression. Women with PPD often blame themselves for feeling depressed and feel they have failed their infant and their partner/family, which negatively affects their self-esteem.
- Assess woman's/partner's/family's relationships. Determines the need for intervention. The partner/family may react with confusion, frustration, anger, or shock. It is necessary to address their needs so that they can offer support and encouragement to the woman. The woman who feels rejected by her family may place even more blame on herself, which further affects her self-esteem negatively.
- Monitor ongoing level of self-esteem. Determines effectiveness of interventions. Continued negative verbalizations of self-worth or deprecating comments may mean that other interventions are necessary; however, changes in self-esteem occur over a relatively long time.

Independent Nursing Actions

- Use a caring, nonjudgmental approach. It is essential to establish trust so that the woman will be open to discussions about her feelings toward herself, infant, and family; be open to receiving information provided; and be motivated to cooperate with treatments.

- Discuss the woman's feelings about herself. Helps identify misconceptions that need to be corrected and allows the nurse to offer reassurance about the woman's future. Reassuring the woman that she is not alone and that other women experience PPD too may help her focus on a more positive future.
- Assist with identification of personal strengths and reinforce identified strengths. Helps the woman gain a more positive and realistic view of herself and her ability as a mother. Reinforcement motivates continuation of same behaviors; e.g., focusing on positive rather than negative behaviors.
- Help the woman set realistic goals for herself and care of her infant. Small goals are more readily achieved than long-range or unrealistic goals. Successes, even when small or seemingly insignificant, demonstrate progress and promote positive self-esteem.
- Assist woman/partner/family with decision making and problem solving. The depressed woman has difficulty concentrating and making decisions effectively. Providing assistance relieves stress and decreases anxiety.

Collaborative Activity

- Refer to support group or counseling as appropriate. Women/families may not be able to cope with their feelings without outside assistance. Reassure them that it is acceptable and desirable to seek outside assistance when needed.

Patient/Family Teaching

- Teach partner/family the importance of their interest and support. The woman is already blaming herself and feeling self-deprecated. Lack of support from the family can increase her depression and further decrease her self-esteem.
- Teach partner/family regarding woman's possible negative reactions. Depression may cause the woman to be overly critical, which makes it difficult for family members to remain supportive. If they understand that this is part of her illness, they may be better able to provide support.
- Teach family the need to maintain prescribed medication schedules. The woman may decide to stop taking medication if she does not feel better right away. It takes up to 4 weeks for medications to reach therapeutic levels and start to have an effect on the person's mood. Mood elevation positively affects self-esteem. Families who understand this can help monitor the woman's compliance with medication regimens and encourage to her to continue taking her medication.

END NOTES

1. Nursing Diagnoses—Definitions and Classification 2009–2011. Copyright © 2009, 2007, 2005, 2003, 2001, 1998, 1996, 1994 by NANDA International. Used by arrangement with Blackwell Publishing Limited, a company of John Wiley & Sons, Inc. In order to make safe and effective judgments using NANDA-I nursing diagnoses it is essential that nurses refer to the definitions and defining characteristics of the diagnoses listed in this work.
2. Nursing Interventions Classification (2009). Copyright Elsevier Science (by permission).

REFERENCES

American College of Obstetricians and Gynecologists (ACOG). (2006). Clinical management guidelines practice bulletin No. 76: Postpartum hemorrhage. *Obstetrics & Gynecology, 108*(4),1039–1047.

Aronoff, D. M., & Zuber, D. M. (2008). Postpartum invasive group A streptococcal disease in the modern era. *Infectious Diseases in Obstetrics and Gynecology.* doi:10.1155/2008/796892

Brown, H. L., & Hiett, A. K. (2010). Deep vein thrombosis and pulmonary embolism in pregnancy: Diagnosis, complications, and management. *Clinical Obstetrics and Gynecology, 53*(2), 345–358.

Bulechek, G. M., Butcher, H. K., & McCloskey, J. (2009). *Nursing interventions classification.* St. Louis, MO: Mosby/Elsevier.

Delatte, R., Cao, H., Meltzer-Brody, S., & Menard, M. K. (2009). Universal screening for postpartum depression: An inquiry into provider attitudes and practice. *American Journal of Obstetrics and Gynecology, 200*(5), 63–64.

Doucet, S., Dennis, C., Letourneau, N., & Blackmore, E. (2009). Differentiation and clinical implications of postpartum depression and postpartum psychosis. *JOGGN, 38*(3), 269–279.

Francois, K. E., & Foley, M. R. (2007). Antepartum and postpartum hemorrhage. In S. G. Grabe, J. R. Niebyl, & J. L. Simpson (Eds.), *Obstetrics: Normal and problem pregnancies* (5th ed., pp. 456–485). New York, NY: Churchill Livingstone.

James, A. H., Jamison, M. G., Brancazio, L. R., & Myers, E. R. (2006). Venous thromboembolism during pregnancy and the postpartum period: Incidence, risk factors, and mortality. *American Journal of Obstetrics and Gynecology, 194,* 1311–1315.

Kamaya, A., Kyung, R., Benedetti, N. J., Chang, P. L., & Desser, T. S. (2009). Imaging and diagnosis of postpartum complications. *Ultrasound Quarterly, 25,* 151–162.

Neiman, S., Carter, S., Sell, S. V., & Kindred, C. (2010). Best practice guidelines for the nurse practitioner regarding screening, prevention, and management of postpartum depression. *Critical Care Nurse Quarterly. 33* (3), 212–218.

North American Nursing Diagnosis Association International (NANDA). (2009). *Nursing diagnoses, 2009–2011: Definitions and classification.* Ames, IA: John Wiley & Sons.

Pawlby, S., Sharp, D., Hay, D., & O'Keane, V. (2008). Postnatal depression and child outcome at 11 years: The importance of accurate diagnosis. *Journal of Affective Disorders, 107*(1–3), 241–245.

Ricci, S. S. (2009). *Essentials of maternity, newborn, and women's health nursing.* Philadelphia, PA: Lippincott.

Smith, J. R., & Brennan, B. G. (2009, September 24). *Postpartum hemorrhage: Treatment.* Retrieved from http://emedicine.medscape.com/article/275038-treatment

RESOURCES

American College of Obstetricians and Gynecologists Committee on Health Care for Underserved Women. (2007). ACOG Committee Opinion 361: Breastfeeding: Maternal and infant aspects. *Obstetrics and Gynecology, 109*(2 Pt 1), 479–480.

Anderson, J. M., & Duncan, E. (2007). Prevention and management of postpartum hemorrhage. *American Family Physician, 75,* 875–882.

Cadwell, K., & Turner-Maffei, C. (2008). *Pocket guide for lactation management.* Sudbury, MA: Jones & Bartlett.

Costantine, M. M., Rahman, M., Ghulmiyah, L., Byers, B. D., Longo, M., Wen, T., & Saade, G. R. et al. (2008). Timing of perioperative antibiotics for cesarean delivery: A meta-analysis. *American Journal of Obstetrics & Gynecology, 199*(3), 301.e1–301.e6.

Ford, A. A. D., & Simpson, L. L. (2008). Breastfeeding. *Postgraduate Obstetrics and Gynecology, 28*(23), 2–6.

Glavin, K., Smith, L., Sorum, R., & Ellefsen, B. (2010). Supportive counselling by public health nurses for women with postpartum depression. *Journal of Advanced Nursing, 6*(6), 1317–1327.

James, A. H. (2009). Venous thromboembolism in pregnancy. *Arteriosclerosis, Thrombosis, and Vascular Biology, 29,* 326–331. doi: 10.1161/ATVBAHA.109.184127

Kendall-Tackett, K., & Hale, T. W. (2010). The use of antidepressants in pregnant and breastfeeding women: A review of recent studies. *Journal of Human Lactation, 26*(2), 187–195.

Lowdermilk, D., Perry, S., & Bobak, I. (2007). *Maternity & Women's Health Care* (9th ed.). St. Louis, MO: Mosby.

Maharaj, D. (2007). Puerperal pyrexia: A review. Part II. *Obstetrical & Gynecological Survey, 62*(6), 400–406.

Mattson, S., & Smith, J. E. (2010). *Core Curriculum for Maternal-Newborn Nursing* (2nd ed.). St. Louis, MO: Mosby.

McComish, J. F., & Visger, J. M. (2009, March–April). Domains of postpartum doula care and maternal responsiveness and competence. *Journal of Obstetric, Gynecologic & Neonatal Nursing, 38*(2), 148–156.

Pillitteri, A. (Ed.). (2010). *Maternal and child health nursing: Care of the childbearing and childrearing family* (6th ed.). Philadelphia, PA: Lippincott.

Smaill, F. M., & Gyte, G. M (2010). Antibiotic prophylaxis versus no prophylaxis for preventing infection after cesarean section. *Cochrane Database of Systematic Reviews.*

Smith, J. R., & Brennan, B. G. (2009, September 24). *Overview: Postpartum hemorrhage.* Retrieved from http://emedicine.medscape.com/article/275038-overview

Society of Obstetrics and Gynecology of Canada. (2008). Postpartum hemorrhage. In *ALARM Manual* (15th ed.). Ontario, Canada: The Association.

Stafford, I., Hernandez, J., Laibl, V., Sheffield, J., Roberts, R., & Wendel, G. (2008). Community-acquired methicillin-resistant *Staphylococcus aureus* among patients with puerperal mastitis requiring hospitalization. *Obstetrics and Gynecology, 112*(3), 533–537.

Varney, H., Kriebs, J. M., & Gegor, C. L. (2004). *Varney's midwifery* (4th ed.). Sudbury, MA: Jones & Bartlett.

Wong, A. W., & Rosh, A. J. (2009). *Pregnancy, postpartum infections.* Retrieved from http://emedicine.medscape.com/article/796892-overview

Wong, A. W., & Rosh, A. J. (2009). *Pregnancy, postpartum infections: Treatment and medications.* Retrieved from http://emedicine.medscape.com/article/796892-treatment

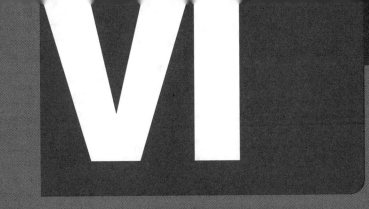

VI

CARE OF THE NEWBORN

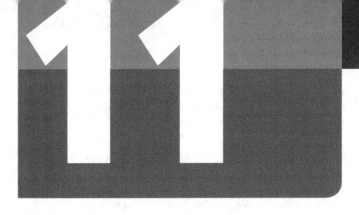

NORMAL NEWBORN CARE

Allison L. Scott

NEWBORN CARE: FIRST 4 HOURS

The physiologic adaptations that occur at birth continue into the first 4 hours of life. Although most newborns make the necessary physiologic adjustments, their well-being depends almost totally on the care they receive from others. The newborn is assessed in the first 4 hours for congenital anomalies, gestational age, and normal functioning. Nurses provide initial care while continually assessing for adaptation to extrauterine life and for potential problems.

∎ Key Nursing Activities

- Assess for and support adjustments to extrauterine life until body systems are stable.
- Assess for congenital anomalies.
- Assess gestational age and birth weight.
- Provide thermoneutral environment and support thermoregulation.
- Promote parent–infant attachment.

∎ Etiologies and Risk Factors

Newborn adaptation to extrauterine life is a normal physiologic event rather than an illness, so risk factors are applicable primarily for infants at high risk. However, factors that increase the risk for a normal newborn's developing problems include exposure to a cold environment, a long labor, cesarean birth, and exposure to certain medications during labor. Underlying maternal illness, such as infection, diabetes, or hypertension, would put the infant into the category of high-risk rather than normal. This is also true for infant conditions such as birth asphyxia, birth trauma, and for a large- or small-for-gestational-age infant.

∎ Signs and Symptoms

Signs and symptoms are not applicable. A normal newborn should not have symptoms of problems. The following are some of the important normal assessment findings.

Weight

- 2,500–4,000 g (5 lb 8 oz to 8 lb 13 oz)
- Initial weight loss of 5–10% of birth weight in the first 3–5 days of life

Length

- 45–55 cm (18–22 in)

Head Circumference

- 32–38 cm (13–15 in)

Heart

- Point of maximal impulse should be noted in the left mid-clavicular line at the fifth intercostal space.
- Apical heart rate 120–160 bpm. May range from as low as 100 during sleep to as high as 180 bpm when crying.
- Murmurs are common during the first few hours as the foramen ovale is closing.

Respirations

- Rate 30–60 breaths/min, shallow and irregular, with apneic periods of 5–10 sec.
- Acrocyanosis may be present.
- During the first hour after birth, crackles may be auscultated while fluid is still being expelled or absorbed.

Temperature

- Axillary temperature: 36.4–37.2°C (97.5–99.0°F)

∎ Diagnostic Studies

Note: These studies are for normal, not high-risk, infants.

- Cord blood for blood type (A, B, AB, O), Rh factor. Negative or positive.
- Cord blood for rapid plasma reagin. Detects congenital syphilis.
- Direct Coombs' test (on cord blood) for the newborn born to a Rh-negative mother. Should be negative for antibodies; if positive, a titer measurement is done.
- Hb (14–24 g/dl) and Hct (44–64%).
- Blood glucose by heel stick (40–60 mg/dl).
- Direct bilirubin, if indicated (0–1 mg/dl).
- Screening for phenylketonuria (phenylketonuria/newborn screening/Guthrie test). Test may differ from state to state.

∎ Medical Management

- Erythromycin or tetracycline ophthalmic ointment to be given in the first 1 hour. Prophylaxis for ophthalmia neonatorum, an eye infection from *Neisseria gonorrhoeae* acquired at birth that can cause blindness.
- Vitamin K (phytonadione) 0.5–1 mg (0.25–0.5 ml) intramuscularly, using 25–30 gauge needle (⅜–⅝ inch needle), within 1 hour of birth. Increases prothrombin production and prevents and treats hemorrhagic disease in the newborn.
- Blood glucose monitoring. Detects hypoglycemia.

- Hepatitis B vaccine intramuscularly within 12 hours of birth or hepatitis B immunoglobulin prophylaxis intramuscularly within the first 12 hr, when the mother is infected, a carrier, or has unknown status. Promotes immunity to hepatitis.
- Circumcision and follow-up care, with parental permission.
- Metabolic screen (phenylketonuria) before discharge.
- Hearing screen before discharge.

▉ *Collaborative Problems*

Potential Complications of Transition to Extrauterine Life

- Hypoglycemia
- Hyperbilirubinemia
- Respiratory distress
- Infection
- Ineffective thermoregulation[1]
- Risk for Injury[1]
- Risk for Impaired Parent–Infant/Child Attachment[1]

COLLABORATIVE (STANDARDIZED) CARE FOR ALL NEWBORNS DURING THE FIRST 4 HOURS AFTER BIRTH

Perform a comprehensive assessment to identify individual needs for parental teaching, emotional support, and physical care of infant.

▉ **Potential Complication of Transition to Extrauterine Life: HYPOGLYCEMIA**

Focus Assessments

- Assess labor and birth record for the length of labor, type of birth, use of instrumentation, fetal distress during labor, maternal fever, length of time from rupture of membranes to birth, and medications administered. All of these are stressors that can cause increased consumption of glucose, depleting the serum level.
- Review prenatal record of maternal screening, including glucose tolerance testing at 28 and 32 weeks' gestation and various intervals throughout the pregnancy, depending on the risk. Determines presence of gestational diabetes.
- Review prenatal and birth record for presence of maternal diabetes. Infants of diabetic mothers are at increased risk for hypoglycemia. Constant exposure to high levels of glucose in utero causes hyperplasia of the fetal pancreas and results in hyperinsulinemia. When the cord is cut at birth, the infant's high insulin level causes the blood glucose level to fall rapidly, resulting in hypoglycemia.

- Assess birth weight. Low-birth-weight and preterm infants are at high risk for hypoglycemia because they have inadequate stores of glucose and fat and decreased muscle protein and other nutrients. Large-for-gestational-age infants are also at risk for hypoglycemia.
- Monitor temperature and respiratory status. Identifies changes so that measures can be taken to prevent hypothermia and respiratory distress, which may lead to hypoglycemia due to increased oxygen consumption and metabolic rate.
- Monitor blood glucose at birth if indicated per hospital protocol. Routine testing at birth should be done for newborns at high risk (i.e., large for gestational age, small for gestational age, or low birth weight). This is often a part of routine care because the glucose level declines during the first hours after birth and hypoglycemia may be asymptomatic. When the cord is cut at birth, the glucose supply from the placenta is abruptly removed.
- Observe for jitteriness, irregular respiratory efforts, cyanosis, apnea, weak cry, feeding difficulty, lethargy, low body temperature, twitching, eye rolling, and seizures. These are signs of low blood glucose, which indicate the need to check the blood glucose and institute corrective measures as needed.

Preventive Nursing Activities

- Institute early feeding; provide supplemental formula to breastfed infants if blood glucose is less than 50 mg/dl. Feeding will usually eliminate hypoglycemia in a low-risk, term infant by providing food, which can be converted to glucose. Note: The definition of hypoglycemia varies by facility. Some facilities define it as blood glucose less than 40 mg/dl. Provide a thermoneutral environment and do not let the infant become chilled. Immediately following birth, the newborn should have skin-skin contact with the mother and be dried and covered with a warm blanket and hat to decrease heat loss. Hypoglycemia is aggravated by hypothermia, which increases the infant's metabolic rate.
- Support respiratory transition to extrauterine life. Hypoglycemia is worsened by respiratory distress.

▉ **Potential Complication of Transition to Extrauterine Life: HYPERBILIRUBINEMIA**

Refer to "Hyperbilirubinemia," beginning on p. 436 in Chapter 12.

Focus Assessments

- Review maternal records for diabetes, intrauterine infections, and medications (e.g., sulfa, salicylates, diazepam, oxytocin). These are factors that predispose the newborn to hyperbilirubinemia.

- Be aware of maternal and fetal blood types. ABO and Rh incompatibility may result in jaundice.
- Review newborn records and assess for pyloric stenosis, sepsis, cephalohematoma, asphyxia neonatorum, hypothermia, and hypoglycemia. These conditions predispose the infant to hyperbilirubinemia.
- Observe for jaundice, especially in the sclera and mucous membranes for early detection. Jaundice occurs first in the head and progresses gradually to the abdomen and extremities. Although jaundice is usually benign, bilirubin may accumulate to dangerous levels. A general rule to estimate bilirubin level in the first week of life is to use the rule of fives, whereby jaundice of the sclera, buccal membranes, and face is approximately a bilirubin level of 5 mg/dl. Jaundice visible to the chest at the nipple line is grossly equal to 10 mg/dl. Yellow skin to the level of the umbilicus usually equates to a bilirubin level of 15 mg/dl. Jaundice extending past the groin suggests a dangerously high bilirubin level of 18 mg/dl or more. This assessment should be reported to the healthcare provider for intervention.
- Assess in daylight. Artificial lighting can distort the actual skin color.
- Differentiate between physiologic and pathologic jaundice. In a normal newborn, jaundice first appears after 24 hrs and disappears by the end of day 7. If jaundice appears during the first 24 hours of life or persists beyond 7 days, it usually is a sign of a pathologic process.
- Review birth records for bilirubin levels. A serum level of unconjugated bilirubin of 2 mg/dl is normal in cord blood. In physiologic jaundice, the level will peak at more than 6 mg/dl by 72 hr of age. No toxicity occurs at these levels.
- Assess to determine if the newborn voided or had a stool since birth. Bilirubin is eliminated in feces and urine.

Preventive Nursing Activities

- Feed infant within the first hour after birth. Helps to prevent hyperbilirubinemia by promoting hydration and stimulating intestinal activity and passage of meconium, helping to keep the serum bilirubin level low (bilirubin is eliminated in the urine and feces).
- Place the crib near a window if possible and practical, but do not overheat infant. Natural sunlight though a window can help reduce bilirubin through the skin.
- Provide thermoneutral environment; prevent cold stress. Cold stress can result in acidosis, which weakens the ability of albumin to bind bilirubin and increases the level of free bilirubin.
- Teach parents how to assess and report jaundice. The infant may be discharged before 48 hours, so jaundice may appear or worsen after the family returns home. One reason for this is that dehydration may occur if the breastfeeding infant is discharged before the mother's milk supply is established.

Potential Complication of Transition to Extrauterine Life: RESPIRATORY DISTRESS

Focus Assessments

- Review the prenatal and labor record for risk factors. The prenatal record contains information about problems during the pregnancy. The labor record contains information about problems occurring during labor and birth that may predispose the infant to respiratory distress.
- Review labor record specifically for types and timing of pain medications given to the mother. Narcotic analgesics cross the placenta. Given too close to the time of birth, they may cause respiratory depression in the newborn. Narcotic antagonists will reverse respiratory depression and restore normal breathing.
- Monitor respirations on admission to newborn nursery and at least every 30 min until stable for at least 2 hr; then every 8 hr or according to facility policy. For early detection and treatment of respiratory distress.
- Auscultate lungs for adventitious sounds, ventilation, respiratory rate and pattern, use of accessory muscles, chest for retractions and symmetrical movement, audible sounds such as grunting, and nasal flaring. Signs of respiratory distress alert the nurse to intervene to prevent complications.
- Assess for other signs of neonatal respiratory distress— tachycardia 170 beats per minute or more, apneic episodes longer than 15 sec, respirations fewer than 25 breaths/min, respirations more than 60 breaths/min, expiratory grunting, crackles, rhonchi or wheezing, nasal flaring, chin tug, sternal retractions, asymmetrical chest movement, and labored breathing. These are signs of respiratory distress. Respiratory insufficiency increases heart rate and oxygen consumption as the heart attempts to compensate for lack of oxygen or poor ventilation/perfusion ratios.

Preventive Nursing Activities

- Keep a bulb syringe with the newborn at all times. Routine suctioning of the newborn at birth is no longer recommended. If the oropharynx and nose become blocked with secretions, the bulb syringe will be readily available for immediate action. Invasive suctioning is only required if the infant is not vigorous.
- Position the newborn in a head down position if suctioning is required. Gravity will assist with the removal of secretions and help prevent aspiration.
- Demonstrate to the mother and family how to position the newborn for feeding, burping, and rest. Place in supine position; do not place prone for sleep. Makes use of gravity to promote drainage of mucus from the mouth. Because

the infant cannot spit out pharyngeal secretions or regurgitated feedings, aspiration may occur. Also, the prone position has been associated with increased incidence of sudden infant death syndrome (SIDS).

- Teach mother and family signs of choking, i.e., gagging, cyanosis, apnea. The mother and family may be with the newborn after the initial assessment period when the newborn chokes. This information will enable them to take immediate actions.
- Teach mother and family how to use the bulb syringe, and keep bulb syringe accessible in crib. After the initial assessment period the nurse may not be present when the newborn needs to be suctioned. During the second period of reactivity there is an increase in mucus production, which can block the airways. The bulb syringe must be compressed before being inserted in the nares or the side of the mouth. Placing the tip of the bulb syringe on the center of the tongue will cause the newborn to gag and will not be effective.
- Inform the mother and family how to contact the nurse in the event of respiratory distress, apnea, or cyanosis. Provides immediate assistance if newborn has a blocked airway.

Potential Complication of Transition to Extrauterine Life: INFECTION

Also refer to the generic NDCP, "Risk for Infection,[1]" which begins on p. 21 in Chapter 2.

Focus Assessments

- Note on the newborn's record if the mother is group B strep positive, hepatitis B positive, human immunodeficiency virus positive, or has active herpes or other infectious diseases or conditions that may increase the risk for postnatal infection. Assists with planning preventive collaborative interventions.
- If the mother is positive for group B strep, determine if she was given antibiotics during labor. Prevents neonatal infection. Note: Maternal antibodies may obscure the interpretation of the infant's cultured blood.
- Assess skin integrity. Loss of skin integrity provides a portal of entry for pathogens. The newborn may have loss of skin integrity due to fetal scalp monitor and birth trauma. The umbilical cord and circumcised penis (for male infants) are other portals of microbial entry. The newborn has passive immunity at birth but has an immature immune system.
- Assess for other signs of an infection; e.g., lethargy, weak cry, poor muscle tone, mottling, pallor, apnea. Because

temperature may be subnormal, labile, or elevated from an infection, the nurse must assess for other signs. Poor feeding and respiratory distress often accompany an infectious process. Drainage (e.g., from eyes or cord), redness, rash, blisters, or warmth at the site are other signs; however, they usually occur later than 4 hours after birth.

Preventive Nursing Activities

- Administer fluids as ordered. Hydration helps to prevent stasis of secretions and infection.
- Wash hands at beginning of shift, from the fingertips to the elbows, for 2–3 minutes with good friction and soap. Removes pathogens and prevents transfer of microbes to newborn. Washing from the fingertips to the elbows covers the hands and arms that come in contact with the newborn. Friction, soap, and water help to remove pathogens.
- Wash hands for at least 15 seconds between newborn contact and contact with other objects or other newborns. Removes pathogens and prevents transfer to newborn.
- Teach good hand-washing techniques to everyone in contact with the newborn. Minimizes the chance that pathogens will be transmitted.
- Wear gloves for any contact with amniotic fluid, blood, urine, stool, or any other body secretions, and wash hands after removing soiled gloves. These are sources of pathogens that might be transferred to or from the infant. Nurses and hospital staff must protect themselves from blood and body fluids. Newborns have blood and amniotic fluid on their bodies immediately after birth until the first bath. Bathing and changing diapers and wet linens require gloves. Gloves may become less protective with time and use. Hand washing after removal adds further protection.
- Avoid transferring objects from one infant's crib or warmer to another's. Pathogens can be transmitted from one crib or warmer to another by objects used for more than one infant. The electronic thermometer is an example of an object that should be held or placed outside of the crib or warmer.
- Clean stethoscope after each newborn assessment, or use a different one for each infant. Prevents transfer of pathogens from one infant to another.
- Treat each crib, self-contained incubator (Isolette), and radiant warmer like a patient room, and wash hands after care and before touching another newborn or parts of the newborn's crib, incubator, or radiant warmer. Removes pathogens, which can be transmitted on objects or hands from one newborn to another.
- Hospital personnel with contagious diseases should not provide newborn care. Helps prevent nosocomial infections. The newborn's immature immune status creates susceptibility to contagious diseases.
- Apply triple dye or other antibiotic or antiseptic solutions to the umbilical cord if ordered. Destroys pathogens.

- Teach parents how to keep the umbilical cord clean and dry. The mother will be caring for the newborn's cord site in the hospital setting and at home. The newborn has an immature immune system and the umbilical cord site provides a portal of entry and a moist environment for growth of pathogens. Teach parents how to care for the circumcised infant and that granulation tissue appears slightly yellow, but does not indicate infection and should not be removed. Promotes healing and prevents infection. The circumcision provides a portal of entry for pathogens. Cleaning is very important for preventing infection. Petroleum jelly or ointment may be recommended by the healthcare provider.

- Teach the mother and family signs and symptoms of infection and when to report it to the healthcare provider. Teaching should be done gradually. During the first 4 hours, one or two aspects may be taught; for example, describe the feeding pattern and explain that poor feeding may be a sign of infection or other problem. Each contact with the mother can be used to continue this teaching.

- Educate the mother about how to assess the infant's feeding and hydration. Fluids are important to prevent dehydration and infections. Colostrum in early milk contains leukocytes that augment immunity and protect the newborn from infection.

- Administer erythromycin or other prescribed antibiotic ointment to each eye in the first 2 hours after birth. Prevents the transmission of pathogens (especially *Chlamydia* and gonorrhea) to the newborn during passage through the birth canal. These can cause blindness in the newborn.

- Obtain signed consent form and administer hepatitis B vaccine, per order. It is recommended that all infants receive hepatitis B vaccine; however, for infants born to healthy women with a low risk of hepatitis B virus or with negative screening (HBsAg screening), the first dose may be given at age 1–2 months.

- Administer hepatitis B immunoglobulin prophylaxis intramuscularly within the first 12 hours when the mother has hepatitis B, is a chronic carrier, or has an unknown prenatal history. The immune globulin provides antibodies and provides protection immediately since it does not require the infant to manufacture antibodies.

- Space newborns at least 4 feet apart in the nursery. Avoids contaminating the space of the adjacent newborns and prevents transfer of pathogens from one infant to another. This spacing meets hospital accreditation standards.

- Encourage having the baby room in with the mother if possible. Optimal protection from infection is to minimize direct contact with and physical proximity to others.

Nursing Diagnosis: RISK FOR IMPAIRED PARENT–INFANT/CHILD ATTACHMENT[1]

Refer to the generic NDCP, "Risk for Impaired Parent–Infant/Child Attachment,[1]" beginning on p. 19 in Chapter 2.

Nursing Diagnosis: RISK FOR INJURY[1]

Related Factors: normal physiologic transition changes from intrauterine life to extrauterine life, relative helplessness of the newborn and dependence on others for basic needs, and physical separation between an infant and his or her mother.

NIC Interventions[2]

Environmental Management: Safety (6486)—Monitoring and manipulation of the physical environment to promote safety.

Fall Prevention (6490)—Instituting special precautions with patient at risk for injury from falling.

Newborn Care (6880)—The management of the neonate during the transition to extrauterine life and subsequent period of stabilization.

Newborn Monitoring (6890)—The measurement and interpretation of the physiologic status of the neonate during the first 24 hours after delivery.

Teaching: Infant Safety (5628)—Instruction on safety during first year of life.

Goals, Outcomes, and Evaluation Criteria

- Parents practice safe infant holding, feeding, burping, bulb syringe use, positioning, and security.
- Parents provide adequate nourishment.
- Parents describe normal characteristics and behavior for a newborn.
- Infant discharged safely from birthing setting with no physical injury.
- Parents arrange to take infant home in an appropriate car seat properly secured in the back seat of the vehicle.

Nursing Activities and Rationales

Assessments

- Check that hospital identification bands are accurate and in place. Matching bands are placed on the mother and infant at birth, before they are separated.
- Monitor temperature, heart rate, and respirations at birth, on admission to the nursery or rooming-in unit, every 30 min until the temperature is stable for a minimum of 2 hr, and then every 8 hr or according to hospital policy. Vital signs are useful for identifying a variety of complications.

- Perform head-to-toe physical assessment in the birth area as well as the newborn nursery. Determines if the newborn has any gross anomalies, birth injuries, or complications that require immediate interventions. A second head-to-toe assessment is made to determine how the newborn is transitioning from intrauterine to extrauterine life and to continue to assess for normal and abnormal functioning.
- Assess circumcised penis for bleeding and infection. Ensures early treatment should complications develop.

Independent Nursing Actions

- Practice hospital security policy for newborns and teach the mother and family the same. Prevents abduction.

Parent/Family Teaching

Teach safety measures that include the following:
- Methods for identification of the newborn while in the birth setting. Safety is an important issue in the hospital environment. The newborn and mother will have matching wrist/ankle bands that are used for identification purposes. In some hospitals the father may also have a matching band. Healthcare providers must always check and compare the names and numbers on the bands to insure safety.
- Normal newborn physical characteristics. Promotes bonding; provides an opportunity for questions and concerns about the newborn; provides reassurance of normal findings; provides an opportunity to reinforce how the newborn responds to the parents; and demonstrates safety measures.
- Cues that newborns send to the mother and caregivers. Cues are a form of communication that helps to ensure that the infant's needs are met. For example, if the newborn is crying, the mother and family can learn to ask themselves the following questions: Does the baby have a wet or soiled diaper? Has the baby regurgitated? Is the baby lying in cold, wet linens? How long has it been since the baby has eaten? Is the baby hungry? Does the baby need burping? Does the baby want to be held and comforted?
- Positions for holding the newborn and supporting the neck and head; teach cradle, football, and upright holding positions. Ensures that the infant's neck and head are supported to prevent injury.
- Methods for feeding the newborn. The newborn should be held at the breast level, slightly inclined, with the bottle held so liquid is covering the nipple opening, to facilitate swallowing, meet nutritional needs, and prevent choking.
- Need for and how to burp the newborn (after each ½ oz of formula or after nursing from one breast). Prevents discomfort and regurgitation with possible aspiration. Elimination of air from the stomach may also help reduce the infant's feeling of fullness and promote better feeding.
- How to position the newborn during feeding as well as in the crib. A nonprone position reduces the risk for aspiration and SIDS. The prone position increases the risk for SIDS.
- How to contact the nurse if parents need immediate assistance with the newborn. After the initial stabilization period, the newborn is placed in an open crib and taken to the mother's room. The mother must be aware of how to contact the nurse in case of an emergency such as choking or apnea.
- Need to keep a bulb syringe always with the newborn. In case of choking or excess mucus.
- How to change the diaper and clean the genitalia; the importance of keeping track of stooling and voiding. Prevents skin irritation. Stooling and voiding (6–10 voidings/day) are an indication of the adequacy of nutrition and hydration. Number of stools passed varies; a breast-fed baby should have at least two bowel movements every 24 hr. In the first 2 weeks, stools of the bottle-fed baby decrease to one or two per day.
- How to know if the newborn is receiving enough to eat. Ensures adequate nutrients, maintains a normal glucose level, and prevents high bilirubin levels.
- When to call the physician for complications. Ensures that necessary interventions are begun promptly.
- How to contact support groups and obtain Women, Infants, and Children (WIC) benefits and other community services. Support groups can help provide assistance at home and help ensure that the infant's needs are met.
- Not to leave infant unattended on bed, tables, or other surfaces without side rails. Prevents newborn from falling. Even a newborn can move enough to fall.

Collaborative Activity

- Provide Vitamin K (phytonadione) 0.5–1 mg (0.25–0.5 ml) intramuscularly, using a 25–30 gauge needle, ⅜–⅝ inch needle, within 1 hour of birth. Increases prothrombin production and prevents hemorrhagic disease in the newborn.

Nursing Diagnosis: INEFFECTIVE THERMOREGULATION[1]

Related Factors: an immature neuroendocrine system; large body surface-to-mass ratio; easy loss of body heat through evaporation, conduction, convection, and radiation; inability to shiver; minimal subcutaneous tissue; and the use of warmers, which can overheat the newborn if not monitored appropriately; overwrapping; and other environmental effects.

Goal, Outcome, and Evaluation Criterion

- Axillary temperature is maintained between 36.5°C and 37°C (97.5–98.6°F); or at 36–36.5°C (96.8–97.7°F) if using a skin probe.

NIC Interventions[2]

Temperature Regulation (3900)—Attaining and/or maintaining body temperature within a normal range.

Nursing Activities and Rationales

Assessments

- Perform a comprehensive physical assessment upon admission to the newborn or mother–baby unit. Provides a baseline and identifies potential problems that can lead to hypothermia or hyperthermia.
- Assess the axillary temperature every 30–60 minutes until stable (or use a thermistor probe to obtain a constant skin temperature reading), every 2 hours for 8 hours, and then every 8 hours or more frequently depending on facility policy. The newborn's temperature is normally unstable initially, requiring frequent monitoring to prevent cold stress or hyperthermia. It should stabilize by the 12th hour after birth. When the newborn is under a radiant warmer, a skin probe constantly monitors the temperature, but an axillary temperature should still be taken to ensure accuracy of the equipment and proper contact with the skin probe.
- Check the newborn's temperature before and after the first bath. The newborn may lose heat during the bath by radiation, evaporation, conduction, and convection and may require rewarming.
- Assess the heart rate and respiratory rate. Temperature fluctuations cause an increase in the respiratory rate, an increased metabolism of brown fat, and an elevated heart rate.
- Assess mother's and family's knowledge and ability to help maintain the infant's normal temperature. The newborn will be staying in the mother's room and can become exposed to cool temperatures if the mother is not aware of the need to maintain the infant's temperature.

Independent Nursing Actions

- A radiant warmer may be used to monitor and help maintain a normal temperature. A radiant warmer provides heat. An automatic sensor keeps the heat within a specified range, usually between 36°C and 37°C (96.8–98.9°F).
- Use radiant warmer when performing procedures (e.g., bathing, assessment). Prevents heat loss and maintains normal body temperatures.
- Place infant away from air drafts. Prevents heat loss by convection.
- Monitor temperatures in the mother's room. Maintains a neutral thermal environment.
- Several methods can be used to help conserve body temperature after birth. The method depends on the mother's and infant's health status, individual situations, facility policy, and the environment. Prevents heat loss by conduction.

- Prewarm the incubator for transport of the newborn from one area to another. Helps prevent heat loss through conduction.
- Prewarm the radiant warmer and the linens. Helps prevent heat loss through conduction.
- Maintain the environmental temperature at 71–75.2°F (21.7–24.0°C) with a relative humidity of 60–65%. Prevents body heat loss to cool air. Temperature standards in the environment are regulated through various agencies. Humidity is an important factor because the newborn has been in a wet environment with a consistent temperature throughout the pregnancy.
- At birth, dry the newborn, place the newborn on mother's chest, and cover both with a warm blanket. Helps prevent heat loss through evaporation. Skin-to-skin contact with the mother provides heat. The warm blanket adds heat and reduces heat loss by convection and evaporation.
- Position the uncovered and unclothed newborn on either side in a radiant warmer. The radiant warmer creates an environment to gain and maintain heat.
- Wrap the newborn in two blankets when moving from the radiant warmer to the open crib. Wrapping in two blankets, one at a time, traps the body heat in the blankets.
- Avoid placing the infant in a drafty area of the room. Convective heat loss can lead to cold stress, which may cause delayed transition to extrauterine life and risk for respiratory distress.
- Postpone the newborn's first bath until temperature is stable and at least 36.5°C (97.7°F) and bathe under radiant warmer. Prevents heat loss by evaporation, radiation, convection, and conduction. Newborns have an immature neurologic system and the environment can increase heat loss. Everyone caring for the newborn must be aware of the mechanisms of heat loss. When the newborn is cold stressed, metabolism increases to raise the body temperature, brown fat is metabolized, glucose becomes depleted, and respirations and heart rate increase. If the newborn becomes acidotic, fatty acids replace bilirubin from the albumin-binding sites and hyperbilirubinemia can result.
- Rewarming the newborn should always be done slowly over a 2–4-hour period. Hyperthermia can happen very quickly in the newborn and cause cerebral damage.

Parent/Family Teaching

- Teach the mother and family to change the diaper, clothing, and linens when wet. Prevents heat loss by evaporation.
- Teach the mother and family the importance of keeping the newborn warm by skin-to-skin contact and blankets or clothing, stocking hat, and double-wrapped blankets during this initial period. Prevents heat loss by convection and evaporation.

Other Nursing Diagnoses

Also assess for the following nursing diagnoses, which are frequently present with this condition:

- Pain[1] related to hospital procedures such as neonatal intramuscular injections, heel sticks for laboratory tests, circumcision, circumcision care, and tape or sensor removal.
- Impaired Skin Integrity[1] related to fetal monitor attachment sites, trauma during birth, cutting the umbilical cord and leaving a stump, scratching self with own nails, denuded skin from tape or temperature sensors, circumcision, lack of normal skin flora, and fragile skin.
- Impaired Parenting[1] related to anxiety over assuming the role of a parent, deficient knowledge of parenting and care of the newborn, hospitalization, and pain interfering with the parenting role.

NEWBORN CARE: 4 HOURS TO 2 DAYS

This section focuses on care of the newborn during the stay in the birthing unit. Use these care plans with those in "Newborn Care: First 4 Hours," which begins on p. 369 of this chapter.

The normal newborn is typically physiologically stable by 4 hours of age. Respirations are well established, body temperature is stable, and the infant is adapting to the extrauterine environment. Circulation is functionally adult, that is, with no extra heart sounds, stable BP, and pink skin color with acrocyanosis. Typically, the initial newborn care and assessment are complete and the infant is ready to stay in the room with mother/family.

Key Nursing Activities

- Assess for and support transition to extrauterine life.
- Promote parent–infant attachment.
- Educate parents regarding infant care.

Etiologies and Risk Factors

Newborn adaptation to extrauterine life is a normal physiologic event, rather than an illness, so risk factors are applicable primarily for high-risk infants.

Signs and Symptoms

Signs and symptoms are not applicable. A normal newborn should not have symptoms of problems. For normal assessment findings, see "Newborn Care: First 4 Hours," which begins on p. 369 in this chapter.

Diagnostic Studies

- Newborn screening tests (e.g., phenylketonuria, galactosemia, hemoglobinopathies, thyroid). Required newborn screening tests vary by state and state protocols should be accessed and

followed. Tests are performed after infant has received at least 24 hrs of feedings to ensure validity. Screening ensures early intervention for identified abnormalities.

Medical Management

See "Newborn Care: First 4 Hours," which begins on p. 369 in this chapter.

Collaborative Problems

Potential complications of newborn status include the following:

- Hyperbilirubinemia
- Infection (umbilical cord, eyes, systemic infection)

Potential complications of circumcision include the following:

- Hemorrhage
- Infection

The following are nursing diagnoses, not collaborative problems. However, they should be a part of the standardized care provided for all newborns:

- Risk for Injury[1]
- Risk for Imbalanced Nutrition: less than body requirements[1]
- Risk for Impaired Parent–Infant/Child Attachment[1]
- Health-Seeking Behaviors[1]

COLLABORATIVE (STANDARDIZED) CARE FOR ALL NEWBORNS 4 HOURS TO 2 DAYS AFTER BIRTH

Perform a comprehensive assessment to identify individual needs for parental teaching and emotional support and infant physical care.

Potential Complication of Newborn Status: HYPERBILIRUBINEMIA

Refer to "Potential Complication of Transition to Extrauterine Life: Hyperbilirubinemia," which begins on p. 370 in this chapter.

Potential Complication of Newborn Status: INFECTION (UMBILICAL CORD, EYES, SYSTEMIC)

Refer to the generic NDCP, "Risk for Infection,[1]" beginning on p. 21 in Chapter 2; also refer to the collaborative care plan, "Potential Complication of Transition to Extrauterine Life: Infection," beginning on p. 372 in, "Newborn Care: First 4 Hours," in this chapter.

Focus Assessments

- Inspect umbilical cord stump for redness or drainage. These are signs of infection. The cord gradually dries up and falls off by the 14th day after birth. Diligent cord care with soap, water, and careful drying prevents infection and helps in drying the cord at the insertion site. The use of alcohol is contraindicated because it slows healing. If the cord has not receded by 2 to 3 weeks of age, the caregiver should notify the healthcare provider. It may be an umbilical granuloma, requiring silver nitrate application.

Preventive Nursing Activities

- Teach parents to avoid exposing the infant to crowds and people with contagious illnesses. Newborns receive some immunoglobulins passively in utero; however, the immune system is immature and incapable of fully reacting until a few weeks after birth.
- Teach parents to recognize signs of upper respiratory infections; e.g., clear mucus in nasal passages. Ensures that proper care will be given by parents, to prevent complications from a simple upper respiratory infection.
- Teach parents ways to care for infant with upper respiratory infection. Increasing fluids, using and cleaning the vaporizer, clearing the nose with bulb syringe, and placing the infant in upright positioning will help liquefy and remove nasal secretions. Newborns are obligate nose breathers and cannot breathe if their nose is not clear. Vaporizers must be cleaned carefully according to instructions because they may provide a medium for bacterial growth, causing a secondary infection.
- Teach parents to consult healthcare provider before medicating the infant; teach to use acetaminophen (Tylenol) instead of aspirin-containing products for pain and fever. Use of aspirin when viral infection is present has been linked to Reye's syndrome.
- Teach signs of sepsis; e.g., poor feeding; decreased muscle tone; frequent vomiting; green, watery stools; fever or hypothermia; fewer than six wet diapers a day; restlessness and irritability; lethargy. These signs may occur after the parents return home with the infant. They must know when to contact the healthcare provider; sepsis can be fatal in a very short period of time.
- Teach parents to inspect palate, inner cheeks, and tongue for white, curdy patches. Gastrointestinal distress and fever may accompany these signs. These are signs of *Candida albicans* (thrush), which may have been acquired during descent through the birth canal. It can also be caused by poor hand washing or contaminated bottles/nipples. Infants with thrush frequently develop diaper dermatitis from this organism. This type of rash is typically very red, raised, and contains satellite lesions. An antifungal oral suspension and skin cream may be needed to prevent further spread of the yeast.
- Inform parents about the benefits of breastfeeding. Human milk conveys passive transfer of maternal immunity to common mucosal pathogens and produces a bacteriostatic effect on *Escherichia coli*.
- Teach the mother and family about the newborn's susceptibility to infections and how to prevent infections during the neonatal period. The mother and family need to understand that the newborn has an immature immune system, and measures must be instituted when they go home in order to prevent and detect infections.

Potential Complications of Circumcision: HEMORRHAGE AND INFECTION

Focus Assessments

- Assess penis for bleeding every 15 minutes during the first hour after the circumcision. Report failure to form clot or continued or heavy bleeding. Thereafter, observe the infant's circumcision site during diaper changes up until at least 2 hours prior to discharge from the hospital. Detects bleeding that might require treatment. Scant bleeding and oozing is normal; however, blood should not saturate the dressing nor persist beyond the first few hours. Persistent bleeding may require treatment (e.g., absorbable gelatin sponge [Gelfoam] or sutures); it may also indicate a clotting disorder.
- Assess penis at each diaper change for redness, edema, or purulent drainage. Timely detection of infection allows for treatment and prevention of sepsis.
- Monitor axillary temperature every 4 hr. Unstable temperature (either high or low) may indicate infection.
- If signs of infection occur, obtain culture of drainage, if any and as ordered. Identifies the specific pathogen and guides medical treatment.
- If signs of infection occur, review ordered platelet and WBC count. Helps to confirm or rule out infection. Normal WBC count for a newborn is $15,000/mm^3$.
- Assess parents' knowledge of circumcision care and complications. Provides data for the nurse to individualize teaching.
- Note and record first voiding after the circumcision. Identifies possible obstruction due to trauma and meatal edema.
- Assess for inadequate urine stream and hematuria. Trauma from the procedure may result in edema of the meatus and urethra, blocking passage of urine.

Preventive Nursing Activities

- Demonstrate changing the dressing, cleansing the penis, and changing the diaper; have parents return demonstration; and explain that if a plastic bell was used, they should observe for displacement and report to healthcare provider if it does not fall off in 7–10 days. Actual practice is the best way to learn a psychomotor skill. Supervising practice ensures that parents know how to perform the procedure correctly and provides opportunity to reinforce their parenting skills.

- Apply petroleum jelly gauze to the circumcision site as recommended by healthcare provider. Prevents bleeding and allows for easy removal and replacement when the gauze becomes soiled. Prevents dried blood from adhering to the diaper and pulling the clot loose.

- If dressing or diaper stick to the penis, do not pull it loose. First, soak with clear, warm water. Avoids pulling the clot loose and causing further bleeding.

- If bleeding is heavy, use sterile gauze pad to apply slight pressure to the site. Mechanically stops bleeding until clot can form.

- If bleeding persists, apply Gelfoam or epinephrine, per order, to the site. Promotes platelet adhesion and clotting.

- Have all personnel having direct contact with the baby scrub for 2–3 min from fingertips to above the elbows, and wash hands vigorously for 15 seconds before and after each contact with the newborn. Advise parents to use antiseptic hand cleaner before touching the baby. Prevents transferring microorganisms to the circumcised penis.

- Teach parents signs of infection and hemorrhage, as needed. Parents need to know that they should report bleeding, infection, and/or difficult or no urination to obtain prompt treatment.

- Teach parents that the yellowish exudate that will form over the site (usually between 24 and 48 hours after the procedure) is normal and that they should not remove it. This information helps them to discriminate between normal healing and what might appear to them to be infected tissue. The exudate is a sign of the granulation process and will disappear spontaneously.

- With diaper change, cleanse penis with warm, sterile water. Removes feces and urine, which may harbor infectious microorganisms.

Nursing Diagnosis: RISK FOR INJURY (ASPIRATION, CARDIAC COMPROMISE, ABO OR Rh INCOMPATIBILITY, AND TRAUMA)[1]

Related Factors: normal dependence of the newborn (e.g., inability to roll over, inability to breathe through the mouth), undetected congenital anomalies, deficient parental knowledge, environmental hazards for suffocation or injury. Also refer to the NDCP, "Risk for Injury,[1]" beginning on p. 373 in "Newborn Care: First 4 Hours," in this chapter.

Goals, Outcomes, and Evaluation Criteria

- Newborn remains free of aspiration.
- Newborn remains free of falls or other injury.
- Parents verbalize and demonstrate safe infant care.

NIC Interventions[2]

Anticipatory Guidance (5210)—Preparation of patient for an anticipated developmental and/or situational crisis.

Fall Prevention (6490)—Instituting special precautions with patient at risk for injury from falling.

Immunization/Vaccination Management (6530)—Monitoring immunization status, facilitating access to immunizations, and provision of immunizations to prevent communicable disease.

Parent Education: Infant (5568)—Instruction on nurturing and physical care needed during the first year of life.

Risk Identification: Childbearing Family (6612)—Identification of an individual or family likely to experience difficulties in parenting and prioritization of strategies to prevent parenting problems.

Surveillance: Safety (6654)—Purposeful and ongoing collection and analysis of information about the patient and the environment for use in promoting and maintaining patient safety.

Nursing Activities and Rationales

Assessments

- Review prenatal and intrapartal records for factors such as maternal diabetes, maternal bleeding, cesarean birth, breech delivery, intrapartal asphyxia, and maternal narcotics or general anesthesia given near time of birth. These conditions/situations decrease the newborn's ability to clear airways of excess fluid, mucus, and aspirated liquids (e.g., feedings).

- Assess for cyanosis (presence, degree, and location). Acrocyanosis, associated with vasomotor instability or mild hypothermia, does not require intervention. Cyanosis and mottling may occur during the second period of reactivity, along with changes in heart and respiratory rates. However, cyanosis that becomes worse with crying or movement may indicate cardiac problems. Cyanosis that improves with crying is usually of respiratory origin, though respiratory-induced cyanosis can also worsen with crying if oxygen reserves are already compromised. Cyanosis not associated with respiratory distress is a sign of congenital heart defect.

- Auscultate heart sounds. Transient systolic murmurs are normal in the early newborn period until the transition to adult circulation is complete. The foramen ovale usually closes 1–2 hours after birth, but the ductus arteriosus remains patent for 3–4 days. Loud, machinery-type murmurs or those associated with an audible or palpable thrill need to be evaluated by a cardiologist.

- Be aware of Rh factor and ABO blood group of newborn and mother (Coombs' test). Identifies Rh or ABO incompatibility, which reduces Hgb levels and oxygen-carrying capacity.
- Inquire about home environment, e.g., running water, heat, supplies for infant care, number of people living in the home. Facilitates identification of conditions/situations that increase the risk for injury to the infant so that appropriate interventions can be planned.
- Assess parents' knowledge of infant care and safety. Identifies teaching needs so that misconceptions can be corrected.

Independent Nursing Actions

- Observe for apnea lasting more than 20 sec, possibly associated with changes in heart rate and skin color. Apnea, which is different from periodic breathing, may require intervention. Periodic breathing is recognized by periods of apnea lasting 5–15 sec and periods of motor activity occurring during sleep; tactile/sensory stimulation converts it to a normal breathing pattern.
- Position the infant supine with his or her head in a neutral position or to the side. Drainage of secretions is enhanced by side positioning of the head.
- Change position of the infant frequently. Expansion of the lungs is enhanced by frequent position changes.

Parent/Family Teaching

Refer to the generic NDCP, "Deficient Knowledge,[1]" which begins on p. 13 in Chapter 2.

- Emphasize the importance of an infant car seat. Proper installation in the car and adjustment of belts are essential for protection of the infant in the car.
- Teach parents the safe method to suction nasopharynx with bulb syringe if needed. Ensures airway clearance without harm to the infant's delicate nasal and oral mucosa. The newborn is an obligate nose breather until about 3–4 weeks of age. Gagging and regurgitation of swallowed mucus are common in the second period of reactivity (2–6 hours after birth); suction will prevent the secretions from being aspirated into the lungs. The newborn's nasal passages are small, so the presence of mucus can easily obstruct them.
- Teach the parents the signs of problems for which they should notify their healthcare provider. During the first week, most hospital readmissions are because of dehydration, jaundice, or sepsis.
- Emphasize the importance of not throwing the infant in the air during play. Risks injury to infant's muscles, joints, bones, and nerves.
- Encourage pacifier use between 4 weeks and 1 year of age while falling asleep. Evidence supported an almost two-thirds reduction in risk of SIDS in infants who used a pacifier when sleeping compared to infants who did not use a pacifier (Hauck, Omojokun, & Siadaty, 2005).

- Advise parents to remove stuffed animals, pillows, blankets, and other objects that could block the infant's nose from the crib, and move crib away from hanging quilts, decorative shelves, or curtains that could pose a risk to the infant in the crib. The infant can burrow under pillows or blankets. Hanging quilts can fall on the baby or cause the baby to become entangled.
- Teach parents to use a firm mattress in the crib. Pliable surfaces such as soft mattresses and sheepskin mattress pads are associated with an increased risk for SIDS.

Nursing Diagnosis: RISK FOR IMPAIRED NUTRITION: LESS THAN BODY REQUIREMENTS[1]

Related Factors: incorrect feeding techniques, ineffective sucking (infant), inexperienced caregivers, maternal nipple/breast soreness, and insufficient breast milk supply. Also see the NDCPs, "Risk for Ineffective Breastfeeding[1]; or Effective Breastfeeding,[1]" beginning on p. 318 in "Postpartum Period: Days 1–2"; and "Risk for Ineffective Breastfeeding[1]; or Effective Breastfeeding,[1]" beginning on p. 325 in "Postpartum Period: First Home Visit," in Chapter 9.

Goals, Outcomes, and Evaluation Criteria

- Newborn loses less than 10% of birth weight during the first 3–5 days.
- Newborn gains 20–29 g/day after day 5.
- Newborn regains birth weight by day 14.
- Newborn has six to eight wet diapers/day.
- Newborn has one bowel movement or more/day.
- Newborn is content after feedings.

NIC Interventions[2]

Bottle Feeding (1052)—Preparation and administration of fluids to an infant via a bottle.
Lactation Counseling (5244)—Use of an interactive helping process to assist in maintenance of successful breastfeeding.
Nutrition Management (1100)—Assisting with or providing a balanced dietary intake of foods and fluids.
Nutrition Monitoring (1160)—Collection and analysis of patient data to prevent or minimize malnourishment.

Nursing Activities and Rationales

Assessments

- Assess infant's weight, number of stools, and number of wet diapers per day. Determines if interventions are needed to maintain homeostasis.

- Compare current weight with birth weight. Infant may lose up to 10% of birth weight during the first 3–5 days. After that, the infant should gain 20–29 g/day and should regain full birth weight by day 14.
- Assess hydration. The most sensitive indicator of dehydration is decreased urine output. Other physical indicators include sticky mucous membranes, jaundice, low-grade fever, and poor skin turgor. A late, uncommon sign of dehydration is sunken fontanels. A well-hydrated infant should have 6–8 wet diapers per day.
- Monitor temperature. Detects infection, which interferes with nutrition by increasing metabolic rate.
- Auscultate infant's bowel sounds and monitor stools. Loose, green stool may indicate infection or excess bilirubin. Hard or dry stool may result from dehydration. Persistent meconium or transition stools after day 4 may indicate insufficient milk transfer.
- Observe parents' feeding techniques. Identifies teaching needs.
- Observe infant while breastfeeding. Facilitates evaluation of positioning, latching on, and suck-swallow reflex.
- Assess adequacy of human milk supply. If problem is with the milk supply, determine whether an insufficient amount is being produced or whether the problem is with transfer to the infant (e.g., let-down).
- If human milk is insufficient, assess for causes. Smoking, stress, fatigue, infection, history of breast surgery, lack of stimulation (minimum of 8 feedings/24 hours), caffeine, or medication use. Insufficient fluid intake can decrease milk supply, for example.

Independent Nursing Actions

- Advise parents about the benefits of breastfeeding. But for those who cannot or choose not to breastfeed, provide reassurance that formula feeding will provide all the nutrients the baby needs, and that feeding times can still be used for close contact and socializing. Some parents fear that the baby will suffer from not being breastfed.
- Assist the mother in improving breastfeeding techniques as needed. Slow weight gain is often caused by inadequate breastfeeding, and the solution is usually to improve feeding techniques. Examples include helping the mother adjust positioning, helping the infant with latching on, or suggesting that the mother add an extra feeding or two per day.
- Consult with a lactation consultant, if available, once ineffective breastfeeding is identified. Facilitates breastfeeding. A lactation consultant is able to work with the mother to improve technique or reduce stress so that breastfeeding becomes effective and enjoyable.
- If breastfed baby is calorie deprived, provide supplementation with a bottle, spoon, nursing supplementer, or cup. The mother may pump her milk between feedings to increase her milk supply. Supplementation is usually needed only for a short time. If there is a latch-on problem, avoid bottles.

Parent/Family Teaching

- Teach waking techniques (rub the baby's back, talk to the baby, sit baby upright, remove baby's clothes). Baby must be awake to feed well.
- Teach parents how to evaluate infant's nutritional status. Breastfed infant should be weighed at 3–5 days and at 2 weeks of age. Feeding problems may not be resolved in the birthing unit or may not even become apparent until the infant returns home.
- Provide information about the infant's fluid requirements; as a rule, neither breastfed nor formula-fed infants need to be fed water. A normal infant needs 80–100 ml of water/kg of body weight per 24 hours. Water may cause the baby to take in less milk, which is needed for calories and nutrients.
- Stress the importance of the first follow-up visit with the heathcare provider. Provides an opportunity to establish a baseline weight and evaluate the infant's nutritional status.
- Demonstrate the method for examining infant's mouth for thrush (infant may bite or gum at breast, may be fussy and gassy, and may have white patches in mouth and on tongue). Monilial infection can interfere with the infant's ability to suck. It can cause maternal sore nipples. Mother and infant are treated simultaneously with an antifungal cream. Bottle-fed babies are also susceptible to monilial infection.
- Teach bottle-feeding technique. Inexperienced parents who are formula feeding usually need teaching and support.
- Explain that newborns may drink as much as they desire. Milk intake increases as a baby adjusts to extrauterine life and the gastrointestinal tract is cleared of meconium.
- Instruct that the newborn should be fed every 3–4 hr, even if that means waking the baby for the feedings. Most newborns need 6–8 feedings in 24 hours.
- Use a flexible schedule for feedings, keeping in mind the need to feed every 3–4 hrs. A rigid schedule may not meet the baby's needs, but the schedule can gradually be adjusted to move feedings to times convenient for the family.
- Never prop the bottle and leave the infant. The baby may choke. This also deprives the baby of interaction during feeding. Feedings provide opportunities to bond with the baby.
- Encourage parent to sit comfortably and hold baby in a semiupright position; hold bottle so that fluid fills the nipple and the air in the bottle does not enter the nipple. Prevents air from entering baby's stomach and causing discomfort.
- Alternate infant's position during feeding; feed for half of feeding holding in one arm, then switch to other arm.

Stimulates infant and promotes development of eye muscles.

- Review formula preparation with the parents; teach safe storage practices; if unsafe sanitary conditions exist in the home, recommend the use of ready-to-feed formula. Prevents infant infections and illness. Improper dilution may cause a sodium imbalance.
- Teach parents to look for cues that the baby is hungry and feed on demand rather than on a rigid schedule. Baby will eat better when hungry. Hunger cues occur even during light sleep and include hand-to-mouth or hand-to-hand movements, sucking motions, rooting, and mouthing. It is best to feed before the baby cries or withdraws into sleep.

Nursing Diagnosis: RISK FOR IMPAIRED PARENT–INFANT/ CHILD ATTACHMENT[1]

Refer to the generic NDCP, "Risk for Impaired Parent–Infant/ Child Attachment,[1]" which begins on p. 19 in Chapter 2. Also see the NDCP, "Impaired Parent–Infant/Child Attachment,[1]" beginning on p. 317 in "Postpartum Period: Days 1–2"; the NDCP, "Impaired Parent–Infant/Child Attachment,[1]" beginning on p. 323 in "Postpartum Period: First Home Visit"; and the NDCP, "Impaired Parent–Infant/Child Attachment,[1]" beginning on p. 316 in "Postpartum Period: Weeks 1–6," in Chapter 9.

Nursing Diagnosis: HEALTH-SEEKING BEHAVIORS[1]

There are no related factors because this is a wellness diagnosis. Also refer to the NDCP, "Health-Seeking Behaviors,[1]" beginning on p. 316 in "Postpartum Period: Days 1–2," in Chapter 9.

Goals, Outcomes, and Evaluation Criteria

The parents:

- Ask questions about health/health promotion (e.g., infant stimulation).
- Implement strategies to eliminate unhealthy behaviors (e.g., smoking).
- Seek information about infant immunizations.
- Seek information about caring for infant and meeting infant's health needs.
- Demonstrate loving and nurturing behaviors with infant.

NIC Interventions[2]

Family Integrity Promotion: Childbearing Family (7104)— Facilitation of the growth of individuals or families who are adding an infant to the family unit.

Health Education (5510)—Developing and providing instruction and learning experiences to facilitate voluntary adaptation of behavior conducive to health in individuals, families, groups, or communities.

Health System Guidance (7400)—Facilitating a patient's location and use of appropriate health services.

Immunization/Vaccination Management (6530)—Monitoring immunization status, facilitating access to immunizations, and provision of immunizations to prevent communicable diseases.

Nursing Activities and Rationales

Assessment

- Assess parents' cultural beliefs and practices when scheduling first follow-up appointment with healthcare provider. In some cultures, the mother and newborn do not leave the home for the first few weeks after birth. This may be a problem if the first visit is scheduled at 3–4 weeks, as is usually the case if a baseline weight check is needed or if there are feeding problems.

Parent/Family Teaching

- Demonstrate how to take an axillary temperature. Helps ensure accurate results. Infant's temperature will fluctuate quickly with changes in environment during the first few days. Finding that the temperature is normal may reassure anxious or inexperienced parents. Taking rectal temperatures may damage fragile rectal mucosa.
- Discuss ways to promote normal body temperature (e.g., be sure bath water is warm, dress appropriately for the room/air temperature, protect from exposure to sunlight, use warm wraps or extra blankets in cold weather). Infant's temperature will fluctuate rapidly in response to environmental changes. A rule of thumb is to dress the infant as the parents dress themselves. Although wrapping snugly in a blanket maintains body temperature and promotes a feeling of security, overdressing in warm temperatures can cause discomfort and prickly heat rash.
- Review infant skin care. Infants have delicate skin, so new clothes should be washed with a mild, nonperfumed hypoallergenic soap before putting them on the infant. Wash clothing with mild detergent and hot water; double rinse to neutralize detergent residue. Do not use petroleum jelly, lotions, or baby powder; there is risk of inhalation from baby powder. It is safe to wash the soft spot on the infant's head.
- Review changes to be expected in color of the stool and normal stool patterns for breast- and/or bottle-fed infants. Stool patterns differ among infants and depend upon the type of feeding. Stools are an indication of fluid and nutrition status, and changes may signal infection or mechanical problems with feeding or stooling.

- Teach to position infant supine to sleep. Facilitates drainage of mucus from mouth, promotes gastric emptying, and helps prevent SIDS.
- Teach to not leave the infant alone on flat surface. Prevents falls because infants can roll and scoot.
- Teach to hold securely with head supported. Infant cannot support erect posture for more than a few moments.
- Stress importance of using a rear-facing car seat from birth to 20 pounds and to age 1 year. Minimizes injury in case of accident or sudden stop.
- Demonstrate bathing and cord care. The diaper should not cover the cord because a wet diaper slows or prevents drying and fosters infection. The bath provides opportunity for arousal and stimulation activities. Sponge baths should be given until umbilical cord falls off and is healed (about 10–14 days).
- Review the schedule for follow-up visits to healthcare provider. This is usually at 1–2 weeks and then every 2 months until 6 months of age, then every 3 months until 18 months of age.
- Review schedule of immunizations with parents and provide written information on the American Academy of Pediatrics recommended immunization schedule. Subsequent scheduling of immunizations can be discussed at healthcare provider visits. Parents will not be likely to remember the complex immunization schedule without written information.
- Stress the importance of follow-up visits to the healthcare provider. To be certain that parents are aware of the need for continued observation of infant's health. Teach strategies for helping to quiet a fussy baby when the cause is not hunger or a soiled diaper. Strategies include placing the infant in a small bed or bassinet, carrying the baby in a front pack or backpack, swaddling snugly in a small blanket, providing nonnutritive sucking (pacifier after breastfeeding is established), placing baby on her/his stomach across parent's lap, patting or rubbing the back while bouncing or swaying legs gently, changing position, holding the infant upright over the parent's shoulder, using skin-to-skin contact, taking baby for a ride in a carriage or in the car, or rocking in rocking chair or cradle. Infants cry to communicate that they are hungry, uncomfortable, wet, ill, or bored—or for no apparent reason. Parents must learn to interpret the cries in order to meet the infant's needs. Parents need reassurance that sometimes babies cry merely to discharge energy, and it is nearly impossible to comfort them at those times.
- Provide written information on developmental milestones. Anticipatory guidance helps parents to understand and enhance the baby's development.
- Explain to parents that the infant will start to have end-of-the-day fussy periods between the ages of 3 and 12 weeks. Allow parents to recognize this is normal.

- Teach ways to stimulate the infant. Interacting with parents is one way in which infants learn about themselves and their environment. Parents can promote the baby's physical, cognitive, and emotional development through massage and other stimulation techniques. It is best to provide gentle stimulation that appeals to one sense at a time (e.g., rocking, singing, visual stimulation, stroking). The autonomic nervous system is immature in the newborn, and the infant may become overstimulated by complex sensory cues.
- Teach parents to recognize infant's cues. For example, positive cues are eye contact, gazing at parent's face, babbling, cooing, smiling, and making smooth movements with arms and legs. Negative cues include pulling away, frowning, turning the head away, arching the back, squirming, flailing arms and legs, and crying. Other avoidance cues may be subtle, for example, yawning, sneezing, averting gaze, and hiccups. The ability to read cues enhances parents' confidence and self-esteem and promotes healthy attachment.

INDIVIDUALIZED (NURSING DIAGNOSIS) CARE PLANS

The care plans in this section were developed to address unique infant needs.

Nursing Diagnosis: PAIN[1]

Related Factors: procedures such as intramuscular injections, heel sticks for laboratory tests, circumcision, tape or sensor removal. . See the generic NDCP, "Pain,[1]" beginning on p. 18 in Chapter 2.

Goal, Outcome, and Evaluation Criterion

- Infant is free from signs of pain.

Nursing Activities and Rationales

Assessments

- Assess for signs of circumcision pain. The foreskin contains many nerve endings. Although in the past there was controversy about the infant's pain experience, they do react to painful stimuli and, of course, cannot verbalize their pain. Acute pain should subside within an hour; however, some behavior changes may be seen for up to 24 hours.
- Assess feeding techniques (parents should burp infant in an upright position before and after feedings; use smaller, more frequent feedings; and be careful not to get air in nipple if bottle-feeding). Improper burping, too rapid feeding, or improper bottle position causes air ingestion, which may result in gas accumulation and pain.

Independent Nursing Actions

- Remove infant from restraints immediately after the procedures. Being unable to move increases the infant's anxiety and, therefore, increases pain.
- Hold and cuddle infant after releasing restraints. Dress and feed him. Speak in a soft, calm voice. Allow parents to hold and comfort baby. Tactile stimuli provide distraction from pain. Cuddling promotes comfort.
- Provide pacifier if bottle feeding and parents do not object. Sucking provides distraction and may be comforting to the infant.
- Feed the infant. Feeding provides opportunity for sucking, which may be comforting and promote relaxation. The baby was probably on nothing by mouth status prior to some procedures and will be hungry and needing the calories.
- Position infant supine following circumcision. Prevents pressure on and irritation to penis.
- Apply petrolatum jelly and gauze dressing to the glans immediately after circumcision and at each diaper change for the first 24 hours as recommended by the healthcare provider. Protects the area from irritation by urine and keeps diaper from sticking to the area.
- Apply diapers loosely and change frequently following circumcision. Keeps diaper from rubbing affected area and prevents burning and irritation from urine and stool.
- Cleanse circumcised area with clear water, avoiding the use of soap when removing feces or urine. Soap causes burning and irritation.

Collaborative Activities

- Administer acetaminophen drops if prescribed. Sometimes prescribed to relieve acute pain after procedures such as circumcism. Some healthcare providers use topical anesthetics (e.g., lidocaine/prilocaine [EMLA] cream) or dorsal penile blocks before circumcision to prevent infant pain.
- Administer sucrose per healthcare provider order, approximately 2 minutes prior to circumcision procedure. Oral sucrose is a safe and effective method of pain management for single pain events.

Parent/Family Teaching

- Teach parents to determine whether there is a pattern in the times the fussiness occurs, or whether it is in relation to feeding times or household activities. Helps identify the cause of the pain.

Nursing Diagnosis: RISK FOR IMPAIRED SKIN INTEGRITY (DIAPER RASH)[1]

Related Factors: irritating effects of ammonia contained in urine; chemical reactions from laundry detergent or diapers; and maceration of skin secondary to prolonged exposure to wet diaper and/or plastic covering.

Goals, Outcomes, and Evaluation Criteria

- Skin intact and free from rash or excoriation.
- Parents verbalize and demonstrate knowledge of proper skin care.

NIC Interventions[2]

Parent Education: Infant (5568)—Instruction on nurturing and physical care needed during the first year of life.
Skin Surveillance (3590)—Collection and analysis of patient data to maintain skin and mucous membrane integrity.

Nursing Activities and Rationales

Assessments

- Assess perineum for redness and/or rash. Identifies the need for interventions. Early intervention may lessen severity of rash.
- Assess parent's knowledge of infant care. Identifies the need for intervention/teaching to prevent diaper rash.

Parent/Family Teaching

- Teach parents to cleanse diaper area with each diaper change. Removes urine and feces, which irritate the skin.
- Advise to not use baby powder or cornstarch. These products may cake when wet and irritate the perineal area and increase the risk for inhalation; cornstarch may promote fungal infection.
- If rash occurs, use barrier ointments such as zinc oxide or A and D ointment. Protects skin from wetness. Other products are available for more severe rashes that have excoriation.
- Teach to use mild, hypoallergenic laundry detergent that is perfume free, double rinse cloth diapers, and dry in the sun. Helps prevent chemical irritation in the newborn with sensitive skin.
- If rash occurs, advise parents to try a different brand of detergent, fabric softener, or disposable diapers. Eliminates possible cause of the rash.
- If rash persists, advise parents to call healthcare provider. Persistent rash may due to a yeast or fungal infection, which will require treatment with an antifungal agent.

Other Nursing Diagnoses

Also assess for the following nursing diagnoses, which are frequently present with this condition:

- Constipation[1] related to insufficient oral fluids, foods eaten by breastfeeding mother.
- Diarrhea[1] related to infection, medications taken by breastfeeding mother.
- Risk for Suffocation/Trauma[1] related to total dependence on caregivers, deficient knowledge of caregivers.

END NOTES

1. Nursing Diagnoses—Definitions and Classification 2009–2011. Copyright © 2009, 2007, 2005, 2003, 2001, 1998, 1996, 1994 by NANDA International. Used by arrangement with Blackwell Publishing Limited, a company of John Wiley & Sons, Inc. In order to make safe and effective judgments using NANDA-I nursing diagnoses it is essential that nurses refer to the definitions and defining characteristics of the diagnoses listed in this work.

2. Bulechek, G. M., Butcher, H. K., Dochterman, J. M. (2008). *Nursing Interventions Classification* (5th ed). St. Louis, MO: Elsevier, by permission.

REFERENCES

Hauck, F. R., Omojokun, O. O., & Siadaty, M. S. (2005, November). Do pacifiers reduce the risk of sudden infant death syndrome? A meta-analysis. *Pediatrics*, 11(5); e716–23.

RESOURCES

Bredemeyer, S. L., Polverino, J. M., & Beeby, P. J. (2007). Assessment of jaundice in the term infant—accuracy of transcutaneous bilirubinometers compared with serum bilirubin levels: Part two. *Neonatal, Paediatric and Child Health Nursing*, 10(1), 5–12.

Carr, S. (2007, February 1). *Evidence summary: Vitamin K (newborn) administration*. Retrieved from Joanna Briggs Institute database.

Caruana, E. (2007, February 9). *Evidence summary: Screening (newborn): Guthrie test*. Retrieved from Joanna Briggs Institute database.

Caruana, E. (2007, April 5). *Evidence summary: Breastfeeding: Feeding according to need*. Retrieved from Joanna Briggs Institute database.

Graham, K. (2007, March 15). *Evidence summary: Breastfeeding: Benefits*. Retrieved from Joanna Briggs Institute database.

James, S. R., & Ashwill, J. W. (2007). *Nursing care of children: Principles & practice* (3rd ed.). St. Louis, MO: Saunders.

McArthur, A. (2008, December 23). *Evidence summary: Breastfeeding: Best practice (successful breastfeeding)*. Retrieved from Joanna Briggs Institute database.

McArthur, A. (2009, April 9). *Evidence summary: Pacifier use*. Retrieved from Joanna Briggs Institute database.

McArthur, A. (2009, April 21). *Evidence summary: Newborn: Immediate care*. Retrieved from Joanna Briggs Institute database.

McCall, E. M., Alderdice, F., Halliday, H., Jenkins J. G., & Vohra, S. (2008). Interventions to prevent hypothermia at birth in preterm and/or low birthweight infants. *Cochrane Database of Systematic Reviews* (I).

McKinney, E. S., James, S. R., Murray, S. S., & Ashwill, J. W. (2009). *Maternal–child nursing* (3rd ed.). St. Louis, MO: Saunders.

Mercer, J. S., Erickson-Owens, D. A., Graves, B., & Haley, M. M. (2007). Evidence-based practices for the fetal to newborn transition. *Journal of Midwifery and Women's Health*, 52(3).

Sexton, S., & Natale, R. (2009, April 15). Risks and benefits of pacifiers. *American Family Physician*, 79(8), 681–685.

Thompson, P. (2008, July 30). *Evidence summary: Neonate pain management: Sucrose*. Retrieved from Joanna Briggs Institute database.

Walker, M. (2008). Principles & practice: Breastfeeding the late preterm infant. *Journal of Obstetric Gynecology and Neonatal Nursing (JOGNN)*, 37(6), 692–701.

Ward, S. L., & Hisley, S. M. (2009). *Maternal–child nursing care*. Philadelphia, PA: F.A. Davis.

Young, C. (Ed.). (2007). *BMJ clinical evidence handbook: Summer 2007*. London, England: BMJ Publishing Group.

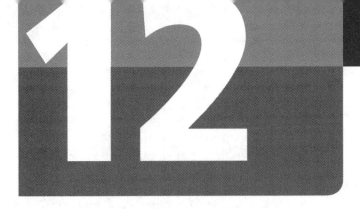

NEONATAL
COMPLICATIONS

Dawn L. Viets

NEONATAL ASPHYXIA

Any condition that decreases oxygen delivery to the fetus can result in asphyxia. Without oxygen, metabolic demands cannot be met, which results in hypoxia, hypercarbia, and metabolic acidosis. Neonatal asphyxia is the most common insult in the perinatal period. Most newborns breathe spontaneously within seconds of delivery and have a regular respiratory pattern by 1 minute of age. However, up to 10% of all newborns require some degree of resuscitation in the delivery room to stimulate spontaneous respirations, and approximately 1% require extensive assistance. Cessation of respirations is the first sign that a baby is oxygen deprived. Infants are considered to be in primary apnea if tactile stimulation resumes breathing. If oxygen deprivation continues during *primary* apnea, the baby enters *secondary* apnea. Assisted ventilation is required to stimulate spontaneous respirations for an infant who is in secondary apnea. Neonatal asphyxia accounts for approximately 20% of all newborn deaths. Infants who do survive birth asphyxia often develop long-term sequelae such as cerebral palsy, intellectual deficiency, or any of numerous other developmental disabilities.

▌ *Key Nursing Activities*

- Early identification of at-risk infants
- Immediate resuscitation of asphyxiated infants
- Continued observation and assessment of resuscitated infants
- Anticipation of diagnostic testing needed to determine etiology
- Physical and emotional support of parents
- Provision of information about and an orientation to the neonatal intensive care unit (NICU)

▌ *Etiologies and Risk Factors*

Neonatal asphyxia can be caused by trauma from a prolonged labor, precipitous birth, multiple gestation, shoulder dystocia, abnormal presentation, or delivery assisted by vacuum or forceps. Fetal hypoxia can also be caused by maternal hypoxia, diabetes, anemia, hypertension, cord compression, or meconium aspiration. Sepsis, congenital malformations, renal anomalies, pulmonary hypoplasia, certain neuromuscular disorders, esophageal atresia, and neural tube defects are additional contributing factors. Infants experiencing hypovolemic shock secondary to placenta previa, placental abruption, and umbilical cord rupture are at increased risk for asphyxia. Other risk factors include medications given to the mother during labor and maternal use of hypnotics, analgesics, anesthetics, narcotics, oxytocin, and street drugs.

▌ *Signs and Symptoms*

Signs of asphyxia include pallor, cyanosis, tachypnea, apnea, gasping respirations, grunting, nasal flaring, retractions, bradycardia, and hypothermia.

▌ *Diagnostic Studies*

Fetal

- Biophysical profile. Assesses biophysical responses to stimuli providing acute and chronic markers of fetal disease.
- Nonstress test. Reflects the functions of the fetal brain stem, autonomic nervous system, and heart.
- Contraction stress test. Assesses fetal heart rate in response to uterine contractions.
- Electronic fetal monitoring. Determines presence of fetal heart tone variations such as decelerations, decreasing baseline variability or increasing baseline rate.
- Scalp blood sampling. Rules out the presence of acidosis, alkalosis, or hypoxia.

Neonatal

- Apgar score. Provides rapid assessment of the need for neonatal resuscitation.
- Chest/abdominal radiograph. Rules out abnormalities/injuries.
- Head ultrasound. Rules out cranial or brain abnormalities/injuries.
- Blood cultures. Rules out the presence of bacteremia (bacteria in bloodstream).
- Urine toxicology screen/meconium drug screen. Determines presence of drugs mother may have used during pregnancy.
- Metabolic screen. Rules out the presence of endocrine or metabolic disorders.

▌ *Medical Management*

Antepartum/Intrapartum Periods

- Prevention of or early intervention for intrauterine asphyxia
- Emergent delivery

Neonatal

- Immediate, effective resuscitation
- Maintenance of neutral thermal environment
- Supportive therapy for hypothermia, hypotension, hypoglycemia, seizures, etc.

Collaborative Problems

- Hypoxia, fetal compromise, and fetal death
- Ischemic brain damage, intraventricular hemorrhage, meconium aspiration (Note: These complications are covered in the NDCP, "Risk for Delayed Development," beginning on p. 387 in this chapter.)
- Necrotizing enterocolitis (NEC) and hypoglycemia (Note: These complications are covered in the NDCP, "Risk for Impaired Nutrition: Less Than Body Requirements,[1]" beginning on p. 388 in this chapter.)

COLLABORATIVE (STANDARDIZED) CARE FOR ALL NEONATES WITH ASPHYXIA

Perform a comprehensive assessment to identify specific family needs for parent teaching and emotional support and infant physical care.

Potential Complications of Neonatal Asphyxia: HYPOXIA, FETAL COMPROMISE, AND FETAL DEATH

Focus Assessments for Antepartum and Intrapartum Periods

- Assess laboratory data (see previous "Diagnostic Studies"). Detects abnormalities that suggest lack of oxygenation or fetal/neonatal compromise.
- Monitor fetal heart rate (FHR) (if less than 100 or greater than 160 beats/min). Determines FHR and variability (increased, decreased, or absent), or late decelerations, which indicate decreased fetal oxygenation. Monitor every 30 min during active labor and every 15 min during second stage of labor.
- Monitor for changes in fetal movement. Increased movement followed by decreased or absent movement is an indication of hypoxia. For the low-risk woman, monitor every 30 min during active labor and every 15 min during second stage of labor. For high-risk women, monitor every 15 min during active phase and every 5 min during second stage.

- Inspect amniotic fluid for meconium (determine whether it is thin, moderate, or particulate). Presence of meconium in the amniotic fluid suggests fetal distress and may lead to neonatal respiratory distress, pneumonitis, pneumothorax, or airway obstruction.
- Perform sterile vaginal exam. Detects prolapsed cord, which is a true obstetric emergency and requires immediate intervention to restore fetal circulation.

Focus Assessments for the Neonatal Period

- Determine Apgar scoring at 1 and 5 minutes. If score at 5 minutes is less than 7, assign score every 5 minutes for up to 20 minutes. The Apgar score does not determine the need for resuscitation or the necessary resuscitative steps. Rather, it gives an overview of the newborn's condition and response to resuscitation. A score between 7 and 10 is considered normal. Scores lower than 7 indicate the need for intervention. The 5- and 10-minute scores are more sensitive prognostic indicators than the 1-minute Apgar score. This method of neonatal assessment in the first minutes of life is useful for monitoring the effectiveness of measures to increase and/or maintain oxygenation.
- Assess cord/arterial blood gases (ABGs). Determines the presence of acidosis related to tissue hypoxia and determines whether asphyxia occurred during intrapartum period or after birth.
- Monitor vital signs (VSs). Detects signs of compromise due to lack of oxygenation including decreased temperature, decreased heart rate (bradycardia), decreased blood pressure (hypotension), and altered respirations (apnea, tachypnea, retractions, grunting, and nasal flaring).
- Monitor color. Detects signs of hypoxia or compromised oxygenation (pallor, cyanosis).
- Monitor muscle tone. Signs of altered oxygenation or hypoxia include decreased tone and depressed or absent reflexes.
- Monitor glucose level and observe for signs of hypoglycemia (e.g., jitteriness, lethargy, cyanosis, apnea, poor feeding, seizures, and high-pitched or weak cry). Ensures euglycemia. Neonates with perinatal asphyxia are at risk for developing hypoglycemia because of the metabolic demands of stress. Less commonly, some infants develop hyperglycemia (high blood sugar) in response to stress.

Preventive Nursing Activities for the Antepartum Period

- Identify women at risk for impaired maternal–fetal circulation. All neonates should be considered at risk for altered tissue perfusion until fully stabilized after birth. However, those with increased risk factors for perinatal asphyxia require vigilant assessment and FHR monitoring. Monitor high-risk women every 15 min during active labor and every 5 min during second stage.

- Teach at-risk pregnant women to monitor fetal movement and report changes in activity. Increased fetal movement may represent compromised oxygenation as the fetus struggles due to hypoxia. Increased movement followed by decreased movement or absence of movement is a sign of severely compromised fetal oxygenation. Decreased fetal movement warrants immediate evaluation.

Preventive Nursing Activities for Labor and Birth

- Position the woman in a lateral position during birth. Enhances uterine perfusion by displacing the uterus off the maternal abdominal aorta.
- During labor, administer oxygen, increase the rate of intravenous (IV) fluids, discontinue oxytocin (if infusing), and notify the care provider when late or variable decelerations or tetanic contractions are noted. Decelerations or tetanic contractions indicate fetal oxygen compromise. When the infant's FHR indicates fetal compromise, the mother typically receives oxygen during the birth process to increase oxygen to the fetus. Increasing hydration improves circulation and delivery of oxygenated blood. Oxytocin stimulates uterine contractions, which can further compromise fetal circulation.
- Assess for possible prolapsed or compressed cord by the presence of severe variable or prolonged late decelerations. Prolapsed cord causes compromise to uteroplacental circulation. This type of poor blood supply and impaired oxygenation can result in life-threatening injury to the infant.
- Have the delivery room equipped with appropriate resuscitation equipment and healthcare team experienced in neonatal resuscitation and airway management during birth. Ensures oxygenation of the infant and prevents permanent injury or death.

Preventive Nursing Activities for the Neonatal Period

- Suction the newborn's oropharynx upon delivery of the head if meconium is present in the amniotic fluid. If the infant is not vigorous, he or she should be taken immediately to the radiant warmer for intubation, tracheal suctioning, and possible resuscitation. Prevents aspiration of meconium. Meconium is a viscous substance that can block the infant's proximal and terminal airways and compromise breathing after delivery.
- Maintain environmental temperatures within the neutral thermal range. Minimizes oxygen consumption and anaerobic glucose metabolism by the newborn from increased metabolic rate.
- Administer oxygen to neonate as ordered. Increases delivery of oxygen to the tissues and organs.
- Maintain a patent airway. Ensures delivery of oxygen to the lungs by positioning infant for maximum respirations and suctioning as needed.

▌ Nursing Diagnosis: RISK FOR DELAYED DEVELOPMENT[1]

Related Factors: ischemic brain damage, intraventricular hemorrhage, and meconium aspiration.

▌ *Goals, Outcomes, and Evaluation Criteria*

- Infant is responsive to stimuli.
- Infant demonstrates smooth, synchronous movements.
- Infant achieves developmental milestones at appropriate age.

▌ *NIC Interventions[2]*

Development Enhancement: Child (7050)—Facilitating or teaching parents/caregivers to facilitate the optimal gross motor, fine motor, language, cognitive, social, and emotional growth of preschool and school-aged children.

Developmental Care (6824)—Structuring the environment and providing care in response to the behavioral cues and states of the preterm infant.

▌ *Nursing Activities and Rationales*

Assessments

- Monitor neurologic status including activity, muscle tone, crying, feeding, and presence of seizure activity. Determines the extent of hypoxic damage, if any. Early recognition of changes facilitates early intervention so that growth and development can be maximized.
- Monitor attainment of developmental milestones. Identifies developmental delays, if any. Delayed attainment of development milestones may be the first indications of fetal asphyxia and resultant injury. The earlier the deficits are recognized and interventions provided, the greater the chance for maximizing growth and development.

Independent Nursing Actions

- Position infant with proper support. Promotes neurobehavioral integration and prevents deformity.
- Promote strategies to facilitate infant attachment. Parents may be grieving the loss of their perfect child and facing issues related to long-term care and quality of life.
- Provide appropriate forms of stimulation according to infant cues and developmental needs. Enhances developmental potential and fosters support of the neonate's capabilities.
- Support family in coping and adaptation to caring for a child with developmental delays and neurologic injury. Raising a child with developmental and neurologic compromise affects the whole family as a unit. The divorce rate is higher in families experiencing this type of stress. Family counseling may be beneficial at some time to facilitate acceptance, communication of feelings, and coping

with the wide array of issues related to a child with special developmental needs.

Collaborative Activities

- Collaborate with physical therapists, occupational therapists, and music-and-play therapists to develop a plan of care. Working with a multidisciplinary team provides opportunities for optimizing the development potential and reinforcing the plan of care.

Parent/Family Teaching

- Teach parents/caregivers to recognize their infant's cues and behavioral states. Facilitates neurobehavioral integration.
- Educate parents/caregivers about normal developmental milestones and associated behaviors (Bulechek, Butcher, & McCloskey, 2009). Provides anticipatory guidance and allows the mother/caregiver to participate in the infant's care.
- Teach and demonstrate activities that promote infant development. Enhances maximal development potential and allows the mother/caregiver an opportunity to participate in care.

Nursing Diagnosis: RISK FOR IMPAIRED NUTRITION: LESS THAN BODY REQUIREMENTS[1]

Related Factors: delayed feedings, NEC, hypoglycemia, and other risk factors.

Goals, Outcomes, and Evaluation Criteria

- Infant tolerates oral/enteral feedings without evidence of gastrointestinal (GI) complications (e.g., feeding intolerance, NEC).
- Maintains glucose within normal levels.

NIC Interventions[2]

Enteral Tube Feeding (1056)—Delivering nutrients and water through a gastrointestinal tube.
Nonnutritive Sucking (6900)—Provision of sucking opportunities for the infant.
Nutritional Monitoring (1160)—Collection and analysis of patient data to prevent or minimize malnourishment.

Nursing Activities and Rationales

Assessments

- Monitor for manifestations of GI complications, such as NEC. Altered intake, apnea, septic appearance, emesis, abdominal distention, decreased or absent bowel sounds,

abdominal tenderness and discoloration, visible loops of bowel, residual feeding in the stomach, and frank or occult blood in stools may indicate NEC.
- Monitor for manifestations of GI complications, such as gastroesophageal reflux. Frequent, small-volume regurgitation, apnea with or without bradycardia, episodes of pallor, or cyanosis may indicate gastroesophageal reflux.
- Monitor glucose levels. Detects hypoglycemia, which may occur within 3 hours of birth from rapid utilization of glucose, reduced glycogen stores, and inadequate gluconeogenesis.

Collaborative Activities

- Notify care provider if hypoglycemia is present and administer feedings/glucose as ordered. Corrects hypoglycemia (see "Monitor glucose levels" under "Assessments," preceding).
- Hold feeding if manifestations of NEC are present and notify care provider. Prevents further gastrointestinal damage due to mechanical irritation. NEC in the newborn can be a life-threatening illness, and treatment must be provided promptly.

Nursing Diagnosis: FEAR[1] OR ANXIETY[1]

Related Factors: maternal fear of infant death or permanent brain damage. See the generic NDCPs, "Anxiety[1]" and "Fear,[1]" beginning on pp. 10 and 15, respectively, in Chapter 2.

Nursing Diagnosis: POWERLESSNESS[1] (PARENTAL)

Related Factors: inability to control the current situation (e.g., to prevent complications of asphyxia or to remove threat to the newborn).

Goals, Outcomes, and Evaluation Criteria

- Parent identifies realistic goals for infant recovery.
- Parent verbalizes feelings of control or lack of control.
- Parent identifies aspects of infant care that are within her control.
- Parent reports adequacy of support systems, including family, financial, community systems.
- Parent participates in decision making with regard to infant care.

NIC Interventions[2]

Mutual Goal Setting (4410)—Collaborating with patient to identify and prioritize care goals, then developing a plan for achieving those goals.

Self-Esteem Enhancement (5400)—Assisting a patient to increase his/her personal judgment of self-worth.

◼ Nursing Activities and Rationales

Assessments

- Assess caregiver's feelings about infant's condition and its effects on the family. Identifies problems that require intervention. Self-esteem can be harmed if the caregiver feels unable to maintain the expected role within the family or that other family members are not being cared for while she is with the sick newborn.
- Assess family support systems. Poor family support during crisis makes it more difficult for caregivers to maintain their own physical and emotional health.

Independent Nursing Actions

- Listen attentively for negative comments about self, feelings of hopelessness, or loss of control. People are not always aware of their true feelings until they have verbally expressed them. Therapeutic listening fosters trust, which is needed when assisting the mother who feels she has little or no control over a situation, or who mistakenly feels that it may be her fault that the baby is ill.
- Offer positive feedback and encouragement for appropriate efforts to participate in decision making and infant care. Demonstrates confidence in the mother's abilities and provides positive reinforcement for continuation of desired behaviors.
- Assure the mother that her infant's outcome was not related to her failure to detect or respond to subtle cues during the pregnancy or during delivery. Feelings of guilt are common when an infant is born with neurological damage related to birth trauma.

Collaborative Activities

- Communicate the emotional needs of the mother/family to her care provider. Nurses spend more time with mother/family than any other healthcare providers do. The information gathered by the nurse is valuable and needs to be shared with other healthcare providers in order to promote continuity of care.

Parent/Family Teaching

- Teach parents to set small, attainable goals for the care of the child/family on a daily basis. Setting goals that are not achievable leads to failure.
- Keep the family well informed about the infant's condition and plan of care. For many people, obtaining information is an effective way to reduce fears and facilitate more effective coping in high-stress situations. Communication with the caregiver can also help to contribute to increased participation in decision making and problem solving.

THE SMALL-FOR-GESTATIONAL-AGE NEWBORN

Newborns are classified as *small for gestational age* (SGA) if they weigh less than two standard deviations below the average for their gestational age or if their length, weight, and/or head circumference falls below the 10th percentile on a growth chart. This means they are smaller than 90% of all other babies of the same gestational age. SGA babies typically weigh less than 2,500 grams (5.5 pounds), which puts them in the *low birth weight* category. A baby born at less than 1,500 grams (3 pounds, 5 ounces) is said to be of *very low birth weight,* and the infant weighing less than 1,000 grams (2 pounds, 3 ounces) is *extremely low birth weight*. When rate of growth varies from expected growth pattern in the SGA infant, it is referred to as *intrauterine growth restriction* (IUGR). Infants who suffer from intrauterine growth restriction have increased morbidity and mortality rates. SGA infants are not always IUGR and IUGR infants are not always SGA.

IUGR is described as symmetrical or asymmetrical. A symmetrically IUGR infant is one who has a poor growth rate of the head, abdomen, and long bones. An infant with asymmetric IUGR has normal growth of head and long bones, but restricted growth of abdomen and internal organs. Typically, IUGR is a continuum from asymmetry in the early stages to symmetry in the late stages of growth and development.

◼ Key Nursing Activities

- Document and compare weight, length, and head circumference.
- Monitor vital signs.
- Maintain thermoregulation.
- Monitor serial blood glucose values.
- Initiate early and frequent feedings.
- Establish intravenous nutrition plan if oral feeds not possible.
- Monitor for signs of polycythemia.
- Offer emotional support and anticipatory guidance to parents.
- Provide information about and an orientation to the NICU.

◼ Etiologies and Risk Factors

Fetal growth is affected by genetic, placental, and maternal factors. Maternal reasons for poor fetal growth include infection, substance abuse, increased blood pressure, chronic renal disease, advanced diabetes, cardiac disease, respiratory disease, malnutrition, and anemia. Poor growth can also be attributed to decreased uteroplacental blood flow, placenta previa, placental abruption, multiple gestation, birth defects, and chromosomal abnormalities.

◼ Signs and Symptoms

Signs include weight, length, and head circumference less than the 10th percentile; a head that is disproportionately large in contrast to the rest of the body; wasted appearance of extremities; reduced subcutaneous fat; decreased breast tissue; scaphoid (sunken) abdomen; widened cranial sutures; decreased muscle tone over buttocks and cheeks; loose skin; and thin umbilical cord.

Diagnostic Studies

- Gestational age assessment. The assessment of physical and neurologic findings to determine maturity.
- Weight and body measurements. Determines if the infant is within or outside the normal range of birth weight.
- Genetic studies. Determines the presence of genetic abnormalities that may affect the infant's growth patterns.
- Metabolic screens (phenylketonuria, thyroid, etc.). Rule out the presence of abnormalities that affect growth patterns.
- Complete blood cell count (CBC). Monitors hemoglobin and hematocrit.
- Blood type. Includes Rh factor and ABO group.
- Point of care glucose (e.g., Dextrostix). Less than 50 mg/dl indicates hypoglycemia. Note: The definition of hypoglycemia varies by agency, some defining it as blood glucose less than 40 mg/dl.
- Serum glucose. Confirms the presence of hypoglycemia.
- TORCH (toxoplasmosis, other, rubella, cytomegalovirus, herpes). Determines if congenital infection is the etiology for poor growth.
- Chest X-ray and arterial blood gas. Help establish differential diagnosis for respiratory distress.
- Blood urea nitrogen, creatinine. Detect impaired kidney function secondary to intrauterine malnutrition and/or asphyxia.

Medical Management

- Supportive care
- Special diet if indicated

Collaborative Problems

Delayed Growth and Development[1] (although this is a nursing diagnosis rather than a collaborative problem, it should be a part of the care given to all SGA infants).

Potential Complications of Small-for-Gestational-Age Infants

- Infection
- Hypoglycemia
- Hypothermia
- Polycythemia
- Meconium aspiration
- Skin excoriation, abrasions, macerations

STANDARDIZED CARE FOR ALL NEWBORNS WHO ARE SMALL FOR GESTATIONAL AGE

Perform a comprehensive assessment to identify individual needs for parent teaching and emotional support and infant physical care.

Nursing Diagnosis: DELAYED GROWTH AND DEVELOPMENT[1]

Related Factors: separation from mother/parents, environmental and stimulation deficiencies, and multiple caregivers.

Goals, Outcomes, and Evaluation Criteria

- Infant remains free of complications (infection, hypoglycemia, and hypothermia).
- Infant's intake is sufficient for consistent growth pattern.
- Infant achieves expected growth norms.

NIC Interventions[2]

Infant Care (6820)—Provision of developmentally appropriate family-centered care to the child under 1 year of age.
Nutrition Therapy (1120)—Administration of food and fluids to support metabolic processes of a patient who is malnourished or at high risk for becoming malnourished.
Nutritional Monitoring (1160)—Collection and analysis of patient data to prevent or minimize malnourishment.
Parenting Promotion (8300)—Providing parenting information, support, and coordination of comprehensive services to high-risk families.

Nursing Activities and Rationales

Assessments

- Weight and length at birth. Determines weight as proportional to length and head circumference for gestational age. A ponderal index, the ratio of weight to length, is used to determine the degree of growth impairment. The risk of perinatal morbidity and mortality are associated with decreased weights for gestational age.
- Head circumference. Determines growth pattern of the brain.
- Monitor parameters of growth over time. Helps determine the presence and degree of growth pattern deviation. Weight gain can be slower in SGA infants because of their increased metabolic needs and reduced distribution of brown fat, which is a source for energy (glycogen) storage. The pattern of growth is a sensitive indicator of the adequacy of nutritional intake.
- Assess for signs of sensory overload. Establishes the appropriate level of stimulation for the infant's size, age, and ability. SGA infants may have altered behavioral responses, decreased activity, or decreased tolerance for stimulation. Sensory overload may be displayed as crying, irritability, restlessness, or facial grimacing. The infant may exhibit avoidance behaviors, such as mottling and pallor, aversion of gaze, hiccups, yawning, and sneezing as a way to shut out external stimulation from environment.
- Monitor caloric intake. Determines if the infant is consuming adequate calories to prevent weight loss and enhance growth.

- Monitor feeding tolerance and signs of GI complications related to feeding. Identifies problems that require further evaluation and intervention (e.g., NEC, intestinal obstruction, gastroesophageal reflux).
- Assess the effectiveness of the infant's suck, swallow, and stamina to sustain effort needed for oral feeding. The inability to suck, swallow, or tolerate feedings will contribute to weight loss.

Independent Nursing Actions

- Encourage frequent feeding (breast, bottle, gavage) every 3–4 hours. Adequate nutrition is essential for growth and development in at-risk infants. Frequent feedings of small amounts are more readily tolerated and help prevent hypoglycemia, which can occur rapidly in the SGA infant. Also helps maintain fluid and electrolyte balance.

Parent/Family Teaching

- Provide information and instruct mother about any special diets ordered. Special diets may be ordered to enhance growth and development and prevent malnutrition or hypoglycemia. Weight loss can occur over time in infants with excessive energy expenditure during feedings. Increased understanding of prescribed diet may enhance compliance.
- Teach parents appropriate stimulation techniques for infant's abilities. Maximizes the infant's development without producing sensory overload. Also assists parents in assuming their role as they move from acute care to home. Due to the immaturity of the autonomic nervous system, the infant is often unable to process multisensory stimulation.
- Teach parents the need to follow up developmental assessments. Helps ensure that future monitoring of the infant will occur in order to maximize the infant's growth and development. Parents who understand the need for follow-up monitoring are more likely to be compliant.

Potential Complication of Small-for-Gestational-Age Infant: INFECTION

Focus Assessments

- Evaluate for maternal history of sexually transmitted infections, TORCH infection, HIV, or premature rupture of membranes. Perinatal infections increase the risk of an infant being SGA.
- Assess for decreased temperature. Temperature regulation is compromised in the SGA infant due to decreased glycogen stores and decreased brown fat. Fever is not necessarily present with neonatal infections.

- Assess heart rate for tachycardia or bradycardia. Neonatal sepsis increases the metabolic demand of the infant, resulting in increased heart rate and bradycardia when compensation is no longer possible.
- Assess respirations for tachypnea, apnea, grunting, retracting, and nasal flaring. Increased oxygen demand associated with sepsis and cold stress result in signs of respiratory distress.
- Assess skin for rash, pustules, petechiae, purpura, and jaundice. Common findings associated especially with the TORCH infections are rashes, petechiae, purpura, and jaundice. Pustules suggest herpes.
- Assess for neurologic signs such as lethargy, jitteriness, irritability, seizures, hypotonia, bulging fontanels, and high-pitched cry. Meningitis and inflammation secondary to TORCH infections result in neurologic changes.
- Assess GI system for poor feeding, vomiting, abdominal distenion, and residuals. Inflammation of the gastrointestinal tract leads to poor feeding, vomiting, abdominal distention, residuals, and irritability due to abdominal cramping. SGA infants are at increased risk for infection and inflammation of the GI tract.
- Assess abdomen for hepatosplenomegaly. Hepatosplenomegaly is a common finding associated with the TORCH infections.
- Monitor CBC for neutropenia and thrombocytopenia. Neutropenia and thrombocytopenia are common neonatal findings in infection due to rapid depletion of the neutrophil storage pool and platelet destruction.
- Review culture reports for positive findings. Cultures are used to identify the etiologic agent associated with the infection.

Preventive Nursing Activities

- Teach pregnant women to avoid contact with people/situations that could lead to TORCH infection, especially in early pregnancy. Decreases risk of exposure.
- Encourage early prenatal care and treatment of STDs. Prevents transmission of pathogens to the neonate.
- Educate pregnant women regarding manifestations associated with rupture of membranes. Prevents development of chorioamnionitis.
- Deliver infants of women with active herpes infections by cesarean birth. Prevents neonatal transmission of herpes virus.
- Practice good hand-washing and infection control measures. Prevents iatrogenic infection of the SGA neonate, who has low resistance to infection due to immaturity and decreased nutritional state.
- Discourage the mother who is HIV positive from breastfeeding. Prevents transmission of the HIV virus from mother to infant.
- Avoid blood transfusion with cytomegalovirus-positive blood during pregnancy. Although cytomegalovirus

does not typically cause significant illness in immune-competent adults, the virus transmitted to an infant during pregnancy can have profound effects on the neurodevelopment of the fetus, including symmetric growth restriction, impaired neurologic function, and pneumonia with respiratory distress.

Potential Complications of Small-for-Gestational-Age Infant: HYPOGLYCEMIA AND HYPOTHERMIA

See the collaborative care plan, "Potential Complication of an Infant of a Diabetic Mother: Hypoglycemia," beginning on p. 399 in "Infant of a Diabetic Mother" in this chapter. Also see the collaborative care plan, "Potential Complication of Postterm Birth: Hypothermia," beginning on p. 433 in "Postterm Newborn," in this chapter.

Focus Assessments

- Monitor temperature. Decreased temperature can be a sign of hypoglycemia. Temperature is difficult to regulate in SGA infants due to decreased muscle mass, decreased subcutaneous fat, limited brown fat stores, increased body surface exposed to the environment, and limited ability to control skin capillaries. Signs of cold stress include apnea, bradycardia, respiratory distress, acidosis, central cyanosis, lethargy, weak cry, abdominal distention, and hypoglycemia. Cold stress increases glucose utilization and intensifies hypoglycemia.
- Monitor heart rate. Tachycardia or bradycardia may occur in response to decreased oxygenation (hypoxia).
- Monitor respirations for tachypnea or apnea. SGA infants typically do not suffer respiratory distress syndrome to the extent that distressed (appropriate weight for age) preterm infants do because of their natural bodily response to accelerate surfactant production. However, depending on the cause of growth restriction in utero, there may be respiratory findings with tachypnea, apnea, hypoxemia, and respiratory acidosis. For example, if the infant is SGA due to TORCH infection, the infant may be showing signs of pneumonia. Additionally, respiratory signs, such as tachypnea, may be associated with problems such as hypoglycemia.
- Monitor neurologic status. Detects neurologic changes that indicate hypoxia, such as jitteriness, seizures, lethargy, weak cry, or tremors. Jitteriness, lethargy, cyanosis, apnea, high-pitched or weak cry, poor feeding, and seizures might also be indicative of hypoglycemia.
- Monitor skin color and perfusion. Cyanosis, pallor, or sweating may indicate hypoxia or hypoglycemia.

- Monitor serum glucose levels; begin point-of-care glucose checks at birth, and continue until glucose values have stabilized. Less than 50 mg/dl indicates hypoglycemia. Intervention is necessary to prevent seizures or death; glucose is the primary source of fuel for the brain. Serum glucose levels help to differentiate between signs of hypoxia, hypothermia, and hypoglycemia. Note: The definition of hypoglycemia varies by agency, some defining it as blood glucose less than 40 mg/dl.
- Monitor for signs of hypoglycemia. Cyanosis, apnea, irregular respirations, tachypnea, flaccidity, high-pitched cry, tremors, jitteriness, and seizures are signs of hypoglycemia. Signs may occur at any time during the first week, but most commonly between 24 and 72 hours after birth.

Preventive Nursing Activities

- Maintain a neutral thermal environment. SGA infants have decreased brown fat, which alters their ability to regulate their body temperature. Maintaining a thermoneutral environment helps to eliminate heat loss through evaporation, conduction, convection, and radiation.
- Initiate breastfeeding or bottle feeding as soon after delivery as condition allows. Prevents hypoglycemia by supplying glucose to meet the increased metabolic needs of the SGA infant.
- Provide nutritional supplements or IV glucose therapy as ordered. Prevents hypoglycemia and helps to maintain fluid and electrolyte balance.
- Correct acidosis, hypoglycemia, hypoxemia, sepsis, and metabolic problems. Eliminates risk factors for hypothermia or corrects conditions contributing to hypothermia.
- Avoid rapid rewarming of infant. Gradual rewarming helps prevent apnea that can occur from rapid rewarming.

Potential Complication of Small-for-Gestational-Age Infant: POLYCYTHEMIA

Focus Assessments

- Assess for signs of polycythemia. Polycythemia is a condition in which the infant's central Hct is greater than 65. Signs include ruddy or pale skin, peripheral cyanosis, lethargy, cardiopulmonary distress (persistent fetal circulation, cyanosis, and apnea), seizures, hyperbilirubinemia, oliguria, hematuria, and gastrointestinal abnormalities. The ruddy appearance is related to the unsaturated Hgb in the blood, which may mask the saturated Hgb.
- Assess for dehydration (e.g., decreased skin turgor, dry mucous membranes, sunken fontanels, decreased urine output, increased urine-specific gravity, and elevated temperature). Dehydration further increases blood viscosity.

The sludging of blood through the small veins can lead to thrombosis of vital organs, such as the kidneys, brain, and intestines, as well as peripheral sites.

- Monitor hemoglobin and hematocrit. Establishes the presence of polycythemia. Hgb greater than 22 mg/dl or Hct greater than 65% indicates polycythemia. Polycythemia increases blood viscosity and may impair circulation. The increased number of red blood cells (RBCs) increases the risk for hyperbilirubinemia due to the increased number of cells that must be hemolyzed. The by-product of RBC breakdown is bilirubin.
- Monitor for jaundice. Jaundice is produced by increased levels of bilirubin. Bilirubin is increased in the infant who must hemolyze a large load of RBCs.
- Note bilirubin level. May be elevated secondary to polycythemia.
- Monitor signs of chronic fetal stress prior to delivery, such as nonreassuring FHTs, low biophysical profile, and decreased fetal movement. In response to chronic hypoxia, erythropoietin production increases, contributing to the development of polycythemia (and subsequent hyperbilirubinemia).

Preventive Nursing Activities

- Identify possible underlying conditions in newborn. For example, hypoxia, hypoglycemia, and hyperbilirubinemia contribute to polycythemia.
- Establish or maintain intravenous access. Fluids may be needed to correct hyperviscosity; or exchange transfusion may be required.
- Prepare infant for plasma exchange if symptomatic and nonresponsive to aggressive IV therapy for hydration. Prevents complications of polycythemia. Plasma exchanges decrease the viscosity of blood and may relieve symptoms.

Potential Complication of Small-for-Gestational-Age Infant: MECONIUM ASPIRATION

See "Meconium Aspiration Syndrome," beginning on p. 441 in this chapter.

Focus Assessments

- Review prenatal and labor/birth records for indications of intrauterine and birth hypoxia. Infants who have suffered chronic intrauterine hypoxia (such as those who are SGA) are at high risk for acidosis and respiratory depression at birth and for persistent fetal circulation after birth, making them less able to cope with the insult of meconium aspiration.
- Assess for meconium-stained amniotic fluid during labor and birth. The presence of meconium in the amniotic fluid

increases the risk for pneumonitis, pneumothorax, and persistent pulmonary hypertension.

- Assess newborn for meconium-stained umbilical cord and nails. Helps establish the presence of meconium in the amniotic fluid, which increases the infant's risk for aspiration.
- Assess for (visualize) meconium below the vocal cords. Helps establish whether or not meconium has been aspirated into the trachea and bronchi.

Preventive Nursing Activities

- Suction the neonate while the head is still on the perineum. Removes meconium from the pharynx at birth to reduce risk for aspiration. After delivery, if the baby is not vigorous, he/she should be taken to radiant warmer for direct visualization of vocal cords and possible tracheal suctioning. A nonvigorous baby is described as having depressed respirations, decreased muscle tone, and/or a heart rate less than 100 beats per minute. A laryngoscope handle and blade; appropriately sized endotracheal tube meconium aspirator device; suction setup; and oxygen bag, mask, and manometer are needed.
- Avoid stimulating respirations in a nonvigorous, meconium-stained infant until the airway is cleared. Decreases the risk for pulmonary aspiration. After meconium has been visualized and aspirated from the trachea, the infant can be stimulated to breathe. Blow-by oxygen or brief continuous positive airway pressure may be needed transiently to aid the infant in adapting to the stress of the procedure.
- Prevent cold stress. Cold stress increases metabolic demands and oxygen needs.

Potential Complications of Small-for-Gestational-Age Infant: SKIN EXCORIATION, ABRASIONS, AND MACERATIONS

Focus Assessments

- Assess skin for areas of redness, excoriation, abrasion, or maceration. A disruption of skin integrity can lead to infection or further skin breakdown.

Preventive Nursing Activities

- Avoid removing vernix. Vernix caseosa is a protective sebaceous coating that protects the intrauterine fetus and continues to protect the skin following birth.
- Avoid using adhesives, tapes, or alcohol on skin. These substances can cause severe irritation and chemical burns in infants. Alcohol is very drying to neonatal skin. Additionally, the bond formed between the adhesive agent

and the epidermis is often stronger than that between the epidermis and the dermis. Additionally, the skin of a newborn is permeable to topical agents and can lead to systemic absorption.

- Reposition every 2 hours as tolerated. Cluster position changes with feedings and other care as much as possible. Prevents pressure on delicate skin that can lead to breakdown or excoriation, especially over bony prominences, since SGA infants have significantly reduced adipose tissue.
- Protect excoriated, abraded, or macerated areas. Transparent coverings or pectin-based barriers protect areas of the skin that are impaired and help prevent infection by providing a barrier against entry of pathogenic organisms and promote healing and maturation of the skin.

INDIVIDUALIZED (NURSING DIAGNOSIS) CARE PLANS

This section includes care plans that were developed to address unique patient needs.

Nursing Diagnosis: IMPAIRED NUTRITION: LESS THAN BODY REQUIREMENTS[1]

Related Factors: increased metabolic rate, decreased nutrient supply, and metabolic disorders such as phenylketonuria, galactose insufficiency, etc.

Goals, Outcomes, and Evaluation Criteria

- Demonstrates normal growth and weight gain.
- Biochemical measures (glucose, calcium, magnesium, and enzymes such as phenylalanine) return to and remain within normal limits.

NIC Interventions[2]

Bottle Feeding (1052)—Preparation and administration of fluids to an infant via a bottle.
Enteral Tube Feeding (1056)—Delivering nutrients and water through a gastrointestinal tube.
Lactation Counseling (5244)—Use of an interactive helping process to assist in maintenance of successful breastfeeding.
Nutritional Monitoring (1160)—Collection and analysis of patient data to prevent or minimize malnourishment.

Nursing Activities and Rationales

Assessments

- Review prenatal records for IUGR, placental deficiency, low weight gain during pregnancy, and oligohydramnios.

Detection of prenatal risk factors for impaired fetal growth in utero may lead to measures for preventing IUGR.

- Monitor intake and output, weight, and laboratory studies indicating nutritional well-being. Detects abnormalities, establishes a basis for intervention, and evaluates the effectiveness of nutritional interventions. SGA infants may already have lost weight in utero and may have reduced fat/glycogen stores; they may not feed well, which predisposes them to hypoglycemia, hypothermia, malnutrition, and fluid and electrolyte imbalances.
- Assess feeding ability (suck-swallow coordination, breastfeeding success). Determines if the infant is capable of adequate feeding to facilitate growth and weight gain.
- Monitor bowel sounds, presence of abdominal distention, gastric residual contents. Determines the infant's ability to tolerate feedings and helps identify the presence of disease or deformity that impedes the infant's ability to take in milk/formula.
- Monitor serum glucose levels. Detects hypoglycemia. SGA infants have increased oxygen demands and an increased metabolic rate, which quickly depletes their glucose stores. They are unable to generate new glucose (gluconeogenesis) due to insufficient fat and muscle (protein). Hypoglycemia can result in permanent central nervous system (CNS) alterations and may increase infant mortality. Adequate intake helps reduce the incidence of hypoglycemia by providing adequate calories, carbohydrates, fats, and protein. Signs of hypoglycemia include irritability/restlessness, lethargy, increased respiratory rate, irregular respiratory pattern, apnea, tachycardia or bradycardia, shrill cry, and seizures.
- Monitor skin temperature. Detects hypothermia. Hypothermia increases metabolic demands and oxygen consumption, which increases the caloric requirements necessary to prevent further weight loss in a compromised infant.
- Monitor serum calcium levels (Note: hypomagnesemia is usually associated with hypocalcemia). A total serum calcium less than 6 mg/dl or ionized calcium less than 2 mg/dl is an indication of hypocalcemia. Calcium is essential for muscle tone and function. Hypocalcemia may produce twitching, tremors, seizures, vomiting, hypotonia, apnea, or cardiac dysrhythmias. SGA infants are at increased risk for hypocalcemia due to risk factors such as prenatal asphyxia and metabolic disorders.
- Assess for signs of hypocalcemia. Tremors, twitching, seizures, hypotonia, vomiting, cyanosis, apnea, cardiac dysrhythmias, and a high-pitched cry are signs of hypocalcemia, which may be a complication of asphyxia in the SGA infant. Symptoms commonly occur between 48 and 72 hours after birth.
- Be aware of electrolyte levels (e.g., sodium, potassium, chloride, phosphorus, and magnesium). Electrolyte

imbalance may result from intrauterine malnutrition. Hypomagnesemia is usually associated with hypocalcemia.

Collaborative Activities

- Gavage feed as needed. Provides nutrients required for growth. Gavage feedings may be necessary to maintain adequate caloric intake until the infant is able to take all feedings by breast or bottle.
- Prevent cold stress (e.g., use radiant warmer, maintain neutral thermal environment). Hypothermia increases metabolic demands, requiring increased intake of calories.

Parent/Family Teaching

- Teach the importance of correcting malnutrition. Malnutrition, particularly protein deficiency, may lead to cerebral dysfunction (e.g., hyperactivity, learning difficulties, short attention span, poor fine-motor coordination, and speech deficits).
- Counsel mother about ways to facilitate breastfeeding. (Refer to the NDCP, "Risk for Ineffective Breastfeeding[1]; or Effective Breastfeeding,[1]" beginning on p. 318 in "Postpartum Period: Days 1–2," in Chapter 9. Also refer to the NDCP, "Risk for Ineffective Breastfeeding[1]; or Effective Breastfeeding,[1]" beginning on p. 325 in "Postpartum Period: First Home Visit," in Chapter 9.) Improves the success of breastfeeding. Infants who do not latch on or suck sufficiently to receive adequate milk are at increased risk for malnutrition and delayed development.
- Begin feedings as soon as possible after birth. The SGA infant may have inadequate body stores of fat and glycogen from experiencing malnutrition in utero and will need calories to support metabolic processes and prevent hypoglycemia.
- Encourage caregivers to feed in an upright position and to burp frequently. Enhances feeding tolerance and prevents aspiration. Infants swallow air as well as formula/milk when nursing. Air fills the stomach and can result in cramping (colic) or vomiting. Frequent burping facilitates the removal of air from the infant's stomach.
- Teach parents of infants with inherited metabolic conditions about the condition, the need for special diets, and resources available. Prevents life-threatening complications due to inadequate feeding or lack of adherence to prescribed diet.
- Educate parents of infants about how to conserve the energy expenditure of the baby in the daily care. Growth can be impaired by activities that cause the infant to utilize more energy, such as excessive multisensory stimulation and overhandling the baby. Prolonged feeding times, whereby the infant tires while trying to take a sufficient volume, can negatively impact the growth rate. Additionally, the infant who is underdressed will consume calories to warm, and conversely, to cool to a normal body temperature.

Nursing Diagnosis: RISK FOR DISORGANIZED INFANT BEHAVIOR[1]

Related Factors: maternal substance abuse, prematurity, hypoxic brain damage (all of which are associated with SGA), pain, invasive/painful procedures, and environmental overstimulation.

▍ Goals, Outcomes, and Evaluation Criteria

- Infant adapts to extrauterine environment.
- Infant establishes sleep-wake cycles.
- Infant demonstrates neurobehavioral integration.
- Parents recognize infant cues and respond appropriately.

▍ NIC Interventions[2]

Developmental Care (6824)—Structuring the environment and providing care in response to the behavioral cues and states of the preterm infant.

Sleep Enhancement (1850)—Facilitation of regular sleep-wake cycles.

▍ Nursing Activities and Rationales

Assessments

- Monitor infant cues and sleep-awake states. Determines if abnormalities exist and establishes a basis for any needed interventions.
- Observe infant for overstimulation (e.g., lack of eye contact, irritability, restlessness). The autonomic nervous system in the newborn infant is immature. Often, newborns are unable to process external stimulation, particularly complex sources, and may exhibit avoidance behaviors in order to avoid sensory overload, which creates a demand on infant's energy.
- Monitor amount and quality of environmental stimuli. Determines the need for environmental controls. Overstimulation due to environmental factors may stress the infant, predisposing him or her to weight loss and delayed development.

Independent Nursing Actions

- Avoid overstimulation and provide periods of time out when the infant displays signs of stress. Allows for neurobehavioral integration. The stressed infant is at risk for complications and delayed growth and development because of increased energy demands created by the stressors.
- Provide boundaries (nests, bunting, swaddling, etc.). Provides a sense of security and reduces stress.
- Position with arms midline. Facilitates hand-to-mouth activities, which enhances development.

- Alter environmental lighting as needed (Bulechek, Butcher, & McCloskey, 2009). Provides diurnal rhythmicity in order to establish normal sleep-wake cycle. Lighting must also be monitored to prevent overstimulation of infant.
- Cluster care and develop routines. Allows uninterrupted periods of sleep that facilitate establishment of sleep-wake cycles.
- Provide for periods of nonnutritive sucking. Promotes neurobehavioral integration and enhances development.

Collaborative Activities

- Refer for early stimulation as appropriate. Some communities offer early stimulation programs to enhance preterm or SGA infant's developmental and behavioral skills.

Parent/Family Teaching

- Teach parents how to identify their infant's capabilities, self-regulatory behaviors, cues, and states. Facilitates parental enhancement of development. Stimulation needs to be consistent with the infant's capabilities in order to prevent stress.
- Demonstrate environmental controls and positioning techniques (see previous "Independent Nursing Actions" list). Enhances neurobehavioral integration, growth, and development.

Nursing Diagnosis: RISK FOR IMPAIRED PARENTING[1]

Related Factors: prolonged separation and newborn hospitalization. See the generic NDCP, "Impaired Parenting,[1]" beginning on p. 16 in Chapter 2. See the NDCP, "Risk for Impaired Parenting,[1]" beginning on p. 85 in "The Pregnant Adolescent" in Chapter 5. See the NDCP, "Risk for Impaired Parent-Infant/Child Attachment,[1]" beginning on p. 329 in "Postpartum Period: Weeks 1–6" in Chapter 9.

Nursing Activities and Rationales

Assessments

- Assess family's response to newborn, hospitalization, separation from newborn, and family's strengths, coping mechanisms, and social support systems. Identifies the presence of problems and establishes a basis for intervention. Parents may be unprepared to care for an infant with special needs. Those with strong support systems and who use coping mechanisms effectively are more likely to adapt to the care of an infant who is at risk for developmental problems. Other parents may need referrals to community agencies as they adjust to caring for their SGA infant.

- Assess family's understanding of newborn's condition. Corrects misconceptions and determines the need for teaching and/or counseling. The parents' perception of their infant's abilities/disabilities will affect their ability to care for their SGA infant.
- Review prenatal records and assess for presence or history of abusive relationships in the home. One cause of IUGR is maternal abuse during pregnancy. It is important to be sure that the infant is not discharged into an unsafe home.

Independent Nursing Actions

- Encourage family to verbalize feelings and concerns. Alleviates anxiety and facilitates coping by allowing parents to place their fears/concerns in perspective.
- Listen with empathy and acceptance. Creates an environment of trust, which facilitates the nurse–patient relationship.
- Encourage parents to call, visit, and provide allowable care. Promotes parent–infant attachment and provides parents with a sense of control.

Collaborative Activities

- Collaborate with social services, pastoral care, psychology to identify resources and support systems. Facilitates parental coping during this time of crisis. Parents may be unaware of resources that are available to them.

Parent/Family Teaching

- Orient the family to the newborn intensive care unit, explain unit rules and visitation procedures. Reduces anxiety and promotes parent–newborn interactions. Parents will feel less fear about leaving their newborn if they are comfortable in the NICU environment and with the care their infant is receiving.
- Inform parents about allowable activities (e.g., touching and caressing infant, changing diapers). Promotes parent–newborn interactions while minimizing newborn stress and allows the parents a sense of control via their ability to participate in their infant's care. Parents who are frightened may be reluctant to interact with their infant unless they are given permission by the nurse or reassured that it is okay.
- Instruct the family about coping mechanisms and time and stress management techniques. Parents who must leave their infants experience considerable stress. The stress the parents experience might be minimized if they have effective coping mechanisms.
- Educate parents about possible complications associated with their SGA infant. For example, intrauterine and neonatal malnutrition may cause impaired intellectual development, hyperactivity, as well as hearing and speech problems.

INFANT OF A DIABETIC MOTHER

The infant of a diabetic mother (IDM) is one born to a mother with type 1, type 2, or gestational diabetes. The IDM is at high risk for a number of health-related complications, especially hypoglycemia. These infants have increased morbidity and mortality in the perinatal period and also experience increased incidence of major congenital anomalies. The most common types of malformations seen in IDMs involve the cardiovascular, skeletal, gastrointestinal, genitourinary, and central nervous systems. IDMs are typically larger than infants of similar gestational age born to nondiabetic mothers. They also tend to have some organomegaly (increased organ weights) and excessive fat deposits on their shoulders and trunks, which predisposes them to the risk of shoulder dystocia at delivery. The infants may also be macrosomic. Macrosomia is defined as a birth weight greater than 4,000 grams or greater than 90% for gestational age after correcting for sex and ethnicity. This excessive growth in IDMs is contributed to chronic exposure of the fetus to high maternal glucose levels that results in an increased fetal insulin response and enhanced intrauterine growth. Following birth, the maternal blood supply with high circulating levels of insulin is abruptly removed from the infant. Hypoglycemia results because fetal insulin levels do not adjust rapidly to the loss of material glucose supply.

In IDM, birth weight is not necessarily a good indicator of maturity. Newborns of mothers without vascular compromise tend to be large for gestational age, while those born to mothers with vascular compromise tend to be small for gestational age. The severity, duration, and control of the maternal diabetes largely determine how the fetus will be affected and the degree of problems the newborn will experience.

▐ Key Nursing Activities

- Early identification of woman at risk for diabetes.
- Prevent hypoglycemia.
- Maintain fluid and electrolyte balance.
- Provide parental support.

▐ Etiologies and Risk Factors

The etiology is a mother with pregestational (type 1 or type 2) or gestational diabetes. Factors that increase a woman's risk of having gestational diabetes include a previous infant with congenital anomaly; history of gestational diabetes or hydramnios in a previous pregnancy; family history of diabetes; maternal age over 35; previous baby weighing greater than 9 pounds (4,000 grams); previous fetal demise or neonatal death of unknown etiology; maternal obesity; hypertension; recurrent yeast infections that don't respond well to treatment; signs and symptoms of glucose intolerance; presence of glucose or protein in the urine; or being of Hispanic, Native American, or African American ethnicity.

▐ Signs and Symptoms

Full, rosy cheeks, a short neck, redundant skin at nape of neck, wide shoulders, distended abdomen, and excessive subcutaneous fat on extremities. Common problems seen in infants of diabetic mothers include macrosomia, respiratory distress syndrome (RDS), hypoglycemia, polycythemia, hypocalcemia, hypomagnesemia, hyperbilirubinemia, and other congenital anomalies.

▐ Diagnostic Studies

- Serum glucose. Detects hyper- or hypoglycemia.
- Hemoglobin and hematocrit. Detects abnormalities such as polycythemia.
- Total bilirubin. Indicates degree of red cell (erythrocyte) breakdown.
- Serum electrolytes. Determines degree of fluid and electrolyte imbalance.
- Weight. Determines if infant is small, average, or large for gestational age.
- Length. Determines if infant is small, average, or large for gestational age.
- Head circumference. Determines if infant is small, average, or large for gestational age.
- Ultrasound. May be done predelivery to detect fetal abnormalities.
- Radiography. Aids in identifying neonatal malformations or anomalies.
- Amniocentesis for lecithin-sphingomyelin ratio. Assesses for fetal lung maturity. Insulin interferes with lecithin synthesis that is needed for fetal lung maturation; there is also a decrease of phospholipid PG, which stabilizes surfactant. This is true for infants of mothers in White's classifications A through C only. (White's classifications distinguish between types of diabetes that existed prior to pregnancy and developed during pregnancy. For more information about White's classifications, refer to a maternity care textbook.)

▐ Medical Management

- Correct hypoglycemia
- Correct hypocalcemia
- Correct hypomagnesemia
- Initiate phototherapy as indicated
- Maintain oxygenation and ventilation

▐ Collaborative Problems

- Risk for Injury[1] (birth trauma). Note: Even though this is not, by definition, a collaborative problem, the nursing diagnosis, "Risk for Injury[1]" is included here because it is a part of the standardized care that should be given to all infants of diabetic mothers.

Potential Complications of Infants of Diabetic Mothers

- Macrosomia
- Prematurity

- Respiratory distress syndrome
- Hypoglycemia
- Polycythemia
- Hyperbilirubinemia
- Congenital anomalies (coarctation of the aorta, atrial and ventricular septal defects, transposition of the great vessels, sacral agenesis, hip and joint malformations, spina bifida, anencephaly, caudal dysplasia, and hydrocephalus)

COLLABORATIVE (STANDARDIZED) CARE FOR ALL INFANTS OF DIABETIC MOTHERS

Perform a comprehensive assessment to identify individual needs for parent teaching and emotional support and infant physical care.

Nursing Diagnosis: RISK FOR INJURY (BIRTH TRAUMA)[1]

Related Factors: birth trauma secondary to macrosomia and possible birth with forceps or vacuum assistance.

Goals, Outcomes, and Evaluation Criteria

- Absence of fractures, bruises, and lacerations.
- Absence of head injury, seizures, and subarachnoid hemorrhage.
- Absence of complications from any birth injuries that do occur.

NIC Interventions[2]

Intrapartal Care: High-Risk Delivery (6834)—Assisting vaginal birth or multiple or malpositioned fetuses.
Resuscitation: Neonate (6974)—Administering emergency measures to support newborn adaptation to extrauterine life.
Risk Identification (6610)—Analysis of potential risk factors, determination of health risks, and prioritization of risk-reduction strategies for an individual or group.
Seizure Precautions (2680)—Care of a patient during a seizure and the postictal state.

Nursing Activities and Rationales

Assessments

- Assess for signs of macrosomia. Signs such as round, chubby face, reddish or flushed appearing skin, organomegaly, increased body fat, and larger than normal placenta and umbilical cord are indications of macrosomia. Macrosomia occurs in up to 50% of infants born to

mothers with gestational diabetes and approximately 40% of infants born to mothers with type 1 diabetes.

- Assess head. Detects complications of macrosomia, including tense, bulging fontanels; cephalohematoma; fractures; and paralysis of the facial nerve.
- Assess cry. A high-pitched cry may indicate birth trauma or fetal hypoxia.
- Assess shoulders/extremities. The presence of asymmetric appearance or posturing, paralysis, or crying with passive movement may indicate birth trauma.
- Assess skin. The presence of bruising may indicate birth trauma; jaundice indicates hemolysis of red blood cells.
- Report signs of hip instability. Macrosomic infants are at a higher risk of developing hip dysplasia (also known as hip dislocation) because of the intrauterine position.

Independent Nursing Actions

- Inform parents that large-for-gestational-age infants who are delivered vaginally commonly have facial, scalp, or body swelling and bruising. Although these are not life threatening, they may frighten the parents. Preparing the parents for any possible deviations from normal will help them adjust to the appearance of their infant and enable them to cope with more serious injuries.
- Encourage family to verbalize feelings and concerns. Alleviates anxiety and facilitates coping by allowing parents to place their fears/concerns in perspective, express concerns, and work through their feelings.
- Listen with empathy and acceptance. Creates an environment of trust, which facilitates the nurse–patient relationship.

Collaborative Activities

- During the intrapartum period, prepare mother for cesarean birth. If the infant of the diabetic mother is too large to deliver vaginally due to cephalopelvic disproportion, cesarean birth will be considered in order to protect the fetus from birth trauma and possible serious injury. The mother who understands that cesarean birth may protect her infant from intrapartum stress may be more likely to support the plan of care.

Parent/Family Teaching

- During the intrapartum period, teach regarding the possible need for cesarean birth if the baby is large for gestational age and the birth outlet is suspected to be too small to allow a vaginal birth. Helps prepare the mother for surgical birth if needed to prevent injury to the fetus during vaginal delivery. Increased understanding decreases anxiety and fosters cooperation on the part of the mother.

Potential Complication of an Infant of a Diabetic Mother: HYPOGLYCEMIA

Focus Assessments

- Monitor blood glucose levels. Detects hypoglycemia, which is associated with blood glucose levels less than 50 mg/dl in term infants (Note: the definition of hypoglycemia varies by agency, some defining it as blood glucose less than 40 mg/dl). Infants exposed to high maternal glucose levels develop pancreatic hyperplasia and resultant hyperinsulinism. When the umbilical cord is severed, the infant is no longer exposed to the high maternal glucose levels. This, in combination with the infant's hyperinsulinism, produces a rapid decrease in blood glucose levels.
- Assess skin. Cyanosis, pallor, and sweating indicate hypoglycemia.
- Assess neurologic status. Tremors, jitteriness, twitches, seizures, lethargy, and poor feeding may indicate hypoglycemia.
- Monitor temperature. Cold stress increases glucose utilization and exacerbates hypoglycemia.

Preventive Nursing Activities

- Initiate early oral feeds with formula or human milk. Encourages glucose homeostasis. Early feedings also reduce hematocrit and promote bilirubin excretion.
- Provide rest period. Decreases energy demand and expenditure, which conserves glucose and glycogen stores.
- Maintain a neutral thermal environment. A thermoneutral environment helps to eliminate heat loss through evaporation, conduction, convection, and radiation, thereby preventing cold stress, which increases metabolic rate and the demand for glucose.

Potential Complication of an Infant of a Diabetic Mother: RESPIRATORY DISTRESS

Focus Assessments

- Assess prenatal fetal lung maturity (e.g., with lecithin-sphingomyelin ratio). Assesses fetal lung maturity. A lecithin-sphingomyelin ratio of 3:1 or greater or the presence of phosphatidylglycerol in amniotic fluid indicates lung maturity in the infant of a diabetic mother.
- Evaluate lung sounds. Allows for early detection of change in respiratory status.

- Continuously monitor oxygen saturations. Determines adequacy of tissue perfusion.
- Monitor respirations. Identifies the presence of tachypnea, grunting, nasal flaring, retractions, and abnormal breath sounds, which are indications of compromised oxygenation. Infants with hyperinsulinism may have delayed synthesis of surfactant in the lung. Respiratory distress syndrome may occur even in the near-term infant who is born to a diabetic mother because of the potential lung immaturity in this population of infants.
- Assess skin. Detects cyanosis and/or pallor and mottling, which indicates compromised oxygenation.
- Monitor temperature. Establishes a baseline for future comparisons.
- Assess blood gases. Determines the presence of acidosis, hypoxemia, or hypercarbia, all of which are complications of respiratory distress syndrome.

Preventive Nursing Activities

- Maintain airway. Ensures that respirations can occur freely. A compromised airway prevents the intake of air (oxygen) and expulsion of carbon dioxide. A baby who is large for gestational age has the appearance of a short neck due to fat deposition. They also tend to have more hypopharyngeal collapse than term average-for-gestational-age infants who are not IDM. A neutral airway position is important, particularly to an IDM baby, to prevent airway obstruction.
- Place in prone position. This position optimizes respiratory status and may help reduce stress.
- Administer oxygen as ordered. Promotes adequate tissue perfusion.
- Reposition every 3–4 hours when hands-on care is provided. Prevents stasis of secretions that can compromise a patent airway or adequate oxygenation.
- Provide chest physiotherapy as needed. Helps clear secretions from the lungs and maintain oxygenation. Percussion is effective in the recruitment of alveoli for improved air–gas exchange. Suctioning mucus from the pharynx also helps to facilitate good air entry for more effective breathing.
- Administer surfactant as needed. Aids in stabilizing lungs until postnatal synthesis of surfactant improves.
- Maintain normal blood glucose levels and a neutral thermal environment. Decreases oxygen consumption.

Potential Complication of an Infant of a Diabetic Mother: POLYCYTHEMIA

See the collaborative care plan, "Potential Complication of Small-for-Gestational-Age Infant: Polycythemia," beginning on p. 392

in "The Small-for-Gestational-Age Newborn," in this chapter. Polycythemia is thought to be caused by the IDM's decreased extracellular volume.

Potential Complication of an Infant of a Diabetic Mother: HYPERBILIRUBINEMIA

Refer to "Hyperbilirubinemia," beginning on p. 436 in this chapter. For IDMs, assess for hyperbilirubinemia, and if it is present, institute that care plan. In the IDM, hyperbilirubinemia may be caused by slightly decreased extracellular fluid volume and hepatic immaturity. If there is birth trauma, enclosed hemorrhages can also cause hyperbilirubinemia.

Potential Complication of an Infant of a Diabetic Mother: HYPOCALCEMIA AND HYPOMAGNESEMIA

Focus Assessments

- Monitor serum calcium (Ca++) levels. A total serum Ca++ of less than 7 mg/dl or ionized calcium less than 2 mg/dl is an indication of hypocalcemia. Hypocalcemia can occur in 50% of infants born to diabetic mothers.
- Assess for signs of hypocalcemia. Hypocalcemia is manifested by tremors, hypotonia, apnea, and a high-pitched cry. Seizures may develop due to the abrupt cessation of maternal transfer of calcium, especially in infants who have experienced birth asphyxia.
- Monitor serum magnesium (Mg+) levels. A serum Mg+ less than 1.5 mg/dl is an indication of hypomagnesemia, which can result in life-threatening cardiac dysrhythmias.
- Monitor respirations. Apnea can be a sign of hypocalcemia.
- Monitor neurologic status. Tremors, convulsions, and high-pitched cry may indicate decreased calcium or magnesium levels.

Preventive Nursing Activities

- Administer Ca++/Mg+ as prescribed. Prevents and/or corrects hypocalcemia and hypomagnesemia.

Potential Complication of an Infant of a Diabetic Mother: CONGENITAL ANOMALIES

Focus Assessments

- Assess for skeletal abnormalities. These are common in IDMs.
- Perform cardiovascular assessment (cyanosis, murmurs, and abnormal heart sounds). Cardiac anomalies such as septal hypertrophy and transposition of the great arteries are common in IDMs born to insulin-dependent mothers. Heart murmurs related to hyperplasia of the ventricular wall are common and benign. This type of ventricular enlargement will usually spontaneously resolve without intervention and should cause no systemic problem.
- Perform neural assessment (abnormal head, limb development). Anencephaly, holoprosencephaly, and sacral agenesis (caudal regression syndrome) are often seen in IDMs whose mothers are poorly controlled and insulin dependent.
- Assess GI system (failure to pass meconium, abdominal distention, and bilious emesis). Duodenal or anorectal atresia and small left colon syndrome are seen more frequently in infants born to diabetic mothers.

Preventive Nursing Activities

- Assess maternal glucose control during pregnancy. Poor maternal glucose control during organogenesis is associated with an increased incidence of congenital anomalies in the infant. Once the infant has been born, of course, congenital anomalies cannot be prevented—only diagnosed and treated.

Potential Complication of an Infant of a Diabetic Mother: PREMATURITY

See the topic, "Preterm Newborn," beginning on p. 412 in this chapter. For IDMs, assess for signs of prematurity, and if the infant is premature, institute the care plan for preterm newborn.

INDIVIDUALIZED (NURSING DIAGNOSIS) CARE PLANS

This section includes care plans that were developed to address unique patient needs.

Nursing Diagnosis: DISABLED FAMILY COPING[1]

Related Factors: feelings of guilt and responsibility for the infant's condition and stress.

Goals, Outcomes, and Evaluation Criteria

- Mother resolves feelings of guilt.
- Mother demonstrates behaviors consistent with parent–infant attachment.

NIC Interventions[2]

Family Integrity Promotion: Childbearing Family (7104)— Facilitation of the growth of individuals or families who are adding an infant to the family.

Nursing Activities and Rationales

Assessments

- Identify family's coping mechanisms and supports. Identifies family strengths, limitations, problems, and potential problems in order to establish a basis for intervention. Lack of effective coping mechanisms or support systems may alter the ability of the family to care for a new infant.
- Determine family understanding of the neonate's condition. Identifies misconceptions, feelings of guilt, fears, concerns, or irrational beliefs so that corrections can be made and interventions planned. The mother may feel that she is the cause of her infant's condition, which may incapacitate her or interfere with her ability to care for the infant.
- Assess for indications of parent–infant attachment. Even though parents may be unable to hold or cuddle their infant, attachment can still occur. Talking or singing to the infant, stroking the infant or holding its hand is a positive indication of attachment. Parents who are unable to look at or focus on their infant may be at risk for impaired attachment.

Independent Nursing Actions

- Encourage verbalization of fears and concerns and listen with empathy. Creates an environment of trust and acceptance that facilitates communication. Verbalizing one's fears allows for correction of misconceptions, helps place fears in perspective with other life events, and promotes adjustment and coping.
- Encourage parents to spend time with other siblings. Allows parents an opportunity to refocus on healthy children and helps reassure siblings that they are valued and important.
- Allow privacy for parents. Provides an opportunity for parents to freely discuss their feelings and concerns with one another and helps them clarify their fears and concerns.

Collaborative Activities

- Refer to social services, counseling, and pastoral care as needed. Provides additional resources for social support, especially for those couples who do not use effective coping mechanisms or those who do not have adequate support systems in place.

Parent/Family Teaching

- Provide the family information about the relationship between maternal diabetes and neonatal consequences. Provides accurate information and helps eliminate fear. Lack of knowledge can increase fears and anxiety. Parents who know what to expect are more likely to effectively cope with their infant's condition and make positive adjustments to the situation. Reassure the mother that she did not cause her infant's condition. Many people need to hear this repeatedly in order not to blame themselves.
- Discuss normal responses to giving birth to a high-risk infant. Facilitates parent understanding and coping. Parents may feel that their feelings are wrong or abnormal and blame themselves even more for their infant's condition. Self-blame is a negative response that interferes with coping, adjustment, and decision making.
- Provide information about constructive coping mechanisms and resources. Facilitates coping. If parents have used coping mechanisms successfully in the past, they are likely to be successful with each new crisis. Parents who have not used coping strategies successfully may need information or resources to help them cope with their current crisis.

Other Nursing Diagnoses

Also assess for the following nursing diagnoses, which are frequently present:

- Anxiety[1] related to infant's prognosis and/or ability to care for an infant with complications.
- Deficient Knowledge[1] (parents) related to inexperience caring for ill infant.

INFANT OF A SUBSTANCE-ABUSING MOTHER

Infants born to women who abuse tobacco, alcohol, or illicit substances are at risk for numerous complications before and following birth. Substances of abuse readily pass the placental barrier, and the fetus may become passively addicted. The fetus is much more vulnerable to drugs because it does not have the developed enzymatic system needed to metabolize drugs. Mothers who present with substance abuse are commonly polysubstance abusers, which is likely to be even more dangerous than abusing a single substance. Substance abuse during pregnancy is associated with miscarriage, premature labor, intrauterine growth restriction of the fetus, placental abruption, low birth weight, neurobehavioral abnormalities, and long-term developmental consequences.

Key Nursing Activities

- Monitor and support the infant experiencing alcohol/drug withdrawal.
- Assess feeding plan to ensure appropriate weight gain.
- Prevent other related complications.
- Promote parent–infant attachment.
- Offer emotional support to parent(s).
- Encourage and support maternal drug rehabilitation.

Etiologies and Risk Factors

Etiologies and risk factors include maternal use/abuse of tobacco, alcohol, or illicit drugs or misuse of prescription medications.

Signs and Symptoms

Signs and symptoms vary with the maternal agent used/abused. Many infants appear normal at birth, but others appear undergrown, jaundiced, or jittery. Signs of withdrawal may be exhibited between birth and 2 weeks of age, but the majority are apparent within the first 72 hours of life. Signs and symptoms include the following:

- Fetal alcohol syndrome/fetal alcohol spectrum disorder. Intrauterine growth restriction, microcephaly, low nasal bridge, hypoplastic philtrum, thin upper lip, short upturned nose, micrognathia, narrow forehead, poor postnatal growth, poor coordination, joint and limb defects, congenital cardiac defects, clinically significant brain abnormalities, delayed cognitive development, and delayed fine and gross motor development.
- Cocaine toxicity. Intrauterine growth restriction, intrauterine fetal distress, seizures, cerebral infarcts, microcephaly, neural tube defects, congenital anomalies (hypospadias, ambiguous genitalia, hydronephrosis, prune belly syndrome), irritability, hypertonicity, increased response to stimuli, gaze aversion, decreased orientation to voice, poor state control as a newborn, hyperactivity, poor concentration, and interpersonal skill deficits.
- Neonatal withdrawal syndrome. Tremors, seizures, hyperreflexia, increased muscle tone, high-pitched cry, disturbed sleep patterns, fever, yawing, mottling, sweating, tachypnea, apnea, poor feeding, frantic sucking/rooting, water loss stools, emesis/projectile vomiting.
- Tobacco/nicotine. Low birth weight, intrauterine growth restriction, sudden infant death syndrome (SIDS), cognitive deficits, and behavioral problems (hyperactivity, inattention, impulsivity).

Diagnostic Studies

- Finnegan abstinence score. A scoring system used to assess for signs of withdrawal. This tool is most reliable in infants exposed to opiates.
- Toxicology screen of infant blood, urine, and meconium; maternal blood and urine. Identifies exposure to specific substances. Urine detects substances recently used and meconium detects substances used over a longer period of time.
- Ultrasound. Identifies fetal anomalies.
- HIV testing. Identifies exposure to HIV.
- Complete blood count. Provides general data to support presence/absence of infection/sepsis (especially group B streptococci) in newborn; platelet count may be decreased due to maternal tranquilizer use.
- Serum calcium. Identifies electrolyte imbalance.
- Serum glucose. Identifies hyper- or hypoglycemia; helps to determine whether infant is experiencing withdrawal or hypoglycemia, as some of the signs are similar.
- Bilirubin levels. Risk of jaundice is increased if mother is a methadone user.
- Serologic tests. Identifies sexually transmitted infections.
- Electroencephalogram. Identifies neurologic alterations due to cerebral irritation (especially if the mother is a cocaine user).

Medical Management

- Supportive care
- Pharmacologic therapy
- Long-term management

Collaborative Problems

Potential Complications of Infants of Substance-Abusing Mothers

- Infectious diseases
- HIV-positive serology
- Multiple drug abuse
- Anemia
- Poor nutritional status
- SIDS
- Prematurity
- Intrauterine growth restriction
- Asphyxia

COLLABORATIVE (STANDARDIZED) CARE FOR INFANTS OF SUBSTANCE-ABUSING MOTHERS

Perform a comprehensive assessment to identify individual needs for parent teaching and emotional support and infant physical care.

Potential Complication of an Infant of a Substance-Abusing Mother: INFECTION

See the generic NDCP, "Risk for Infection,[1]" beginning on p. 21 in Chapter 2. See the generic collaborative care plan, "Potential Complication: Infection," beginning on p. 29 in Chapter 3.

Focus Assessments

- Assess maternal history. Identifies risky behaviors, STIs, HIV, group B streptococcus, or prolonged rupture of membranes, which increase the infant's risk for infection. Realize that the mother/family may not provide accurate detail about her drug use.
- Assess laboratory data. Identifies abnormalities of the blood and cerebrospinal fluid; bacterial growth from tracheal, urine, and surface cultures; and identifies substances being abused.

Preventive Nursing Activities

- Discourage maternal breastfeeding if HIV infection is suspected. Prevents the transfer of HIV virus to infant via human milk. Human milk does contain the virus and it can be transmitted to the infant.

Potential Complication of an Infant of a Substance-Abusing Mother: NEONATAL ABSTINENCE SYNDROME

Focus Assessments

- Assess for signs of neonatal abstinence syndrome (NAS). Early identification allows for early initiation of treatment. Metabolic, vasomotor, and respiratory signs include increased respiratory rate greater than 60 breaths/min, nasal flaring, nasal congestion, frequent sneezing, diaphoresis, skin mottling, excessive yawning, apnea, and fever. Signs of central nervous system dysfunction include tremors, seizures, hyperactive reflexes, restlessness, hypertonic muscle tone, shrill, high-pitched cry and sleep pattern disturbances. Signs of gastrointestinal dysfunction include poor feeding, frantic sucking or rooting, loose stools, regurgitation, and projectile vomiting. Acute symptoms may last for several weeks, but subacute symptoms (irritability, sleep disturbances, hypertonia, and feeding difficulties) can persist for 4–6 months.
- Monitor for seizure activity. Seizure activity includes abnormal eye movements, jerking of extremities, tongue thrusting, etc.
- Monitor for changes in condition/status. Determines the effectiveness of interventions.

Preventive Nursing Activities

- Decrease ambient noise, dim nursery lights, use calm, gentle approach when handling newborn. Decreases external stimuli that may cause CNS irritability and seizures.
- Swaddle infant tightly in flexed position with arms midline. Helps to reduce self-stimulation behaviors that may increase CNS irritability and precipitate seizures. Provides a sense of security for the infant and prevents skin abrasions.
- Rock gently in vertical position. Helps reduce irritability, decreases the risk for seizures, and counters depressed interactive behaviors.
- Provide opportunities for nonnutritive sucking. Use of a pacifier helps satisfy the increased need for sucking, calms the infant, and facilitates behavior organization.
- Feed small quantities in upright position and burp frequently. Minimizes vomiting and regurgitation and the potential for aspiration.
- Keep infant's chin tucked downward and support chin or chin and cheeks. Facilitates suck-swallow coordination and decreases the risk for aspiration should vomiting occur.
- Encourage kangaroo care. Provides sense of security and has a calming effect on the infant.
- Cluster care of infant. Minimizes handling and stimulation of infant and decreases the potential for seizures related to overstimulation.
- Provide skin care. Apply barrier dressings to elbows and knees to prevent excoriation related to increased activity.
- Reposition infant every 3–4 hours. Prevents development of pressure areas on infant's tender skin.
- Administer medications as prescribed for seizures, CNS stimulation, or insomnia. Paregoric controls narcotic withdrawal seizures more effectively than phenobarbital. Phenobarbital is effective at controlling narcotic withdrawal symptoms of irritability, fussiness, and hyperexcitability. Other agents used to manage neonatal drug withdrawal are tincture of opium, chlorpromazine, clonidine, and diazepam.

Potential Complication of an Infant of a Substance-Abusing Mother: SUDDEN INFANT DEATH SYNDROME

Focus Assessments

- Assess maternal history. Determines if the mother used/abused cocaine, heroin, methadone, or tobacco, which are risk factors for SIDS.
- Determine the infant's sleep position. The incidence of SIDS is greatest among infants who sleep prone or are born to mothers who received inadequate prenatal care, have low maternal age, or smoked during the prenatal and postnatal periods.
- Assess for family history of SIDS, especially in siblings of SIDS infants. It has not been proven that subsequent

siblings of one SIDS victim are at increased risk; however, increased awareness of the possibility may cause parents to be proactive in implementing strategies to reduce the risk for SIDS.

- Monitor respirations. Prolonged sleep apnea is a condition associated with SIDS; however, it is not the cause of SIDS. Apnea can also occur from excessive periodic breathing, impaired responsiveness to increased carbon dioxide levels, or decreased oxygen, all of which may be associated with SIDS.

- Assess infant behavior. Detects poor self-protective mechanisms such as the inability to move the head from side to side, which increases the risk for airway obstruction.

Preventive Nursing Activities

- Position the infant supine to sleep. The incidence of SIDS has dropped significantly since the implementation of the "Back to Sleep" campaign. Infants sleeping prone and/or on soft bedding may not be able to protect their airway by moving their head side to the side, placing them at increased risk for suffocation and rebreathing of carbon dioxide, which leads to hyperventilation and apnea.

- Never leave an infant alone except in its crib. Cribs should be free of stuffed toys, crib pads, and extra blankets while the infant is sleeping. It is also important to pay attention to the proximity of the crib to window treatments, decorative shelf units, and wall hangings that could fall onto infant. Prevents accidental airway obstruction from clothing, blankets, or stuffed toys.

- Teach parents to avoid smoking crack, tobacco, or marijuana around the infant. These substances interfere with oxygenation, which may increase the risk for SIDS in infants who are predisposed to the condition.

- Teach parents about proper positioning and avoiding the use of water beds, pillows, and other soft bedding materials. Prevents suffocation.

- Discourage parents from sleeping with infant. Prevents suffocation.

- Instruct parents in CPR procedures. Prepares the parents for intervention if their infant is not breathing. Allows the parents to feel more comfortable caring for an at-risk infant if they know how to intervene should it become necessary.

▌ Potential Complication of an Infant of a Substance-Abusing Mother: PREMATURITY

See "Preterm Newborn," beginning on p. 412 in this chapter.

▌ Potential Complication of an Infant of a Substance-Abusing Mother: INTRAUTERINE GROWTH RETARDATION

See "The Small-for-Gestational-Age Newborn," beginning on p. 389 in this chapter.

▌ Potential Complication of an Infant of a Substance-Abusing Mother: ASPHYXIA

See "Neonatal Asphyxia," which begins on p. 385 in this chapter.

INDIVIDUALIZED (NURSING DIAGNOSIS) CARE PLANS

The care plans in this section were developed to address unique patient needs.

▌ Nursing Diagnosis: IMBALANCED NUTRITION: LESS THAN BODY REQUIREMENTS[1]

Related Factors: uncoordinated suck and swallow, vomiting, regurgitation, diarrhea, and failure to wake for feedings. See the NDCP, "Impaired Nutrition: Less Than Body Requirements,[1]" beginning on p. 394 in "The Small-for-Gestational-Age Newborn" in this chapter.

▌ *Nursing Activities and Rationales*

Independent Nursing Actions

- Wake infant as needed for feeding. NAS infants may be sedated in order to prevent overstimulation and seizures. It may be necessary to wake the infant for feeding in order to ensure adequate intake.

- Feed small quantities in upright position and burp frequently. Helps minimize regurgitation and vomiting; helps prevent aspiration.

- Keep infant's chin tucked downward and support chin and/or cheeks as necessary. Facilitates suck-swallow coordination and prevents aspiration.

Collaborative Activities

- Provide nutritional supplements or high-calorie formulas as ordered. Ensures that infant is receiving adequate nutrition. Infants with NAS are at increased risk for nutritional deficits due to poor feeding, irritability, and increased motor activity.

- Refer to occupational or speech therapy. Provides opportunity for specialized assistance with techniques that promote suck-swallow coordination and successful feeding positions.

Parent/Family Teaching

- Instruct parents on techniques to enhance suck-swallow coordination. Facilitates infant's ability to coordinate sucking and swallowing. Infants with NAS have increased sucking reflex but are often poor feeders. Strategies to insure adequate intake help reduce the risk for malnutrition or fluid volume deficit.

Nursing Diagnosis: DIARRHEA[1]

Related Factors: neonatal abstinence syndrome.

Goals, Outcomes, and Evaluation Criteria

- Infant maintains fluid/electrolyte balance.
- Infant maintains acid/base balance.
- Absence of diarrhea.
- Absence of irritation, rash, or excoriation at perineal area.

NIC Interventions[2]

Acid/Base Monitoring (1920)—Collection and analysis of patient data to regulate acid-base balance.

Diarrhea Management (0460)—Management and alleviation of diarrhea.

Electrolyte Monitoring (2020)—Collection and analysis of patient data to regulate electrolyte balance.

Fluid Monitoring (4130)—Collection and analysis of patient data to regulate fluid balance.

Nursing Activities and Rationales

Assessments

- Monitor frequency and characteristics of bowel movements. Determines persistence of diarrhea. Massive amounts of fluids and electrolytes can be eliminated through the bowel. Persistent diarrhea predisposes the infant to fluid and electrolyte imbalance, fluid volume deficit, altered tissue integrity, and weight loss.
- Monitor fluid and electrolyte status. Detects fluid and electrolyte imbalances; determines need for corrective action.
- Monitor acid/base status. Detects acid-base disturbance; determines appropriate action to be taken.
- Monitor hydration status. Detects dehydration related to fluid losses through diarrhea. Poor skin turgor, weight loss, dry oral mucous membranes, sunken fontanels, and

increased urine-specific gravity are indications of fluid volume deficit/dehydration.

- Monitor skin in perianal area for irritation and ulceration (Bulechek et al., 2009). Diarrhea has a high acid content and can be excoriating to skin and mucous membranes.

Independent Nursing Actions

- Maintain nothing-by-mouth status as ordered. Rests the gastrointestinal tract in order to reduce peristalsis and diarrhea.
- Administer oral and parenteral fluids as prescribed. Replaces fluid lost in diarrhea stools and prevents fluid volume deficit. Fluid intake should approximate output. Infants are at much greater risk for dehydration secondary to fluid volume deficit than older children or adults.
- Apply protective creams to excoriated perineum/buttocks. Protects newborn's skin from irritation. Liquid stool has a high acid content that is irritating to the skin, producing redness and excoriation.

Collaborative Activities

- Administer antidiarrheal medications as prescribed. Decreases the frequency of watery bowel movements and prevents fluid volume deficits, altered tissue integrity, and electrolyte imbalance.

Nursing Diagnosis: RISK FOR ASPIRATION[1]

Related Factors: frequent regurgitation, vomiting, poor suck-swallow coordination, and abdominal distention.

Goal, Outcome, and Evaluation Criterion

- Infant remains free of pulmonary aspiration.

NIC Interventions[2]

Aspiration Precaution (3200)—Prevention or minimization of risk factors in the patient at risk for aspiration.

Nonnutritive Sucking (6900)—Provision of sucking opportunities for the infant.

Nursing Activities and Rationales

Assessments

- Monitor ability to coordinate sucking and swallowing and track incidents of regurgitation. Poor suck-swallow coordination, frequent regurgitation, and vomiting are risk factors for aspiration.
- Monitor pulmonary status. Frequent choking or coughing indicates possible aspiration. Lung crackles, difficulty

breathing, fever, and cough are signs of aspiration pneumonia. Frequent apnea or bradycardia may indicate injury to the lungs or gastroesophageal reflux.

Independent Nursing Actions

- Feed small quantities in upright position and burp frequently. Minimizes vomiting. Small quantities are more easily digested. Burping removes air from the stomach and decreases the risk of vomiting and aspiration.
- Keep infant's chin tucked downward and support chin or chin and cheeks. Facilitates suck-swallow coordination. The infant who is unable to suck and swallow properly is at increased risk for aspiration. This technique opens the esophagus and protects the airway during swallowing.
- Keep head elevated for at least 30 minutes after feeding (e.g., may place in infant car seat). Prevents regurgitation by allowing the stomach to partially empty. A full stomach increases intragastric pressure and contents are more likely to be regurgitated when the infant is lying down due to pressure on the lower esophageal sphincter.
- Keep suction equipment at bedside. To clear airway of foods and fluids if regurgitation occurs, to prevent aspiration.

Collaborative Activities

- Refer to occupational or speech therapy. Provides opportunity for specialized assistance with techniques that promote suck, suck-swallow coordination, and proper feeding positions.
- Thicken human milk or formula with cereal or thickening agent as prescribed (this is controversial in some areas). Prevents regurgitation. Thickened fluids are less easily regurgitated than thin fluids, which can be easily aspirated.

Parent/Family Teaching

- Teach parents positioning and feeding techniques. Facilitates suck-swallow coordination and helps prevent regurgitation or vomiting.
- Teach parents how to use the bulb syringe. A bulb syringe can be used to aspirate milk or thick secretions in order to maintain a patent airway and ensure oxygenation.
- Teach parents CPR. Parents are likely to be present if the infant aspirates. Knowing how to clear the infant's airway and restore breathing may increase their comfort level in caring for an infant at risk for aspiration.

Nursing Diagnosis: DISTURBED SLEEP PATTERN[1]

Related Factors: maternal alcohol or illicit substance use.

▌ *Goal, Outcome, and Evaluation Criterion*

- Establishes regular, efficient sleep-wake cycle for developmental age.

▌ *NIC Interventions[2]*

Developmental Care (6824)—Structuring the environment and providing care in response to the behavioral cues and states of the preterm infant.

Sleep Enhancement (1850)—Facilitation of regular sleep-wake cycles.

▌ *Nursing Activities and Rationales*

Assessments

- Monitor periods of sleep-wake cycles. Determines presence of or lack of an efficient sleep-wake cycle so that corrective actions can be planned and initiated.
- Evaluate contribution of environmental stimuli to disturbed sleep pattern. NAS infants are hyperactive and easily stimulated. External noise and lights may contribute to the infant's hyperactive state and inability to maintain a normal sleep cycle.

Independent Nursing Actions

- Provide white noise and decrease environmental stimuli. Calms infant and helps ensure adequate sleep. NAS infants are readily stimulated and have difficulty sleeping; therefore, noise and lights need to be minimized to enhance sleep.
- Swaddle infant tightly in flexed position with arms midline. Calms infant and provides a sense of security in order to promote sleep.
- Rock gently in vertical position. Decreases irritability, counters decreased interactive behaviors, and facilitates infant's ability to sleep.
- Provide opportunities for nonnutritive sucking. NAS infants have an increased suck reflex. Pacifiers calm the infant and facilitate sleep.
- Cluster care. Minimizes handling and stimulation of infant, who is prone to hyperactivity and irritability, in order to facilitate sleep.

Parent/Family Teaching

- Teach parents about infant sleep needs. Increases awareness about appropriate sleep behavior in their infant and helps ensure that parents will recognize sleep alterations in their infant and implement actions to enhance sleep.

Nursing Diagnosis: RISK FOR DISORGANIZED INFANT BEHAVIOR[1]

Related Factors: maternal alcohol or illicit substance use. See the NCDP, "Risk for Disorganized Infant Behavior,[1]" beginning on p. 395 in "The Small-for-Gestational-Age Newborn" in this chapter.

▌ *Goals, Outcomes, and Evaluation Criteria*

- Infant tolerates stimulation.
- Infant controls autonomic and motoric systems.
- Infant modulates between sleep-wake states.
- Infant demonstrates self-regulation.

▌ *NIC Intervention[2]*

Temperature Regulation (3900)—Attaining and/or maintaining body temperature within a normal range.

▌ *Nursing Activities and Rationales*

Assessments

- Monitor skin color, temperature, heart rate, and blood pressure. Identifies extent of autonomic nervous system control.
- Monitor infant for cues related to stress. Provides a basis for intervention.

Independent Nursing Actions

- Decrease environmental stimuli. Calms infant and decreases irritability.
- Swaddle infant tightly in flexed position with arms midline. Calms infant and promotes self-regulating behaviors.
- Rock gently in vertical position. Decreases CNS irritability.
- Cluster care. Minimizes sleep disruption.
- Provide appropriate forms of stimulation (massage, touch, music, mobiles). Enhances development.

Parent/Family Teaching

- Provide parents with information on how to provide developmentally appropriate forms of stimulation. Enhances the developmental potential.
- Teach parents quieting techniques. Equips parents to help infant control behavior.

▌ **Nursing Diagnosis: RISK FOR IMPAIRED PARENTING[1]**

Related Factors: maternal substance use, extended newborn hospitalization, unrealistic expectations and lack of knowledge about infant care needs, and an irritable newborn with poorly established sleep-wake cycles. See the NDCP, "Risk for Impaired Parenting,[1]" which begins on p. 85 in "The Pregnant Adolescent" in Chapter 5. Also see the NDCP, "Risk for Impaired Parent–Infant/Child Attachment,[1]" which begins on p. 329 in "Postpartum Period: Weeks 1–6" in Chapter 9.

▌ *Nursing Activities and Rationales*

Assessments

- Assess the mother's understanding of her substance dependency. Determines if the mother has a realistic and accurate view of her own situation and allows for appropriate intervention.
- Monitor extent of parental involvement in infant's care. Identifies cues to impaired parenting. A mother who abuses substances during pregnancy is at increased risk for doing so following birth. An impaired mother may be unable or uninterested in meeting the special needs of her NAS infant. She may not tolerate the infant's irritability and increased motor activity or have the attention needed to feed a baby who might be a difficult feeder.
- Determine parental understanding of infant needs. Determines if teaching or other interventions are needed to enhance parents' understanding of the special needs of the substance-exposed infant.
- Assess mother's perception of her ability to provide for infant. Women who abuse substances have control and self-esteem issues and may be ill equipped to care for a newborn. The mother's perceptions of her own abilities will influence the degree to which she will be able to participate in her infant's care.
- Assess for social supports. Determines the needs of the parents for assistance in caring for their NAS infant. If parents are impaired they may need greater support and assistance than usual or may be incapable of caring for their infant.

Parent/Family Teaching

- Teach parents about the special needs of their infant. Helps equip parents to meet their infant's needs and to help ensure the infant's safety once discharged. Special-needs infants can tax the patience and ability of any parent, but they may overtax the ability of the impaired parent to meet the infant's needs.
- Approach mother in a nonjudgmental manner. Helps establish trust and increases the mother's comfort with verbalizing her fears about care of her newborn and her substance-abuse problem.
- Reinforce mother's desires and attempts to participate in her infant's care. The mother may feel guilty over her addiction problem and feel unworthy of caring for her infant. Reinforcement of positive efforts helps build the mother's self-confidence and helps ensure that those behaviors will be repeated.
- Encourage mother to enter or consider entering a substance abuse treatment program. The mother who is substance dependent may have the desire to change her behaviors but not the will or support necessary to do so. The support and guidance provided in treatment programs may make the difference in allowing the mother to keep her baby versus the NAS infant being placed in foster care services.

Nursing Diagnosis: RISK FOR IMPAIRED PARENT–INFANT/CHILD ATTACHMENT[1]

Related Factors: maternal substance abuse. See the generic NDCP, "Risk for Impaired Parent–Infant/Child Attachment,[1]" beginning on p. 19 in Chapter 2.

Nursing Diagnosis: RISK FOR IMPAIRED TISSUE INTEGRITY[1]

Related Factors: rubbing, diarrhea, vomiting, mechanical factors (shearing, rubbing, and pressure), excretions/secretions, alterations in skin turgor (elasticity), and poor nutritional status.

Goal, Outcome, and Evaluation Criterion

- Skin remains intact.

NIC Intervention[2]

Skin Surveillance (3590)—Collection and analysis of patient data to maintain skin and mucous membrane integrity.

Nursing Activities and Rationales

Assessments

- Monitor skin status. Identifies scratches, excoriation, poor skin turgor, or other alterations related to diarrhea, poor nutritional status, or fluid volume deficits so that appropriate interventions can be planned.
- Monitor hydration status. Infants who have fluid volume deficits from lack of eating or diarrhea are at increased risk for impaired tissue integrity.
- Monitor nutritional status. NAS infants are often poor feeders, which interferes with their nutritional status. Poor nutrition predisposes the infant to decreased healing and loss of tissue integrity.

Independent Nursing Actions

- Apply barrier dressings to knees, elbows, etc. Protects bony prominences from excoriation. Infant's knees and elbows are in frequent contact with items such as sheets, blankets, and diapers. NAS infants are hyperactive and move their extremities constantly. Frequent rubbing and shearing place them at increased risk for skin breakdown.
- Change diaper frequently. Prevents irritation from urine or diarrhea stools, which are highly acidic and increase the infant's risk for rashes and skin excoriation.
- Immediately clean emesis and stool from skin. Prevents skin irritation and breakdown. Emesis and stool, especially diarrhea stools, contain acids, which are very irritating to the infant's tender skin.
- Expose excoriated buttocks to air. Allows drying and promotes healing. Skin that is irritated from stool or urine is further irritated by cloth and paper diapers.

INFANT EXPOSED TO HIV/AIDS

The HIV/AIDS pandemic has affected the health of women and children in all parts of the world unlike any other infection. An estimated 2.4 million infected women give birth annually. More than 90% of pediatric-acquired HIV infections occur late in pregnancy or during delivery. Therefore, special care needs to be given, prenatally, to mothers with known HIV infections and postnatally to the infants of these mothers.

Key Nursing Activities

- Protect the infant from further exposure to maternal blood or body fluids.
- Implement and maintain treatment regimens for HIV infection.
- Teach mother about care of the HIV-exposed infant, including prophylactic antiviral therapy.
- Provide emotional support.

Etiologies and Risk Factors

An HIV-infected mother can transmit the virus to her baby before the onset of labor, during labor and delivery, and through breastfeeding. Studies have demonstrated that the time of highest risk is during the peripartum period. After delivery, human milk is responsible for up to 16% of infections transmitted to babies who were not prenatally infected (Nduati et al., 2000). Any infant born to a high-risk mother is at increased risk of contracting the disease. High-risk mothers include IV drug users, spouses of bisexual males, and women from areas where the disease is more prevalent among heterosexuals, hemophiliacs, and spouses of hemophiliacs.

Signs and Symptoms

Clinical manifestations of HIV infection are rarely seen in the neonatal period but begin to develop during infancy and early childhood. Signs and symptoms of neonatal HIV infection include low birth weight, weight loss, failure to thrive, recurrent upper respiratory infections, otitis media, sinusitis, oral thrush, and invasive bacterial infections.

Diagnostic Studies

- HIV DNA polymerase chain reaction. Preferred test to diagnose HIV-1 infection in children less than 18 months of age. High sensitivity (95%) and specificity (97%) in infants from 1 month to 36 months. The majority of infants will have detectable HIV-1 DNA by 2 weeks of age. Infants born to

HIV-infected mothers should be tested during the first 48 hours of life to identify in utero transmission.

- HIV RNA polymerase chain reaction. Not recommended for routine testing. Useful in identifying non-B subtype HIV-1 infections. Can be used to quantify the amount of virus present as a predictor of disease progression.
- Enzyme immunoassays. Enzyme immunoassay, enzyme-linked immunoassay, and Western blot test. The enzyme immunoassay or enzyme-linked immunoassay detects serum HIV antibodies, which can then be confirmed by the Western blot test. Highly sensitive and specific; however, HIV antibody testing is not useful in determining the HIV status of neonates immediately following birth because maternal HIV antibodies transfer to the fetus via the placenta. Virologic assays (HIV culture, HIV DNA PCR, or HIV RNA polymerase chain reaction) are used to confirm diagnosis of HIV status.
- HIV p24 antigen. Detects the p24 antigen in the newborn. Less sensitive than the HIV-1 DNA polymerase chain reaction. High occurrence of false-positive results in samples taken from infants at less than 1 month of age. This test is no longer recommended for neonates.
- Viral culture. Determines the presence of HIV and helps distinguish between infant and maternal HIV infection. Limited availability, expensive, and requires up to 28 days for positive results.
- Complete blood count. Monitors for immune system compromise as well as anemia associated with administration of zidovudine (AZT, Retrovir).
- CD4+ lymphocyte count. CD4+ lymphocyte is a type of white blood cell. The count determines how HIV infection is affecting the immune system.

Medical Management

The goal of medical management is the diagnosis of HIV early in pregnancy and initiation of appropriate interventions to prevent mother-to-child transmission. The three primary measures to achieve this goal include antiretroviral prophylaxis, cesarean section before labor and rupture of membranes, and avoidance of breastfeeding. Oral administration of zidovudine should be initiated at 14 weeks' gestation and continued throughout pregnancy. During labor, intravenous zidovudine should be given to the mother, and following delivery, oral zidovudine should be given to the infant for the first 6 weeks of extrauterine life. When used, this regimen has demonstrated a significant reduction in disease transmission.

Collaborative Problems

Potential Complication of Exposure to HIV

- HIV infection

Potential Complications of HIV Infection

- Opportunistic infections
- Transmission of infection to others

COLLABORATIVE (STANDARDIZED) CARE FOR ALL INFANTS EXPOSED TO HIV/AIDS

Perform a comprehensive assessment to identify individual needs for parent teaching and emotional support, and infant physical care.

Potential Complication of Exposure to HIV: HIV INFECTION

Focus Assessments

- Assess the mother for risk factors/behaviors for HIV disease. Identifies those neonates at risk for HIV infection by obtaining and reviewing the maternal history. Effective antiretroviral agents are available for treating the mother and preventing the transmission of HIV infection from the mother to the fetus. Perinatal transmission rates are as high as 35% without intervention, but below 5% when appropriate care is given and antiretroviral treatment regimen is prescribed and when the woman adheres to the treatment.
- Assess infant lymph nodes. Lymphadenopathy (enlarged lymph nodes greater than 0.5 cm at more than two sites) in an infant who has been exposed to HIV may indicate the presence of HIV infection. According to the Centers for Disease Control and Prevention classification system for HIV in children younger than 13 years of age, if lymphadenopathy is coupled with one other condition such as hepatomegaly, splenomegaly, dermatitis, parotitis, sinusitis, otitis media, and/or recurrent or persistent respiratory infection, the infant meets the criteria for category A: mildly symptomatic.
- Assess spleen and liver. The presence of hepatomegaly or splenomegaly may indicate HIV infection in infants exposed to maternal HIV infection.
- Assess laboratory data. See previous "Diagnostic Studies" list. Detects changes in infant status and may detect altered humoral immune status.

Preventive Nursing Activities

- Implement standard precautions. The use of standard precautions for all patients prevents the transmission of HIV and other pathogens and reduces the risk of infection to the neonate and healthcare providers. Infants born to HIV-positive mothers are not always HIV positive. Strict standard precautions should be used by healthcare providers to interrupt mother-to-child transmission of HIV. HIV is transmitted by the direct contact of body fluids, so all body fluids must be considered a source of HIV transmission.
- Bathe the neonate with mild soap and water. Bathing the neonate minimizes the risk of infection with HIV or other

contaminants due to contact with maternal blood and body fluids.

- Monitor for signs and symptoms of local or systemic infection. Signs of systemic infection include elevated temperature, lethargy, and elevated white blood cell count. Signs of localized infection include erythema, swelling, tenderness, and warmth.

Nursing Diagnosis: RISK FOR INFECTION (OPPORTUNISTIC)[1]

Related Factors: HIV/AIDS.

Goals, Outcomes, and Evaluation Criteria

- Infant is free of signs of opportunistic infections.
- Infant has a normal growth curve.
- Infant demonstrates normal activity.
- Infant has a normal physical assessment.

NIC Interventions[2]

Infection Control (6540)—Minimizing the acquisition and transmission of infectious agents.

Infection Protection (6550)—Prevention and early detection of a patient at risk.

Newborn Care (6880)—Management of the neonate during the transition to extrauterine life and subsequent period of stabilization.

Risk Identification (6610)—Identification of an individual or family likely to experience difficulties in parenting and prioritization of strategies to prevent parenting problems

Nursing Activities and Rationales

Assessments

- Assess growth measurements (i.e., head circumference, length, and weight). Deviations from expected growth patterns may be an indication of HIV infection. Growth delay is a frequent, early finding in untreated perinatal HIV infection.
- Assess for signs and symptoms of opportunistic infections. Infection in HIV-infected newborns can be extremely serious and even life threatening. It is important to note the course and frequency of infectious episodes. Opportunistic infections can be bacterial, viral, fungal, or protozoal.
- Assess perianal area for rash. The presence of a red, raised rash, sometimes with white cottage cheese–like discharge, may indicate the presence of *Candida albicans*.
- Assess neurologic development. Detects changes that may indicate altered development or presence of opportunistic infection related to HIV infection. Encephalopathy is a

frequent manifestation of HIV infection in children prior to initiation of aggressive antiretroviral therapies.

- Assess bowel function and intolerance of feedings. The presence of loose, watery stools, which are recurrent or chronic, may indicate the presence of a protozoal infection with cryptosporidia. Prolonged diarrheal disease often leads to severe wasting.
- Assess respiratory status. An infant who presents with an acute respiratory illness, hypoxemia, and an atypical chest X-ray may have *Pneumocystis jiroveci* (formerly called *Pneumocystis carinii*). A dramatic reduction in the incidence and severity of *P. jiroveci* has been seen since the introduction of guidelines for *P. jiroveci* prophylaxis in HIV-exposed infants and HIV-infected children by the World Health Organization and the Joint United Nations Programme on HIV/AIDS (UNAIDS) in 2000.
- Monitor laboratory data. Establishes baseline and allows trending of data that might prove useful in detecting the presence of anemia, infection, and humoral immune dysfunction.

Parent/Family Teaching

- Maintain medical and surgical asepsis. Infants born to HIV-infected mothers may be infected with HIV; therefore, they are at increased risk for developing opportunistic infections.
- Thoroughly clean skin prior to administering vitamin K to prevent the introduction of pathogens. Prevents the introduction of microorganisms that may result in infection if the child is immunocompromised due to HIV infection.
- Teach mother signs and symptoms of opportunistic infection. Initially the HIV-infected newborn will not likely shows signs of infection. The mother needs to know how to recognize the signs of infection so that treatment can be implemented before the infant becomes severely ill. Signs of infection include fever, chills, restlessness, lethargy, cough, diarrhea, vomiting, white crusty patches in the mouth, or erythema of perineal area.
- Teach the mother the need for complying with HIV diagnostic testing of her infant. Virologic assays should be performed within the first 48 hours of birth, at 14 days of age, between 1 and 2 months of age, and again at 3–6 months of age. Follow-up testing should include two negative enzyme-linked immunoassays between 6 and 18 months of age or one negative enzyme-linked immunoassay between 18 and 24 months of age. Helping the mother understand the importance of monitoring her infant for HIV infection may increase her compliance with infant testing.
- Teach the mother about prescribed antiretroviral therapy for her infant. Antiretroviral drugs are prescribed for infants who are born to HIV-positive mothers in order

to prevent HIV infection. The drugs have numerous side effects, and schedules must be maintained in order to prevent drug resistance and maximize drug effectiveness. Understanding that maintaining prescribed drug regimens may prevent HIV infection in the infant may increase maternal compliance with infant's treatment regimen. The mother needs to know which side effects are expected and which ones need to be reported so that drug therapy can be adjusted if needed.

- Inform the mother/parents of the need for maintaining normal immunization schedules. HIV-infected infants should be immunized according to the Recommended Childhood and Adolescent Immunization schedule. Routine polio schedule should be administered as intramuscular inactivated polio vaccine. Influenza vaccines should be given annually and the pneumococcal vaccine given at 2 years of age. Children receiving intravenous immunoglobulin prophylaxis may not respond to measles, mumps, and rubella vaccine. Children who have symptomatic HIV infection have a poor immunologic response to vaccines. If HIV-infected children are exposed to a vaccine-preventable disease, they should be considered susceptible and treated with immune globulin.

▌ Nursing Diagnosis: RISK FOR TRANSMISSION OF INFECTION (HIV)

Related Factors: lack of knowledge regarding infection transmission and lack of motivation. See the generic NDCP, "Risk for Infection,[1]" beginning on p. 21 in Chapter 2.

▌ Goals, Outcomes, and Evaluation Criteria

The mother/parent(s):

- Keep scheduled appointments.
- Maintain prescribed drug dosages and schedules.
- Describe perinatal transmission of HIV.
- Describe methods to reduce perinatal transmission of HIV.
- Describe methods to prevent contracting opportunistic infections.
- Consume nutritious, well-balanced diet and adequate fluids.

▌ NIC Interventions[2]

High–Risk Pregnancy Care (6800)—Identification and management of a high-risk pregnancy to promote healthy outcomes for mother and baby.

Infection Control (6540)—Minimizing the acquisition and transmission of infectious agents.

Infection Protection (6550)—Prevention and early detection of infection in a patient at risk.

Nutrition Management (1100)—Assisting with or providing a balanced dietary intake of foods and fluids.

Teaching: Disease Process (5602)—Assisting the patient to understand information related to a specific disease process.

Teaching: Prescribed Medications (5616)—Preparing a patient to safely take prescribed medications and monitor for their effects.

▌ Nursing Activities and Rationales

Assessments

- During pregnancy, assess mother's understanding of HIV/AIDS and the risks it poses to the developing fetus. Identifies teaching needs and corrects misconceptions about transmission of HIV infection to her fetus.
- Assess understanding of her prescribed medications, dosages, and potential side effects. Determines teaching needs and identifies possible reasons why the mother may not comply with drug regimen.
- Monitor laboratory data (CD4 lymphocyte count, HIV RNA viral load, CBC and differential). Pregnancy is a stress response that may serve as an activating cofactor for viral replication, placing the mother at increased risk for disease progression and opportunistic infections.

Parent/Family Teaching

- Teach parents about HIV/AIDS and its implications on the newborn. The mother may be unaware of the potential risk for HIV infection of her infant. Teaching needs to include routes of pre-, intra-, and postnatal transmission so that the mother will cooperate with procedures implemented to reduce the risk of transmission to the infant.
- Teach mother the importance of maintaining zidovudine prophylaxis. Decreases the risk of prenatal transmission of HIV to the infant. Adherence to medication schedules and dosages is essential to maximize drug effectiveness in preventing transmission of the virus.
- Teach the mother the dose, frequency, side effects, and duration of zidovudine therapy. Knowledge of the medication regimen and its expected effects may increase compliance. The mother also needs to know expected side effects of the drug and those that need to be reported should they occur.
- Teach parents regarding the risk for HIV transmission through human milk and other body fluids. Reduces the risk of transmission of HIV to the infant. An HIV-infected mother who understands that her milk contains HIV and poses a risk to her infant's safety is more likely to accept the idea that she cannot safely breastfeed her infant.

Independent Nursing Actions

- Emphasize the importance of keeping all prenatal appointments. It is essential that the mother is closely monitored throughout pregnancy for disease progression and development of opportunistic infections. Pregnancy can cause an exacerbation of the disease process. Therefore, it is important to monitor the pregnant mother for signs of perinatal complications. Close follow-up will ensure early recognition of problems associated with HIV infection (e.g., weight loss, fatigue, drug side effects).

- Demonstrate support with a nonjudgmental attitude to convey concern and acceptance. Trust is essential to the helping relationship. The mother's fears or concerns may escalate in response to the nurse's approach in the absence of trust.

- Encourage verbalization of fears and concerns regarding transmission of HIV infection to newborn. Recognition and verbalization of fears often help reduce them.

- Encourage expression of factors that magnify feelings of fear (e.g., lifestyle changes, fetal well-being, financial changes, family functioning, and personal safety). A sense of greater self-control and adequacy in confronting danger reduces fear. Awareness of factors that intensify fears increases control and reduces fear when the reality of a situation is confronted.

INDIVIDUALIZED (NURSING DIAGNOSIS) CARE PLANS

This section includes care plans that were developed to address unique patient needs.

Nursing Diagnosis: INEFFECTIVE MANAGEMENT OF THERAPEUTIC REGIMEN, FAMILY[1]

Related Factors: knowledge deficit, fatigue, and complexity of the regimen.

Goals, Outcomes, and Evaluation Criteria

The mother/parent(s):

- Describes the rationale for the treatment regimen.
- Avoids behaviors associated with increased risk for infection.
- Complies with the prescribed plan of care.
- Describes the drug regimen and its side effects.

NIC Interventions[2]

Health System Guidance (7400)—Facilitating a patient's location and use of appropriate health services.

High-Risk Pregnancy Care (6800)—Identification and management of a high-risk pregnancy to promote healthy outcomes for mother and baby.

Teaching: Disease Process (5602)—Assisting the patient to understand information related to a specific disease process.

Nursing Activities and Rationales

Assessments

- Review history for past episodes of opportunistic infections. Determines if mother has asymptomatic HIV infection or AIDS. As immunosuppression begins to occur, opportunistic infections will arise, which qualifies the individual for the diagnosis of AIDS.

- Assess mother's understanding of her disease, the potential for opportunistic infections, and prescribed medications. Provides a baseline for teaching. Encourages early detection, which can promote early intervention. Stress the importance of compliance with prescribed antiretroviral drug therapy to prevent disease progression and improve resistance.

Parent/Family Teaching

- Teach mother about her HIV infection/AIDS. The mother may be unaware of the risk of perinatal transmission. She should also be counseled to avoid breastfeeding since HIV can be transmitted via human milk.

- Inform the mother about home care needs, including medication administration and side effects, restrictions in physical and sexual activity, and diet and hydration needs. Explain safe sex practices and appropriate birth control options to prevent disease transmission. Encourage rest periods throughout the day. Refer to nutritionist if necessary to ensure understanding of what constitutes a well-balanced diet that promotes health and helps prevent infection.

Other Nursing Diagnoses

Also assess for the following nursing diagnoses, which are frequently present:

- Impaired Parent–Infant/Child Attachment[1] related to mother's illness and complexity of therapeutic regimens, feelings of guilt, inability to care for the infant, and fear of transmitting illness to the infant.

- Spiritual Distress[1] (mother) related to feelings of guilt, despair over her own condition, and potential effects on the infant.

PRETERM NEWBORN

Infants born before the completion of 37 weeks' gestation are considered preterm. While the national birth average has been declining, the number of preterm births continues to climb. Prematurity is the leading cause of death during the first month of life and the second leading cause of all neonatal deaths. Preterm infants can be classified as small for gestational age (SGA), average for gestational age, or large for gestational age.

Because preterm infants do not stay in utero long enough, every one of their body systems may be immature, which might affect their ability to transition from intrauterine to extrauterine life.

Key Nursing Activities

- Differentiate between preterm and SGA infant.
- Monitor for and prevent complications (e.g., hypothermia, hypoglycemia, respiratory distress syndrome, hyperbilirubinemia).
- Provide neutral thermal environment.
- Monitor and support nutritional status.
- Provide appropriate developmental care.
- Provide parents with information about and an orientation to the NICU.

Etiologies and Risk Factors

The exact etiology of premature birth is not known in all circumstances. There are many associated risk factors with preterm labor and birth, but some of the more common ones include African American race, maternal age less than 16 years or greater than 40 years, low socioeconomic status, alcohol and/or drug use, cigarette smoking, insufficient prenatal care, multiple gestation, previous history of preterm birth, poor maternal nutrition, and maternal diabetes or hypertension.

Signs and Symptoms

- Birth weight less than 5.5 pounds, scrawny appearance, head circumference greater than chest circumference, decreased muscle tone, minimal subcutaneous fat, undescended testes, abundant lanugo, poorly formed ear pinnae, fused eyelids, soft and pliable skull bones, absent or diminished palmar and plantar creases, minimal scrotal rugae in males, prominent labia and clitoris in females, thin and transparent skin, underdeveloped breast tissue/nipples, and abundant vernix caseosa.
- Preterm infants continue to be at high risk for neurodevelopmental disorders, intraventricular hemorrhage, congenital anomalies, neurosensory impairment, behavioral issues, and chronic lung disease.

Diagnostic Studies

During Pregnancy

- Lecithin-sphingomyelin (L:S) ratio. Performed on amniotic fluid to estimate fetal lung maturity. A lecithin-sphingomyelin ratio of greater than or equal to 2.1 indicates mature lungs.
- Phosphatidylglycerol. Substance found in amniotic fluid that increases with gestational age. Can be useful in determining fetal lung maturity, although this test is less commonly used today than L:S ratio.
- Ultrasound. Can be helpful in predicting size and gestational age. Early sonography is more reliable than ultrasounds performed later in pregnancy.

Newborn

- Gestational age assessment. The Ballard and Dubowitz gestational age assessment tools estimate gestational age.

The more premature, the more likely that complications will occur.

- Point of care glucose monitoring. Detects hypoglycemia.
- Serum glucose. Confirmatory test for hypoglycemia when point-of-care glucose testing reveals blood glucose less than 50 mg/dl. Note: The definition of hypoglycemia varies by agency, some defining it as blood glucose less than 40 mg/dl.
- Serum calcium. Detects hypocalcemia.
- Evaluate serum bilirubin concentrations. Detects hyperbilirubinemia.
- CBC. Detects anemia and infection.
- Serum electrolyte levels. Determines serum levels of sodium, potassium, chloride, and carbon dioxide.
- C-reactive protein. An elevated C-reactive protein indicates an inflammatory process. C-reactive protein tests are most reliable at 24 hours of age and greater. Useful for trending purposes.
- Arterial blood gases (ABGs). Determines oxygenation status as well as acid-base balance.
- Fibrinogen levels. A decrease may indicate disseminated intravascular coagulation (DIC); an increase may occur with injury or inflammation.
- Blood and/or body fluid cultures. Identify the presence of infectious organisms.
- Urinalysis, culture, and specific gravity. Assess hydration and detect infection and/or renal injury; specific gravity greater than 1.015 is indicative of dehydration.
- Stool analysis. Detects occult blood, which may be a sign of NEC.
- Cranial ultrasound. Detects periventricular or intraventricular hemorrhage.
- Fibrin split products. Determines coagulation status if DIC occurs.
- Chest X-ray. Useful in establishing differential diagnosis for respiratory distress (e.g., respiratory distress syndrome vs. aspiration vs. transient tachypnea of the newborn vs. pneumonia).
- Lumbar puncture. Helpful in evaluating for sepsis. Might also be beneficial in managing intraventricular hemorrhage with communicating hydrocephalus.
- Computerized tomography scanning. Evaluates extent of intraventricular hemorrhage (IVH).

Medical Management

- Maternal betamethasone administration. Hastens fetal lung development when preterm birth is anticipated.
- Artificial surfactant administration. Premature infants lack surfactant in their lungs, predisposing them to RDS.
- Promote oxygenation.
- Maintain thermal regulation.
- Promote nutrition and fluid balance.
- Prevent infection; adequately treat if infection present.

- Prevent complications (RDS, IVH, chronic lung disease, retinopathy of prematurity, hyperbilirubinemia, anemia, necrotizing enterocolitis [NEC], hypoglycemia, infection, delayed growth and development.
- Provide appropriate stimulation.
- Manage pain.
- Promote adequate growth and development.
- Promote parental coping.
- Prepare for discharge (discharge planning starts at admission).

▋ Collaborative Problems

Potential Complications of Preterm Birth

- Respiratory distress syndrome
- Apnea and bradycardia
- Acidosis
- Anemia
- Hypocalcemia
- Hyponatremia
- Hyperkalemia
- Hypothermia
- Hyperbilirubinemia and bilirubin encephalopathy
- Hypoglycemia, hyperglycemia
- Periventricular/intraventricular hemorrhage
- Patent ductus arteriosus
- Retinopathy of prematurity
- Seizures
- Infection

Note: the three following nursing diagnoses should be included in the standardized care for all preterm infants.

1. Risk for Disorganized Infant Behavior[1]
2. Risk for Impaired Skin Integrity[1]
3. Risk for Imbalance Nutrition: Less Than Body Requirements[1]

COLLABORATIVE (STANDARDIZED) CARE FOR PRETERM INFANTS

Perform a comprehensive assessment to identify individual needs for parent teaching and emotional support and infant physical care.

▋ Potential Complication of Preterm Birth: RESPIRATORY DISTRESS SYNDROME

Focus Assessments

- Carefully assess gestational age and risk factors for respiratory distress syndrome. The more immature the infant, the more likely he/she will develop RDS. The incidence is inversely proportional to gestational age and birth weight. Statistically, white males are more susceptible to RDS than female infants, and Caucasian infants are more susceptible than African American infants.
- Assess respirations (normal is 30–60 breaths/min without assisted ventilation). Detects RDS. Preterm infants are born with numerous underdeveloped alveoli, which limit pulmonary blood flow and decrease the production of surfactant. The absence or deficiency of surfactant in the immature lung leads to decreased lung compliance and increased work of breathing. As exhaustion increases, neonates are able to open fewer and fewer alveoli, leading to atelectasis. Signs of respiratory decompensation or increased workload include tachypnea, grunting, nasal flaring, and retractions.
- Assess skin color and perfusion (capillary refill). Hypoxia due to RDS causes poor tissue perfusion with resulting changes in skin color (pale, gray, cyanotic). Cyanosis is a late sign of hypoxia and does not appear until oxygen saturation is as low as 75–85% and PO_2 levels are less than 40 mmHg. Cyanosis is an indication for prompt intervention.
- Analyze ABGs. Determines the effectiveness of ventilation. Atelectasis leads to hypoxemia and retained carbon dioxide, resulting in a respiratory acidosis. Hypoxemia, hypercapnia, and acidosis further reduce surfactant production in the immature lung, increasing the likelihood and severity of RDS.
- Obtain pulse oximetry (oxygen saturation should be about 88–92%). Evaluates severity of RDS and effectiveness of air/gas exchange and systemic absorption of oxygen in the bloodstream. Oxygen saturation (the amount of oxygen available to the tissues) and ultimately tissue perfusion decrease because of decreased gas exchange within the lungs and/or because of apnea and bradycardia.
- Review chest radiograph. Typical radiographic findings are consistent with hypoaeration, underexpansion, ground glass appearance, and visible air bronchograms.
- Monitor hydration and provide IV fluids in prescribed range. Dehydration causes mucus to become thick, making it difficult to clear the airways. Overhydration contributes to pulmonary edema.
- Monitor for complications related to oxygen therapy (e.g., retinopathy of prematurity). The developing retinal vessels in the premature infant are sensitive to high PaO_2 levels, which leads to the overgrowth of blood vessels in the retina. Secondary changes leading to visual impairment are due to retinal vessel constriction and buckling of the retina, which can lead to retinal detachment. Oxygen toxicity coupled with barotrauma from mechanical ventilation injures lung cells leading to chronic lung disease. Administering oxygen at concentrations over 70% increases the risk of pulmonary edema and retinopathy by creating a very high PaO_2. These complications are likely to

occur if blood oxygen saturation becomes greater than 100 mmHg for prolonged periods. Conversely, when the oxygen saturation/PaO$_2$ is low, the infant can suffer sequelae related to hypoxia, which affects all body systems.

Preventive Nursing Activities

- Administer antenatal steroids (betamethasone) to the mother when premature birth (34 or fewer weeks' gestation) is anticipated. Betamethasone is a corticosteroid that crosses the placenta to the fetus and stimulates fetal lung maturation. May also help prevent IVH and NEC.
- Administer artificial surfactant to neonate if RDS is confirmed by clinical symptoms, blood gas interpretation, and radiographic findings. Improves gas exchange and decreases the need for supplemental oxygen and ventilation. Fetal lungs do not produce adequate surfactant until after 34 weeks' gestation. Therefore, lung compliance (the ability of the lung to easily fill with air) is decreased and greater inspiratory pressure is needed to expand the lungs and fill the collapsed alveoli. This results in decreased gas exchange and hypoxia.
- Place infant in prone position. Facilitates chest expansion and improves air entry and oxygenation.
- If supine position must be used, slightly elevate the infant's head and place a small roll under shoulders to maintain head position. Facilitates inspiration and drainage of mucus or regurgitated formula. The bronchi and trachea are quite narrow and easily obstructed. The hypopharyngeal area is more collapsible in the preterm infant, which can lead to obstruction of the upper airway. The newborn has weak chest and abdominal muscles, making it difficult to raise the chest. Accessory muscles of respiration are underdeveloped, and the soft rib cartilage tends to collapse on expiration. The newborn has weak neck muscles and cannot control head movement.
- Maintain a neutral thermal environment. Reduces oxygen consumption. If infant becomes hypothermic, the metabolic rate increases in an effort to maintain body temperature; this increases oxygen consumption and may further inhibit surfactant production or accelerate utilization of endogenous surfactant.
- Cluster activities to provide rest periods and minimize stimulation. Reduces oxygen consumption.
- If RDS occurs:
  - Administer oxygen and ventilate as ordered to maintain adequate oxygen saturations and PaO$_2$. Relieves hypoxemia. If not treated immediately, hypoxemia can lead to metabolic acidosis.
  - Perform chest physiotherapy (percussion, vibration, and postural drainage) and suction as needed. Mobilizes secretions and maintains a patent airway.
  - Provide heated, humidified oxygen. Liquefies secretions, prevents drying of mucosa, and prevents cold

stress. Cold stress increases metabolism and further compromises the available oxygen supply.

Potential Complications of Preterm Birth: APNEA AND BRADYCARDIA

Focus Assessments

- Review records for maternal history of narcotic administration during labor. Identifies risk for RDS. Narcotics given close to the time of birth cause respiratory depression that may lead to neonatal apnea and bradycardia. A narcotic antagonist, such as naloxone (Narcan), may be necessary to reverse the respiratory depressant effects of the maternal narcotic analgesics.
- Assess respirations; monitor apneic episodes (cessation of breathing lasting more than 20 seconds). Many preterm infants have episodes of periodic breathing, but true apnea lasts more than 20 seconds and is accompanied by circumoral cyanosis, compromised perfusion, and most of the time, bradycardia with or without desaturation. Apnea is primarily a result of neuronal immaturity; however, it may occur because of hypoxia and CO$_2$ retention and decreased pH. It may be a sign of complications such as sepsis, RDS, cold stress, intracranial hemorrhage, hypoglycemia, and PDA.
- Assess cardiovascular status. Auscultate for regular rate and rhythm and for the presence of murmurs. The most likely audible murmur in a preterm infant is a patent ductus arteriosus (PDA) unless the infant has congenital heart disease. Infants born prematurely might also have a very active precordium.
- Monitor temperature. Assess temperature at least hourly until stable. Preterm babies have little to no brown fat and are not able to use nonshivering thermogenesis for heat production. Signs of cold stress include respiratory distress, central cyanosis, hypoglycemia, lethargy, weak cry, abdominal distention, apnea, bradycardia, and acidosis.
- Assess skin color and perfusion. Apnea and bradycardia cause tissue hypoxia, leading to poor tissue perfusion with resulting changes in skin color (pale gray, cyanotic, poor perfusion). Cyanosis is a late sign of hypoxia and does not appear until oxygen saturation is as low as 75–85% and PO$_2$ levels are less than 40 mmHg. Cyanosis indicates the need for prompt intervention.
- Obtain appropriate laboratory samples. Preterm infants are at higher risk for hypoglycemia secondary to depleted glycogen stores, so frequent monitoring of blood glucose values is essential. Infants of low birth weight also have increased insensible body fluid losses and immature

renal function, so they have increased fluid requirements and are at increased risk for electrolyte disturbances. Hypoglycemia and electrolyte disturbances can lead to apnea and bradycardia.

- Obtain appropriate cultures if infection is suspected. Preterm infants are often born infected or have come from an infected environment. Appropriate cultures should be obtained and antibiotic therapy should be initiated. Oftentimes, infection presents with apnea and bradycardia episodes.

Preventive Nursing Activities

- Maintain neutral thermal environment. Prevents cold stress, which can lead to apnea. Refer to the collaborative care plan, "Potential Complication of Preterm Birth: Hypothermia," beginning on p. 418 in this chapter.
- Correct underlying problems, such as respiratory distress, infection, hypoglycemia, anemia, and hypothermia. Prevents /treats apnea and bradycardia.
- If apnea develops:
  - Stimulate by stroking back. Promotes inspiration and ventilation. Stimulating the CNS promotes spontaneous resumption of breathing during apneic episodes.
  - Face-mask continuous positive airway pressure (CPAP) or bag-mask ventilation. Recruits alveoli and facilitates gas exchange.
  - Administer naloxone (Narcan). Counteracts narcotic-induced respiratory depression.
  - Administer respiratory stimulants. Preterm infants are at high risk for apnea of prematurity, which can be treated with theophylline, caffeine, or doxapram. If respiratory stimulant therapy is not effective, intubation and mechanical ventilation may be necessary.

Potential Complication of Preterm Birth: ACIDOSIS

Focus Assessments

- Assess ABGs. Blood gases provide information about the functional status of alveolar and capillary diffusion, alveolar ventilation, pulmonary circulation, pulmonary gas exchange, and acid-base balance. Low pH (normal 7.35–7.45), normal to increased bicarbonate (normal 22–26 mEq/L), and high $PaCO_2$ (normal 35–45 mmHg) indicate respiratory acidosis, which occurs from decreased alveolar ventilation and retention of CO_2 secondary to surfactant deficiency and atelectasis. In addition to respiratory acidosis, the preterm infant is susceptible to metabolic acidosis (decreased pH, decreased bicarbonate [HCO_3], and normal to decreased $PaCO_2$) because the immature kidneys have poor buffering capacity (they require a

longer time to excrete the lactic acid that accumulates during hypoxia or other insult), and the preterm baby is susceptible to cold stress, which leads to metabolic acidosis as the infant attempts to compensate by conserving heat and increasing heat production.

- Assess base excess (negative). A negative base excess is indicative of acidosis.
- Assess anion gap (greater than 20 mEq). Determining the specific type of acidosis is important for effective treatment. An elevated anion gap is associated with metabolic acidosis caused by excess acid instead of a rise in chloride levels. Acidosis of respiratory origin is primarily corrected with ventilation and oxygenation whereas metabolic acidosis is initially treated with bicarbonate solution to increase the pH. The major component of the anion gap is albumin. Hypoalbuminemia is very common in critically ill neonates.
- Assess urine pH (less than 7). Urine pH reflects the kidney's ability to regulate acid-base balance. In both respiratory and metabolic acidosis, excess lactic acid must be excreted in the urine.
- Assess blood chemistries (calcium, potassium, carbon dioxide). Identifies the type and severity of acidosis. Several electrolyte imbalances are associated with acidosis. Acidosis causes potassium to be driven out of the cells. When calcium is incorporated into bone, hydrogen ions are released, leading to acidosis. In metabolic acidosis, bicarbonate and bases are used to neutralize excess acids, resulting in a loss of carbon dioxide.
- Assess respirations. Tachypnea is a symptom of acidosis. In an attempt to compensate for high levels of carbonic acid, the respiratory rate increases to expire excess CO_2.

Preventive Nursing Activities

- Have all basic equipment readily available and resuscitate immediately after birth if necessary. Resuscitation measures include stabilization, ventilation, chest compressions, and administration of medications. The decision to progress from one action to another is based on clinical assessment of infant's respirations, heart rate, and color. Prevents respiratory and metabolic acidosis, respectively. Because most preterm infants have an immature pulmonary capillary bed to absorb oxygen as well as an insufficient amount of endogenous lung surfactant, they have difficulty maintaining adequate respirations at birth to meet bodily needs. When an infant does not have sufficient surfactant in the lungs, the air sacs collapse and air/gas exchange is impaired. A great deal of energy is used merely to inflate the alveoli with each breath. Demonstrate good thermoregulation principles during resuscitation efforts. If not kept warm, the infant must increase the metabolic rate to maintain body temperature; this requires energy (and oxygen) expenditure, leading quickly to irreversible acidosis.

- Maintain oxygenation and ventilation. Facilitates the elimination of carbon dioxide. Increasing oxygenation may correct acid-base balance and eliminate the need for bicarbonate administration.
- Administer bicarbonate as ordered. Corrects metabolic acidosis. Immature kidneys excrete bicarbonate at a lower serum level, so it is easily depleted; they excrete acid more slowly, so it tends to build up. Increasing oxygenation may correct acid-base balance and eliminate the need for bicarbonate administration.
- Maintain a neutral thermal environment. A neutral thermal environment is the environmental temperature that minimizes heat loss, which in turn decreases oxygen consumption and decreases metabolic stress.

Potential Complication of Preterm Birth: ANEMIA

Focus Assessments

- Assess skin color and perfusion. Pallor and cyanosis reflect decreased oxygen-carrying capacity with low hemoglobin. Capillary refill greater than 3 seconds indicates impaired circulatory perfusion. In neonates, a change in perfusion is a sensitive indicator of cardiorespiratory stability.
- Monitor heart rate. Tachycardia or bradycardia can be indicative of anemia. To compensate for decreased oxygenation and hypoxia, the heart rate increases above baseline. However, with severe anemia, when the oxygen-carrying capacity is diminished to the point at which hypoxemia and tissue compromise occur, then the infant may experience apnea and bradycardia.
- Monitor respirations (tachypnea, apnea, grunting, retractions, and nasal flaring). Respiratory effort increases to compensate for hypoxia secondary to decreased oxygen-carrying capacity of the RBCs, leading to signs of respiratory distress.
- Monitor neurologic status. An infant with anemia often experiences lethargy because of reduced oxygen delivery to the body systems and tissues.
- Assess abdomen for enlarged liver. Hepatosplenomegaly is associated with extramedullary hematopoiesis.
- Monitor CBC. Anemia is indicated by a low hemoglobin/hematocrit and red blood cell count.
- Note reticulocyte count. Red blood cell production increases to compensate for anemia, resulting in the increased presence of immature reticulocytes. This may not be apparent in infants born at less than 32 weeks' gestation because the bone marrow does not increase its production until approximately 32 weeks. Reticulocyte counts are also not reliable in infants who have been recently transfused.

- Note ferritin levels. Decreased ferritin levels are associated with decreased stores of iron, common in the preterm infant.
- Guaiac test stools. Positive test indicates occult blood in the stools, possibly as a result of feeding intolerance or necrotizing enterocolitis.

Preventive Nursing Activities

- Identify infants at risk because of obstetric accidents, internal hemorrhage, twin-to-twin transfusion, Rh or ABO incompatibility, infection, or inherited metabolic conditions. Detects anemia so that it can be treated before it becomes severe.
- Monitor and record volumes of blood obtained for lab work. Prevents iatrogenic anemia and identifies the need for blood replacement. In the preterm infant normochromic normocytic anemia with low RBC count occurs because (1) RBC production is decreased and the bone marrow does not increase its production until about 32 weeks' gestation; (2) RBC destruction is increased and the infant has a low level of vitamin E, which normally protects RBCs from destruction; (3) the infant has inadequate iron stores; (4) red cells have a shorter life span; (5) there is increased tendency to bleed (prolonged prothrombin and partial thromboplastin time); and (6) capillaries are friable. Anemia of prematurity is typically most common in infants born at less than 35 weeks' gestation and appears between 2 and 6 weeks of age.
- If anemia occurs:
  - Determine most likely etiology and treat accordingly. Anemia can be treated with volume expanders, iron, folic acid, vitamin E, and recombinant erythropoietin. Promotes erythropoiesis (stimulation of red blood cells' production by the bone marrow) and restores blood volume.
  - Transfuse with blood products as ordered. Replaces blood components, especially RBCs.

Potential Complications of Preterm Birth: HYPOCALCEMIA AND HYPOPROTEINEMIA

Focus Assessments

- Monitor serum chemistries and report abnormalities. Determines physiologic status; serum calcium less than 7 mg/dl indicates hypocalcemia. Low levels of calcium, magnesium, protein, and albumin may occur, as stores are inadequate at birth (two thirds of calcium stores are deposited in the third trimester). The preterm newborn requires a larger amount of nutrients than the mature infant because the body attempts to maintain the rapid growth that would be occurring if still in utero. If nutrients are not supplied, hypocalcemia and hypoproteinemia (low protein level in the blood) develop. Because about 50% of calcium is protein bound, low total protein and albumin levels also affect the storage of calcium in the body. Deficits in magnesium are associated with low calcium levels.

- Monitor glucose levels. Differentiates between hypoglycemia and hypocalcemia. Clinical signs of hypoglycemia are similar to those of hypocalcemia. Also, hypocalcemia often occurs with hypoglycemia.
- Perform a neurologic assessment. Detects clinical signs of hypocalcemia (irritability, tremors, poor feeding, muscle twitches, jitteriness, high-pitched cry, and seizures), which occur because calcium level is not adequate for normal nerve impulse transmission.
- Monitor respirations (for apnea). Apnea, a sign of hypocalcemia, may occur because calcium is important in neuromuscular function, including the muscles of respiration.
- Monitor heart rate (for bradycardia). Bradycardia is a sign of hypocalcemia. Calcium is important in cardiac impulse conduction.
- Monitor blood pressure (for hypotension). Helps detect hypocalcemia. Calcium is important in cardiac muscle contraction; forceful contraction is essential for maintaining the blood pressure.
- Monitor serum protein levels. Detects hypoproteinemia. Sufficient protein is required for calcium binding, transport, and utilization.

Preventive Nursing Activity

- Administer vitamin D and calcium gluconate as ordered. Vitamin D naturally increases calcium levels by facilitating calcium absorption and bone reabsorption; calcium gluconate provides supplemental calcium.

Potential Complication of Preterm Birth: HYPONATREMIA

Focus Assessments

- Assess blood chemistry (for sodium). Low serum sodium may occur due to inadequate intake, decreased renal absorption, overhydration (dilutional hyponatremia), or dehydration.
- Assess serum osmolality (to see if it is low). Since sodium is the major determinate of osmolality, low concentrations of sodium will result in low osmolality.
- Perform a neurologic assessment. Hyponatremia may cause cerebral edema, which may lead to lethargy and seizures.
- Monitor respirations (for apnea). Apnea is a clinical sign of hyponatremia.

- Monitor for vomiting. Electrolyte losses through emesis can lead to hyponatremia.
- Maintain and monitor intake and output. Detects dehydration or overhydration, which can cause hyponatremia. Sodium is the most abundant cation in extracellular fluid; thus, changes in sodium concentration are a reflection of fluid balance. Sodium levels decrease whether the total fluid volume decreases or increases (e.g., through dilution in overhydration).

Preventive Nursing Activities

- If hyponatremia occurs, administer sodium as ordered. Restores normal levels.
- Correct underlying problems (e.g., renal insufficiency, vomiting). Prevents further sodium loss.

Potential Complication of Preterm Birth: HYPOTHERMIA

Focus Assessments

- Monitor temperature with skin probe (should be 36–37°C [96.8–97.7°F]). Detects hypothermia. Ineffective thermoregulation is a common and serious problem for preterm infants related to immaturity of the hypothalamus, which is the temperature regulation center in the brain. An infant servo-controlled skin probe provides continuous monitoring and regulation of environmental temperature support for more stable thermoregulation in the infant. Temperature changes are reflected first in the skin and later, in the body core. Preterm infants produce little heat because they have limited glycogen stores (glycogen stores are laid down mainly during the third trimester), and limited stores of brown fat can be metabolized for heat production; muscle mass is small, and muscular activity is limited. Heat loss is increased because the preterm infant has a high ratio of body surface to body weight (heat loss in a 1,500-g infant is five times per unit of body weight more than in an adult), thin, permeable skin, minimal subcutaneous fat to serve as insulation (heat is lost from the blood vessels, which lie close to the skin), poor muscle tone, greater surface area exposed to the environment, decreased ability to vasoconstrict superficial blood vessels, and an immature temperature regulation center in the brain. Preterm infants often have other complications, such as hypoglycemia and hypoxia, that may lead to hypothermia as a result of metabolic changes and the need for more oxygen than the lungs can supply. Other conditions, such as hyperbilirubinemia, are caused or aggravated by hypothermia.
- Take axillary temperature periodically. Be sure skin probe is securely adhered to the skin. Ensures accuracy of skin probe and functioning of warming unit. If skin probe

detaches, warmer-induced hyperthermia may occur. Keep in mind, a skin protectant is essential to prevent damage to the stratum corneum layers of skin in the preterm infant.

- Review intrapartum records for maternal medications and/or fetal distress or hypoxia. Hypoxia and maternal meperidine (Demerol) impair metabolism of brown fat, possibly interfering with the infant's ability to maintain body temperature. Administration of MgSO4 to the mother during labor can cause neonatal vasodilation, contributing to heat loss.

- Monitor heart rate for tachycardia or bradycardia. These are clinical signs of hypothermia. In hypothermia, the heart rate increases as a result of increased metabolism that occurs as the body attempts to produce heat. If the heart cannot compensate or hypothermia is sustained, bradycardia occurs (decompensation).

- Monitor respirations (tachypnea, apnea, grunting, retractions, nasal flaring). These are clinical signs of hypothermia. Hypoxia and acidosis associated with hypothermia lead to respiratory distress.

- If hypothermia occurs, monitor ABGs for metabolic acidosis. Detects complications of hypothermia. In hypothermia, as brown fat is metabolized to generate heat, fatty acids are released, resulting in metabolic acidosis.

- Monitor serum glucose (to see if it has decreased). Brown fat requires glucose. Hypoglycemia can be associated with hypothermia.

- Assess skin (for coolness, poor perfusion, pallor, cyanosis, mottling, and acrocyanosis). These are clinical signs of hypothermia. Peripheral vasoconstriction occurs as the body shuts blood away from the periphery to increase circulation to and oxygenation of vital organs. Decreased circulation to the skin coupled with decreased core body temperature decreases extremity perfusion and produces cool, discolored extremities.

- Assess neurologic status (check for restlessness, lethargy, hypotonia, weak cry, and poor feeding). The metabolism of brown fat by a hypothermic infant requires glucose and oxygen; therefore, there is a lack of glucose and oxygen for use by the central nervous system, which can result in neurologic compromise, particularly in the preterm infant who is prone to brain injury and other central nervous system damage.

Preventive Nursing Activities

- Maintain neutral thermal environment. An ambient nursery temperature of 25°C (77°F) is a rule of thumb; however, the ambient room temperature may require adjustment depending on the infant's core or surface temperature. Minimizes oxygen consumption expended in maintaining a normal core temperature and prevents cold stress. Cold stress (hypothermia) increases oxygen and calorie needs and may lead to hypoxia and acidosis and/or further inhibit surfactant production. Cold stress can occur in an infant even when environmental temperatures are normal.

- Place infant in double-walled incubator or under radiant warmer. Use heat shield over very small infants. Prevents heat loss via convection.

- Use warmed, humidified oxygen and do not blow it over the face. Prevents heat loss via convection; increases oxygen consumption. Oxygen should be at 31–34°C (88–93°F).

- Do not place baby on cold surfaces (e.g., scales, X-ray plates, metal treatment tables); pad cold surfaces and place under radiant warmer during procedures; warm hands before touching the baby. Prevents heat loss via conduction and radiation.

- Keep dry (e.g., change damp linens immediately); place cap on baby's head. Prevents heat loss by evaporation and radiation. The head is very vascular, with vessels lying close to the skin, and makes up a proportionately large area of the infant's body; therefore, a great deal of heat can be lost through the scalp.

- Warm formula or stored human milk before feeding. Prevents heat loss by conduction.

- Keep crib away from windows and cold walls and out of drafts. Prevents heat loss via radiation and convection.

- Correct acidosis, hypoglycemia, hypoxemia, sepsis, and metabolic problems that may compromise thermoregulation. Because such conditions increase metabolism, they deplete oxygen and brown fat stores that are needed for maintaining temperature.

- If infant requires warming, gradually rewarm infant using hats, clothing, blankets, and external sources such as incubator, radiant warmer); check temperature every 15 min during rewarming. Rapid rewarming causes excessive oxygen consumption, leading to apnea. Never use hot water bottles, hot water-filled gloves, or warm blankets in a microwave oven.

- Encourage kangaroo care. Facilitates maintenance of the premature infant's body temperature.

- Support respiratory efforts; provide oxygen as needed. Hypoxia decreases the oxygen needed for the increased metabolism that occurs in an effort to maintain body temperature and can, therefore, lead to cold stress. Conversely, if hypothermia exists, it reduces the infant's ability to cope with hypoxia and hypercapnia.

Potential Complications of Preterm Birth: HYPERBILIRUBINEMIA AND BILIRUBIN ENCEPHALOPATHY

Refer to "Hyperbilirubinemia," which begins on p. 436 in this chapter. Note that, as a result of increased ability of bilirubin to cross the blood–brain barrier, preterm infants tend to develop bilirubin encephalopathy at lower serum bilirubin levels than full-term infants do. Causes of hyperbilirubinemia include overproduction, undersecretion, a combination of overproduction/undersecretion, breastfeeding/human milk jaundice, and a few other miscellaneous causes such as hypothyroidism and galactosemia. Infants of diabetic mothers also tend to be at increased risk for hyperbilirubinemia as a result of an expanded red blood cell mass and hypovolemia.

Preventive Nursing Activities

- Correct hematologic problems (e.g., administer vitamin E); support nutrition (tube feed, if necessary). Preterm infants are at risk for hyperbilirubinemia because of increased destruction of their RBCs secondary to a low level of vitamin E, which normally protects RBCs from destruction; their red cells have a shorter-than-normal life span; their immature livers cannot convert bilirubin to a form that can be excreted; and they may have delayed feeding so that bilirubin is not eliminated sufficiently in the stool.
- Prevent or correct dehydration. Allows bilirubin to be excreted in the urine. Preterm infants are at risk for dehydration because of their relatively thin skin and poor oral intake. When the infant is not well hydrated, the bilirubin tends to increase further. In addition, kidney function is immature, which leads to fluid volume imbalance.
- Institute early enteral feedings as tolerated. Use of the intestine for enteral feedings will prevent the uptake of bilirubin from the gut back into the bloodstream. Stooling is an effective way to eliminate bilirubin.
- Closely monitor the infant who is at risk for hyperbilirubinemia. Early intervention prevents bilirubin encephalopathy. Infants at risk are those who are less than 37 weeks' gestation; are born to a mother with Coombs'-positive blood, incompatible blood type, and antibody in the serum; have sepsis; have a viral infection or neonatal hepatitis; have delayed enteral feedings; have cephalohematoma and/or extensive bruising; receive twin-to-twin transfusion or maternal–fetal transfusion; have delayed cord clamping; have maternal diabetes mellitus; have a genetic syndrome (trisomy 21 or Beckwith-Wiedemann syndrome); have polycythemia; or have conditions associated with hemolytic anemia (e.g., spherocytosis, elliptocytosis, or G6PD).

Potential Complication of Preterm Birth: HYPOGLYCEMIA

See the collaborative care plan, "Potential Complication of an Infant of a Diabetic Mother: Hypoglycemia," beginning on p. 399 in "Infant of a Diabetic Mother," in this chapter. Brain damage may

occur when serum glucose is less than 30 mg/dl. Preterm infants are at risk for hypoglycemia because they have inadequate stores of glycogen (which is not built up until about 32 weeks' gestation) and because the immature liver does not store or release glycogen well. Note that the preterm infant's kidneys begin excreting glucose at a lower than normal serum glucose level, so glycosuria is not unusual.

Focus Assessments

- Assess blood chemistries for hypocalcemia (serum calcium less than 7 mg/dl). Hypocalcemia is often present with hypoglycemia; it may lead to seizures and/or apnea.

Potential Complication of Preterm Birth: PERIVENTRICULAR/ INTRAVENTRICULAR HEMORRHAGE

Focus Assessments

- Note birth weight. Determines risk for periventricular hemorrhage (bleeding into the tissue surrounding the ventricles) and intraventricular hemorrhage (bleeding into the ventricles), which occur in about 50% of very-low-birth-weight infants. IVH is the most common type of intracranial hemorrhage in preterm infants of less than 34 weeks' gestation or those weighing less than 1,500 g. Before 35 weeks, the brain ventricles are highly susceptible to hypoxia (e.g., as in RDS and birth asphyxia). The germinal matrix is very vascular and the blood vessels are fragile, so they rupture easily in the presence of changes in cerebral blood pressure, such as occurs with hypoxia, IV infusion, ventilation, and pneumothorax. In addition, premature infants have prolonged bleeding times, making them even more susceptible to hemorrhage. The biggest majority of bleeding events occur in the first 72 hours of life. In neonates, intraventricular hemorrhages are classified as grade I, II, III, or IV. Grade I is a germinal matrix hemorrhage with little or no intraventricular hemorrhage, grade II has blood in 10–50% of the ventricular area, grade III has intraventricular blood in greater than 50% of the area, and a grade IV bleed has blood extending beyond the ventricles into the surrounding parenchyma.
- Assess the infant's overall activity level and muscle tone, check for change in level of consciousness, full fontanels with increased separation in the sagittal suture, pallor or compromised perfusion, seizure activity, and lack of papillary change to light. Bulging or tense fontanels may be the first sign of IVH or increased intracranial pressure (ICP).
- Monitor vital signs. Detects ICP. Most commonly, the

preterm infant will develop increased frequency and severity of apnea and bradycardia episodes. For severe hemorrhage, Cheyne-Stokes respirations may occur in response to the lowering of PaO_2 levels and increasing $PaCO_2$ levels.

- Monitor Hgb and Hct. A sudden decrease in Hct may be the first indicator of IVH.
- Monitor blood gases for metabolic acidosis. Although metabolic acidosis is a nonspecific finding, it almost invariably occurs with grade II–IV IVH/periventricular hemorrhage.
- Assess for signs of overstimulation (flaccidity, yawning, irritability, crying, and staring). Allows infant to rest by minimizing stimulation and possibly preventing ICP.
- Monitor for signs of pneumothorax. Pneumothorax often precedes periventricular hemorrhage/IVH in preterm infants.

Preventive Nursing Activities

- Prepare the infant and parents for the cranial ultrasound. This is a noninvasive screening procedure that can be performed at the infant's bedside at most level II, III, and IV nurseries. The scan is obtained through the anterior fontanel and takes a short amount of time for imaging.
- Monitor and support respiratory function (e.g., administer oxygen, as needed). The brain is very vascular and blood vessels are friable, so they rupture easily in the presence of hypoxia.
- Limit the amount of stimulation the infant receives. Decreases stress response to prevent ICP.
- Institute pain control methods. Decreases stress response to prevent ICP.
- Avoid hypertonic solutions and medications. These increase ICP by increasing cerebral blood flow.
- Elevate head of bed 15–20 degrees, and position head in midline. Makes use of gravity to decrease ICP.
- Administer corticosteroids prenatally when preterm birth is expected prior to 33 weeks' gestation. Reduces the incidence of periventricular hemorrhage/IVH.

Potential Complication of Preterm Birth: PATENT DUCTUS ARTERIOSUS

Focus Assessments

- Assess skin color (it should be pink). Because preterm infants lack surfactant, their lungs are noncompliant and it is difficult for them to move blood from the pulmonary artery into the lungs. Because of pulmonary artery hypertension, underdeveloped pulmonary arteriole musculature, and hypoxemia, the ductus arteriosus fails to close. However, patent ductus arteriosus (PDA) is a left-to-right

shunt, so cyanosis is typically not present. If cyanosis is present, it is likely to be of respiratory origin rather than a symptom of PDA.

- Assess the cardiovascular system (listen for tachycardia, continuous machine-like murmur, active precordium, and bounding pulses). Systolic murmur is best heard at the second or third intercostal space at the upper left sternal border, often with radiation to left axilla and back. The blood flow through a PDA is primarily from the aorta to the pulmonary artery (left-to-right shunt). Turbulence is often present, especially if the PDA is closing. Many times, the smaller the opening, the louder the noise. The shunt also increases pulmonary vascular resistance, leading to pulmonary congestion, congestive heart failure, tachycardia, an active precordium, and bounding pulses.
- Assess respirations (check for apnea, tachypnea, grunting, retractions, nasal flaring, crackles, rhonchi, and RDS). Increased pulmonary congestion and pulmonary hypertension associated with a PDA lead to alveolar and bronchiolar edema, resulting in the signs of respiratory distress.
- Evaluate ABGs for hypercapnia and metabolic acidosis. The PDA itself does not change the arterial blood gas values. However, with associated respiratory distress syndrome, blood gas results may demonstrate hypercapnia and metabolic acidosis.
- Review chest radiograph. With small shunts, chest radiograph examination should reveal normal cardiac size and shape. With larger shunts, there will likely be cardiac enlargement with evidence of increased pulmonary vascularity.
- Daily weight. Weight is increased with fluid retention, decreased with increased cardiac work. Congestive heart failure increases the metabolic needs because of increased workload of the heart, leading to weight loss and failure to thrive.

Preventive Nursing Activities

- If PDA occurs, asymptomatic infants generally do not require medical or surgical management but should be closely monitored for evidence of congestive heart failure, failure to thrive, increasing oxygen requirements, or other associated complications. Care should be provided as follows:
  - Restrict fluids. Prevents congestive heart failure and pulmonary edema, prevents increasing blood pressure, including pulmonary artery pressure, and intensifying the pathophysiology of the PDA. Note: Medical management with fluid restriction is not always highly successful.
  - Administer indomethacin as prescribed. Medically closes the patent ductus. Indomethacin blocks the effects of the arachidonic acid products on the ductus and causes the PDA to constrict. It can be administered orally or

intravenously for a total of three doses. It is not as effective after 7 days of age and probably has no effect if treatment is initiated beyond 14 days of age. Urine output must be closely monitored and indomethacin should be stopped if there is a dramatic decrease in output. Contraindications to indomethacin therapy include severe renal impairment or failure, active CNS or gastrointestinal tract bleeding, and NEC.

- Administer ibuprofen as prescribed. Ibuprofen is a prostaglandin synthetase inhibitor that has similar effects on ductal closure and possibly reduced renal side effects. It is also given for a total of three doses.
- Administer diuretics as prescribed. Removes excess fluid and prevents/relieves congestive heart failure and pulmonary edema. Hypervolemia causes leakage of plasma fluid across pulmonary capillary membranes into the lungs and increases the workload of the heart. When the heart can no longer pump the increased volume, contractility will diminish (heart failure) and fluid will back up into the lungs (pulmonary edema). Osmotic diuretics pull fluid from interstitial spaces into the vascular space where it can be eliminated by the kidneys. Loop diuretics prevent the reabsorption of water at the renal tubules, promoting fluid elimination.

- Maintain oxygenation and ventilation as needed, based on ABG values. Prevents hypoxia and corrects acid-base imbalances.

Potential Complication of Preterm Infants: SEIZURES

Seizures are the most frequent and sometimes the only clinical sign of central nervous system dysfunction in the neonate. They are caused by a variety of acute and chronic stressors on the brain (electrolyte disturbances, hypoglycemia, metabolic conditions, infection, intracranial hemorrhage, congenital malformations, drug withdrawal, bilirubin encephalopathy, etc.). Seizures prompt urgent medical attention.

Focus Assessments

- Assess temperature (note whether it has increased or decreased). Identifies risk for or symptoms of seizures. Hypothermia and hyperthermia may lead to seizures. Also, because of the increase in metabolism seen in seizures, body temperature may increase.
- Assess heart rate (check for bradycardia). Bradycardia may be seen secondary to hypoxia and hypoglycemia, conditions that can lead to seizures.
- Assess respirations (check for apnea). Evaluates effects of seizures on respiratory functioning. Repeated seizures lead to hypoventilation and apnea secondary to hypoxia and hypoglycemia.

- Observe for lethargy, eye rolling, bulging fontanels, hypotonia, hyperreflexia, apnea, high-pitched cry, and opisthotonos. These indicate altered CNS function (e.g., from increased ICP, intracranial hemorrhage, hypoxemia, and hypoglycemia), which may precede seizure activity.
- Obtain CBC. A CBC may suggest an etiology for the seizures, such as infection, anemia, hemorrhage, or hyperviscosity. Any condition that reduces the oxygen-carrying capacity of the blood or that affects oxygenation and tissue perfusion affects the CNS and can lead to seizures.
- Monitor blood glucose and observe for symptoms of hypoglycemia (e.g., jitteriness, tremors, lethargy, high-pitched cry). Identifies risk factor for seizures. Because of the metabolic demands present in preterm infants, hypoglycemia is common, as is hypoxia. Seizures occur when there is a lack of oxygen and glucose in the brain cells.
- Monitor bilirubin levels; observe for jaundice. Detects bilirubin encephalopathy, which can cause seizures. Preterm infants develop bilirubin encephalopathy at lower serum bilirubin levels than full-term infants.
- Report abnormalities in serum chemistries (such as abnormal levels of sodium, calcium, and magnesium). Identifies risk factor or etiology of seizures. Hypocalcemia, which often accompanies hypoglycemia, may result in seizures, as can hyponatremia. Serum chemistries are also used to rule out metabolic and electrolyte disturbances as the etiology of CNS symptoms.
- If seizures occur, assist with or review the results of the following:
  - Lumbar puncture. Cerebrospinal fluid should be examined for red blood cells, white blood cells, glucose, protein, and microorganisms. Meningitis is a dangerous but treatable cause of seizures.
  - Cultures (blood, urine, cerebrospinal fluid, pharyngeal or tracheal aspirate). Seizures can occur secondary to underlying infection.
  - Electroencephalogram. The EEG is the only way to detect paroxysmal electrical discharge associated with seizures.
  - Neurologic assessment (note decorticate posturing, clonic jerking, horizontal deviation of eyes, nystagmus, drooling, sucking, smacking, tongue thrusting, pedaling, rowing, or swimming movements, eye blinking or fluttering, and normal size, shape, and reactivity of pupils). Assesses effects of seizure activity on the central nervous system. Neural damage and dysfunction due to inflammation, alterations in blood flow, hypoglycemia, and hypoxia lead to a variety of nonspecific manifestations associated with paroxysmal electrical activity that occurs with seizures.
  - CT scan. Identifies areas of brain injury and dysfunction.
  - Cranial ultrasound examination. Identifies brain pathology. Seizures may result from increased intracranial pressure and brain hemorrhaging.

- Skull radiograph. Skull radiographs may be used to detect IVH or skull fractures.
- Liver function studies (including those for alanine aminotransferase, aspartate aminotransferase, and ammonia). Rules out metabolic encephalopathy.

Preventive Nursing Activities

- Identify and correct underlying problems associated with seizure activity (e.g., hypoglycemia, fluid/electrolyte imbalances, meningitis, hypothermia). If caused by underlying pathophysiology, seizures may be halted without CNS damage. Some permanent seizure disorders result directly from neurologic defects or damage.
- Provide supplemental oxygen, as needed. Hypoxemia can cause seizures; if seizures are caused by another condition, hypoxemia increases the risk of permanent CNS damage.
- When seizures occur:
  - Maintain patent airway. Prevents worsening hypoxia. Placing the infant on its side facilitates mucus drainage, helps maintain a patent airway, and prevents aspiration.
  - Avoid moving or forcefully restraining infant during seizure. Protects the infant from injury. Once the seizure has started it cannot be halted and the seizure should be allowed to end without interference.
  - Assess for breathing immediately following seizure. Identifies the need for rescue breathing if spontaneous respirations do not return following seizure activity.
  - Administer anticonvulsants as ordered. Arrests seizure activity.
  - Provide fluid replacement or maintain fluid restrictions, as appropriate. Adequate fluid volume is needed for cerebral perfusion; however, fluid restriction may be necessary when there is cerebral edema or increased cranial pressure.

Nursing Diagnosis: RISK FOR INFECTION[1]

Newborns are more susceptible to infection because their immune systems are immature and slow to react, which make preterm infants even more susceptible. The mortality rate of newborns with sepsis may be as high as 50% if untreated, and it is a major cause of death during the first month of life. Newborn infections are generally classified as congenital, early onset, or late onset. Major risk factors include premature rupture of membranes, premature onset of labor, chorioamnionitis, recent maternal illness, maternal fever during the peripartum period, maternal urinary tract infection, rupture of membranes greater than 18 hours, and instrumentation at delivery. The preterm infant is also at increased risk secondary to poor skin integrity, invasive procedures, exposure to numerous caregivers, and an environment that is conducive to bacterial colonization.

Goals, Outcomes, and Evaluation Criteria

- Infant remains free of infection, as evidenced by temperature stable at 36.5°C (97.6°F) (axillary) and no signs of infection (poor growth, poor muscle tone, low activity level, poor feeding or feeding intolerance, abdominal distention, pallor, poor perfusion, increase in severity and/or frequency of apnea and bradycardia, or jaundice).

NIC Interventions[2]

Infection Control (6540)—Minimizing the acquisition and transmission of infectious agents.

Infection Protection (6550)—Prevention and early detection of infection in a patient at risk.

Nursing Activities and Rationales

Assessments

- Review antepartum and intrapartum records for maternal infections, especially group B Streptococcus, rubella, sexually transmitted infections, TORCH, and hepatitis. Identifies risk for infection, enables preventive measures, and enables the nurse/practitioner to anticipate possible interventions should infection occur.
- Review birth records to determine whether there was maternal fever, maternal history of urinary tract infection, or viral illness prior to delivery; presence of prolonged, premature, preterm rupture of membranes; prolonged labor; and whether resuscitation was required. Infants who have undergone invasive procedures are more likely to have been exposed to pathogens. Premature rupture of membranes and preterm labor may have been caused by an infectious process, which the infant may have acquired in utero.
- Assess gestational age and assess for IUGR. Infants born prior to 28 weeks' gestation are at higher risk for infection. IUGR further increases the risk.
- Assess nutritional status. Malnutrition predisposes to infection.
- Monitor and observe for signs of infection (temperature alone is not an adequate means of assessing infection in the preterm infant) using the following cues:
  - Temperature instability (usually decreased, but can be increased). Temperatures usually decrease in newborns due to an immaturity of the febrile mechanism.
  - Heart rate (tachycardia, bradycardia, poor perfusion, hypotension). Heart rate abnormalities are common. The heart rate increases with an increased metabolism, which occurs in infection, and bradycardia is seen with decompensation.
  - Respirations (tachypnea, apnea, grunting, retractions, nasal flaring). These are signs of respiratory distress and aids in diagnosis of possible pneumonia.
  - Gastrointestinal problems (poor feeding, abdominal distention, vomiting, diarrhea, glucose instability,

bloody stools). Abdominal distention and poor feeding are often associated with NEC.

■ C-reactive protein level. Will most likely be elevated in the presence of anti-inflammatory response to infection. The C-reactive protein level is a valuable adjunct in diagnosing sepsis, monitoring the response to treatment, and serving as a guide to length of treatment.

■ Bicarbonate and base excess. Metabolic acidosis is a common sign of infection.

■ CNS changes (lethargy, irritability, seizures). Meningitis, hypoglycemia, hyperglycemia, and hypoxia associated with sepsis may lead to lethargy and seizures in the neonate.

■ CBC with differential (neutropenia, anemia, thrombocytopenia, sudden increase or decrease in white blood cell count). An abnormally high or low white blood cell count is worrisome. A WBC < 6,000/mcg or > 30,000/mcg in the first 24 hours of life is abnormal. However, the total white blood cell count may vary on a daily basis, so it is not a reliable diagnostic indicator.

■ Platelet count (increased or decreased). May be indicative of sepsis. Platelet count generally decreases in the presence of bacterial infection but might be increased during viral illness. The platelet count should be greater than 100,000, and it is important to follow laboratory trends, but a decreased platelet count is very nonspecific and usually a late sign of infection.

• If infection occurs:

■ Obtain/review cultures of blood, stool, urine, umbilical cord, and any drainage. Identifies the causative organism and associated sensitivities to antimicrobials.

■ Obtain/review chest radiographs. Diagnoses or rules out pneumonia.

■ Review serum chemistries (hypoglycemia, hypocalcemia, hyponatremia). Infection may lead to a number of metabolic and electrolyte abnormalities.

■ Obtain ABGs (metabolic acidosis). Initiation of the inflammatory response often leads to decreased tissue perfusion, lactic acid buildup, and metabolic acidosis.

■ Observe for signs of septic shock or disseminated intravascular coagulation (DIC) (e.g., listlessness, bradycardia, hypotension, petechiae, bleeding, or erythema). These are complications of septicemia.

Independent Nursing Actions

• Maintain a neutral thermal environment. Minimizes metabolic expenditures, which are increased in the presence of infection.

• Encourage the mother to pump and provide human milk for feedings, if possible. Human milk contains IgA and some of the white blood cells the infant lacks but needs to fight infection.

• Perform cord care according to agency protocol. Cleaning or antimicrobials per protocol or order might help retard growth of pathogens.

• Use strict aseptic practices when changing IV tubing and solutions and performing other sterile procedures (e.g., suctioning); discard irrigation/humidification fluids after 24 hr. Prevents the introduction of microorganisms directly into bloodstream or lungs.

• Maintain universal precautions (reverse isolation, if indicated). Prevents the spread of microorganisms to or from infant.

• Keep linen and equipment clean; have separate supplies for each infant; provide a minimum of 3 feet spacing between infant bed sides in nursery. Helps prevent cross-contamination.

• Strictly enforce hand-washing and gowning procedures. Prevents microorganism transmission. Hand washing is the single most important measure for preventing iatrogenic infections. Many intensive care units require a 3-min hand scrub with iodine antibacterial solutions to reduce the possible spread of infection.

• Limit visitors, and monitor visitors and staff for fever, skin lesions, respiratory infection symptoms, and draining wounds. Remember that caregivers (e.g., staff, parents) must be free from infection. Prevents direct or indirect transmission of infectious organisms.

• Preserve skin integrity. See the NDCP, "Risk for Impaired Skin Integrity,[1]" beginning on p. 426 in this topic. Intact skin is the body's first line of defense against infection.

Collaborative Activities If Infection Occurs

• Administer antimicrobials as ordered (usually IV). Controls the infectious process. Broad-spectrum antibiotics are usually given pending results of cultures.

• Administer IV immunoglobulin as ordered. Improves survival rate in septic infants and may be given prophylactically for infants weighing less than 1,500 g.

• Monitor drug levels and kidney function. Immature kidneys do not excrete drugs well, so toxicity can occur sooner and at lower levels than in full-term infants.

• Treat complications (e.g., hypothermia/hyperthermia, shock, hypoxemia, acidosis, electrolyte imbalances). These conditions may be as life threatening as the infection itself.

• Maintain oxygenation and ventilation. Prevents worsening of hypoxia.

Parent/Family Teaching

• Explain the importance of appropriate hand-washing techniques. Pathologic organisms are primarily spread from person to person by the hands. Correct hand washing remains the single most important activity for limiting the spread of microorganisms and decreasing the spread of infection.

Nursing Diagnosis: RISK FOR DISORGANIZED INFANT BEHAVIOR[1]

Related Factors: pain, invasive/painful procedures, lack of containment/boundaries, prematurity of CNS, environmental over-stimulation, and separation from parents.

Goals, Outcomes, and Evaluation Criteria

- Infant exhibits age-appropriate neurobehavioral functioning.
- Infant demonstrates increasing ability to adapt to stimuli.
- Infant maintains appropriate sleep-wake cycles.
- Infant exhibits no evidence of maladaptive behaviors.
- Infant integrates physiologic and behavioral functions.

NIC Interventions[2]

Developmental Care (8250)—Structuring the environment and providing care in response to the behavioral cues and states of the preterm infant.

Environmental Management: Comfort (6482)—Manipulation of the patient's surroundings for promotion of optimal comfort.

Kangaroo Care (6840)—Promoting closeness between parent and physiologically stable preterm infant by preparing the parent and providing the environment for skin-to-skin contact.

Newborn Monitoring (6890)—Measurement and interpretation of physiologic status of the neonate the first 24 hours after delivery.

Nonnutritive Sucking (6900)—Provision of sucking opportunities for the infant.

Pain Management (1400)—Alleviation of pain or a reduction in pain to a level of comfort that is acceptable to the patient.

Positioning (0840)—Deliberative placement of the patient or a body part to promote physiologic and/or psychologic well-being.

Nursing Activities and Rationales

Assessments

- Monitor for erratic or prolonged sleep. Rest may be the single most important environmental change. Studies show a direct correlation between hypoxemia and sleep disruption.
- Assess skin (check for duskiness, mottling, and cyanosis). A stressed infant is unable to control autonomic responses, resulting in various skin-color changes.
- Assess developmental behaviors using specifically designed scale, such as the Assessment of Preterm Infant Behavioral scale. Assesses autonomic, motor, state organization, attention, and self-regulation systems.
- Assess infant's behavioral reactions to stimulation (e.g., sighing, looking away, hiccuping, gagging, regurgitating food, or respiratory changes that indicate overstimulation). Enables the planning of specific developmental interventions to meet the individual needs of the infant. Some preterm infants are not able to deal with more than one sensory input at a time. The goal is to reduce detrimental stimuli as much as possible and still provide opportunities for development.

- Assess vital signs (indicators of infant's ability to regulate all physical and behavioral systems), including the following:
  - Temperature. An immature ability to regulate temperature predisposes the infant to low skin temperatures.
  - Heart rate. Bradycardia is a common response to stress.
  - Respirations. Tachypnea, apnea, and periodic respirations are common reactions to stress.
- Assess neurologic behaviors (tremors, startles, twitches, yawning, gagging, spitting up, hiccupping, sneezing, coughing, flaccidity, hypertonicity, finger splays, facial grimacing, putting his or her hands on his or her face, fisting, fussiness, irritability, averting gaze, and exhibiting a worried or glassy-eyed alertness). Neonates display a number of neurologic behaviors when unable to integrate stimuli and control autonomic, motor, state, and self-regulatory systems.

Independent Nursing Activities

- Assign the same nurse each day if possible. Ensures continuity of care that is essential for infant's developmental agenda. Multiple caregivers can confuse the infant by providing too many cues for the infant to learn. Minimal caregivers offer a greater ability to assess and revise infant's care plan and add consistency and continuity for the parents.
- Recognize cues and infant states. Minimizes stress and identifies optimal times for interacting with the infant. Preterm infants do not exhibit the same behavioral states as term infants. They are unable to attend as well to objects in the environment and to the human face.
- Plan nursing care around the times when infant is awake and alert and maximize rest periods. Maximizes infant's ability to appropriately interact with surrounding environment. Rest periods of less than 60 minutes are ineffective and insufficient for the preterm newborn to complete a normal sleep cycle.
- Reduce environmental stimuli (e.g., silence alarms; keep conversations quiet and away from the baby's crib; dim the lights; place a "Quiet" sign in the nursery). Minimizes stress. Noise levels of 45–85 decibels are not unusual in NICUs; an incubator alone produces a constant noise level of 60–80 db. A constant db level of 90 can damage hearing. Preterm infants are easily overstimulated because of autonomic nervous system immaturity. Dim lights may encourage infants to open their eyes and better interact with their parents and caregivers.
- Cluster care around feeding schedule if possible. Minimizes handling and stimulation while providing longer periods of uninterrupted sleep.

- Position flexed on side with hands midline. Promotes flexion and hand-to-mouth activities, which promote neurobehavioral organization.
- Swaddle tightly with extremities in flexed position, being sure that hands can reach the face, and place in bunting or create a nest by placing blanket rolls next to infant's sides and feet. Facilitates self-consoling and soothing activities and inhibits disorganized behavior; provides containment, preserves energy, and promotes growth. Hands should be free for hand-to-mouth activities to promote neurobehavioral organization.
- Place on soft foam, gel pillows/mattresses, or approved waterbed. Provides tactile input and prevents skin abrasions; to simulate the kinesthetic stimulation of the intra-uterine environment.
- Provide objects to grasp, suck. Promotes neurobehavioral organization.
- Encourage nonnutritive sucking with a pacifier. Serves as a source of self-consolation and self-regulation that will facilitate the introduction of nutritive sucking by organizing suck-swallow coordination. Improves oxygen saturation, decreases body movements, improves sleep, and increases weight gain.
- Hold over shoulder to burp. The ventral position enhances orientation and visual stimulation.
- Contain limbs during interventions (e.g., during suctioning). Use of body containment during stressful procedures decreases the physiologic and behavioral responses.
- Provide comfort measures (e.g., remove painful stimuli, prevent hunger, change wet or soiled clothing). Normally, infants acquire a sense of trust as they learn the feel, sound, and smell of their caregivers. Painful procedures should be minimized to those absolutely medically indicated, and it is essential to provide containment, comfort measures, and adequate pain relief during this time.
- Provide black and white mobiles or decals when the infant is ready for stimulation; change occasionally. For best visual stimulation, place about 8 in. from face. Preterm infants attend best to black and white objects. Infant can become habituated to the same stimulus over a period of time.
- Allow for recovery after interventions. Enables the infant to regain control of physiologic state.
- Change position every 2 to 4 hours when providing care (e.g., feedings). Because of neuromuscular immaturity, the infant cannot move about or change positions easily. Tactile stimulation associated with repositioning infant is beneficial to the infant for a variety of reasons. It provides neurosensory input to aid in the maturation of the central and autonomic nervous systems, prevents skin breakdown, reduces muscular changes associated with immobility, and offers the opportunity for personal interaction between caregiver and baby.

- Provide kangaroo care (skin-to-skin holding). Provides direct interaction with the parent; improves thermoregulation and oxygenation; decreases episodes of apnea; meets developmental needs by fostering neurobehavioral development.

Parent/Family Teaching

- Teach parents to recognize infant cues and states. Teaching optimal times for interaction (i.e., when infant is alert) enhances the infant's ability to attend to the parent(s) and fosters attachment and infant development. Ability to read visual cues allows parents to move at the infant's pace when providing stimulation. In addition, knowledge of infant behaviors prepares parents to meet the infant's needs. Nurses can be excellent role models for parents.
- Teach parents activities for stimulation, while approaching one sense at time, e.g., rocking, cuddling, quiet talking or singing, gentle pressure without stroking, mobiles, and en face interaction. Although the preterm infant should not be overstimulated, it is important to provide developmental stimuli, as the infant is able to tolerate them, as a part of the baby's care.

Nursing Diagnosis: RISK FOR IMPAIRED SKIN INTEGRITY[1]

Related Factors: immobility, invasive procedures (e.g., IV insertion), hypothermia or hyperthermia, prematurity, altered metabolic state, altered circulation or tissue perfusion, or impaired nutrition.

Goal, Outcome, and Evaluation Criterion

- Skin remains intact, with no irritation or injury.

NIC Interventions[2]

Positioning (0840)—Deliberative placement of the patient or a body part to promote physiologic and/or psychologic well-being.

Pressure Management (3500)—Minimizing pressure to body parts.

Skin Surveillance (3590)—Collection and analysis of patient data to maintain skin and mucous membrane integrity.

Nursing Activities and Rationales

Assessments

- Monitor skin condition (redness, rash, excoriation, transparency, stripping, bruising, infiltration, blisters). Enables early treatment of complications if they occur. The premature infant's skin is thin, low in resilience, and prone to epidermal stripping and infection. The premature infant has minimal subcutaneous fat to protect areas over bony prominences.

- Monitor electrode, IV catheter, and other insertion sites for signs of infection, skin breakdown, or extravasation of fluid. The preterm infant undergoes invasive therapies that expose the skin to injury.
- Monitor fluid status (intake and output, skin turgor and moisture, sunken fontanels). The thinness of the premature infant's skin increases the risk of dehydration. Skin dryness, in turn, increases the risk for impaired skin integrity.
- Monitor use of thermal devices (e.g., heating pads, warmers). Prevents burns.

Independent Nursing Actions

- Avoid removal of vernix. Vernix protects and lubricates the skin.
- Bathe with warm water and low-alkaline soap (or no soap) infrequently. Alkaline soaps temporarily destroy the acid mantle of the skin, a defense mechanism against bacteria.
- Provide appropriate skin care to edematous areas. Edema decreases circulation in the affected area and thus increases the risk of skin breakdown and subsequent risk of infection.
- Remove antibacterial solutions immediately after a procedure. Prevents transdermal absorption and systemic toxicity and prevents loss of protective epidermal barrier.
- Use creams, lotions, and emollients cautiously, and only if alcohol-free and without perfumes, dyes, and artificial substances that can be absorbed into the bloodstream. Although moisturizing agents may be needed to prevent skin dryness, it is important to avoid those that may change the skin pH or be absorbed through the infant's permeable skin. The chemical additives used for fragrance, color, or other consumer appeal can irritate and dry the baby's skin.
- Avoid use of adhesives, adhesive skin preps, and adhesive removers; use transparent dressings for securing IV lines. Prevents stripping of the epidermal layer. The bond between the adhesive and the epidermal layer is often stronger than the bond that exists between the epidermal and dermal layers of the skin.
- Use protective transparent covering over joints. Prevents skin tears. The preterm infant has little subcutaneous tissue between bony prominences and the skin.
- Use pectin-based barriers under adhesives. Minimizes skin excoriation.
- Use limb electrodes when possible. Prevents epidermal stripping.
- Apply transparent polyurethane film over areas of skin breakdown. Promotes healing. Transparent films promote air circulation and maintain moisture but are impermeable to water and bacteria.
- Place on soft foam, waterbed, or sling and monitor baby closely. Prevents pressure-related tissue necrosis.
- Change infant's position often (every 2–4 hours), perform range-of-motion exercises, use water- or gel-filled mattress. Prevents pressure area breakdown of delicate skin.

Skin is the body's first line of defense against infectious microorganisms.

- Monitor IVs hourly and discontinue if infiltration suspected. Infiltration decreases tissue circulation and causes necrosis.
- Maintain fluid/electrolyte balance. Minimizes edema and promotes tissue perfusion.

Nursing Diagnosis: RISK FOR IMBALANCED NUTRITION, LESS THAN BODY REQUIREMENTS[1]

Related Factors: small stomach capacity; weak abdominal muscles; decreased ability to digest protein; decreased ability to absorb nutrients; uncoordinated sucking and swallowing secondary to neurologic immaturity; inadequate intake secondary to feeding difficulty, illness, or fatigue; immature cardiac sphincter that allows regurgitation to occur; and so forth.

Goals, Outcomes, and Evaluation Criteria

- Infant receives adequate nutrients for growth.
- Infant's weight and ponderal index are normal for age. (The ponderal index is the proportion of weight to height [length] and indicates how well proportioned the baby is overall.)
- Infant has weight loss of 15% or less in first 3 days of life and continues to gain weight after that.
- Infant has good skin turgor.
- Infant maintains positive nitrogen balance and stable electrolytes, calcium, phosphorus, and other biochemical indices of nutritional well-being.

NIC Interventions[2]

Enteral Tube Feeding (1056)—Delivering nutrients and water through a gastrointestinal tube.

Feeding (1050)—Providing nutritional intake for a patient who is unable to feed himself or herself.

Nutrition Therapy (1120)—Administration of food and fluids to support metabolic processes of a patient who is malnourished or at high risk for becoming malnourished.

Nutritional Monitoring (1160)—Collection and analysis of patient data to prevent or minimize malnourishment.

Total Parenteral Nutrition (TPN) Administration (1200)—Preparation and delivery of nutrients intravenously and monitoring of patient responsiveness.

Weight Gain Assistance (1240)—Facilitating gain of body weight.

Nursing Activities and Rationales

Assessments

- Assess suck-swallow coordination. Decreased coordination affects intake; adequate suck-swallow coordination indicates readiness for oral feedings.

- Auscultate bowel sounds. If peristalsis is present and infant is stable, infant can be fed within a few hours after birth.
- Observe for abdominal distention. Abdominal distention may be seen with gastrointestinal inflammation and decreased motility.
- For infants receiving TPN, periodically assess readiness for oral feedings (strong suck, swallow, and gag reflexes; and continued weight gain of 20–30 g/day). Evaluates readiness for transition from TPN to oral feeding.
- Observe skin color and other signs of respiratory distress, especially after feeding. The infant's small stomach predisposes to distention, which can inhibit lung expansion and cause respiratory distress. Oral feedings cannot be given if respiratory distress occurs. Changes in color and perfusion may indicate GI complications.
- Daily weight. Calculate daily intake and daily caloric intake. Appropriate weight gain is a good indicator of nutritional status.
- Assess gavage feedings. Gavage tube placement should be confirmed, and stomach contents should be aspirated prior to each feeding to ensure infant digested food. Acceptable ranges of gastric residuals vary among practitioners and should be individualized to each baby. Gastric residual food can indicate feeding intolerance. Repeated discarding of larger volume gastric residuals can lead to hyponatremia and other electrolyte imbalances due to the high sodium content in the gastric aspirates. Progressive worsening of residual volumes, accompanied by other signs and symptoms, might be associated with NEC.
- Assess skin turgor. While assessment is warranted for many reasons, the nurse should be aware that skin turgor is not a good indicator of fluid status in the preterm infant because of the decreased elasticity of premature skin.
- Monitor serum chemistries. Identifies nutrients that need replacement/supplementation to prevent complications.
- For infants receiving TPN, monitor for infection, venous thrombosis, and fluid overload. *Candida septicemia* accounts for about half of the complications associated with TPN. Dyspnea may be a symptom of fluid overload.

Independent Nursing Actions

- Encourage nonnutritive sucking. Facilitates suck-swallow coordination and gastric motility, strengthens the gag reflex, and provides oral satisfaction for infants not receiving oral feeding.
- Feed small amounts and gradually increase based on infant's feeding tolerance. Prevents stomach distention and regurgitation because of small stomach capacity and immature cardiac sphincter.
- Use a small, slow flow, soft nipple for bottle feedings. Conserves energy.
- Elevate the head while feeding. Prevents regurgitation and aspiration. Gag reflex is not intact until 32 weeks' gestation.

- Keep infant's chin tucked downward and support chin or chin and cheeks. Facilitates suck-swallow coordination and coordinates with effective breathing. The hypopharynx in the preterm infant tends to be collapsible and can lead to feeding-related apnea.
- Position on right side after feeding. Facilitates gastric emptying and prevents reflux.
- Gavage feed if respiratory distress or tachypnea is present or infant is too tired to complete feeding. Provides for nutritional needs and prevents aspiration. The gag reflex is not intact before 32 weeks' gestation; therefore, infants born before that age are usually started on gavage feedings.
- Begin feedings by gavage, breast, or bottle as soon as infant is able to tolerate them. Prevents deterioration of the intestinal villi and depletion of nutrient reserves. Breastfeeding may be tolerated by the stable, preterm infant.
- Hold feedings if abdominal distention, absent bowel sounds, or increasing gastric residuals occur. Prevents GI complications related to feedings, such as NEC.
- Feed with manually expressed human milk or assist with breastfeeding, if possible. Human milk has immunologic properties that help to prevent GI complications, such as NEC or rotavirus. Preterm infants can maintain higher transcutaneous oxygen pressures and regulate body temperature better when breastfed than when bottle fed.
- Use flexible feeding schedule. Feeding and overall rate of growth improve if infant can nurse during alert times and have uninterrupted periods of sleep between feedings.
- Maintain thermal-neutral environment. Hypothermia increases the metabolic rate and uses calories that are needed for weight gain.

Collaborative Activities

- Provide high-calorie formulas, dextrose-containing IV fluids, TPN, as ordered. Provides fluids and nutrients needed for maintenance needs and growth. With early administration of IV fluids to prevent hypoglycemia and supply fluids, oral feedings can be delayed until infant's respiratory status is stable. Preterm infants need 110–140 cal/kg body weight per day, compared to the 100–110 cal/kg/day needed by term infants. Protein requirements are also higher. Typical preterm infant formulas range from 20 to 24 cal/oz. Some infants may require as much as 30 cal/oz formula.
- Advance volume and concentration of formula (oral feedings) as infant tolerates. Prevents feeding intolerance.
- Provide supplements of vitamin D, vitamin E, vitamin A, and calcium. Replaces inadequate and depleted stores. Vitamin D enhances retention of calcium; vitamin E is necessary for preventing hemolytic anemia; vitamin A is needed for healing and perhaps reducing incidence of lung disease.
- Consider obtaining milk from human milk bank. This is a costly alternative, but many NICUs are resorting to the use of human milk banks because human milk is easy to digest

and reduces the potential for NEC. In addition, human milk contains immune globulins that the preterm infant cannot produce.

INDIVIDUALIZED (NURSING DIAGNOSIS) CARE PLANS

The care plans in this section were developed to address unique patient needs.

Nursing Diagnosis: RISK FOR FLUID VOLUME DEFICIT[1]

Related Factors: thin epidermis, increased metabolism, losses through lungs (tachypnea), environmental heat sources (e.g., radiant warmer, phototherapy), and large insensible water loss due to large body surface as compared to total body weight.

Goals, Outcomes, and Evaluation Criteria

- Infant maintains fluid/electrolyte balance.
- Infant's intake approximately equals output.
- Infant's urine-specific gravity is within normal limits for age.
- Infant has good skin turgor.
- Infant is without sunken eyes or fontanels.
- Infant has moist mucous membranes.

NIC Interventions[2]

Fluid Management (4120)—Promotion of fluid balance and prevention of complications resulting from abnormal or undesired fluid levels.

Fluid Monitoring (4130)—Collection and analysis of patient data to regulate fluid balance.

Temperature Regulation (3900)—Attaining and/or maintaining body temperature within a normal range.

Nursing Activities and Rationales

Assessments

- Calculate infant's fluid requirements. A preterm infant's immature kidneys cannot concentrate urine and conserve fluid effectively. In addition, more fluid is lost via the skin than in full-term infants. Fluid requirements are based on the infant's weight and postnatal age, as well as environmental factors, and range from 80 to 100 ml/kg/day on day 1 up to 150 ml/kg/day on day 3. Amounts may be increased up to 200 ml/kg/day for very small infants, those under a radiant warmer, or those receiving phototherapy. Fluid requirements may be less if the environment is humid or if a heat shield is used.
- Weigh daily. Daily weights are the most sensitive indicator of fluid losses or gains, as well as growth progress.

Insufficient fluid and calories may cause dehydration, acidosis, and weight loss. Overhydration may cause nonnutritional weight gain, pulmonary edema, and heart failure.

- Monitor intake and output. Prevents the possibility of excess fluid losses.
- Assess skin turgor, fontanel status, mucous membranes. Establishes the need for intervention. If infant has a fluid deficit, skin will be dry, fontanels sunken, and mucous membranes sticky. Even small fluid losses or shifts can lead rapidly to dehydration. Skin turgor is, however, a poor indicator of fluid status in the premature infant.
- Monitor temperature. Establishes the need for correction of environmental temperature. If environmental temperature is too high, fluid loss increases in an effort to cool the body by evaporation.
- Assess for complications/conditions indicating the need for increased fluids (e.g., fever, hypovolemic shock, sepsis, asphyxia, and hypoxia). The preterm infant is prone to multisystem problems, which increase metabolism and cause fluid loss.
- Monitor electrolytes (especially potassium, sodium, and chloride). Determines the need for electrolyte replacement. Electrolytes can be a good indicator of overall fluid balance.
- Monitor amount and specific gravity of urine and weigh diapers instead of using collection bags. Immature kidneys do not concentrate urine well, so specific gravity is low. Oliguria may occur secondary to hypoxia and hypotension. Collection bags can cause skin breakdown and may also leak.
- Monitor Hct. Elevated hematocrit may be a sign of dehydration.
- Monitor blood urea nitrogen, creatinine, and uric acid levels. Assesses for renal function.

Independent Nursing Actions

- Maintain temperature within neutral thermal range and dress infant in clothing appropriate to the environment. Minimizes insensible water loss. The preterm infant's thin skin with blood vessels close to the surface increases the potential for fluid loss through the skin.
- Humidify oxygen. Minimizes insensible water loss.
- Administer IV fluids by continuous infusion pump. Ensures constant infusion rate and prevents accidental fluid overload.
- Use ambient humidity. Minimizes insensible water loss to the environment.
- Prevent infection (refer to the NDCP, "Risk for Infection,[1]" beginning on p. 423 in this topic). Infection increases fluid loss by increasing metabolism and possibly causing fever.

Collaborative Activities

- Administer fluids and electrolytes as ordered. Maintains fluid/electrolyte balance. When feedings cannot be given orally, IV fluids are ordered and administered to fulfill fluid requirements and maintain glucose homeostasis.

- Avoid hypertonic fluids and undiluted medications. Prevents excess solute load on immature kidneys.

Nursing Diagnosis: INTERRUPTED FAMILY PROCESSES[1]

Goal, Outcome, and Evaluation Criterion

Mother/parents:

- Integrate infant into the family.

Nursing Activities and Rationales

Assessments

- Identify family's strengths, coping mechanisms, and support systems. Establishes a basis for intervention. Strengths should be integrated into the plan of care to help the family focus on behaviors that have been effective in the past, rather than on their problems.
- Determine whether feelings of guilt or failure are present. Determines the need for intervention and support. Parents, realistically or not, may feel that they have done something to cause the infant's prematurity and/or illness.

Independent Nursing Actions

- Encourage and provide opportunities for sibling visits if possible. Otherwise, provide pictures, "notes from the baby," and so on. Promotes family involvement, helps siblings resolve fears, and promotes understanding and acceptance of the new infant into the family.
- Encourage parents to limit the number of visitors once the infant returns home and to alter environmental temperature as needed. Anticipatory guidance will help parents to adjust the home environment to accommodate the needs of the infant.

Collaborative Activities

- Refer to social services, counseling, pastoral care, and/or support groups as needed. Provides additional resources for social support. Counseling may be needed in order to maintain family integrity. Make appropriate referrals to local and state agencies as necessary.

Parent/Family Teaching

- Discuss normal responses to giving birth to a high-risk infant. Facilitates parent understanding and coping. It is reassuring to know that one's responses and feelings are shared by others and, therefore, are normal. Parents may

experience anticipatory grieving over the potential loss of an ill baby; or they may be experiencing grief and depression over failure to give birth to a healthy, term infant.

- Provide information about constructive coping mechanisms and resources. Enhances coping and feelings of self-confidence with infant care activities as well as role within the parent–child dyad.
- Provide information about sibling adjustment to a new family member and the role change for all members of the family. Equips the family to handle sibling needs and concerns. Once the infant goes home, siblings may be confused and angry at the disproportionate amount of parental time spent on the newborn.

Nursing Diagnosis: RISK FOR IMPAIRED PARENT–INFANT/CHILD ATTACHMENT[1]

Refer to the generic NDCP, "Risk for Impaired Parent–Infant/Child Attachment,[1]" beginning on p. 19 in Chapter 2.

Goals, Outcomes, and Evaluation Criteria

Mother/parent:

- Visits/calls the NICU regularly.
- Participates in newborn care as able.
- Is attentive to the newborn.
- Interacts appropriately with the newborn, including facial expression, eye contact, posture, and handling.

NIC Intervention[2]

Environmental Management: Attachment Process (6481)— Manipulation of the patient's surroundings to facilitate the development of the parent–infant relationship.

Nursing Activities and Rationales

Assessments

- Assess parents' psychologic responses to the infant's condition and needs. Parents of a preterm infant must accomplish some psychologic tasks before effective parenting can occur. For example, when a critically ill baby is admitted to a NICU, the parents must experience and work through anticipatory grief over the potential loss of the infant. Anticipatory grief allows them to plan and feel more in control of the situation. Some family members, however, may detach from the infant and other family members in an effort to protect themselves from the pain of loss. As the baby's condition improves, family members resume the process of relating to the infant and developing attachment.

- Monitor parental interest in infant (calls, visits). Establishes the need for intervention.

Independent Nursing Actions

- Before their first visit to the NICU, explain to the parents what to anticipate (e.g., the infant's appearance and function of the equipment). Preparation will help reduce fear and shock at unexpected sights and sounds.
- Keep parents informed about infant's care and condition; encourage questions. Helps alleviate anxiety about the unknown and unexpected; promotes trust and communicates caring.
- Encourage visits to the NICU, and provide uninterrupted opportunities for parent–infant interaction. Allows parents time to get to know infant and to form an emotional bond.
- Encourage holding, touching, or caressing infant as condition allows; encourage the bringing of personal items (e.g., blankets, family pictures, a stuffed toy). Promotes emotional attachment.
- If separated, keep parents informed of infant's status; provide pictures, memorabilia, footprint; provide toll-free phone number to out-of-town parents, and encourage calling at least daily. Provides a connection to the infant.
- Encourage involvement in infant care. Decreases feelings of helplessness and reinforces the parent role.
- Reinforce and praise parents' efforts to be involved and participate in care. Increases self-confidence, reduces anxiety. Parents may be afraid of harming the infant, who appears small and fragile.
- Encourage kangaroo care. Fosters a sense of closeness to infant.
- Provide opportunities for rooming in and infant-care activities. Provides the parents with an opportunity for assumption of care responsibilities in a safe environment.

Parent/Family Teaching

- Identify infant characteristics, their similarities to the parents (e.g., eyes, shape of face), and infant behaviors. Facilitates identification of infant as own, parent–infant interaction, and reciprocity.
- Provide information about support groups and services. Empowers the family to seek help as desired/needed.
- Stress the importance of follow-up care on discharge; refer to social services or visiting nurses for follow-up if there is evidence of attachment problems. Although parents of most preterm infants do form emotional bonds with them, the incidence of physical and emotional abuse is greater in preterm or ill infants who are separated from their parents for a time after birth. Parents may become emotionally detached because they unconsciously rejected the infant in order to protect themselves from grieving over a potential loss. The infant may represent a financial burden or a threat to self-esteem. If attachment problems are diagnosed in the hospital, further problems may be prevented.

▌ Other Nursing Diagnoses

Also assess for the following nursing diagnoses, which are frequently present with this condition:

- Delayed Growth and Development[1] related to premature birth, physiologic insults (e.g., from asphyxia or intracranial hemorrhage), and long-term hospitalization.
- Risk for Delayed Development[1] related to premature birth, physiologic insults (e.g., from asphyxia or intracranial hemorrhage), long-term hospitalization.
- Pain[1] related to invasive procedures.

POSTTERM NEWBORN

An infant born after completion of 42 weeks' gestation is considered postterm. Postterm newborns can be *large for gestational age, small for gestational age* (SGA), or *dysmature*. Dysmature infants weigh less than the established normal parameters for gestational age (they are IUGR), depending on placental function. Approximately 10% of pregnancies are prolonged. The placenta gradually loses its ability to provide adequate oxygenation and nutrients to the fetus beyond 42 weeks, which leads to increased perinatal mortality and morbidity from asphyxia, hypoglycemia, and respiratory distress. Anticipating the need for newborn resuscitation for this group of infants must be a top priority. While the cause of postterm birth is poorly understood, infants with certain congenital conditions, such as anencephaly and neonatal hypothyroidism, are almost always postterm. The terms *postterm* or *postdate* refer to the infant who is born after 42 weeks' gestation. The term *postmature* refers to the infant born after 42 weeks of gestation who shows the effects of progressive placental insufficiency.

▌ Key Nursing Activities

- Monitor for and detect complications related to placental insufficiency.
- Assess for birth trauma.
- Prevent complications of birth trauma.
- Maintain neonate's body temperature.
- Offer emotional support to mother/partner.
- Maintain a patent airway with suction apparatus for infant born with meconium-stained amniotic fluid.

▌ Etiologies and Risk Factors

The etiology of postterm birth is unknown. Women with a history of prolonged pregnancies, primiparas, obesity, and maternal age between 30 and 40 seem to be at greatest risk (Caughey, Stotland, & Washington, 2009). Altered fetal adrenocortical activity has also been implicated. Postterm delivery may also be a function of incorrect pregnancy dating.

▌ Signs and Symptoms

Postterm Infant—Greater than 42 weeks' gestation.

Postmature Infant—Infants with postmaturity syndrome are typically small for gestational age; have dry, cracked, parchment-like wrinkled skin; have wide-eyed alert expression; have long, thin extremities; have long nails; have profuse scalp hair; are devoid of vernix and lanugo; and have meconium-stained skin. There usually is a history of oligohydramnios and cord compression.

Diagnostic Studies

Antepartum/Intrapartum

- Biophysical profile. Evaluates fetal well-being.
- Nonstress test. Reflects the function of the fetal brain stem, autonomic nervous system, and heart.
- Contraction stress test. Assesses fetal heart rate in response to uterine contractions.
- Doppler flow studies. Identifies fetal heart and great vessel abnormalities and variations in blood flow.
- Electronic fetal monitoring. Identifies presence of fetal heart tone variations such as decelerations, decreasing baseline variability, or increasing baseline rate.
- Fetal scalp gases. Rules out the presence of acidosis, alkalosis, or hypoxia.
- Metabolic/hormone assays. Rules out the presence of endocrine or metabolic disorders that may have influenced postterm birth.

Newborn

- Gestational age assessment. Determines if the neonate is preterm, term, or postmature.
- Complete blood count. Identifies infection, anemia, or other hematologic abnormalities.
- Serum glucose. Detects hyper- or hypoglycemia.
- Bilirubin. Detects hemolytic anemia (erythroblastosis fetalis) or congenital icterus.

Medical Management

- Induction of labor.
- Cesarean birth if cephalopelvic disproportion is present.
- Supportive care for infant.

Collaborative Problems

Potential Complications of Postterm Infant

- Birth trauma secondary to macrosomia
- Hypothermia
- Polycythemia
- Hypoglycemia
- Meconium aspiration
- Hyperbilirubinemia
- Persistent pulmonary hypertension
- Risk for Impaired Gas Exchange.[1] (Note: Although this is a nursing diagnosis, it should be a part of the standardized care for all postterm newborns.)

COLLABORATIVE (STANDARDIZED) CARE FOR ALL POSTTERM NEWBORNS

Potential Complication of Postterm Birth: BIRTH TRAUMA SECONDARY TO MACROSOMIA

Focus Assessments

- Assess neonate's head. Identifies injuries such as cephalohematoma (collection of blood beneath the periosteum and skull surface), subgaleal hemorrhage, linear or depressed fractures, increased intracranial pressure, or subdural hematoma.
- Assess for subarachnoid hemorrhage. Signs of intracranial hemorrhage may include shrill cry, bulging fontanels, blood cells in cerebrospinal fluid, irritability or depression, refractory seizures, poor muscle tone, and poor feeding. Cerebrospinal fluid evaluation will show gross blood with normal proportion of white blood cells.
- Assess face and eyes. Identifies injuries. Localized erythema, ecchymoses, petechiae, abrasions, lacerations, edema, and facial paralysis (flattened affected side, nonresponsive to grimace) are signs of trauma related to birth process or use of instruments (forceps, vacuum).
- Assess shoulders/extremities. Signs of injury include asymmetric appearance or posturing, flaccid arm with elbow extended and hand rotated inward (brachial paralysis), absence of Moro's reflex on affected side, loss of sensation over lateral portion of arm, or crying with passive movement.
- Assess trunk. Localized erythema, ecchymoses, petechiae, abrasions, lacerations, and edema are indications of birth trauma.
- Assess abdomen. Tenderness with palpation or rigid, distended abdomen are signs of liver or spleen laceration and bleeding.

Preventive Nursing Activities (Antepartum and Intrapartum)

- Estimate gestational age. Gestational age greater than 42 weeks places the infant at increased risk for macrosomia. A large fetus is more likely to suffer birth trauma than the smaller, less mature fetus. Placental insufficiency increases the postterm fetus's risks for birth trauma.
- Prepare woman for cesarean birth. If the infant is too large to deliver vaginally due to cephalopelvic disproportion, cesarean birth will be considered in order to protect the fetus from birth trauma and possible serious injury. The

woman who understands that cesarean birth may protect her infant is more likely to support the plan of care.

Potential Complication of Postterm Birth: HYPOTHERMIA[1]

Focus Assessments

- Assess skin temperature. Identifies hypothermia and cold stress. Cold stress is detrimental to the newborn because it increases oxygen consumption and alters acid-base balance. The infant's skin temperature is used as the point of reference when warmers are used. An initial skin temperature of 36°C (96.8°F) is not uncommon for newborns but should stabilize around 36.6°C (97.8°F) within 12 hours.
- Assess heart rate and respirations. Identifies abnormalities so that corrective actions can be implemented. Signs of hypothermia include bradycardia (less than 90 beats/min), tachypnea (60 or more breaths/min), crackles, wheezing, grunting, retractions, expiratory grunt, and nasal flaring. Apnea can occur from rapid cooling or rapid rewarming.
- Assess for cyanosis. Determines the presence of cold stress. Cold stress increases oxygen demands and may lead to hypoxia, which is manifest as cyanosis. Acrocyanosis is normal in the first 2–3 days of life and is not a sign of hypoxemia.
- Assess arterial blood gases. Identifies metabolic acidosis. Metabolic acidosis results from an imbalance between oxygen supply and oxygen consumption. Hypothermia increases oxygen consumption and therefore increases oxygen demands and acidosis.
- Assess serum glucose. All stressed infants, including those who are cold stressed, are at increased risk for hypoglycemia. A blood glucose level less than 50 mg/dl is hypoglycemia in a full-term (or postmature) infant. Note: The definition of hypoglycemia varies by agency, some defining it as blood glucose less than 40 mg/dl.
- Assess skin. Signs of hypothermia include cool skin, poor tissue perfusion, pallor, cyanosis, mottling, and acrocyanosis (blue discoloration or cyanosis).
- Assess neurologic status. Signs of hypothermia include restlessness, lethargy, hypotonia, weak cry, and poor feeding. Uncorrected hypothermia can lead to apnea.

Preventive Nursing Activities

- Eliminate sources of heat loss. Heat can be lost through evaporation, conduction, convection, or radiation. Placing the infant on the mother's abdomen, drying the infant immediately after birth, wrapping the infant in a warm blanket, placing a knit cap on the infant's head, and keeping the delivery room temperature between 25°C and 28°C (77°F and 82.4°F) helps maintain the infant's temperature.

- Correct acidosis, hypoglycemia, hypoxemia, sepsis, and metabolic problems. Prevents further heat loss by eliminating factors that are causing heat loss or by correcting conditions that are contributing to it.
- Gradually rewarm the infant. Knit hats, clothing, blankets, and external sources (incubator, radiant warmer, etc.) can be used to gradually raise the neonate's temperature. Rapid warming may cause apneic spells and acidosis.
- Place infant in incubator or on radiant warmer until body temperature stabilizes. Prevents heat loss and development of hypothermia. The control panel is generally maintained between 36°C and 37°C (96.8°F–98.6°F) in order to maintain the infant's skin temperature around 36.5°C (97.7°F).

Potential Complication of Postterm Newborns: POLYCYTHEMIA

See the collaborative care plan, "Potential Complication of Small-for-Gestational-Age Infant: Polycythemia," beginning on p. 392 in "The Small-for-Gestational-Age Newborn" in this chapter.

Preventive Nursing Activities

- Assess the mother for diabetes mellitus. Infants born to mothers who have diabetes mellitus are at increased risk for development of hypoglycemia due to hyperinsulinism and polycythemia secondary to intrauterine hypoxia due to placental insufficiency from maternal diabetes.
- Provide adequate hydration of neonate. Helps decrease the viscosity of the neonate's blood. Fluid volume deficit due to inadequate fluid intake potentiates the increased blood viscosity. Aggressive hydration may be needed to prevent complications such as thrombosis.

Potential Complication of Postterm Newborns: MECONIUM ASPIRATION

See "Meconium Aspiration Syndrome," beginning on p. 441 in this chapter.

Focus Assessments

- Review prenatal and labor/birth records for indications of intrauterine and birth hypoxia. Infants who have suffered chronic intrauterine hypoxia (such as those who are postterm) are at high risk for acidosis and respiratory depression at birth, and persistent fetal circulation after birth, making them less able to cope with the insult of meconium aspiration.

- Assess for meconium-stained amniotic fluid during labor and birth. The presence of meconium in the amniotic fluid increases the risk for aspiration and associated complications, such as pneumonitis, pneumothorax, and persistent pulmonary hypertension.
- Assess newborn for meconium-stained umbilical cord and nails. This helps establish the presence of meconium in the amniotic fluid, which increases the infant's risk for aspiration.
- Assess for (visualize) meconium below the vocal cords. This decreases risk of meconium being aspirated into trachea.

Preventive Nursing Activities

- Suction the neonate while the head is still on the perineum. After birth when the baby cries, the infant is more likely to breathe in meconium from the pharyngeal area. Removal of meconium from the upper airway reduces the risk for pulmonary aspiration.
- Avoid stimulating respirations in a meconium-stained infant. Decreases the risk for aspiration. Once meconium has been visualized and aspirated from the lungs, the infant can be stimulated to breathe.
- Prevent cold stress. Cold stress increases metabolic demands and oxygen needs and development of acidosis.
- Review labor and birth records for indications of hypoxia. Infants who have suffered chronic intrauterine hypoxia (such as those who are postterm) are at high risk for acidosis and respiratory depression at birth and persistent fetal circulation after birth.

Potential Complication of Postterm Newborns: HYPERBILIRUBINEMIA

Refer to "Hyperbilirubinemia," beginning on p. 436 in this chapter. Assess for hyperbilirubinemia, and if it is present, institute that care plan.

Potential Complication of Postterm Newborns: NEONATAL ASPHYXIA

Refer to "Neonatal Asphyxia," beginning on p. 385 in this chapter. Assess for asphyxia, and if it is present, institute that care plan.

Potential Complication of Postterm Newborns: HYPOGLYCEMIA

Focus Assessments

- Monitor serum glucose levels; begin glucose monitoring at birth and continue until glucose values have stabilized. Less than 50 mg/dl in the full-term newborn indicates hypoglycemia. Intervention is necessary to prevent seizures or death; glucose is the primary source of fuel for the brain. Serum glucose levels help to differentiate between signs of hypoxia, hypothermia, and hypoglycemia. The definition of hypoglycemia varies by agency, some defining it as blood glucose less than 40 mg/dl.
- Assess neurologic status. Tremors, jitteriness, seizures, lethargy, and poor feeding may indicate hypoglycemia.
- Monitor temperature. Cold stress increases glucose utilization and intensifies hypoglycemia.
- Monitor for signs of hypoglycemia. Jitteriness is the most common symptom in the infant with a low blood sugar level. If the serum glucose is less than 25 mg/dl, the infant is at risk for seizures. Other symptoms of hypoglycemia include irritability, hypotonia, lethargy, high-pitched cry, hypothermia, poor suck, tachypnea, cyanosis, apnea, and seizures. Symptoms may occur at any time during the 1st week but most commonly occur between 24 and 72 hours after birth.

Preventive Nursing Activities

- Feed neonate as early as possible or administer glucose containing IV solution. Counters or prevents hypoglycemia.
- Decrease energy requirements. Conserves glucose and glycogen stores. Glucose is required for energy, which further depletes glycogen stores.
- Maintain a neutral thermal environment. A thermoneutral environment helps to eliminate heat loss through evaporation, conduction, convection, and radiation, thereby preventing cold stress; cold stress can cause or exacerbate hypoglycemia.

Potential Complication of Postterm Newborns: PERSISTENT PULMONARY HYPERTENSION

Focus Assessments

- Assess for risk factors for persistent pulmonary hypertension. Risk factors include perinatal asphyxia, meconium aspiration, metabolic acidosis, sepsis, congenital diaphragmatic hernia, hypothermia, or respiratory distress within 24 hours of birth. Recognition of risk factors allows for appropriate care planning.
- Assess for signs of persistent pulmonary hypertension. Signs include marked cyanosis, tachypnea, grunting, retractions, decreased peripheral perfusion, loud pulmonary component of second heart sound, and systolic ejection murmur. Recognition of signs allows for early intervention and helps prevent injury to major organs or death.
- Monitor for bleeding following extracorporeal membrane oxygenation (ECMO). Bleeding is the major complication when infusing blood that has been anticoagulated with heparin.

Preventive Nursing Activities

- Early recognition and management of conditions that contribute to hypoxia. Hypoxic stress increases pulmonary vascular resistance, which results in a return to fetal cardiopulmonary circulation (right-to-left shunting of blood through the foramen ovale and ductus arteriosus) and pulmonary vasoconstriction.
- Administer prescribed oxygen. Reduces hypoxia and decreases pulmonary vasoconstriction.
- Administer prescribed vasodilators. Decreases pulmonary vascular resistance, which reduces right-to-left shunting and increases cardiac output.
- Prepare for assisted ventilation. Increases oxygenation when hypoxia is severe.
- Administer prescribed sodium bicarbonate or tromethamine. Restores and/or maintains acid-base balance.
- Assist with nitrous oxide administration. Reverses pulmonary vascular vasoconstriction.
- Prepare for ECMO. Shunts blood from right atrium or right internal jugular vein through a heat exchanger and membrane lung and back into the systemic circulation via the carotid artery or aortic arch, which allows the lungs to rest and recover.
- Prepare for high-frequency ventilation therapy if baby is unresponsive to conventional ventilation. This form of oscillatory breathing is used to promote air/gas exchange at an extremely rapid rate, whereby the infant does not have inspiratory and expiratory phases of ventilation.
- Decrease external stressors on infant. External stimuli (e.g., handling, IV puncture, environmental noise, and lights) causes stress, which increases metabolic rate and oxygen utilization, increasing the risk of hypoxia.

- Cluster nursing activities. Maximizes the infant's rest, decreases metabolic demands and oxygen utilization, and decreases the risk of hypoxia.
- Administer prescribed intravenous fluids. Replaces/maintains fluid balance, prevents relative hypovolemia and supports cardiac output.
- Offer emotional support to parents. Parents need reassurance about their infant's condition, progress, and response to treatment. Knowledge decreases fear and anxiety and helps the parents better cope with the illness of their infant and cooperate with treatment plans.

INDIVIDUALIZED (NURSING DIAGNOSIS) CARE PLANS

Nursing Diagnosis: RISK FOR IMPAIRED GAS EXCHANGE[1]

Related Factors: meconium aspiration, polycythemia, hypothermia, and hypoglycemia.

Goals, Outcomes, and Evaluation Criteria

- Infant is free of adventitious lung sounds.
- Infant has an absence of dyspnea, nasal flaring, substernal retraction, and cyanosis.
- PaO_2 and $PaCO_2$ are within normal limits for a neonate.
- Respiratory rate is within normal limits for a neonate.
- There is an absence of respiratory rhythm abnormalities.
- Infant has a serum blood glucose level greater than 50 mg/dl.
- Infant's skin temperature is greater than 36.5°C (97.7°F).
- Infant's blood pressure is within normal limits for a neonate.

NIC Interventions

Acid-Base Management (1910)—Promotion of acid-base balance and prevention of complications resulting from acid-base imbalance.
Airway Management (3140)—Facilitation of patency of air passages.
Oxygen Therapy (3320)—Administration of oxygen and monitoring of its effectiveness.
Resuscitation: Neonate (6974)—Administering emergency measures to support newborn adaptation to extrauterine life.

Nursing Activities and Rationales

Assessments

- Assess arterial blood gases. Detects abnormalities that suggest lack of oxygenation or increased oxygen consumption, hypoxia, or metabolic acidosis secondary to hypoglycemia or hypothermia.

- Assess temperature. Neonatal skin temperatures below 36.5°C (97.7°F) may indicate development of hypothermia. Temperatures of 36°C (96.8°F) are not uncommon for newborns, but should stabilize within 12 hours.
- Assess respirations and heart rate. Bradycardia (fewer than 90 beats/min), tachypnea (greater than 60 breaths/min), crackles, wheezing, grunting, retractions, and nasal flaring may indicate respiratory or cardiac compromise secondary to hypoglycemia or hypothermia. Apnea can occur from hypothermia or rapid rewarming of infant.
- Monitor appearance of amniotic fluid during birth. The presence of meconium in the amniotic fluid suggests fetal distress, which is increased in postterm infants.
- Perform Apgar assessment immediately upon delivery. An Apgar assessment score between 7 and 10 is considered normal. Scores less than 7 indicate the need for intervention. Postterm neonates are at increased risk for respiratory complications due to placental insufficiency after 42 weeks' gestation.
- Assess cord/arterial blood gases. Determines the presence of acidosis related to tissue hypoxia.
- Monitor color. Detects signs of hypoxia or compromised oxygenation (pale, cyanotic appearance).
- Monitor neonate's muscle tone. Signs of altered oxygenation or hypoxia include limp, depressed, or absent reflexes.

Independent Nursing Actions

- Identify infants at risk. Postterm neonates should be considered at risk for altered tissue perfusion due to placental insufficiency after 42 weeks' gestation.
- Maintain environmental temperatures within the neutral thermal range. Minimizes oxygen consumption and nutrient use by the newborn due to increased metabolic rate.
- Administer oxygen to neonate as ordered. Ensures adequate delivery of oxygen to prevent tissue hypoxia.
- Maintain a patent airway. Ensures delivery of oxygen to the lungs by positioning infant for maximum respirations and suctioning as needed.

Collaborative Activities

- Correct fluid volume deficit. Prevents development of polycythemia and subsequent respiratory or cardiac compromise.

HYPERBILIRUBINEMIA

Hyperbilirubinemia, an elevated level of bilirubin (a yellow bile pigment produced during the destruction of red blood cells) in the blood, may be physiologic or pathologic. There are two types of hyperbilirubinemia: conjugated (direct) and unconjugated (indirect). *Jaundice* (yellowing of the body tissues and fluids) results when there is an imbalance between the rate of bilirubin production and bilirubin elimination.

Physiologic jaundice is a common newborn phenomenon, occurring in 60–80% of term infants and virtually all preterm infants. Physiologic jaundice does not usually appear until the 3rd to 4th day of life due to the limitations and abnormalities of bilirubin metabolism. Treatment is dependent on the age and gestation of the infant, feeding method, family ethnicity, and fluid and electrolyte status of the infant.

Pathologic jaundice occurs when total bilirubin levels increase by more than 5 mg/dl/day, exceed 17 mg/dl in a term infant or 10–14 mg/dl in preterm infants, and produce visible jaundice within the first 24 hours following birth. Unconjugated bilirubin is highly toxic to neurons; therefore, the infant with severe hyperbilirubinemia is at increased risk for *bilirubin encephalopathy,* which is associated with total bilirubin levels of greater than 25 mg/dl in normal term infants.

▋ *Key Nursing Activities*

- Assess for risk factors that may increase bilirubin levels (prematurity, hypoglycemia, infection, hypothermia, significant bruising, delayed cord clamping, family history of jaundice, inadequate feeding, delayed stooling, male gender, and ethnicity).
- Provide adequate treatment (phototherapy, adequate nutrition, fluid therapy, or exchange transfusion).
- Provide parental education and support.
- Provide parents with information about and an orientation to the NICU.

▋ *Etiologies and Risk Factors*

Etiologies and risk factors include physiologic jaundice of the newborn, hemolytic anemia (e.g., G6PD, ABO incompatibility, Rh incompatibility, infection), polycythemia, blood extravasation, defects of conjugation (Crigler-Najjar syndrome, Lucey-Driscoll syndrome), breastfeeding and human milk jaundice, metabolic disorders (galactosemia, hypothyroidism), increased enterohepatic circulation of bilirubin and substances or disorders that affect the binding of bilirubin to albumin (drugs, asphyxia, acidosis, infection, hypothermia, and hypoglycemia).

▋ *Signs and Symptoms*

Signs and symptoms include elevated total and direct serum bilirubin levels, jaundice, icteric sclera, lethargy, and poor feeding.

▋ *Diagnostic Studies*

- Blood type. Determines blood type and Rh status of infant in the event exchange transfusion is necessary.
- Direct Coombs' test. Establishes diagnosis of hemolytic disease in newborn; positive result indicates infant's RBCs have been sensitized (coated with antibodies).

- Indirect Coombs' test. Measures the amount of Rh-positive antibodies in the mother's blood.
- Total and direct bilirubin. Establishes diagnosis of hyperbilirubinemia. The Bhutani hour-specific nomogram is widely use as a predictive indicator of hyperbilirubinemia in the term and preterm infant. Serum bilirubin levels alone do not predict the risk for brain injury due to bilirubin kernicterus, although it is associated with levels of more than 25 mg/dl in normal, term infants.
- Complete blood count with differential. Detects hemolysis, infection, anemia (Hgb less than 14 g/dl), or polycythemia (Hct greater than 65%). Hct less than 40% (cord blood) indicates severe hemolysis.
- Total serum protein. Detects reduced binding capacity (less than 3.0 g/dl).
- Serum glucose. Detects hypoglycemia (less than 50 mg/dl). Note: The definition of hypoglycemia varies by agency, some defining it as blood glucose less than 40 mg/dl.
- Kleihauer-Betke test. Test performed on mother to detect fetal erythrocytes in maternal blood.
- Reticulocyte count. Increased count is consistent with increased hemolysis.

Medical Management

- Increase maintenance intravenous fluids if applicable.
- Perform serial bilirubin testing (approximately every 6–12 hours).
- Early feeding or frequent breastfeeding. Prevents enterohepatic circulation.
- Phototherapy.
- Phenobarbital. Reduces serum bilirubin level by increasing hepatic glucuronosyltransferase activity and bilirubin conjugation.
- Exchange transfusion.
- Correction of underlying problems (sepsis, acidosis, etc.).

Collaborative Problems

Potential Complications of Hyperbilirubinemia

- Bilirubin encephalopathy
- Complications of phototherapy
- Altered body temperature
- Diarrhea
- Eye damage
- Fluid deficit
- Risk for Impaired Skin/Tissue Integrity.[1] (Note: Although it is not a collaborative problem, this nursing diagnosis is included because it should be a part of the standard care given to all newborns having phototherapy.)

Potential Complications of Exchange Transfusion

- Acid-base imbalances
- Hypovolemia
- Fluid/electrolyte imbalances
- Infection

COLLABORATIVE (STANDARDIZED) CARE FOR INFANTS WITH HYPERBILIRUBINEMIA

Perform a comprehensive assessment to identify individual needs for parent teaching and emotional support and infant physical care.

Potential Complication of Hyperbilirubinemia: BILIRUBIN ENCEPHALOPATHY

Focus Assessments

- Assess for factors that promote development of bilirubin encephalopathy. Metabolic acidosis, lowered serum albumin levels, intracranial infections (meningitis), abrupt increases in blood pressure, fetal distress, hypoxia, hypothermia, and hypoglycemia are factors that contribute to bilirubin neurotoxicity.
- Assess maternal and fetal blood types. ABO and Rh incompatibilities increase the risk for jaundice. Maternal antibodies cross the placenta in Rh-negative women who have been previously sensitized due to Rh-positive infant. Antibodies attach to fetal RBCs and increase the risk for hemolysis.
- Assess infant for jaundice. Facilitates early detection. Jaundice occurs because RBCs in newborns have short life spans, the liver has a slower uptake, there are no intestinal bacteria, and hydration is not well established. Jaundice is best observed by assessing the infant's skin, sclerae, and mucous membranes. Gently pressing over bony prominences (tip of nose, sternum) causes blanching and allows yellow stain to be more readily observed. Jaundice begins on the head and gradually progresses to the abdomen and extremities. Jaundice appearing within the first 24 hours following birth indicates the need for assessment of bilirubin level.
- Assess infant in daylight. Prevents distortion of actual skin color by artificial lighting.
- Monitor temperature. Detects hypothermia or fever, both of which contribute to development of jaundice and the risk for bilirubin encephalopathy.
- Differentiate between physiologic and pathologic jaundice. Jaundice appearing during the first 24 hours of life or persisting beyond 7 days is a sign of a pathologic process, which predisposes the infant to bilirubin encephalopathy.

- Assess bilirubin levels. If the serum bilirubin increases more than 5 mg/dl per day, hyperbilirubinemia exists. Bilirubin levels alone are not good predictors of brain injury.
- Assess neurologic status. Detects nervous system depression or irritability due to bilirubin encephalopathy. Initially, the infant may have lethargy, decreased activity, irritability, or poor feeding. As encephalopathy continues, the infant will develop rigid extension of extremities, fever, irritable cry, opisthotonos, and seizures. Infants who survive this condition may be mentally impaired, have attention deficit or other behavioral disorders, hearing loss, or abnormal motor activity (ataxia or athetosis).
- Assess infant/maternal nutritional status. Inadequate nutrition can cause hypoproteinemia and subsequent jaundice. One gram of albumin has the capacity to bind approximately 16 mg of unconjugated bilirubin. Decreased albumin results in increased circulating bilirubin and increases the risk for encephalopathy.
- Assess serum bilirubin levels every 6–12 hours after phototherapy is initiated. Evaluates the effectiveness of phototherapy. After phototherapy is initiated, visual assessment of jaundice alone is not considered valid.

Preventive Nursing Activities

- Place unclothed infant in servo-controlled incubator or under radiant warmer. Eyes should be protected and genitals covered. Initiate phototherapy as ordered. Light promotes bilirubin excretion by altering the structure of bilirubin to a soluble form (photoisomerization) so that it can be eliminated readily in feces and urine. The infant's skin must be fully exposed in order for lights to be effective. However, phototherapy may produce DNA strand breaks and possible mutations, so the genitals must be protected.
- Turn every 2 hours under phototherapy. Maximizes exposure and enhances effectiveness of light therapy.
- Turn off phototherapy and remove eye shields for feedings. Maximizes treatment effectiveness and allows infant to interact with surrounding environment.
- Correct acidosis, hypoproteinemia, and hypoxia. Prevents and/or relieves factors that contribute to development of bilirubin encephalopathy.
- Avoid use of medications that compete for albumin-binding sites. Prevents further reduced binding capacity.
- Maintain neutral thermal environment. Hyperthermia (fever) and hypothermia enhance the penetration of bilirubin to the brain and increase the risk for bilirubin encephalopathy.
- Estimate albumin–bilirubin binding capacity obtained by dividing total bilirubin by serum protein. Estimates the risk for bilirubin encephalopathy, which increases as binding capacity decreases.
- Encourage early feedings and frequent breastfeeding. Reduces unconjugated bilirubin and promotes GI excretion through the stools. Feeding promotes intestinal motility, decreases enterohepatic shunting, and increases normal flora within the bowel, which facilitates elimination of unconjugated bilirubin in the feces and may reduce the risk for encephalopathy.
- Administer phenobarbital as prescribed. Promotes synthesis of hepatic glucuronyl transferase, which increases conjugation of bilirubin and clearance of bile pigment by the liver.
- Monitor stool for consistency and frequency. Bilirubin stools are typically loose and green.
- Avoid administration of intravenous glucose and sodium bicarbonate in acutely ill infants. These substances produce a rapid rise in serum osmolarity and have been implicated in development of encephalopathy.
- Assist with exchange transfusion. Exchange transfusion may be necessary for reducing bilirubin levels that are dangerously high to prevent neurotoxicity. The infant's sensitized RBCs are removed and replaced with Rh-negative blood of the infant's blood type so that lysing of RBCs does not occur. Exchange transfusion also removes bilirubin and increases available albumin, facilitating binding of bilirubin.
- Provide meticulous skin care. Skin might be dry and/or irritated secondary to the dehydrating effects of phototherapy. Acidic stools may cause excoriation of buttocks.
- Offer emotional support to parents. Parents need reassurance about their infant's condition, progress, warmth, and comfort. Parents who understand the need for procedures will be less anxious and more likely to agree with the treatment plan.
- Discuss the need for continued follow-up care. Infants with severe bilirubin encephalopathy may suffer permanent neurologic damage. Infants should be monitored frequently in order to detect complications and implement interventions early. Parents who understand the need for close follow-up care are more likely to agree and cooperate with long-term plans.

Potential Complications of Phototherapy: ALTERED BODY TEMPERATURE, DIARRHEA, EYE INJURY, AND FLUID DEFICITS

Focus Assessments

- Monitor temperature. Hypothermia or fever (secondary to infection) may be the etiology of the hyperbilirubinemia;

treating the underlying cause may alleviate the hyper-bilirubinemia. Fever may indicate progression of bili-rubin toxicity to the brain or dehydration secondary to phototherapy.

- Assess stool characteristics and frequency. Phototherapy enhances the excretion of unconjugated bilirubin in feces, which will have a greenish appearance. Loose stools may be present and indicate accelerated excretion of bilirubin. Absence of stooling due to intestinal obstruction is a con-traindication for phototherapy because bilirubin cannot be excreted.
- Assess eyes at least once per shift by turning off photo-therapy and removing eye patches. Identifies discharge, excessive pressure on eyelids, or corneal irritation that may develop from use of eye shield. Also allows infant to inter-act with caretakers and surrounding environment.
- Monitor weight. Detects weight loss related to increased fluid excretion in stools or inadequate fluid intake. Infants receiving phototherapy sleep for longer periods, which increases their risk for fluid volume deficits.
- Monitor intake and output. Detects decreased output related to decreased intake or dehydration. Fluid intake should be slightly greater than output in the newborn because of insensible water losses.
- Monitor urine-specific gravity. Urine-specific gravity increases with dehydration and fluid volume deficit and indicates the need for rehydration.

Preventive Nursing Activities

- Protect eyes during phototherapy. Prevents eye injury. Shield the infant's eyes with an opaque mask to prevent exposure to the light. The mask should cover the eyes com-pletely without occluding the nares. Close the infant's eyes prior to applying the mask to prevent corneal excoriation. Pressure on the eyes must be avoided.
- Remove eye mask with nursing assessments and feedings. Facilitates examination of the eyes for pressure, drainage, or corneal irritation and to allow for visual and sensory stimulation.
- Cleanse eyes with sterile water. Removes debris and pre-vents bacterial growth.
- Replace eye mask according to agency protocol. Prevents bacterial growth, which may cause infection.
- Administer enteral or parenteral fluids as prescribed. Compensates for insensible and intestinal fluid vol-ume losses and supplies nutrients if feedings are with-held during phototherapy for infants with severe hyperbilirubinemia.
- Document phototherapy. Documentation includes infor-mation pertaining to the times phototherapy was initiated and stopped, shielding of eyes, manufacturer of florescent lamp, number of lamps used, distance between lamps and infant (should not be closer than 18 inches), photometer

of light intensity, use of incubator or crib, and any side effects noted.

■ Nursing Diagnosis: RISK FOR IMPAIRED TISSUE INTEGRITY[1]

Related Factors: phototherapy, pressure from eye mask, corneal irritation, loose stools, and fluid volume deficit.

■ Goals, Outcomes, and Evaluation Criteria

- Absence of skin excoriation.
- Absence of eye injury.
- Absence of corneal irritation, drainage.

■ NIC Interventions[2]

Fluid Management (4120)—Promotion of fluid balance and pre-vention of complications resulting from abnormal or unde-sired fluid levels.

Skin Surveillance (3590)—Collection and analysis of patient data to maintain skin and mucous membrane integrity.

Nutrition Management (1100)—Assisting with or providing a bal-anced dietary intake of foods and fluids.

■ Nursing Activities/Rationales

Assessments

- Assess skin for dehydration, drying, rash, excoriation related to hyperbilirubinemia and phototherapy treat-ment. Detects alterations so that treatment can be imple-mented. Phototherapy can cause dehydration and skin drying, which predisposes to excoriation and break-down. Burns can occur if the lamps are positioned too close to the infant. Loose stools may produce perianal excoriation. Tanning (bronzing) can occur from light exposure but generally resolves when phototherapy is discontinued.

Independent Nursing Actions

- Reposition approximately every 2 hours, clustered with other nursing care. Equalizes exposure to phototherapy and reduces risk for skin breakdown due to pressure.
- Cleanse perianal area with sterile water. Removes highly acidic stool, which is irritating to skin and increases the risk for excoriation and breakdown.
- Avoid use of lotions or oils. Prevents tissue injury related to the quality of oil and the burning effect that could occur with phototherapy use.
- Monitor intensity of light source; maintain between 6 and 8 m. Prevents burning, skin rash, and excoriation.

Potential Complications of Exchange Transfusions: ACID-BASE IMBALANCE, FLUID AND ELECTROLYTE IMBALANCE, CARDIOVASCULAR COMPROMISE, AND INFECTION

Focus Assessments

- Monitor blood pressure, heart rate, and rhythm. Detects possible cardiac compromise that can occur following exchange transfusion so that corrective interventions can be implemented.
- Monitor temperature. Increased temperature (fever) may indicate infection from contamination of cord or infused blood; decreased temperature occurs with hypothermia, which increases metabolic needs and oxygen consumption. Fever (infection) and hypothermia are risk factors for hyperbilirubinemia and subsequent kernicterus.
- Assess tissue perfusion. Detects complications of transfusion indicated by poor capillary refill and cool or mottled extremities.
- Monitor hemoglobin and hematocrit. Evaluates effectiveness of transfusion and determines need for second exchange. Decreasing levels following transfusion indicate the need for a second exchange.
- Monitor complete blood count. Detects complications of exchange transfusion such as neutropenia, anemia, or thrombocytopenia. Approximately 85% of the neonate's blood is replaced if two exchanges are done, increasing the risk for complications.
- Assess weight change. Detects weight gain related to fluid overload. Fluid overload can cause cardiac and respiratory compromise.
- Assess for edema. Periorbital, dependent, and extremity edema are indications of fluid volume overload.
- Assess neurologic status. Detects signs of hyperkalemia or hypocalcemia such as irritability, jitteriness, twitching, seizures, or neurotoxicity from jaundice.
- Monitor serum electrolytes. Donor blood containing citrate (anticoagulant) binds calcium, increasing the risk for hypocalcemia (serum calcium less than 7 mg/dl) and subsequent cardiac dysrhythmias. Hyperkalemia (serum potassium greater than 7 mEq/L) can occur if infused blood is over 2 days old; red blood cell destruction is occurring and potassium is released. Hyperkalemia can cause cardiac arrest.
- Assess blood gases for acidosis. The infant may be unable to metabolize citrate used to anticoagulate donor blood resulting in metabolic acidosis.
- Monitor for umbilical cord bleeding following transfusion. Infused blood has been anticoagulated with heparin or citrate, increasing the risk for bleeding for up to 6 hours following infusion. Less risk occurs when citrate is countered with calcium gluconate during the infusion process.
- Assess for signs of infection following transfusion. Blood is transfused directly into the umbilical vein, placing the infant at increased risk for infection. Fever, periumbilical redness, tachycardia, and lethargy are signs of infection. Infection increases the risk for bilirubin encephalopathy/kernicterus.

Preventive Nursing Activities

- Use heparin-preserved blood if possible. Prevents hypocalcemia and metabolic problems associated with infusing citrate.
- Ensure correct umbilical line placement and patency. Drying of the umbilical cord may hamper placement. If drying has occurred, saline soaks can be applied for an hour prior to attempting transfusion to ensure access and patency.
- Check accuracy of blood type and cross-match. Prevents complications arising from ABO and Rh incompatibilities in the already-compromised infant. The majority of compatibility problems arise from human error.
- Avoid overheating of blood prior to infusion. Heating promotes hemolysis and release of potassium, which causes hyperkalemia.
- Monitor blood aliquots removed and infused. Prevents fluid volume overload from excessive infusion or fluid volume deficit from inadequate replacement.
- Screen donor blood for potassium level before administration. Determines degree of hemolysis. As blood ages, RBCs deteriorate, releasing potassium into the serum. Infusing blood with increased levels of potassium increases the neonate's risk for hyperkalemia and cardiac arrest.
- Administer calcium, glucose, and albumin as prescribed. Corrects hypocalcemia, hypoglycemia, and hypoalbuminemia.
- Maintain the rate of exchange at 2 to 4 ml/minute. Rate of exchange depends on the weight of the infant. Time is allotted following each 100 ml of blood to infuse calcium gluconate if needed to prevent hypocalcemia if infant is receiving blood anticoagulated with citrate phosphate.
- Administer calcium gluconate or protamine sulfate as prescribed. Calcium gluconate corrects hypocalcemia related to infusion of blood anticoagulated with citrate. Protamine sulfate counteracts anticoagulation with heparin to prevent bleeding.
- Maintain absolute sterility. Blood infuses directly into the infant's umbilical vein; therefore, absolute sterility is essential to prevent infection.
- Administer antimicrobials as prescribed. Prevents and/or treats infection.

INDIVIDUALIZED (NURSING DIAGNOSIS) CARE PLANS

This section includes care plans that were developed to address unique patient needs.

Nursing Diagnosis: ANXIETY[1]

Related Factors: Parents' anxiety about their infant being undressed and masked, restricted handling, and fear of outcome for the infant. Refer to the generic NDCPs, "Anxiety[1]" and "Fear,[1]" beginning on pp. 10 and 15, respectively, in Chapter 2.

Goals, Outcomes, and Evaluation Criteria

Mother/parents:

- Acknowledge understanding of exposure and restricted handling.
- Express fears and concerns.
- Participate in plan of care.

Nursing Activities and Rationales

Independent Nursing Actions

- Encourage parents to verbalize their concerns. Displays interest and empathy. Recognition and verbalization of fears often help reduce them.
- Encourage parents to visit during feeding times. Allows parents an opportunity to participate in their infant's care, promotes parent–infant attachment, and provides visual and sensory stimulation for the infant.

Parent/Family Teaching

- Teach parents the need for exposing their infant to phototherapy. Promotes understanding, alleviates fear and anxiety, and involves them in care planning. The benefits of phototherapy and measures taken to protect the infant's safety should be stressed to reassure the parents that their infant is being well cared for.
- Inform parents about ways to interact with their infant while under phototherapy. Touch is an example of a way to promote parent–infant attachment and provide sensory stimulation.
- Teach mother/parents how to assess infant for jaundice. The infant may be discharged from the hospital prior to developing jaundice. The parents will be monitoring the infant at home and need to recognize jaundice, assess for worsening or resolution of jaundice, and recognize changes that indicate the need for medical intervention. Knowledge will increase their confidence and ability to care for their infant, thereby reducing anxiety.
- Teach home care for their infant. Facilitates care of the infant at home and continued treatment for hyperbilirubinemia and helps prevent development of unrecognized complications. Knowledge will increase their confidence in their ability to care for their infant, thereby reducing anxiety. They may fear that the baby will become ill at home.
- Teach mother about breastfeeding jaundice and encourage frequent breastfeeding. Decreases woman's anxiety regarding jaundice and prevents prolonged hospitalization of jaundiced infant, needless discontinuance of breastfeeding, and unnecessary phototherapy. Breastfeeding jaundice may be related to decreased milk intake before the mother's milk supply is well established, since feeding facilitates hepatic clearing of bilirubin. Early breastfeeding jaundice begins in the first few days of life; late breastfeeding jaundice usually peaks between 1 and 2 weeks of age. Breastfeeding may be discontinued for 1–2 days if bilirubin levels reach dangerous levels. Formula substitution during this time usually results in a prompt decline of bilirubin levels. Home phototherapy treatment may be necessary.

MECONIUM ASPIRATION SYNDROME

Meconium is a viscous green substance composed of water and gastrointestinal secretions that can be noted in the fetus as early as 10–16 weeks' gestation. Meconium is passed when the anal sphincter relaxes as a result of hypoxic stress and the fetus then sucks or swallows the meconium-stained amniotic fluid in utero or upon taking the first breath after birth. Meconium staining with the possibility of aspiration happens in up to 20% of all term pregnancies. The presence of meconium in the trachea can cause airway obstruction and a chemical pneumonitis, which can lead to severe respiratory distress. When meconium is aspirated into the lungs, it creates a ball-valve effect whereby air is inspired into the alveoli but can't be fully expired because the diameter of the airways is reduced and the existing surfactant is inactivated. Worsening respiratory distress is often followed by persistent pulmonary hypertension, right-to-left shunting of blood and patent ductus arteriosus. Babies with meconium aspiration syndrome may require conventional ventilation, extracorporeal membrane oxygenation (ECMO), nitric oxide therapy, or high-frequency or liquid ventilation.

Key Nursing Activities

- Prevent infant from aspirating meconium-stained amniotic fluid
- Early identification of meconium aspiration
- Emotional support for parents
- Prevention of complications
- Information about and orientation to the NICU for parents

▮ Etiologies and Risk Factors

Etiologies and risk factors include postterm pregnancy, breech presentation, forceps or vacuum extraction births, prolonged or difficult labor associated with fetal distress, maternal hypertension or diabetes, oligohydramnios, IUGR, prolapsed cord, or acute or chronic placental insufficiency.

▮ Signs and Symptoms

Signs and symptoms include yellow or green amniotic fluid, meconium-stained cord, infant with meconium-stained skin and nails, meconium visualized beyond the glottis, intrauterine growth restriction, patchy infiltrates, pulmonary interstitial emphysema, pneumothorax on radiograph, hypoxemia, hypercarbia, acidosis, tachypnea and increased respiratory effort, cyanosis, decreased peripheral perfusion, systolic murmur, pulmonic ejection click, split S_2, and prominent right ventricular impulse.

▮ Diagnostic Studies

- Postnatal intubation and visualization of trachea. Identifies presence of meconium in the trachea.
- Chest radiograph. Identifies the presence of pneumonitis, pneumothorax, infiltrates, hyperexpansion, and atelectasis.
- Blood gases. Detects hypoxia and metabolic/respiratory acidosis.

▮ Medical Management

- Early identification of the compromised fetus
- Suctioning of the oropharynx while the head is still on the perineum
- Intubation and suction of the trachea after complete delivery and before the first breath
- Oxygen therapy
- Assisted ventilation (conventional or high frequency)
- Nitric oxide therapy
- Antibiotics
- Extracorporeal membrane oxygenation (ECMO)
- Vasopressors
- Volume expanders
- Correction of acidosis
- Paralyzing agents

▮ Collaborative Problems

Potential Complications of Meconium Aspiration

- Air leaks
- Atelectasis
- Pneumonitis (Note: The preceding complications will all be covered in the next NDCP, "Impaired Gas Exchange.[1]")
- Persistent pulmonary hypertension

COLLABORATIVE (STANDARDIZED CARE) FOR ALL INFANTS WITH MECONIUM ASPIRATION SYNDROME

Perform a comprehensive assessment to identify individual needs for parent teaching and emotional support and infant physical care.

▮ Nursing Diagnosis: IMPAIRED GAS EXCHANGE[1]

Related Factors: meconium aspiration, episode of intrauterine asphyxia, air leaks, atelectasis, pneumonitis, and pneumothorax.

▮ Goals, Outcomes, and Evaluation Criteria

- Infant maintains a patent airway.
- Infant has an absence of complications (pneumonitis, atelectasis, pulmonary hypertension).
- Infant has an absence of hypoxia.
- Infant has an absence of acid-base imbalances.

▮ NIC Interventions[2]

Airway Management (3140)—Facilitation of patency of air passages.

Airway Suctioning (3160)—Removal of airway secretions by inserting a suction catheter into the patient's oral airway and/or trachea.

Aspiration Precautions (3200)—Prevention or minimization of risk factors in the patient at risk for aspiration.

Oxygen Therapy (3320)—Administration of oxygen and monitoring of its effectiveness.

Respiratory Monitoring (3350)—Collection and analysis of patient data to ensure airway patency and adequate gas exchange.

Resuscitation: Neonate (6974)—Administering emergency measures to support newborn adaptation to extrauterine life.

▮ Nursing Activities and Rationales

Assessments

- Review prenatal and labor/birth records for indications of intrauterine and birth hypoxia. Infants who have had chronic intrauterine hypoxia (such as those who are SGA and/or are exposed to maternal substance abuse) are at high risk for meconium aspiration, because they are likely to have passed meconium in utero. They are also at high risk for acidosis and respiratory depression at birth and persistent fetal circulation after birth, making them less able to cope with the insult of meconium aspiration.
- Note and report meconium-stained amniotic fluid during labor and birth. The presence of meconium in the amniotic fluid increases the risk of aspiration.

- Assess newborn for meconium-stained umbilical cord and nails. Helps establish the presence of meconium in the amniotic fluid, which increases the infant's risk for aspiration.
- Assess for (visualize) meconium below the vocal cords. Helps establish whether meconium has been aspirated into the trachea and bronchi.
- Assess skin color and perfusion. Detects pallor and cyanosis, which are indications of respiratory distress because of inadequate oxygenation or decreased oxygen/carbon dioxide exchange. Cyanosis is associated with low oxygen saturation, which occurs as inflamed lung tissue is less able to exchange gases. Pallor is seen with decreased perfusion and peripheral vasoconstriction secondary to hypoxia. A gray hue is associated with shock and occurs from impaired circulation.
- Assess respirations (pattern, effort, and rate). Detects respiratory distress. Tachypnea, apnea, grunting, retractions, nasal flaring, crackles, rhonchi, decreased or absent breath sounds, increased anterior–posterior diameter, or asymmetric chest expansion indicate respiratory distress. Aspiration of meconium into the lungs causes pneumonitis (localized lung inflammation), which disrupts surfactant production and decreases lung compliance (elasticity). Pneumonitis prevents the lungs from fully expanding, causing atelectasis. Both conditions inhibit the exchange of oxygen and carbon dioxide and ultimately intensify the work of breathing.
- Assess heart rate and blood pressure. Detects tachycardia, bradycardia, a shift in point of maximal impulse, and hypotension. Heart rate increases as it attempts to compensate for the hypoxia. Bradycardia occurs with decompensation. A shift in the point of maximal impulse is associated with pneumothorax. Low blood pressures may be associated with asphyxia and shock or as a result of decreased cardiac output secondary to pneumothoraces.
- Monitor ABGs. Detects hypoxemia, hypercapnia, respiratory and/or metabolic acidosis. Atelectasis and air trapping decrease gas exchange, leading to decreased oxygenation, increased carbon dioxide retention, and acid-base imbalance.
- Review chest radiograph report if available. Chest radiograph examination may demonstrate air trapping, hyperexpansion, and hyperinflation. Bilateral, diffuse, coarse, patchy infiltrates might also be noted. Air leaks are depicted as pockets of air in the mediastinum, intrapleural, or intracardiac spaces. Atelectasis causes lung tissue to become dense and appear white on radiograph.
- Monitor pulse oximetry. Detects changes in oxygenation that indicate decreased saturation. If oxygen saturation is not adequately maintained and carbon dioxide levels increase, mechanical ventilation may be necessary.
- Assess temperature. Detects fever or hypothermia. Both fever and hypothermia increase metabolic rate and oxygen consumption, which places the infant at increased risk for hypoxia.

Independent Nursing Actions

- Suction the neonate while the head is still on the perineum. Removes meconium from the mouth, which reduces the risk for aspiration.
- Avoid stimulating respirations in a meconium-stained infant until after removal of particulate meconium or green-stained mucus from the pharyngeal area. Decreases risk for aspiration. Once cords have been visualized and any meconium aspirated, the infant can be stimulated to breathe.
- Prevent cold stress. Cold stress increases metabolic demands and oxygen needs.
- Cluster neonatal care. Prevents oxygen consumption due to increased activity and stress.
- Avoid high inflating pressures to ventilate infant. High pressures increase the risk of airway trauma and air leaks.
- Administer paralytic agents or sedatives as prescribed, if needed. Prevents infant from fighting assisted ventilation to maximize ventilation and oxygenation.
- Perform chest physiotherapy and suctioning as needed. Maintains a patent airway and prevents further respiratory compromise.

Collaborative Activities

- Administer oxygen as prescribed. Provides adequate oxygen to the tissues, reduces hypoxia, and prevents accumulation of lactic acid.
- Maintain hydration and humidify oxygen. Helps to mobilize secretions by keeping them thin so they can be coughed out or suctioned. Thick secretions can block the area and contribute to development of hypoxia.
- Perform chest physiotherapy. Helps mobilize secretions so they do not block the airway and contribute to hypoxia.
- Suction as needed. Removes secretions to maintain a patent airway and enhances oxygenation.
- Provide a neutral thermal environment. Increased environmental temperature contributes to increased body temperature, which increases metabolic demands and oxygen consumption. The same is true for an environmental temperature that is too cool.
- Correct acid-base imbalances and metabolic disorders. Facilitates perfusion and oxygenation of tissues.
- Administer sedatives (or paralytic agents if not responsive to sedatives). Decreases or removes infant's ability to fight the ventilator, hopefully leading to improved ventilation and oxygenation. The use of paralytic agents is controversial but may be reasonable for use in those few infants who do not respond to sedation and appear to be fighting the ventilator.
- Administer vasopressors, pulmonary vasodilators, and volume expanders. Promotes circulation in the presence of persistent fetal circulation.

- Administer antibiotics as prescribed. Prevents infection from retained meconium in the lung. Meconium is a waste product that irritates the lung parenchyma and leads to lung inflammation (pneumonitis) and infection from retained secretions and inadequate alveolar expansion. Prevention or elimination of infection reduces inflammation and prevents hypoxia.

Potential Complication of Meconium Aspiration: PERSISTENT PULMONARY HYPERTENSION

Focus Assessments

- Assess for signs of persistent pulmonary hypertension. Signs include marked cyanosis, tachypnea, grunting, retractions, decreased peripheral perfusion, loud pulmonary component of second heart sound, and systolic ejection murmur. Recognition of signs allows for early intervention and helps prevent injury to major organs or death.
- Monitor for bleeding following ECMO. Bleeding is the major complication when infusing blood that has been anticoagulated with heparin.
- Monitor ABGs. Pulmonary hypertension decreases gas exchange, leading to hypoxemia, hypercapnia, and acidosis.

Preventive Nursing Activities

- Hyperventilate. Helps decrease $PaCO_2$.
- Hyperoxygenate. Vasodilates the pulmonary vascular bed and enhances pulmonary circulation.
- Administer prescribed oxygen. Reduces hypoxia and decreases pulmonary vasoconstriction.
- Administer prescribed vasodilators. Decreases pulmonary vascular resistance, which reduces right-to-left shunting and increases cardiac output.
- Prepare for assisted ventilation. Increases oxygenation when hypoxia is severe.
- Administer prescribed sodium bicarbonate or tromethamine as prescribed. Restores and/or maintains acid-base balance.
- Assist with nitrous oxide administration. Reverses pulmonary vascular vasoconstriction.
- Prepare for ECMO if needed. Shunts blood from right atrium or right internal jugular vein through a heat exchanger and membrane lung and back into the systemic circulation via the carotid artery or aortic arch, which allows the lungs to rest and recover.
- Decrease external stressors on infant. Noxious stimuli cause stress, which increases metabolic rate and oxygen utilization, increasing the risk for hypoxia.

- Cluster nursing activities. Maximizes the infant's rest, decreases metabolic demands and oxygen utilization, and decreases the risk for hypoxia.
- Administer prescribed intravenous fluids. Replaces/maintains fluid balance, prevents relative hypovolemia, and supports cardiac output.
- Offer emotional support to parents. Parents need reassurance about their infant's condition, progress, and response to treatment. Knowledge decreases fear and anxiety and helps the parents better cope with the illness of their infant and cooperate with treatment plans.

INDIVIDUALIZED (NURSING DIAGNOSIS) CARE PLANS

This section includes care plans that were developed to address unique patient needs.

Nursing Diagnosis: INTERRUPTED FAMILY PROCESSES[1]

Related Factors: hospitalization of the newborn, separation of the mother from the infant, and disrupted routines.

Goals, Outcomes, and Evaluation Criteria

The family will:

- Balance responsibilities.
- Integrate the infant into the family.

NIC Interventions[2]

Family Integrity Promotion: Childbearing Family (7104)— Facilitation of the growth of individuals or families who are adding an infant to the family unit.

Family Support (7140)—Promotion of family values, interests, and goals.

Nursing Activities and Rationales

Assessments

- Assess degree of family disruption, lifestyle change, or financial burden infant's illness places on parents/family. Helps identify the extent of family disruption taking place so that a plan of action can be created. Ordinary stressors may be greatly magnified by an infant's illness or the financial burden created by an extended hospitalization.
- Assess for verbal and nonverbal cues or behaviors that indicate decreased family functioning. Parents may verbalize negative feelings toward the infant, each other, or the situation. Behaviors such as anger, withdrawal, crying,

poor eating, or substance abuse may indicate decreased ability to cope with the situation.

- Determine family's understanding of the neonate's condition. Identifies feelings of guilt or irrational beliefs so that misunderstandings can be corrected. Parents may blame themselves or each other for their infant's condition, which impedes their ability to relate to one another or cope with their current situation.

Independent Nursing Actions

- Provide information about and an orientation to the NICU. Decreases anxiety and facilitates parental adaptation, which will foster their ability to cope with their current stressful situation and function more effectively as a family unit. Ineffective coping can lead to family disintegration.
- Encourage verbalization of fears and concerns and listen with empathy. Creates an environment of trust and acceptance and displays interest and empathy. Families who recognize and verbalize their fears are better able to cope with the family stressors created by a sick infant.
- Provide opportunities for sibling visits. Helps siblings resolve fears and promote understanding. Children who feel included are less likely to display negative attention-seeking behaviors.

Collaborative Activities

- Refer to social services, counseling, and pastoral care as needed. Provides additional resources for social support. Adequate support is needed during stressful situation. Counseling may be needed in order to maintain family integrity.

Parent/Family Teaching

- Teach parents the need for close infant monitoring, prolonged hospitalization, and invasive procedures. Promotes understanding, alleviates fear and anxiety, and involves them in plan of care. The benefits of protecting the infant's safety should be stressed to reassure the parents that their infant is being well cared for.
- Inform parents about ways to interact with their infant while hospitalized. Touch and an audiotape of parents reading a book are examples of ways to promote parent–infant attachment and provide sensory stimulation.
- Explain how to assess infant for signs of respiratory distress. The parents will be monitoring the infant at home eventually and need to recognize hypoxia or respiratory distress so that immediate interventions can be implemented. Knowledge increases confidence in the parents' ability to care for their infant, thereby reducing anxiety and enhancing family functioning.
- Teach home care for their infant. Facilitates care of the infant at home and prepares parents to recognize

complications. Knowledge gives parents the confidence to care for their baby independently and hopefully reduces the associated anxiety, if present. They may fear that the baby will become ill at home, which may negatively affect family processes.

Nursing Diagnosis: RISK FOR IMPAIRED PARENT–INFANT/ CHILD ATTACHMENT[1]

Related Factors: parent–infant separation at birth and a life-threatening condition. See the generic NDCP, "Risk for Impaired Parent–Infant/Child Attachment,[1]" beginning on p. 19 in Chapter 2.

Nursing Activities and Rationales

Independent Nursing Actions

- Provide uninterrupted opportunities for parent–infant interaction when feasible. Fosters parent–infant attachment. Constant interruptions increase stress and may decrease the parent's ability to relate to their infant in a comfortable manner.
- If separated, keep parents informed of infant's status; provide pictures, memorabilia, footprint. Provides a connection from parent to infant in order to facilitate attachment.
- Encourage involvement in infant care. Decreases feelings of helplessness and reinforces the parent role.

Parent/Family Teaching

- Teach parents about infant's condition. Increases their understanding of the need for treatments and procedures, corrects misconceptions, and alleviates fears and anxiety.
- Provide information about support groups and services. Empowers the family who may be unfamiliar with community resources or services.

ABO INCOMPATABILITY

ABO incompatibility is an immune reaction that happens when the mother has type O blood and the fetus has type A, B, or AB blood. ABO hemolytic anemia is more common but less severe than Rh hemolytic disease. The hemolytic process begins in utero secondary to the placental transport of maternal antibodies. This causes an immune reaction with the A or B antigen on fetal red blood cells. Clinical disease usually does not present until after birth and is characterized by a compensated mild hemolytic anemia with reticulocytosis, microspherocytosis, and early-onset unconjugated hyperbilirubinemia.

Key Nursing Activities

- Monitor cord blood for blood type and antibody titer (direct Coombs' test).
- Monitor bilirubin levels.
- Observe for clinical and serological signs of hyperbilirubinemia.
- Provide phototherapy if needed.
- Maintain adequate hydration.
- Evaluate for potentially aggravating factors (sepsis, drug exposure, metabolic disturbance).
- Prepare for exchange transfusion as indicated.

Etiologies and Risk Factors

Etiologies and risk factors include maternal type O blood with paternal type A, B, or AB blood. ABO incompatibility is caused when antigens present on the red blood cell surface of each blood type react with antibodies found in the plasma of different blood types. When a conflicting antibody enters the circulation, hemolysis may occur. A mother with type O blood has anti-A and anti-B antibodies. If the fetus inherits the father's blood type, the conflicting antibodies may cause hemolysis of fetal red blood cells.

Signs and Symptoms

Signs and symptoms include early-onset jaundice (within the first 24 hours of life), anemia, hepatosplenomegaly (rare), and hydrops fetalis (rare).

Diagnostic Studies

- Maternal and infant blood type and Rh factor. Determines the possibility of incompatibility.
- Direct Coombs' test (on cord blood). Detects antibodies attached to circulating erythrocytes of affected infant; helps differentiate between Rh and ABO incompatibility. With ABO incompatibility, results may be weakly positive or even negative, even though the indirect Coombs' (maternal blood) is strongly positive. Infants with a positive Coombs' result are more likely to have hyperbilirubinemia.
- Direct (conjugated) and indirect (unconjugated) bilirubin levels. Detects elevated bilirubin levels, which indicate hemolysis. Cord bilirubin level is usually less than 4 mg/dl. Direct bilirubin should be less than 1.5–2.0 mg/dl. Pathologic jaundice occurs when total bilirubin levels (the sum of direct and indirect bilirubin) increase by more than 5 mg/dl per day. There are no specific numbers to guide treatment. It is most important to follow bilirubin level trends and utilize an hour-specific nomogram to guide management and duration of therapy.
- CBC with differential. Detects hemolysis and anemia (Hct less than 40%).
- Reticulocyte count. Elevated values after adjusting for gestational age and degree of anemia support the diagnosis of hemolytic anemia. For term infants, the normal range is 4–5%, and for preterm infants (30–36 weeks' gestation), it is 6–10%.

- Total serum protein. Detects reduced capacity to bind bilirubin.
- Serum glucose. Detects hypoglycemia (less than 50 mg/dl). If anemia is present, the infant must use body stores to maintain metabolism in the presence of anemia. This can cause hypoglycemia; however, severe anemia is rare in ABO incompatibility. The definition of hypoglycemia varies by agency. Some define it as blood glucose less than 40 mg/dl.
- Kleihauer-Betke test (on maternal blood). Determines the amount of fetal blood in maternal circulation.
- Indirect Coombs' test. Detects antibody titers in maternal circulation.
- Blood smear. Typically demonstrates microspherocytes, polychromasia, and normoblastosis.

Medical Management

- Phototherapy (if clinically indicated)
- Possible exchange transfusion (rarely needed)
- Administration of intravenous immunoglobulin

Collaborative Problems

Potential Complication of ABO Incompatibility

- Hyperbilirubinemia

Potential Complications of Phototherapy

- Altered body temperature
- Diarrhea
- Eye damage
- Fluid deficit
- Risk for Impaired Skin/Tissue Integrity.[1] (Note: Although it is not a collaborative problem, this nursing diagnosis is included because it should be a part of the standard care given to all newborns receiving phototherapy.)

COLLABORATIVE (STANDARDIZED) CARE FOR ALL INFANTS WITH ABO BLOOD INCOMPATIBILITIES

Perform a comprehensive assessment to identify individual needs for parent teaching and emotional support and infant physical care.

Potential Complication of ABO Incompatibilities: HYPERBILIRUBINEMIA

See "Hyperbilirubinemia," beginning on p. 436 in this chapter. Assess for presence of hyperbilirubinemia, and if it is identified, implement that care plan.

Focus Assessments

- Assess for risk factors. Mothers with type O blood have anti-A and anti-B antibodies in their blood. If the father's blood is type A, B, or AB, the potential for incompatibility exists. Previous pregnancies with blood type incompatibility indicate an antibody exposure and risk for subsequent response.

Preventive Nursing Activities

- Early recognition of ABO hemolytic disease. Ensures early intervention. Jaundice within the first 24 hours, elevated serum bilirubin levels, red cell spherocytosis, and increased erythrocyte production are indications of ABO hemolytic disease.
- Institute early phototherapy, if pathologic jaundice occurs. Reduces hyperbilirubinemia and associated complications.

Potential Complications of Phototherapy: ALTERED BODY TEMPERATURE, DIARRHEA, EYE DAMAGE, AND FLUID DEFICIT

Refer to the collaborative care plan, "Potential Complications of Phototherapy: Altered Body Temperature, Diarrhea, Eye Injury, and Fluid Deficits," beginning on p. 438 in "Hyperbilirubinemia" in this chapter.

Nursing Diagnosis: RISK FOR IMPAIRED SKIN/TISSUE INTEGRITY[1]

Refer to the NDCP, "Risk for Impaired Tissue Integrity,[1]" beginning on p. 439 in "Hyperbilirubinemia" in this chapter.

INDIVIDUALIZED (NURSING DIAGNOSIS) CARE PLANS

This section includes care plans that were developed to address unique patient needs.

Nursing Diagnosis: DEFICIENT KNOWLEDGE[1]

Related Factors: lack of exposure, information, misinterpretation, and unfamiliarity with information resources. See the generic NDCP, "Deficient Knowledge,[1]" beginning on p. 13 in Chapter 2.

▌ *Nursing Activities and Rationales*

Parent/Family Teaching

- Teach parents about ABO incompatibility. Increases their knowledge of the disease and risks to their infant. The hemolytic disease from ABO incompatibility is generally less severe than that which occurs from Rh incompatibility. ABO incompatibility may occur with the first pregnancy or any subsequent pregnancy and is most commonly associated with an O blood group mother and an A or B blood group infant. Jaundice is treated with phototherapy.
- Provide information about phototherapy treatment for ABO incompatibility. Decreases fears, instills hope, and corrects misconceptions about the disease process and treatment. The parent who is well informed is more likely to cooperate with treatment plans and participate in plan of care.
- Inform parents about the risks of blood transfusions if necessary. Parents should be reassured that blood transfusion is rarely needed to treat ABO incompatibility. If it is needed, the risks are primarily related to thrombosis or infection. Knowledge often reduces fear and anxiety.
- Teach parents about potential long-term outcomes of bilirubin encephalopathy. Helps parents monitor for and recognize changes that may need future intervention.

NEONATAL INFECTION

Infection is a significant cause of infant mortality and morbidity during the first month of life. Neonates are highly susceptible to infection because their immune system is immature and reacts more slowly to pathogens. Neonatal sepsis is invasive infection with the presence of bacterial, viral, or fungal microorganisms in the blood or other tissues. The diagnosis of neonatal sepsis is often difficult to confirm because the symptoms are often nonspecific. Neonatal infections are typically grouped into one of three categories: congenital, early onset, or late onset. The greatest majority of newborn infections present in the first 2 days of life.

▌ *Key Nursing Activities*

- Maintain standard isolation precautions.
- Evaluate and monitor for sepsis.
- Maintain hydration.
- Monitor and support nutritional status.
- Obtain cultures as ordered.
- Administer antibiotics; monitor for therapeutic effects as well as adverse side effects.

▌ *Etiologies and Risk Factors*

Infection can be acquired in utero by vertical transmission before birth (congenital), by vertical transmission either shortly before or during birth (early onset), or by horizontal transmission in the nursery or home setting (late onset). The most common causative agent is group B streptococcus followed by Gram-negative enteric microorganisms (*Escherichia coli*). Other common pathogens seen in the neonatal period include *Listeria monocytogenes*, *Staphylococcus*, other streptococci (enterococci), anaerobes, and *Haemophilus influenzae*. Organisms responsible for hospital-acquired infection vary in each nursery, but the more common ones are *Staphylococcus epidermidis* and Gram-negative rods (*Pseudomonas, Klebsiella, Serratia,* and *Proteus*). *Candida* species are the most common fungal infections seen in the newborn period.

Common maternal risk factors for neonatal infection include:
- Premature rupture of membranes
- Prolonged rupture of membranes
- Maternal peripartum fever (> 38°C); chorioamnionitis, urinary tract infection, and group B streptococcus colonization
- Meconium-stained or foul-smelling amniotic fluid
- History of sexually transmitted infection

▌ Signs and Symptoms

A variety of specific and nonspecific signs and symptoms is seen, depending on the type of infection. These include but are not limited to temperature instability, lethargy, seizures, hypotonia, feeding intolerance, irritability, hypoglycemia, hyperglycemia, respiratory distress, apnea, bradycardia or tachycardia, hypotension, hypertension, pallor, rash, petechiae, and metabolic acidosis.

▌ Diagnostic Studies

- Complete blood count with differential. Detects anemia, leukocytosis, or leukopenia.
- Radiographs. Chest X-ray if respiratory distress present; abdominal X-ray if feeding tolerance and suspicion of necrotizing enterocolitis.
- C-reactive protein level. Increases in the presence of inflammation caused by infection.
- Cultures. Blood, urine, and cerebrospinal cultures are indicated to help identify type and location of infection. Other cultures that are sometimes useful include tracheal, gastric aspirate, wound, and skin surface cultures.

▌ Medical Management

- Antibiotic therapy
- Respiratory support
- Cardiovascular support
- Fluid and electrolyte management
- Nutritional support
- Immunotherapy
- Hematologic support
- Central nervous system support (seizure prevention)
- Pain control

▌ Collaborative Problems

Potential Complications of Neonatal Infection
- Sepsis
- Hypoglycemia and/or hypothermia[1]
- Hypotension/shock

COLLABORATIVE (STANDARDIZED) CARE FOR ALL INFANTS WITH NEONATAL INFECTION

Perform a comprehensive assessment to identify individual needs for parent teaching, emotional support, and infant physical care.

▌ Potential Complication of Neonatal Infection: SEPSIS

See the collaborative care plan, "Potential Complication: Infection (Umbilical Cord, Eyes, Systemic)," beginning on p. 376 in "Newborn Care: 4 Hours to 2 Days," in Chapter 11.

Focus Assessments

- Assess for risk factors (see previous "Etiologies and Risk Factors"). The presence of maternal risk factors is associated with an increase in neonatal infection. If risk factors are known, measures can be taken to reduce the risk for exposing the newborn to infectious agents. High-risk infants have a higher incidence of neonatal infection than normal term infants. Nosocomial infections are prominent in the hospital environment and neonates are at especially high risk of acquiring these due to their immature immune systems. Prevention is the first and best treatment for infection.
- Monitor temperature. Temperature instability, as opposed to fever, commonly indicates sepsis in the neonate, along with other vague, nonspecific signs.
- Monitor heart rate. Tachycardia is often a late sign of sepsis.
- Monitor respirations. Identifies tachypnea, apnea in excess of 20 seconds, nasal flaring, retractions, or grunting with expiration, all of which may suggest sepsis.
- Monitor oxygen saturation. Episodes of desaturation may indicate neonatal sepsis. Oxygen therapy may be needed to maintain adequate perfusion of oxygen to vital organs and tissues.
- Monitor blood pressure. Identifies hypotension, which tends to be a late sign of infection. Sepsis produces vasodilatation and resultant hypotension.
- Assess feeding tolerance. One of the earliest signs of neonatal infection and subsequent sepsis may be poor feeding and poor weight gain. Inadequate intake, vomiting, gastric residuals, and inadequate stooling may indicate sepsis.

- Monitor urine output. Detects changes in fluid volume due to sepsis. Sepsis produces vasodilatation and relative hypovolemia. The body compensates by retaining water in order to increase blood pressure, thus decreasing urine output.
- Monitor neurologic status. Detects change in behavior such as lethargy, irritability, or change in muscle tone.
- Assess skin. Detects possible signs of sepsis, such as poor peripheral perfusion, cyanosis, mottling, pallor, petechiae, rashes, sclerema, or jaundice.
- Assess for glucose instability. Infection increases metabolic rate and may deplete glucose stores, resulting in hypoglycemia. A stress-induced hyperglycemia might also be seen in the presence of infection.
- Monitor laboratory data. The presence of neutropenia in an infant with sepsis is a very serious sign because it indicates that the infant has no reserves to fight infection. It is commonly associated with high mortality.
- Assess for effects of prolonged antibiotic usage. Prolonged use of antibiotics can destroy intestinal flora responsible for synthesis of vitamin K and may alter blood coagulability. They may also predispose the infant to development of secondary fungal infections, such as thrush (*Candida albicans*). Additionally, infants may develop resistance to antibiotics.
- Monitor for complications. Facilitates the initiation of early treatment to prevent meningitis and septic shock, which are potentially fatal complications of sepsis.

Preventive Nursing Activities

- Early recognition, diagnosis, and treatment. Decreases morbidity and mortality rates. The mortality rate from newborn sepsis can be as high as 50% if not treated and accounts for 13–15% of all neonatal deaths.
- Administer antibiotics as prescribed. Rapid empiric antibiotic therapy is recommended whether causative agent is or is not known to decrease infant morbidity and mortality.
- Maintain strict medical and surgical asepsis. Decreases the risk for secondary infections due to cross-contamination. The infant with sepsis is at increased risk for secondary infections due to breaches in sterility or asepsis. Other infants, personnel, or objects in the environment may be sources of secondary infection in the acutely ill infant.
- Use good hand-washing techniques. The single most important measure for preventing cross-contamination and transfer of pathogenic organisms is good and frequent hand washing.
- Administer oxygen as prescribed. Prevents and/or treats respiratory distress or hypoxia. Sepsis increases metabolic rate and oxygen consumption, predisposing the infant to hypoxia.
- Administer fluids as prescribed. Sepsis and resultant septic shock produce profound vasodilation and relative

hypovolemia. Careful fluid replacement helps support circulation and prevents hypotension and reduced renal blood flow.
- Correct acid-base imbalance. Prevents metabolic acidosis, an outcome of impaired tissue perfusion due to hypoxia.
- Administer fresh, irradiated granulocytes or polymorphonuclear leukocytes as prescribed. Treats bacterial sepsis by introducing bacterial-fighting immune cells into neonatal circulation.
- Administer IV immunoglobulin therapy as prescribed. Provides immediate immune protection and helps eliminate causative organisms. Infants are not able to produce their own antibodies until about their 2nd month of life. Gamma globulin is beneficial in protecting the acutely ill infant from some infections.
- Decrease environmental stressors. Stress increases metabolic demand and oxygen consumption, which increases hypoxia and hypoglycemia and increases the infant's risk for secondary infections and mortality from sepsis.

Potential Complications of Neonatal Infection: HYPOGLYCEMIA AND/OR HYPOTHERMIA[1]

Focus Assessments

- Monitor temperature. Decreased temperature is a sign of infection and negatively impacts blood glucose levels. Cold stress increases glucose utilization and intensifies hypoglycemia.
- Monitor heart rate. Tachycardia or bradycardia may occur in response to decreased oxygenation (hypoxia) secondary to infection or sepsis.
- Monitor respirations for tachypnea or apnea. Sudden episodes of apnea and unexplained desaturation episodes in a newborn may indicate infection, especially in preterm or SGA infants.
- Monitor neurologic status. Detects neurologic changes that indicate hypoxia, such as jitteriness, seizures, lethargy, weak cry, or tremors. Sepsis and septic shock intensify hypoxia.
- Monitor skin. Cyanosis, pallor, or sweating may indicate hypoxia or hypoglycemia. Pale, cyanotic, mottled, acrocyanotic, or cool skin indicates hypothermia, which can arise secondary to infection and sepsis.
- Monitor serum glucose levels. Begin glucose monitoring at birth and continue until glucose values have stabilized. Blood glucose values less than 50 mg/dl indicate hypoglycemia. Intervention is necessary to prevent seizures or death; glucose is the primary source of fuel for the brain.

Serum glucose levels help to differentiate between signs of hypoxia, hypothermia, and hypoglycemia. The definition of hypoglycemia varies by agency, with some defining it as blood glucose less than 40 mg/dl.

- Monitor for signs of hypoglycemia. Cyanosis, apnea, irregular respirations, tachypnea, flaccidity, high-pitched cry, tremors, jitteriness, and seizures are symptoms of hypoglycemia. Infection increases metabolic rate and facilitates development of hypoglycemia.

Preventive Nursing Activities

- Maintain a neutral thermal environment. Thermoneutral environment helps to eliminate heat loss through evaporation, conduction, convection, and radiation. Hypothermia is common in infected infants.
- Provide optimal nutrition. Prevents weight loss, hypoglycemia, or fluid and electrolyte imbalances. Sick neonates may be on nothing by mouth status and will need to receive adequate fluid/calories via parenteral nutrition. Once the infant is stabilized and appropriate therapy is established, feeding may be resumed.
- Correct acidosis, hypoglycemia, hypoxemia, sepsis, and metabolic problems. Eliminates risk factors for hypothermia or corrects conditions contributing to hypothermia.
- Avoid rapid rewarming of infant. Gradual rewarming prevents possible adverse side effects from rewarming infant too rapidly.

INDIVIDUALIZED (NURSING DIAGNOSIS) CARE PLANS

This section includes care plans that were developed to address unique patient needs.

Nursing Diagnosis: IMBALANCED NUTRITION: LESS THAN BODY REQUIREMENTS[1]

Related Factors: poor feeding or feeding intolerance secondary to infection and/or sepsis. See the NDCP, "Impaired Nutrition: Less Than Body Requirements,[1]" beginning on p. 394 in "The Small-for-Gestational-Age Newborn" in this chapter.

❚ *Nursing Activities and Rationales*

Assessments

- Assess feeding tolerance and weight gain. Poor feeding (e.g., poor suck, inability to latch on to the breast, lethargy) and failure to gain weight are signs of infection in the newborn.

Independent Nursing Actions

- Supplement fluid intake. Infants with sepsis are at increased risk for actual hypovolemia due to inability to suck and relative hypovolemia due to vasodilation. Fluids must be supplemented to prevent septic shock and dehydration.

Collaborative Activities

- Maintain appropriate antibiotic therapy regimen. To adequately treat infection, the right drug must be given at the right time and according to the correct weight-based dose.

Nursing Diagnosis: RISK FOR INTERRUPTED FAMILY PROCESSES[1]

Related Factors: hospitalization of the newborn, separation of the mother from her infant, and disrupted routines.

❚ *Goals, Outcomes, and Evaluation Criteria*

The mother/family will:

- Balance responsibilities.
- Participate in decision making.
- Use effective coping measures.
- Maintain contact with the infant (if hospitalized).

❚ *NIC Interventions[2]*

Family Integrity Promotion: Childbearing Family (7104)—Facilitation of the growth of individuals or families who are adding an infant to the family unit.

Family Support (7140)—Promotion of family values, interests, and goals.

❚ *Nursing Activities and Rationales*

Assessments

- Assess degree of family disruption, lifestyle change, or financial burden infant's illness places on parents/family. Helps identify the extent of family disruption taking place so that a plan of action can be created. Ordinary stressors may be greatly magnified by an infant's illness or the financial burden created by an extended hospitalization.
- Assess for verbal and nonverbal cues or behaviors that indicate decreased family functioning. Parents may verbalize feelings of guilt or blame or negative feelings toward each other while stressed by the infant's illness. Behaviors such as anger, withdrawal, crying, poor eating, or substance abuse may indicate decreased ability to cope with the situation.
- Assess family's understanding of the infant's condition. Identifies feelings of guilt or irrational beliefs so that

misunderstandings can be corrected. Parents may feel out of control or may irrationally blame themselves or each other for their infant's infection. This may impede their ability to relate to one another or appropriately cope with the child's illness.

Independent Nursing Actions

- Provide information about and an orientation to the NICU. Decreases anxiety and facilitates parental adaptation, which will foster their ability to cope with their current stressful situation and function more effectively as a family unit. Ineffective coping can lead to family disintegration.
- Encourage verbalization of fears and concerns; listen empathetically. Creates an environment of trust and acceptance and displays interest and empathy. Families who recognize and verbalize their fears are better able to cope with the family stressors created by a sick infant.
- Instill hope for a favorable outcome. Most infections are treatable. Parents are better able to cope with a child's illness if there is realistic hope that the child will recover without long-term problems.
- Be honest about the infant's progress. If the prognosis is not good or the infant is not responding to treatment, the parents should be prepared for the infant's death. False hope may make it more difficult for them to cope if the infant does not recover.
- Provide opportunities for sibling visits. Helps siblings resolve fears and promotes understanding. Children who feel included are less likely to display negative, attention-seeking behaviors.

Collaborative Activities

- Refer to social services, counseling, and pastoral care as needed. Provides additional resources for family/social support.

Parent/Family Teaching

- Teach parents the need for close infant monitoring, prolonged hospitalization, and invasive procedures. Promotes understanding, alleviates fear and anxiety, and involves them in care planning. The benefits of protecting the infant's safety should be stressed to reassure the parents. Reassurance helps reduce fear and increase family coping.
- Inform parents about ways to interact with their infant while hospitalized. Human touch or an audiotape of parents reading a book are examples of ways to promote parent–infant attachment, provide infant sensory stimulation, and allow the parents some sense of control.
- Teach mother/parents how to assess infant for signs of infection. The parents will be monitoring the infant at home eventually and need to recognize infection so that immediate interventions can be implemented. Knowledge increases confidence in the parents' ability to care for their infant, thereby reducing anxiety and enhancing family functioning.

- Discuss home care for their infant. Facilitates care of the infant once discharged. Knowledge will increase the parents' confidence in their ability to care for the infant, thereby reducing anxiety. They may fear that the baby will become ill at home, which may negatively affect family processes.

Nursing Diagnosis: POWERLESSNESS (PARENTS)[1]

Related Factors: parents' inability to control situation (infant's infection/sepsis). See the NDCP, "Powerlessness (Parental),[1]" beginning on p. 388 in "Neonatal Asphyxia" in this chapter.

Nursing Diagnosis: FEAR (PARENTS)[1]

Related Factors: parents' fear of infant compromise from infection/sepsis or unknown outcome. See the generic NDCP "Fear,[1]" beginning on p. 15 in Chapter 2.

END NOTES

1. Nursing Diagnoses—Definitions and Classification 2009–2011. Copyright © 2009, 2007, 2005, 2003, 2001, 1998, 1996, 1994 by NANDA International. Used by arrangement with Blackwell Publishing Limited, a company of John Wiley & Sons, Inc. In order to make safe and effective judgments using NANDA-I nursing diagnoses it is essential that nurses refer to the definitions and defining characteristics of the diagnoses listed in this work.
2. Bulechek, G. M., Butcher, H. K., Dochterman, J. M. (2008). *Nursing Interventions Classification* (5th ed). St. Louis, MO: Elsevier, by permission.

REFERENCES

Bulechek, G. M., Butcher, H. K., & McCloskey, J. (2009). *Nursing interventions classification.* St. Louis, MO: Mosby/Elsevier.

Caughey, A. B., Stotland, N. E., & Washington, A. E. (2009, April 19). Who is at risk for prolonged and postterm pregnancy? *American Journal Obstetrics & Gynecology, 200*(6), 683.e1–683.c5. Retrieved from http://www.ncbi.nlm.nih.gov/pubmed/19380120

North American Nursing Diagnosis Association International (NANDA). (2009). *Nursing diagnoses, 2009–2011: Definitions and classification.* Ames, IA: John Wiley & Sons.

RESOURCES

American Academy of Pediatrics. (2009). Recommendations for care of children in special circumstances. In L. K. Pickering, C. J. Baker, D. W. Kimberlin, & S. S. Long (Eds.), *Red book: 2009 report of the committee on infectious diseases* (28th ed., pp. 131–149). Elk Grove Village, IL: Author.

American Academy of Pediatrics and the American College of Obstetricians and Gynecologists. (2007). *Guidelines for perinatal care* (6th ed.). Elk Grove Village, IL: American Academy of Pediatrics.

American Heart Association/American Academy of Pediatrics. (2006). *Neonatal resuscitation textbook* (5th ed). Elk Grove Village, IL: American Academy of Pediatrics.

Andersen-Berry, A .L., & Bellig, L. L. (2007). Neonatal sepsis. *WebMD/ eMedicine.* Retrieved from http://www.emedicine.com/ped/ topic2630.htm

Association of Women's Health, Obstetric, and Neonatal Nurses. (2007). *Neonatal skin care: Evidence-based clinical practice guidelines* (2nd ed.). Washington, DC: Author.

Blackburn, S. (2007). *Maternal, fetal and neonatal physiology: A clinical perspective* (3rd ed.). St. Louis, MO: Saunders/Elsevier.

Bloom, R. S. (2006). *Neonatal resuscitation textbook* (5th ed.). Elk Grove Village, IL: American Heart Association/American Academy of Pediatrics.

Gardner, S. L., Carter, B., Enzman-Hines, M. I., & Hernandez, J. A. (2010). *Merenstein & Gardner's handbook of neonatal intensive care* (7th ed.). St. Louis, MO: Mosby/Elsevier.

Gomella, T. L., Cunningham, M. D., Eyal, F. G., & Tuttle, D. (2009). *Neonatology management, procedures, on-call problems, diseases and drugs* (6th ed.). New York, NY: McGraw-Hill.

Gunn, V., Nechyba, C., & Barone, M. (Eds.), for the Johns Hopkins Hospital. (2008). *The Harriet Lane handbook: A manual for pediatric house officers* (18th ed.). St. Louis, MO: Mosby/Elsevier.

Jazayeri, A. (2010, February 4). Macrosomia. *WebMD/eMedicine.com.* Retrieved from http://emedicine.medscape.com/ article/262679-overview

Karlsen, K. (2006). *The S.T.A.B.L.E. program* (5th ed.). Elk Grove Village, IL: American Academy of Pediatrics.

Kenner, C., & Lott, J. W. (2007). *Comprehensive neonatal care: An interdisciplinary approach* (4th ed.). St. Louis, MO: Saunders/Elsevier.

Kenner, C., & McGrath, J. (2004). *Developmental care of newborns & infants.* St. Louis, MO: Mosby/Elsevier.

Nduati, R., Grace, J., Mbori-Ngacha, D., Richardson, B., Overbaugh, J., Mwatha, A., Ndinya Achola, J., Bwayo, J., Onyango., Hughes, J., & Kreiss, J. (2000). Effect of breastfeeding and formula feeding on transmission of HIV-1: A randomized clinical trial. *Journal of the American Medical Association, 283(9),* 1167–1174. doi:10.1001/ jama.283.9.1167

Potter, C. F., & Kicklighter, S. D. (2009, June 9). Infant of diabetic mother. *WebMD/eMedicine.com.* Retrieved from http://emedicine.medscape. com/article/974230-overview

Remington, J., Klein, J., Wilson, C., & Baker, C. (2006). *Infectious diseases of the fetus and newborn infant* (6th ed.). Philadelphia, PA: Saunders/ Elsevier.

Ricci, S. (2009). *Essentials of maternity, newborn, and women's health nursing* (2nd ed.). Philadelphia, PA: Wolters Kluwer Health/Lippincott Williams & Wilkins.

Springer, S. C., & Annibale, D. J. (2008, September). Kernicterus. *WebMD/eMedicine.com.* Retrieved from http://emedicine.medscape .com/article/975276-overview

Steinhorn, R. H. (2007). Pulmonary hypertension, persistent—newborn. *WebMD/eMedicine.* Retrieved from http://www.emedicine .com/ped/topic2530.htm

Taeusch, H. W., Ballard, R., & Gleason, C. (2005). *Avery's disease of the newborn* (8th ed.). Philadelphia, PA: Saunders/Elsevier.

Volpe, J. (2008). *Neurology of the newborn* (5th ed.). Philadelphia, PA: Saunders/Elsevier.

INDEX

A

ABO incompatibility, neonatal, 445–447
    complications, 446–447
    injury risk, 378–379
Abortion
    classification, 197
    elective/induced, 211–216
        decisional conflict, 214–215
        first trimester, 212–213
        medical *vs.* surgical, 213
        pain, 215
        second trimester, 213
        spiritual distress, 215–216
    spontaneous (*See* Spontaneous
        abortion)
Abrasions
    facial/scalp, 301
    small-for-gestational age newborn,
        393–394
Abruptio placentae, 179–180
    from amniotomy, 247
    complications, 182–184
    medical management, 181
    premature rupture of membranes and,
        209
    signs/symptoms, 180
Abscess formation
    mastitis and, 357
    with postpartum infection, 348–349
Acid-base imbalance, from exchange
    transfusions, 440
Acidosis, in preterm birth, 416–417
Acquired immunodeficiency syndrome.
    See HIV/AIDS
Activity intolerance, nursing diagnosis
    care plans, 3, 9–10
    for HIV/AIDS patients, 133–134
    for maternal cardiac disease, 124–125
    for multigestational pregnancy, 170

for normal pregnancy, 45–46
ADA (American Diabetes Association
    Classification System), 102
Adolescent, pregnant, 82–91
    collaborative care plans, 83–85
    etiologies/risk factors, 82
    key nursing activities, 82
    nursing diagnosis care plans, 85–91
Alcohol abuse, prenatal, 92. *See also*
    Substance abuse, prenatal
Alpha-fetoprotein, 48, 75, 103
American Diabetes Association
    Classification System (ADA), 102
American Nurses Association (ANA),
    definition of nursing, 3
Amniocentesis, 61, 75, 76
Amnioinfusion, 297–299
Amniotic fluid
    analysis, 31
    embolism, 62–63
        collaborative care plan, 247
        precipitous labor/birth, 269–270
    loss, from fetoscopy, 63
Amniotomy, 246–248
ANA (American Nurses Association),
    definition of nursing, 3
Analgesia
    epidural, 248–253
    selection of agents for, 19
Anaphylaxis, epidural anesthesia/
    analgesia, 249
Anemia
    from abruptio placenta or placenta
        previa, 184
    adolescent pregnancy and, 84
    collaborative care plan, 25–26
    from ectopic pregnancy, 152
    multigestational pregnancy and, 166
    prenatal, 114–117
    from preterm birth, 417
Anesthesia, epidural, 248–253
Anoxia
    fetal, precipitous labor/birth, 269–270

from forceps- or vacuum-assisted birth,
    301
Antepartum care, normal
    first trimester, 39–48, 42*t*
    second trimester, 48–54, 50*t*, 51*t*
    third trimester, 54–65, 57*t*
Anxiety, nursing diagnosis care plans, 10–11
    for abruptio placenta or placenta
        previa, 184–185
    for amniotomy, 248
    for cervical insufficiency, 158
    for cesarean section, 282
    for diabetic pregnancy, 113–114
    for dystocia/dysfunctional labor, 267–268
    for FHR monitoring, 245–246
    for genetic disorders, 77–78
    for HIV/AIDS, 132
    for hyperbilirubinemia, 440
    for hyperemesis gravidarum, 146–147
    for hypertensive disorders of
        pregnancy, 179
    for labor induction/augmentation, 259
    for precipitous labor/birth, 270–271
    for preeclampsia, 277
    for premature rupture of membranes,
        210–211
    for spontaneous abortion/preterm
        labor, 202–203
    for surgery during pregnancy, 137–138
    for third trimester, 58, 63–64
    for thrombophlebitis, 355–356
    for vaginal birth after cesarean, 286
Aortic stenosis, 121
Apnea, neonatal, 385, 415–416
Appendicitis, 135
Artificial rupture of amniotic membranes
    (AROM), 246–248
Asphyxia, neonatal, 385–389
Aspiration risk
    after cesarean birth, 281–282
    for infants of substance-abusing
        mothers, 405–406
    neonatal, 378–379